MEDICAL RADIOLOGY
Diagnostic Imaging

Editors:
A. L. Baert, Leuven
K. Sartor, Heidelberg

Emilio Quaia (Ed.)

Contrast Media in Ultrasonography

Basic Principles and Clinical Applications

With Contributions by

T. V. Bartolotta · G. Bellissima · G. Bianchi Porro · M. J. K. Blomley · G. Brancatelli
A. Calgaro · F. Calliada · P. Capelli · G. Caruso · R. Chersevani · D. Cioni · D. O. Cosgrove
M. Cova · D. Dalecki · M. D'Onofrio · R. Eckersley · C. Exacoustos · M. Falconi
G. Ferrandina · E. Fruscella · C. J. Harvey · S. Kalvaitis · A. Klauser · R. Lagalla · R. Lencioni
H. D. Liang · A. K. P. Lim · M. Lynch · G. Maconi · M. Malaggese · R. Malagò · G. Mansueto
E. Martone · M. Midiri · A. Nicosia · A. Palumbo · F. Pozzi Mucelli · R. Pozzi Mucelli
E. Quaia · G. Ralleigh · R. J. Ramey · G. Rizzatto · S. Rossi · L. Rubaltelli · G. Salvaggio
G. Scambia · M. Schirmer · S. Siracusano · F. Sorrentino · R. Stramare · E. Stride · A. C. Testa
A. Tregnaghi · M. Ukmar · K. Wei · T. A. Whittingham · G. Zamboni

Foreword by
A. L. Baert

With 310 Figures in 880 Separate Illustrations, 223 in Color and 11 Tables

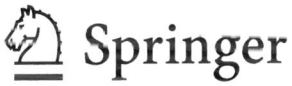

Emilio Quaia, MD
Assistant Professor of Radiology
Department of Radiology
Cattinara Hospital
University of Trieste
Strada di Fiume 447
34149 Trieste
Italy

Medical Radiology · Diagnostic Imaging and Radiation Oncology
Series Editors: A. L. Baert · L. W. Brady · H.-P. Heilmann · M. Molls · K. Sartor

Continuation of Handbuch der medizinischen Radiologie
Encyclopedia of Medical Radiology

Library of Congress Control Number: 2004115720

ISBN 3-540-40740-5 Springer Berlin Heidelberg New York

This work is subject to copyright. All rights are reserved, whether the whole or part of the material is concerned, specifically the rights of translation, reprinting, reuse of illustrations, recitations, broadcasting, reproduction on microfilm or in any other way, and storage in data banks. Duplication of this publication or parts thereof is permitted only under the provisions of the German Copyright Law of September 9, 1965, in its current version, and permission for use must always be obtained from Springer-Verlag. Violations are liable for prosecution under the German Copyright Law.

Springer is part of Springer Science+Business Media

http//www.springeronline.com
© Springer-Verlag Berlin Heidelberg 2005

The use of general descriptive names, trademarks, etc. in this publication does not imply, even in the absence of a specific statement, that such names are exempt from the relevant protective laws and regulations and therefore free for general use.

Product liability: The publishers cannot guarantee the accuracy of any information about dosage and application contained in this book. In every case the user must check such information by consulting the relevant literature.

Medical Editor: Dr. Ute Heilmann, Heidelberg
Desk Editor: Ursula N. Davis, Heidelberg
Production Editor: Kurt Teichmann, Mauer
Cover-Design and Typesetting: Verlagsservice Teichmann, Mauer

Printed on acid-free paper – 21/3150xq – 5 4 3 2 1 0

This book is dedicated to

Lorenza
and *Benedetta*

Foreword

The advantages and the diagnostic potential of microbubble-based contrast agents for ultrasonography have become more and more clear in recent years. Numerous large-scale, multicenter clinical studies have proven that the application of these contrast agents in combination with modern ultrasonographic techniques such as harmonic imaging offers substantial advantages for better management of patients. Indeed, contrast-enhanced ultrasonography allows better tumor characterization in various visceral organs and also improves the study of heart kinetics and vessels patency. The use of microbubble-based contrast agents is now firmly established in routine clinical practice.

This volume covers comprehensively the principles and physical basis of contrast-enhanced ultrasonography as well as its actual clinical applications. The eminently readable text is complemented by superb diagrams and illustrations.

The editor, E. Quaia, is a renowned expert who has lectured and published widely on the topic of ultrasonographic contrast agents .The authors of individual chapters were invited to contribute because of their long-standing experience and their major contributions to the radiological literature on the topic.

I would like to thank the editor and the authors most sincerely and congratulate them for the superb efforts that have resulted in this outstanding volume.

This book will be of great interest for general and specialized radiologists who want to increase their familiarity with this exciting new development in imaging. I am confident that it will meet the same success with readers as the previous volumes published in this series.

Leuven   ALBERT L. BAERT

Preface

Microbubble-based contrast agents for ultrasound were introduced some time ago, although their clinical application has become widespread only in recent years. Since color and power Doppler reveal overt artifacts after microbubble injection due to the peculiar features of harmonic signals produced by insonation of microbubbles, dedicated contrast-specific modes of US were introduced to optimize the registration of such signals. In the past few years numerous reports have described the effectiveness of microbubble-based agents in many fields of clinical imaging, and the utility of microbubble-based agents in routine clinical practice is now under evaluation. The preliminary results are interesting and it seems that microbubble-based agents deserve an important place in the US field.

The most important obstacle to the widespread employment of microbubble-based agents has been the reluctance of many sonologists to accept this new way of performing US scanning. The preparation and the intravenous injection of microbubbles involve a significant increase in the examination time, which seems to negate the traditional advantages of US, such as the feasibility and the rapidity of the diagnostic procedure. Microbubble-based agents have to be considered as a necessary adjunct to baseline US which allows one to solve many diagnostic problems directly in the US unit, avoiding contrast material-enhanced CT or MR examinations in many clinical situations.

The principal areas of employment of microbubble-based agents are the large vessels, the heart and the parenchymal organs. This is because these agents allow assessment of vessel patency, evaluation of heart chamber kinetics and identification and characterization of tumors. Moreover, many other interesting applications have been identified, including the use of microbubble-based contrast agents in the quantification of organ perfusion and in gene therapy.

The offer of Professor Albert Baert to edit a comprehensive textbook on the physical basis and clinical applications of microbubble-based US contrast agents was a wonderful opportunity to describe these new substances and their capabilities in radiologic and clinical practice. Each chapter was written by well-recognized experts in the field, and the principal effort of the editor was to ensure excellent illustrations and literature revision, besides text quality. After a preliminary introduction to the principles and physical basis, this book provides a comprehensive review of the recognized clinical applications of microbubble-based agents. Special attention was also dedicated to practical aspects, such as the preparation of microbubble-based agents and the correct employment of the different contrast-specific techniques after microbubble injection. As reflected by the authors of the chapters, including radiologists, gastroenterologists and physicists, this book is not exclusively intended for the radiology community but also for clinicians and academics. I hope that this book will help to provide for microbubble-based agents a secure place in the daily clinical practice of US.

I would like to express my sincere thanks to my previous department heads, Professor Ludovico Dalla Palma and Professor Roberto Pozzi Mucelli, and to my present director, Professor Maria Cova, for giving me the opportunity and the resources to work in this field of diagnostic imaging. My heartfelt appreciation also goes to all the authors and co-authors who contributed to the realization of this book and to Daniela Curzio and Marc Engelhardt from Bracco Imaging for essential aid with the illustrations.

My sincere gratitude to Professor Baert and to Ms Ursula Davis of Springer for their continuous support and belief in this work. A note of thanks also to other staff of Springer for the editorial work.

Trieste   EMILIO QUAIA

Contents

Basic Principles 1

1. Classification and Safety of Microbubble-Based Contrast Agents
   EMILIO QUAIA 3

2. Physical Basis and Principles of Action of Microbubble-Based Contrast Agents
   EMILIO QUAIA 15

3. Characterization and Design of Microbubble-Based Contrast Agents Suitable for Diagnostic Imaging
   ELEANOR STRIDE 31

4. Contrast Specific Imaging Techniques: Technical Point of View
   THOMAS ANTHONY WHITTINGHAM 43

5. Contrast-Specific Imaging Techniques: Methodological Point of View
   EMILIO QUAIA and ALESSANDRO PALUMBO 71

6. Biological Effects of Microbubble-Based Ultrasound Contrast Agents
   DIANE DALECKI 77

Vascular Applications 87

7. Cerebral Vessels
   GIUSEPPE CARUSO, GIUSEPPE SALVAGGIO, FORTUNATO SORRENTINO, GIUSEPPE BRANCATELLI, ANTONIO NICOSIA, GIUSEPPE BELLISSIMA, and ROBERTO LAGALLA 89

8. Carotid Arteries
   EMILIO QUAIA, FABIO POZZI MUCELLI, and ANTONIO CALGARO 101

9. Detection of Endoleak after Endovascular Abdominal Aortic Aneurysm Repair
   EMILIO QUAIA 111

10. Renal Arteries
    EMILIO QUAIA 117

Abdominal Applications: Liver and Spleen 123

11. Characterization of Focal Liver Lesions
    EMILIO QUAIA, MIRKO D'ONOFRIO, TOMMASO V. BARTOLOTTA, ALESSANDRO PALUMBO, MASSIMO MIDIRI, FABRIZIO CALLIADA, SANDRO ROSSI, and ROBERTO POZZI MUCELLI 125

12 Detection of Focal Liver Lesions
   Emilio Quaia, Maja Ukmar, and Maria Cova 167

13 Guidance and Assessment of Interventional Therapy in Liver
   Riccardo Lencioni and Dania Cioni 187

14 Applications of Ultrasound Microbubbles in the Spleen
   Christopher J. Harvey, Adrian K. P. Lim, Madeline Lynch,
   Martin J. K. Blomley, and David O. Cosgrove 205

Abdominal Applications: Kidneys 221

15 Characterization and Detection of Renal Tumours
   Emilio Quaia 223

16 Detection of Renal Perfusion Defects
   Emilio Quaia and Salvatore Siracusano 245

17 Quantitative Analysis of Renal Perfusion at Contrast-Enhanced US
   Emilio Quaia 255

Cardiac Applications 265

18 Assessment of Regional Myocardial Blood Flow
   Saul Kalvaitis and Kevin Wei 267

19 Assessment of Myocardial Blood Volume
   Kevin Wei 277

Special Topics 293

20 Abdominal Trauma
   Emilio Quaia 295

21 Breast
   Giorgio Rizzatto, Roberta Chersevani, and Gita Ralleigh 301

22 Lymph Nodes
   Leopoldo Rubaltelli, Alberto Tregnaghi, and Roberto Stramare 315

23 Female Pelvis
   Antonia Carla Testa, Erika Fruscella, Gabriella Ferrandina,
   Marinella Malaggese, Giovanni Scambia, Caterina Exacoustos,
   and Emilio Quaia 323

24 Vesicoureteral Reflux
   Emilio Quaia 331

25 Pancreatic Pathology
   Mirko D'Onofrio, Giulia Zamboni, Roberto Malagò, Enrico Martone,
   Massimo Falconi, Paola Capelli, and Giancarlo Mansueto 335

26 Intestinal Pathology
   Giovanni Maconi and Gabriele Bianchi Porro 349

27 Contrast-Enhanced Ultrasound of the Prostate
   Robert J. Ramey 359

28 Contrast-Enhanced Ultrasound in Rheumatic Joints Diseases
   Andrea Klauser 365

Research Perspectives 381

29 Quantitative Analysis of Parenchymal Flow at Contrast-Enhanced US
   David O. Cosgrove, Robert J. Eckersley, and Martin J. K. Blomley 383

30 Therapeutic Application of Microbubble-Based Agents
   Hai-Dong Liang, Martin J. K. Blomley, and David O. Cosgrove 393

Subject Index 403

List of Contributors 407

Basic Principles

1 Classification and Safety of Microbubble-Based Contrast Agents

Emilio Quaia

CONTENTS

1.1 Introduction 3
1.2 Chemical Composition and Classification of Microbubble-Based Contrast Agents 3
1.2.1 Carbon Dioxide Microbubbles 5
1.2.2 Air-Filled Microbubbles 5
1.2.4 Sulphur Hexafluoride-Filled Microbubbles 11
1.3 Pharmacokinetics and Clearance of Microbubble-Based Contrast Agents 11
1.4 Orally Administered US Contrast Agents 12
1.5 Safety of Microbubble-Based Contrast Agents in Humans 12
References 13

1.1 Introduction

The use of microbubble-based ultrasound (US) contrast agents is not a recent development in radiology. The application of microbubbles to increase the backscattering of blood was firstly described in 1968 (Gramiak and Shah 1968) when contrast phenomena in the aorta during cardiac catheterization following injection of saline solution were observed. This was caused by air microbubbles produced by cavitation during the injection of the solution (Bove and Ziskin 1969; Kremkau et al. 1970). From that time on, enormous efforts were dedicated to developing clinically relevant microbubble-based US contrast agents.

The first problem was the low stability of air filled microbubbles in the peripheral circulation, and in the high-pressure environment of the left ventricle, which was progressively solved by the introduction of more stable bubbles covered by galactose-palmitic acid or a phospholipid shell. The second problem was to make the microbubbles capable of passing through the lung circulation after intravenous injection, which requires that microbubbles have a diameter smaller than 8–10 μm.

Free air-filled microbubbles exhibited very limited persistence and efficacy, while aqueous solutions, colloidal suspensions, and emulsions did not meet with the required efficacy and safety profile compatible with US. The physical and chemical properties of the more recently introduced microbubble-based contrast agents are superior to those of the initial agents, and stabilized microbubbles offer both excellent stability and safety profiles, as well as acceptable efficacy.

Microbubble-based agents are injectable intravenously and pass through the pulmonary capillary bed after peripheral intravenous injection, since their diameter is below that of red blood cells (Fig. 1.1). Microbubble-based agents are isotonic to human plasma and are eliminated through the respiratory system. With the advent of the new-generation of perfluorocarbon or sulphur hexafluoride-filled microbubbles, the duration of contrast enhancement has increased up to several minutes which provides sufficient time for a complete study of the vascular bed using slow bolus injections or infusions.

1.2 Chemical Composition and Classification of Microbubble-Based Contrast Agents

Microbubble-based contrast agents may be defined as exogenous substances which can be administered, either in the bloodstream (Kabalnov et al. 1998a and 1998b) or in a cavity, to enhance ultrasonic backscattered signals (de Jong et al. 1992; Forsberg and Tao Shi 2001). Moreover, microbubbles which are prepared to be injected intravenously must be distinguished from oral compounds which are employed to remove the interposing bowel gas limiting the evaluation of organ parenchymas (Goldberg et al. 1994).

E. Quaia, MD
Assistant Professor of Radiology, Department of Radiology, Cattinara Hospital, University of Trieste, Strada di Fiume 447, 34149 Trieste, Italy

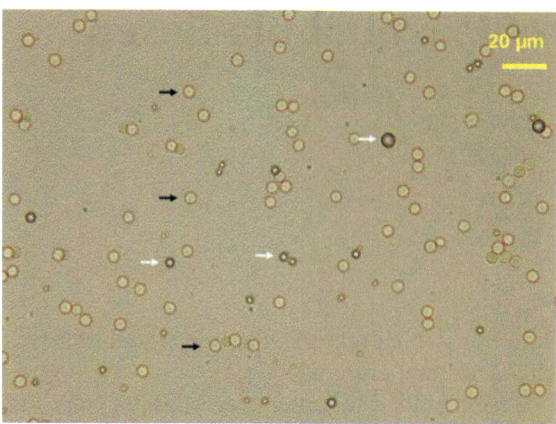

Fig. 1.1. Two-dimensional microscopic photo of SonoVue (*white arrows*) microbubbles (20× magnification; optical microscope) compared to red blood cells (*black arrows*). (Image courtesy of Peter JA Frinking, PhD, Bracco Research, Geneva, Switzerland)

The physical properties of microbubble-based contrast agents are closely related to their gas content and shell composition, besides the frequency of the US beam, the pulse repetition frequency and the employed acoustic power of insonation. At high acoustic power, the microbubbles are disrupted releasing a large amount of acoustic energy rich in harmonic components. At low acoustic power, specific pulse sequences (MEUWL et al. 2003; SHEN and LI 2003) driving the microbubbles to resonance are applied for real-time imaging, producing harmonic frequencies which may be selectively registered.

Microbubble-based contrast agents (diameter 3–10 μm) are smaller than red blood cells (Fig. 1.1) and are composed by a shell of biocompatible material such as a protein, lipid or polymer. The ideal microbubble contrast agents should be inert, intravenously injectable, by bolus or infusion, stable during cardiac and pulmonary passage, persisting within the blood pool or with a well-specified tissue distribution, provide a duration of effect comparable to that of the imaging examination, have a narrow distribution of bubble diameters and respond in a well-defined way to the peak pressure of the incident US. Nowadays, only a few microbubble-based contrast agents have been approved for human use, even though this number may soon increase as several agents are currently undergoing the approval procedure.

Two principal ways were developed to increase microbubble stability and persistence in the peripheral circle: external bubble encapsulation with or without surfactants and selection of gases with low diffusion coefficient. Microbubble-based contrast agents are encapsulated (Fig. 1.2) or otherwise stabilized using a sugar matrix, such as galactose, or microspheres with albumin, lipids (Fig. 1.3), or polymers. The shell is also designed to reduce gas diffusion into the blood and may be stiff (e.g. denatured albumin) or more flexible (phospholipid), while the shell thickness may vary from 10 to 200 nm. Low-solubility and low-diffusibility gases, such as perfluorocarbons and sulphur hexafluoride gas (Fig. 1.3), have also been found to dramatically improve microbubble persistence in the peripheral circle. Microbubbles may be filled by air, perfluorocarbon or sulphur hexafluoride inert gas. The ideal filling gas should be inert and should present a high vapour pressure and the lowest solubility in blood. Air presents high solubility in blood, while perfluorocarbon and sulphur hexafluoride gases present a low diffusibility through the phospholipid layer and a low solubility in blood allowing a longer persistence in the bloodstream. The limited solubility in blood determines an elevated vapour concentration in the microbubble relative to the surrounding blood and establishes an osmotic gradient that opposes the gas diffusion out of the bubble. The stability of a microbubble in the peripheral circle is related to the osmotic pressure of filling gas which counters the sum of the Laplace pressure (surface tension) and blood arterial pressure (CHATTERJEE and SARKAR 2003).

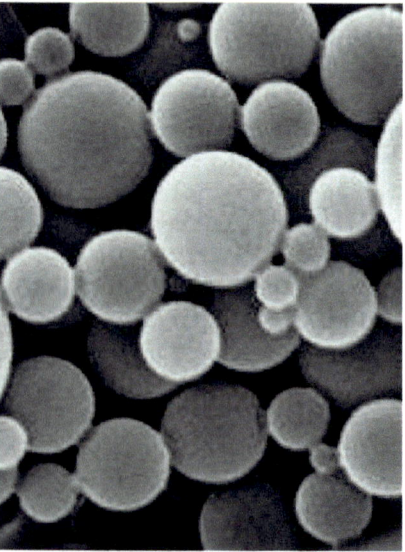

Fig. 1.2. Scanning-electron micrograph photo of SonoVue microbubbles which represents the variability in microbubble diameter. (Image courtesy of Peter JA Frinking, PhD, Bracco Research, Geneva, Switzerland)

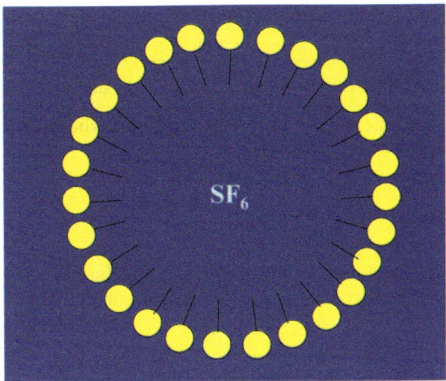

Fig. 1.3. Scheme of a SonoVue microbubble with the peripheral phospholipids monolayer filled by sulphur hexafluoride (SF6) gas. (Image courtesy of Peter JA Frinking, PhD, Bracco Research, Geneva, Switzerland)

The different microbubble-based contrast agents (see also WHEATLEY 2001) are reported in Tables 1.1–1.3. Different microbubble-based contrast agents (Figs. 1.4 and 1.5) present different methods of preparation according to their different composition (Figs. 1.6–1.8).

1.2.1
Carbon Dioxide Microbubbles

Carbon dioxide microbubbles are prepared by vigorously mixing 10 ml of carbon dioxide, 10 ml of heparinized normal saline and 5 ml of patient's blood (KUDO et al. 1992a,b). The size and the density of gas microbubbles are affected by many factors, including mixing times, volume ratio of gas and liquid and the species of gas and liquid (MATSUDA et al. 1998). Blood increases the surface tension and viscosity of solution with an increased stability and smaller diameter of microbubbles. Carbon dioxide microbubbles were employed to detect hepatocellular carcinomas and to characterize focal liver lesions after injection through a catheter placed within the hepatic artery as for selective hepatic angiography (KUDO et al. 1992a,b). Carbon dioxide microbubbles are readily cleared from the lungs.

1.2.2
Air-Filled Microbubbles

1.2.2.1
Air-Filled Microbubbles with a Galactose Shell

1.2.2.1.1
Echovist

Echovist (SH U454; Schering, Berlin, Germany) was the first microbubble-based contrast agent marketed in Europe in 1991. Echovist was approved for echocardiography to opacify right heart cavities and to detect cardiac shunts. The air-filled microbubbles are stabilized within a galactose matrix corresponding to the peripheral shell. Even though the mean diameter of these microbubbles is approximately 2 µm with a relatively narrow size distribution (97% < 6 µm), Echovist stability is not sufficient to allow the microbubbles to cross the lungs after a peripheral intrave-

Table 1.1. Microbubble-based ultrasound contrast agents for intravenous injection

Trademark name	Code name	Manufacturer	Formulation: shell/filling gas
Albunex		Mallinckrodt	Human albumin/air
Bisphere	PB127	Point Biomedical	Polymer bilayer – albumin/air
Definity	MRX-115 DMP-115	Bristol-Myers Squibb	Phospholipid/perfluoropropane
Echogen[a]	QW3600	Sonus Pharmaceutical	Surfactant dodecafluoropentane
Echovist	SH U454	Schering	Galactose/air
Filmix		Cavcon	Lipid/air
Imavist (Imagent)	AFO150	Imcor Pharmaceuticals	Surfactant/perfluorohexane-air
Levovist	SH U508A	Schering	Galactose-palmitic acid/air
Myomap	AIP 201	Quadrant Healthcare	Recombinant albumin/air
Optison	FS069	Amersham Health Inc., Princeton, NJ	Perflutren protein-type A/perfluorobutane
Perflubron	PFOB	Alliance pharmaceuticals	Perfluorooctyl bromide
Quantison		Quadrant Healthcare	Recombinant albumin/air
Sonavist[a]	SH U563A	Schering	Polymer/air
Sonazoid	NC100100	Amersham Health	Lipid/perfluorobutane
SonoGen	QW7437	Sonus Pharmaceuticals	Surfactant/dodecafluoropentane
SonoVue	BR1	Bracco	Phospholipid/sulphur hexafluoride

[a] Withdrawn from the market

Table 1.2. Ultrasound contrast agents for oral administration

Trade name	Manufacturer	Formulation
SonoRx	ImaRx Pharmaceuticals	Simethicone-coated cellulose
Oralex	Molecular Biosystems	Polydextrose solution

Table 1.3. Microbubble-based ultrasound contrast agents under development

Code Name	Manufacturer	Formulation: shell/gas
AI-700	Acusphere	Polymer/perfluorocarbon-nitrogen
BR14	Bracco	Phospholipid/perfluorobutane
BY 963	Byk-Gulden	Lipid/air
PESDA	Porter	Albumin/perfluorocarbon
MP1550	Mallinckrodt	Lipid/perfluorobutane
MP1950	Mallinckrodt	Phospholipid/decafluorobutane
MP2211	Mallinckrodt	Lipid/perfluorobutane
MRX-408	ImaRx Pharmaceuticals	Oligopeptide/perfluoropropane
SH U616A	Schering	Galactose/air

nous injection. This property of Echovist has been employed to detect cardiac and extracardiac right-to-left shunts that predispose to paradoxical embolism (DROSTE et al. 2004a,b) with Doppler interrogation of the mean cerebral artery. The other use of Echovist is in hysterosalpinx contrast-sonography to assess tubal patency (CAMPBELL et al. 1994).

1.2.2.1.2
Levovist

Levovist (SH U508 A; Schering AG, Berlin, Germany) was the first microbubble-based contrast agent approved in Europe and Canada for radiology applications, and nowadays is licensed for use in more than 60 countries worldwide. Levovist is available in vials of 2.5 and 4 g of galactose and 1 g of sterile powder (Fig. 1.4) contains 999 mg of galactose and 1 mg of palmitic acid. Concentrations of 200, 300, and 400 mg are reconstituted by adding specific amounts of sterile water to the galactose powder followed by vigorous shaking of the vial. The 200-mg concentration is recommended for contrast-enhanced transcranial Doppler studies. The 300-mg concentration provides sufficient Doppler signal enhancement for most other applications. Both 300- and 400-mg concentrations can be used with nonlinear imaging sequences to enhance the echostructure of several organs (liver, kidney, heart).

When the sugar matrix dissolves within the plasma, the microbubbles are released and coated by a thin monolayer of palmitic acid (FRINKING 1999). Levovist is characterized by air-filled microbubbles with a mean diameter of 2–3 µm and with 99% of microbubbles smaller than 7 µm covered by biodegradable galactose and palmitic acid shell. Palmitic acid is a fatty acid which increases the stability of the microbubbles to allow multiple recirculations. Microbubbles are stable enough to pass through capillary beds and produce systemic enhancement of Doppler signals for 1–5 min (CORREAS et al. 2001; HARVEY et al. 2001). Microbubbles can be administered after a short resting period of 2 min.

After blood pool clearance, Levovist has been shown to have a late hepatosplenic-specific parenchymal phase and can accumulate within the liver and the spleen up to 20 min after intravenous injection once

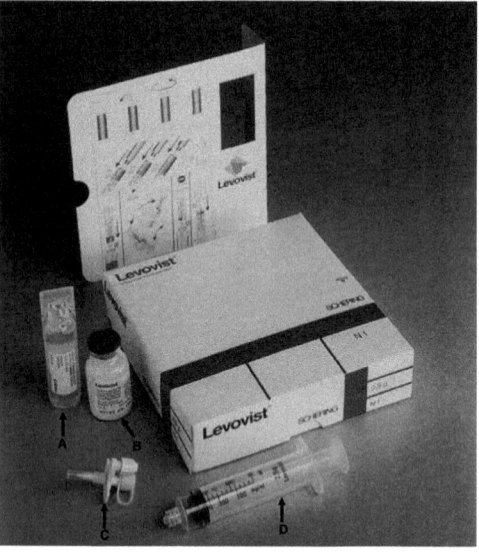

Fig. 1.4. Package of the commercial agent Levovist (Schering, Berlin, Germany) consisting in air-filled microbubbles covered by galactose and palmitic acid shell. Sterile saline solution (A), lyophilisate powder (B), plastic vial (C) and syringe (D)

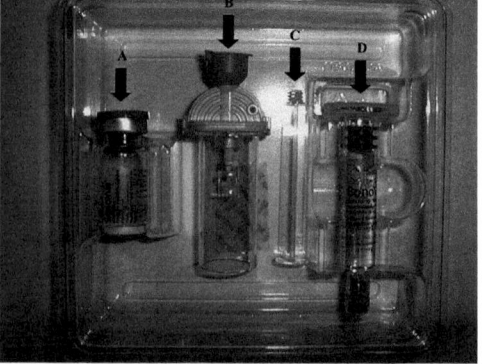

Fig. 1.5. Package of the commercial microbubble-based agents SonoVue (Bracco, Milan, Italy). Lyophilisate powder (A), plastic vial (B), piston of the syringe (C) and syringe filled with sterile saline solution (D)

Classification and Safety of Microbubble-Based Contrast Agents

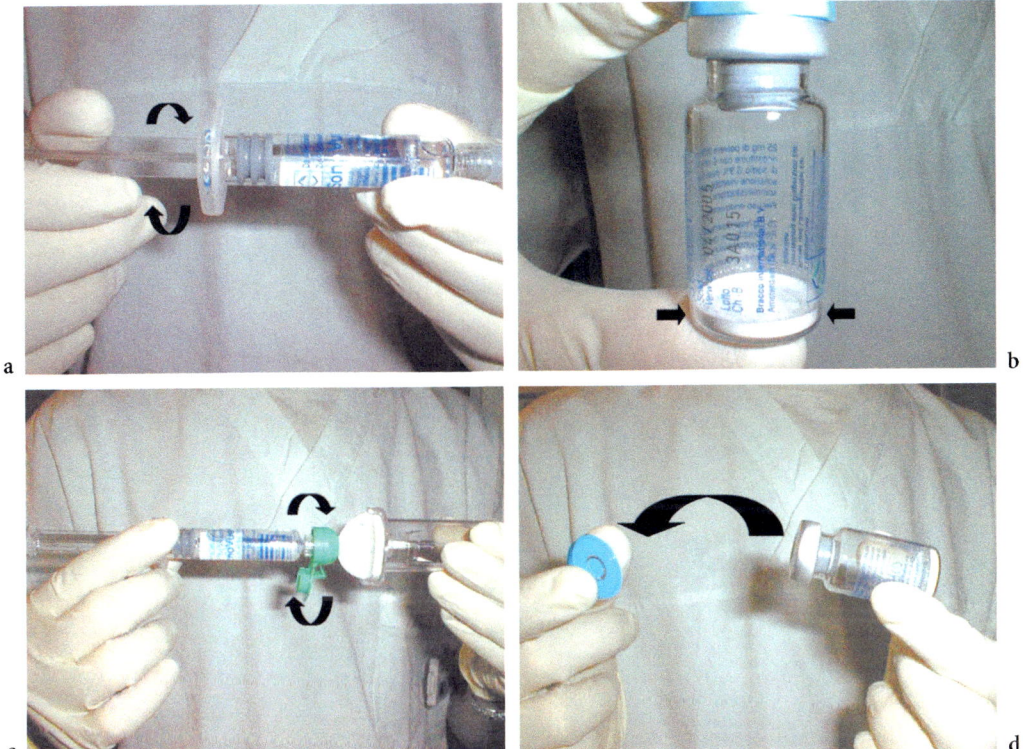

Fig. 1.6a–d. Method of preparation of SonoVue vial preparation. The piston of the syringe is screwed on the plastic support (**a**). The lyophilisate powder containing phospholipids is laid on the bottom of the bottle (**b**). The syringe is screwed on the plastic connection (**c**). The plug of the vial is removed (**d**)

it has disappeared from the blood pool (Blomley et al. 1998; Kitamura et al. 2002; Maruyama et al. 2004). The underlying mechanism of the selective late uptake of Levovist by hepatic and splenic parenchyma is not fully understood. One possible explanation is that the accumulation may be mediated by the reticuloendothelial system (Hauff et al. 1997; Kono et al. 2002; Quaia et al. 2002), or that microbubbles are entrapped in the liver sinusoids.

1.2.2.2
Air-Filled Microbubbles with Albumin Shell

1.2.2.2.1
Albunex

Albunex (developed by Molecular Biosystems, San Diego, CA, USA; distributed by Mallinckrodt, St Louis, Mo, USA) was the first transpulmonary microbubble-based agent which reached the market in 1993 but it is not longer in production. Albunex is produced by sonicating 5% of human albumin to obtain air-filled microbubbles stabilized with a thin shell of human albumin of 3–5 μm. The microbubble concentration is $3-5\times10^8$ microspheres/ml (Killam and Dittrich 1997). The mean diameter is 3.8 μm with a standard deviation of 2.5 μm; however, the distribution of the microbubble population is quite large. Albunex microbubbles are very sensitive to pressure changes and their half-life is very short (<1 min). After an intravenous peripheral injection, the microbubbles can pass through the pulmonary capillary bed and reach the left ventricle.

1.2.2.2.2
Quantison

Quantison (Quadrant Ltd, Nottingham, UK) consists of air-filled microbubbles encapsulated by a relatively thick (200–300 nm) and rigid shell of recombinant albumin. Imaging demonstrated that the liver was the organ with the highest uptake, with a mean uptake of 41.8% (SD 10.4%) of the administered dose 1 h following intravenous administration (Perkins et al. 1997).

1.2.2.2.3
Myomap

Myomap (AIP 201, Quadrant Ltd, Nottingham, UK) consists of an air-filled microbubbles encapsulated

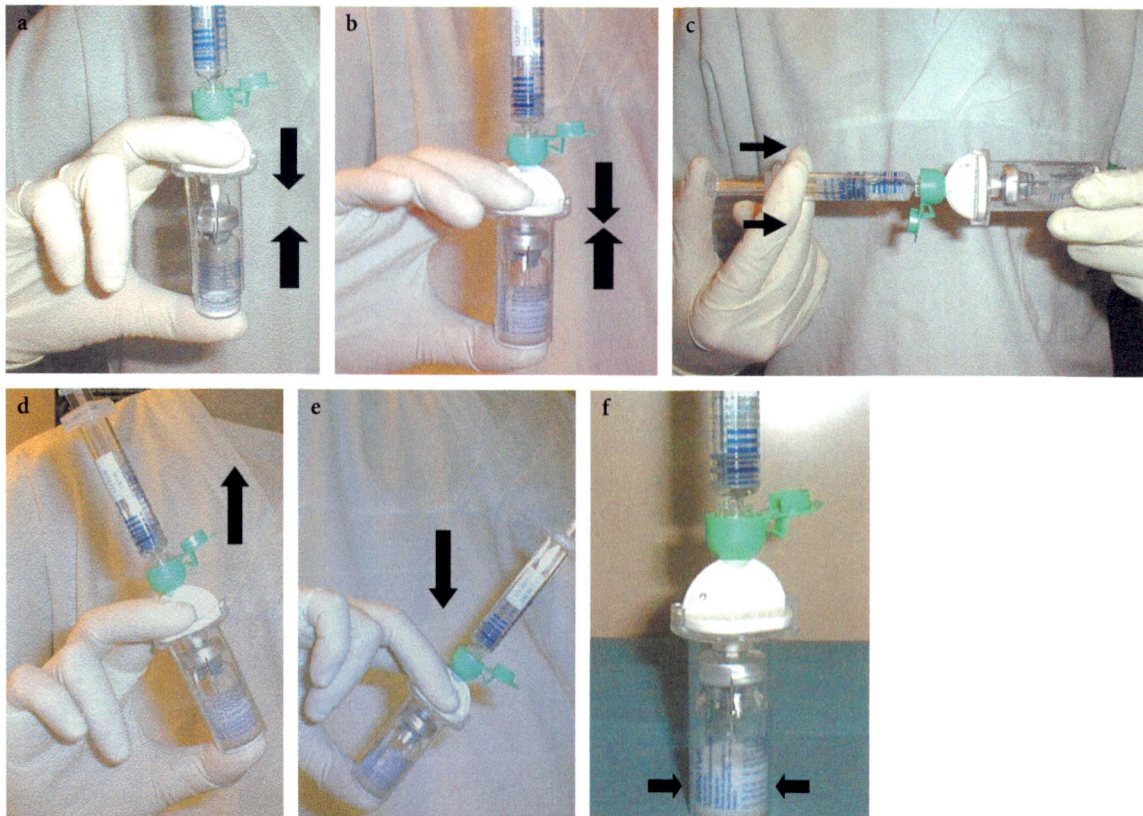

Fig. 1.7a–f. Method of preparation of SonoVue: mixture of the powder with saline solution. The plastic connection is pressed on the bottle (**a,b**). Lyophilisate powder is mixed with water and the mixture has to be shaken for about 10 s (**d,e**). The obtained milky suspension of microbubbles has to remain at rest for about 1 min to promote macrobubbles breaking up (**f**)

by recombinant albumin shell which is more than three times thicker (600–1000 nm) than the Quantison shell (FRINKING 1999). The microbubble mean size is 10 µm (range 1.46–23.5 µm).

1.2.2.3
Air-Filled Microbubbles with Cyanoacrylate Shell

1.2.2.3.1
Sonavist

Sonavist (SH U563A, Schering AG, Berlin, Germany) consists of air-filled microspheres with a mean diameter of 2 µm (BAUER et al. 1999) produced by emulsion polymerization. The shell of the microspheres is formed by a 100-nm thick layer of a biodegradable n-butyl-2-cyanoacrylate polymer. The microspheres are pre-formed as a powdery substance which is suspended by shaking in physiological saline for a few seconds before injection. This suspension is isotonic and remains stable in the vial for several hours. Unlike free gas bubbles and most other microbubble enhancers, the microspheres of SH U563A circulate in the blood pool intact for up to 10 min after intravenous injection. The particles are eventually taken up by the reticuloendothelial system during the late phase (HAUFF et al. 1997; BAUER et al. 1999), principally the Kupffer cells of the liver, which gives them a diagnostic potential similar to that of microparticles of Iron oxide.

1.2.3
Perfluorocarbon-Filled Microbubbles

1.2.3.1
Perfluorochemical

Perfluorochemicals (perflubron emulsion; Alliance Pharmaceutical Corporation, San Diego, USA) are inert compounds with a low surface tension which are immiscible with water and can be intravenously injected if emulsified (MATTREY and PELURA 1997). Perfluorochemicals accumulate in human tissues when inhaled, ingested or given intravenously.

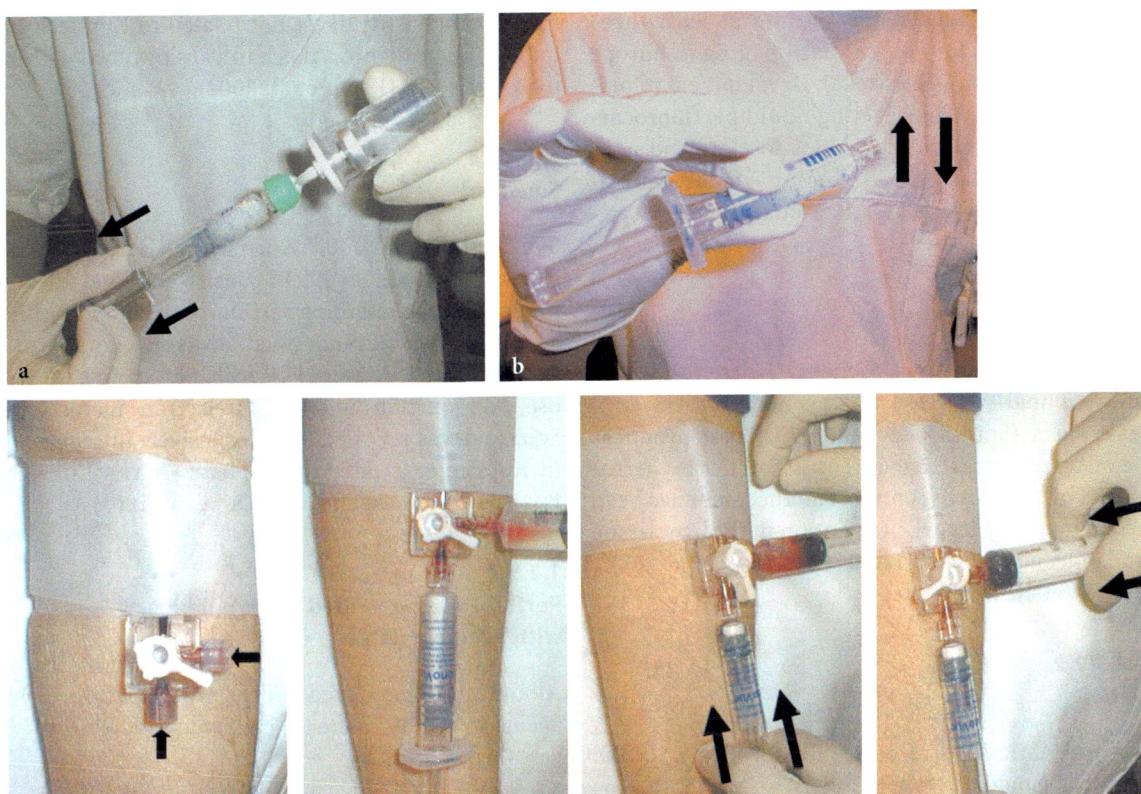

Fig. 1.8a-f. Method of preparation of SonoVue and microbubble injection. The milky microbubble suspension is withdrawn from the bottle (a) and still has to be gently shaken before injection to avoid microbubble sedimentation (b). A three-way stop-cock (c) should be employed and connected to a 16–18 Gauge intravenous cannula. The left arm is preferable since this does not hamper liver scanning during microbubble injection. The first port is connected to the intravenous cannula, the second to the syringe with microbubbles and the third to the syringe with saline solution (d). Needles should be avoided since microbubbles may be destroyed at the end of the needle during injection for the turbulence by Venturi phenomenon. Microbubbles are than injected (e) followed by saline flush (f) to avoid microbubble persistence in the vial and in the vein

Perfluorooctyl bromide (perflubron) is a liquid perfluorocarbon emulsion with particle size ranging from 0.06 to 0.25 µm which is composed of carbon and bromine atoms. Perfluorooctyl bromide circulates in blood with a half-life of hours and is an effective microbubble-based contrast agent which is also radiopaque at plain film X-ray and computed tomography. Perfluorochemical emulsions act as simple scatterers since they present a higher density (1.9 g/ml) and a lower acoustic velocity (600 m/s) than tissues with a difference in acoustic impedance of about 30% (ANDRE et al. 1990; MATTREY and PELURA 1997). Perfluorooctyl bromide accumulates in the reticuloendothelial cells and leaks from inflammatory or tumoral capillaries into the interstitial space where the emulsion particles are phagocytosed by local macrophages (MATTREY et al. 1982; MATTREY and AGUIRRE 2003). The accumulation of a large number of particles within each macrophage results in an aggregate capable of reflecting US.

From the observation that liquid perfluorocarbon vapour in a contained space expanded the space by attracting air because of an osmotic gradient and differential partial pressure, the development of microbubbles that already contained perfluorocarbon vapour and surviving to circulation was proposed (MATTREY et al. 1994; SCHUTT et al. 2003).

1.2.3.2
Perfluorocarbon-Filled Microbubbles with a Phospholipid Shell

Perfluorocarbon-filled microbubbles are currently the most important research field in microbubble-based agents development. There are at least five different perfluorocarbon-filled agents approved for cardiac imaging in the US and at least three agents approved for non-cardiac imaging in Europe (MATTREY and AGUIRRE 2003). Development efforts have also focused on targeting liquid perfluorocarbon emulsion and microbubbles to clots and activated endothelial cells becoming visible only if attached to their target (LANZA et al. 1996).

1.2.3.2.1
BR14

BR14 (Bracco Research, Geneva, Switzerland) is a phospholipid-stabilized third-generation US contrast agent (SCHNEIDER et al. 1997) that produces persistent contrast enhancement of tissue perfusion. This persistent contrast enhancement has been attributed to its transient retention in the liver tissue and spleen microcirculation (BASILICO et al. 2002; FISHER et al. 2002).

1.2.3.2.2
Definity

Definity (MRX 115, DMP115, Bristol-Myers Squibb Medical Imaging, North Billerica, MA) contains octafluoropropane (perflutren)-filled phospholipid microbubbles coated with a single layer of phospholipids and with a mean diameter of 2.5 µm (UNGER et al. 1997; MARUYAMA et al. 2000, 2003, 2004). The microbubbles are formed after a 45-s mechanical shaking and may be injected. The vial contains a clear, colourless, sterile, non-pyrogenic, hypertonic liquid which, upon activation, provides a homogeneous, opaque, milky white injectable suspension of perflutren lipid microspheres.

1.2.3.2.3
Imavist or Imagent

Imagent (AFO-150; Imcor Pharmaceutical, San Diego, CA, USA) consists of a lipid-shell microbubble containing perfluorohexane gas. The microspheres are composed by water-soluble structural agents, surfactants, buffers and salts (MATTREY and PELURA 1997). After reconstitution with sterile water, a suspension of perfluorohexane-filled microbubbles with a surfactant membrane is formed. The perfluorohexane presents a very low solubility in blood and this improves microbubble stability. Like Levovist, Sonavist and Sonazoid, Imavist showed a late hepato-specific phase 3–5 min after injection, suggesting a specific liver entrapment (KONO et al. 2002). However, the late liver parenchymal enhancement of Imavist is likely not related to Kupffer cell uptake, but rather to a mechanical slowdown within liver sinusoids (KONO et al. 2002).

1.2.3.2.4
Sonazoid

Sonazoid (NC100100, Amersham Health, Oslo, Norway) (MARELLI 1999) consists of lipid-coated microbubbles containing perfluorocarbon and within a well-defined size range (median diameter of approximately 3 µm). Sonazoid is prepared as an easy-to-use, non-toxic formulation. At electron microscopy, Sonazoid was revealed to be exclusively internalized in Kupffer cells during late phase (MARELLI 1999; FORSBERG et al. 2002; KINDBERG et al. 2003).

1.2.3.3
Perfluorocarbon-Filled Microbubbles with Albumin Shell

Albumin is employed in perfluorocarbon-filled agents to further increase microbubble stability.

1.2.3.3.1
Optison

Optison (FS069; developed by Molecular Biosystems Inc., San Diego, CA, USA; distributed by Amersham Health Inc., Princeton, NJ) consists of perfluorobutane (perflutren)-filled microbubbles coated by 15-nm thick human albumin shell which are prepared directly in solution. The vial contains a clear liquid lower layer and a white upper layer that, after resuspension by gentle mixing, provides a homogeneous, opaque, milky-white suspension for intravenous injection. This microbubble-based agent should be kept in refrigerated and shaken before use. The mean diameter of the microbubbles ranges from 1.0 to 2.25 µm, with 93% less than 10 µm, and the mean concentration ranges from 5 to 8×10^8 microspheres per millilitre. No immune reaction has been associated with the presence of the human serum albumin. Optison was recently approved in Europe, Canada, and the US for cardiac applications in the case of inconclusive echocardiography to provide opacification of cardiac chambers and to improve left ventricular endocardial border delineation. The recommended dose varies from 0.5 to 3.0 ml. Human albumin shell-covered microbubbles have been shown to be captured and phagocytosed by activated neutrophils while their acoustic properties for ultrasound are preserved (LINDNER et al. 2000).

1.2.3.4
Phase Shift Perfluorocarbon-Filled Microbubbles

Phase shift transition is a phenomenon in which the material changes physical form, such as from liquid to gas (CORREAS et al. 1997).

1.2.3.4.1
EchoGen

EchoGen (QW3600; produced by Sonus Pharmaceuticals, Bothell, WA, USA) is a perflenapent liquid-in-liquid emulsion which contains dodecafluoropentane liquid in the dispersed phase which shifts to a gas phase at body temperature forming microbubbles of 3–8 µm in diameter. Dodecafluoropentane is a perfluorocarbon gas with a low boiling point (28.5°C), low diffusibility, and low solubility in plasma. The emulsion contains particles with a mean diameter of approximately 0.4 µm (CORREAS et al. 1997, 2001). Following intravenous administration, microdroplets form a distribution of microbubbles of dodecafluoropentane with a mean diameter of 2–5 µm. The dodecafluoropentane microbubbles persist in solution much longer than similar sized microbubbles of air. The phase transition from liquid to gas state is achieved by producing a hypobaric pressure followed by an intense shock within the syringe immediately prior to administration or by injecting the emulsion as a bolus through a filter which induces a drop in pressure (CORREAS et al. 1997, 2001). EchoGen obtained a European approval for cardiac indications but was withdrawn from the market in 2000 by Sonus Pharmaceuticals.

1.2.4
Sulphur Hexafluoride-Filled Microbubbles

1.2.4.1
SonoVue

SonoVue (BR1, Bracco imaging, Milan, Italy) is a sulphur hexafluoride-filled microbubble contrast agent encapsulated by a flexible phospholipid shell which is prepared as a lyophilisate powder (Fig. 1.5) (SCHNEIDER et al. 1995; MOREL et al. 2000; CORREAS et al. 2000, 2001). A white, milky suspension of sulphur hexafluoride microbubbles is obtained by adding 5 ml of physiological saline (0.9% sodium chloride) to the powder (25 mg), using standard clinical aseptic techniques, followed by hand agitation (Figs. 1.6, and 1.7). The obtained microbubble density is 2×10^8 microbubbles per millilitre (mean diameter 3 µm, 90% of the microbubbles <8 µm). The microbubbles are stabilized with several surfactants, such as polyethylene glycol, phospholipids and palmitic acid, and are stable in the vial for a few hours (<6 h). However, after standing for more than 2 min buoyancy causes microbubbles to rise to the surface and the vial has to be gently agitated in a top-to-bottom manner to obtain a homogeneous suspension before intravenous injection (Fig. 1.8). SonoVue shows an elimination half-life of 6 min and more than 80% of the compound is exhaled through the lungs in 11 min (MOREL et al. 2000).

Recently SonoVue obtained European approval for both cardiac and liver applications. The advantages of sulphur hexafluoride-filled compared to air-filled microbubbles is the high and prolonged stability in the peripheral blood, due to the low solubility of the gas and to stability of the phospholipids shell, and the uniformity of the microbubble diameter which improves the backscattering and harmonic behaviour at low acoustic power insonation (GORCE et al. 2000).

1.3
Pharmacokinetics and Clearance of Microbubble-Based Contrast Agents

After preparation of microbubble solution, it is always advisable to perform microbubble injection via a flexible venous indwelling cannula (Fig. 1.8) of sufficiently large calibre (18 Gauge). An immediate after-injection flush of about 5–10 ml physiological saline solution is also advisable to wash out microbubbles remaining in the cannula and in the proximal vein tract after injection. The use of a three-way tap open to all sides is recommended so that the saline solution can be injected without delay (Fig. 1.8). Microbubble-based contrast agents may be injected as a bolus or as a slow infusion.

Bolus injection is simple to perform even though the increase in backscattering is brief. For bolus injection, time-intensity curve exhibits a rapid first pass followed by a slower washout and contrast enhancement exhibits a linear relation with the dose (CORREAS et al. 2000). The principal drawback of bolus injection is the possible presence of artefacts during the high peak value of microbubbles.

In slow infusion microbubble administration the enhancement is stable with a plateau-like pattern from 1 to 2 min from injection (CORREAS et al.

2000). Slow infusion may be performed by a dedicated automatic injector and it is mandatory in the quantitation of parenchymal perfusion since stationary levels of microbubbles are necessary. Infusion of microbubble-based agents is easily achieved and allows the duration of enhancement to be increased as long as desired.

After intravenous injection microbubble-based contrast agents present a pure intravascular distribution in the peripheral circle and are defined blood pool agents. After this preliminary vascular phase tissue specific agents are defined, some agents, such as Levovist, Sonavist and Sonazoid, present a late hepatosplenic-specific phase (Hauff et al. 1997; Blomley et al. 1998; Bauer et al. 1999; Forsberg et al. 1999, 2000, 2002; Quaia et al. 2002). This phenomenon is not completely understood but is probably determined by the adherence and selective pooling of the microbubbles in the hepatic sinusoids or by the selective uptake from the circulation by phagocytic cells of the reticuloendothelial system in the liver and spleen (Walday et al. 1994; Forsberg et al. 1999, 2000, 2002; Hauff et al. 1997; Quaia et al. 2002).

Typically, the gas content is eliminated through the lungs while the stabilizing components are filtered by the kidney and eliminated by the liver. Perfluorocarbons and sulphur hexafluoride are inert gases which do not undergo metabolism in the human body and are exhaled, such as air, via the lungs after a few minutes. Sulphur hexafluoride is eliminated for 40%–50% of the injected gas volume 2 min after intravenous injection while 80%–90% is eliminated in 11 min (Morel et al. 2000).

The phospholipids of the shell enter in the normal metabolism. The galactose-based microbubbles are quickly dissolved as a result of the concentration gradient. The galactose becomes dispersed in the extracellular space and is subjected to the glucose metabolism. Galactose is stored primarily in the liver through the formation of galactose-1-phosphate, or is metabolised and broken down to CO_2 after isomerisation to glucose-1-phosphate. If the plasma galactose level exceeds about 50 mg/100 ml and, therefore, the elimination rate of the liver, galactose is eliminated via the kidneys. The elimination rate in patients with liver disease is about one third lower than in healthy subjects, in whom the plasma galactose level falls by 10% per minute. Total clearance is about 40% lower in patients with liver disease. Galactose has a half-life of about 10–11 min in adults and of about 7–9 min in children.

1.4
Orally Administered US Contrast Agents

US imaging of the abdomen often is compromised by artefacts due to adjacent bowel gas since the US beam is almost completely reflected when the acoustic interface bowel gas–parenchyma is encountered. Orally administered US contrast agents (Table 1.2) were introduced to reduce bowel gas interposition between the US beam and the parenchymal organs by filling the bowel lumen with a transonic solution. Different attempts to decrease gas artefacts and improve US image quality were performed with poor results since a high inter-individual variability was found. Recently, a simethicone-coated cellulose suspension, called SonoRx (ImaRx Pharmaceuticals, Tucson/Bracco Princeton, NJ, USA) was introduced with improvement of the visualization of bowel and abdominal anatomy with reduction of gas artefacts (Lund et al. 1992).

1.5
Safety of Microbubble-Based Contrast Agents in Humans

In humans, microbubbles showed an excellent safety profile with no specific renal, liver or cerebral toxicity (Correas et al. 2001). The adverse reactions are rare, usually transient, and of mild intensity (Claudon et al. 2000; Correas et al. 2001). A transitory sensation of pain, warmth or cold and tissue irritation may occur in the vicinity of the injection site or along the draining vein during or immediately after administration. Due to the hyperosmolarity of microbubble solution, a transitory aspecific irritation of vessels endothelium may be observed.

Individual cases of dyspnea, chest pain, hypo- or hypertension, nausea and vomiting, taste alterations, headache, vertigo, warm facial sensation, general flush and cutaneous eruptions have been described (Rott 1999; Correas et al. 2001).

Short-lasting tingling, a feeling of numbness, sensations of taste and dizziness have been reported. No hypersensitivity reactions to the administration of microbubble have so far been reported (Correas et al. 2001). Even though the impaired cardiopulmonary function – including congestive heart failure (New York Heart Association Class II–IV) with or without pulmonary hypertension, moderate or severe chronic obstructive pulmonary disease, and patients with diffuse interstitial pulmonary fibrosis

– is not a contraindication for the administration of microbubble-based agents (Kitzman and Wesley 2000; Correas et al. 2001), the benefits must be weighed very carefully against the risk in this clinical situation.

Recently, general guidelines for the safe employment of microbubble-based contrast agents were proposed (Claudon and Jager 2004; Albrecht et al. 2004). These guidelines include an initial general chapter describing the fundamentals of microbubble-based contrast agents, paying special attention to safety, and will be subject to changes that reflect future advances in scientific knowledge within the rapidly evolving field of US technology (Claudon et al. 2002). The main part of the present text details the guidelines recommended for the evaluation of liver lesions (Albrecht et al. 2004) and, in the next future, guidelines will be directed to the employment of microbubble-based agents in the kidneys.

References

Albrecht T, Blomley M, Bolondi L et al (2004) Guidelines for the use of contrast agents in ultrasound. Ultraschall Med 25:249-256

Andre M, Nelson T, Mattrey RF (1990) Physical and acoustical properties of perfluorooctyl bromide, an ultrasound contrast agent. Invest Radiol 25:983-987

Basilico R, Blomley MJ, Cosgrove DO (2002) The first phase I study of a novel ultrasound contrast agent (BR14): assessment of safety and efficacy in liver and kidneys. Acad Radiol 9 [Suppl 2]:S380-S381

Bauer A, Blomley MJK, Leen E, Cosgrove D, Schlief R (1999) Liver-specific imaging with SHU 563 A: diagnostic potential of a new class of ultrasound contrast media. Eur Radiol 9 [Suppl 3]:S349-S352

Blomley MJK, Albrecht T, Cosgrove DO et al (1998) Stimulated acoustic emission in liver parenchyma with Levovist. Lancet 351:568-569

Bove A, Ziskin M (1969) Ultrasonic detection of in vivo cavitation and pressure effects of high speed injection through catheters. Invest Radiol 3:236-241

Campbell S, Bourne TH, Tan SL, Collins WP (1994) Hysterosalpingo contrast sonography (HyCoSy) and its future role within the investigation of infertility in Europe. Ultrasound Obstet Gynecol 4:245-253

Chatterjee D, Sarkar K (2003) A Newtonian rheological model for the interface of microbubble contrast agents. Ultrasound Med Biol 29:1749-1757

Claudon M, Jager KA (2004) It is time to establish guidelines for the use of ultrasound contrast agents. Ultraschall Med 25:247-248

Claudon M, Plouin PF, Baxter G et al (2000) Renal arteries in patients at risk of renal arterial stenosis: multicenter evaluation of the echo-enhancer SH U 508A at color and spectral Doppler US. Levovist Renal Artery Stenosis Study Group. Radiology 214:739-746

Claudon M, Tranquart F, Evans AH et al (2002) Advances in Ultrasound. Eur Radiol 12(1):7-18

Correas JM, Kessler D, Worah D, Quay SC (1997) The first phase shift ultrasound contrast agent: EchoGen. In: Goldberg BB (ed) Ultrasound contrast agents. Dunitz, London, pp 101-120

Correas JM, Burns PN, Lai X, Qi X (2000) Infusion versus Bolus of an ultrasound contrast agent: in vivo dose-response measurements of BR1. Invest Radiol 35:72-79

Correas JM, Bridal L, Lesavre A et al (2001) Ultrasound contrast agents: properties, principles of action, tolerance, and artifacts. Eur Radiol 11:1316-1328

de Jong N, Hoff L, Skotland T, Bom N (1992) Absorption and scatter of encapsulated gas filled microspheres: theoretical considerations and some measurements. Ultrasonics 30:95-103

Droste DW, Lakemeier H, Ritter M et al (2004a) The identification of right-to-left shunts using contrast transcranial Doppler ultrasound: performance and interpretation modalities, and absence of a significant side difference of cardiac micro-emboli. Neurol Res 26:325-330

Droste DW, Schmidt-Rimpler C et al (2004b) Right-to-left-shunts detected by transesophageal echocardiography and transcranial Doppler sonography. Cerebrovasc Dis 17:191-196

Fisher NG, Christiansen JP, Leong-Poi H et al (2002) Myocardial and microcirculatory kinetics of BR14, a novel third-generation intravenous ultrasound contrast agent. J Am Coll Cardiol 39:530-537

Forsberg F, Tao Shi W (2001) Physics of contrast microbubbles. In: Goldberg B, Raichlen JS, Forsberg F (eds) Ultrasound contrast agents: basic principles and clinical applications. Dunitz, London, pp 15-23

Forsberg F, Goldberg BB, Liu JB et al (1999) Tissue specific US contrast agent for evaluation of hepatic and splenic parenchyma. Radiology 210:125-132

Forsberg F, Liu JB, Merton DA et al (2000) Gray scale second harmonic imaging of acoustic emission signals improves detection of liver tumors in rabbits. J Ultrasound Med 19:557-563

Forsberg F, Piccoli CW, Liu JB et al (2002) Hepatic tumor detection: MR imaging and conventional US versus pulse-inversion harmonic US of NC100100 during its reticuloendothelial system-specific phase. Radiology 222:824-829

Frinking PJA (1999) Ultrasound contrast agents: acoustic characterization and diagnostic imaging. Optima Grafische Communicatie, Rotterdam, The Netherlands

Goldberg BB, Liu JB, Forsberg (1994) Ultrasound contrast agents: a review. Ultrasound Med Biol 20:319-333

Gorce JM, Arditi M, Schneider M (2000) Influence of bubble size distribution on the echogenicity of ultrasound contrast agents: a study of SonoVue. Invest Radiol 35:661-671

Gramiak R, Shah PM (1968) Echocardiography of the aortic root. Invest Radiol 3:356-366

Harvey CJ, Blomley MJK, Eckersley RJ, Cosgrove DO (2001) Developments in ultrasound contrast media. Eur Radiol 11:675-689

Hauff P, Fritsch T, Reinhardt M et al (1997) Delineation of experimental liver tumors in rabbits by a new ultrasound contrast agent and stimulated acoustic emission. Invest Radiol 32:94-99

Killam A, Dittrich HC (1997) Cardiac applications of Albunex and FS069. In: Goldberg BB (ed) Ultrasound contrast agents. Dunitz, London, pp 43-55

Kindberg GM, Tolleshaug H, Roos N, Skotland T (2003) Hepatic clearance of Sonazoid perfluorobutane microbubbles by Kupffer cells does not reduce the ability of liver to phagocytose or degrade albumin microspheres. Cell Tissue Res 312:49-54

Kitamura H, Kawasaki S, Nakajima K et al (2002) Correlation between microbubble contrast-enhanced color Doppler sonography and immunostaining for Kupffer cells in assessing the histopathologic grade of hepatocellular carcinoma: preliminary results. J Clin Ultrasound 30:465-471

Kitzman DW, Wesley DJ (2000) Safety assessment of perflenapent emulsion for echocardiographic contrast enhancement in patients with congestive heart failure or chronic obstructive pulmonary disease. Am Heart J 139:1077-1080

Kabalnov A, Klein D, Pelura T et al (1998a) Dissolution of multicomponent microbubble in the blood stream: 1. Theory. Ultrasound Med Biol 24:739-749

Kabalnov A, Bradley JA, Flam S et al (1998b) Dissolution of multicomponent microbubble in the blood stream: 2. Experiment. Ultrasound Med Biol 24:751-760

Kono Y, Steinbach GC, Peterson T et al (2002) Mechanism of parenchymal enhancement of the liver with a microbubble-based US contrast medium: an intravital microscopy study in rats. Radiology 224:253-257

Kremkau FW, Gramiak R, Cartensen EL, Shah PM, Kramer H (1970) Ultrasonic detection of cavitation at catheter tips. AJR Am J Roentgenol 110:177-183

Kudo M, Tomita S, Tochio H et al (1992a) Sonography with intraarterial infusion of carbon dioxide microbubbles (sonographic angiography): value in differential diagnosis of hepatic tumors. Am J Roentgenol 158:65-74

Kudo M, Tomita S, Tochio H et al (1992b) Small hepatocellular carcinoma: diagnosis with US angiography with intraarterial CO2 microbubbles. Radiology 182:155-160

Lanza GM, Wallace KD, Scott MJ et al (1996) A novel site-targeted ultrasonic contrast agent with broad biomedical application. Circulation 94:3334-3340 (erratum in Circulation 1997, 95:2458)

Lindner JR, Dayton PA, Coggins MP et al (2000) Noninvasive imaging of inflammation by ultrasound detection of phagocytosed microbubbles. Circulation 102:531-538

Lund PJ, Fritz TA, Unger EC et al (1992) Cellulose as a gastrointestinal US contrast agent. Radiology 185:783-788

Marelli C (1999) Preliminary experience with NC100100, a new ultrasound contrast agent for intravenous injection. Eur Radiol 9 [Suppl 3]:S343-S346

Maruyama H, Matsutani S, Saisho H et al (2000) Grey-scale contrast enhancement in rabbit liver with DMP115 at different acoustic power levels. Ultrasound Med Biol 26:1429-1438

Maruyama H, Matsutani S, Saisho H et al (2003) Extra-low acoustic power harmonic images of the liver with perflutren. Novel imaging for real-time observation of liver perfusion. J Ultrasound Med 22:931-938

Maruyama H, Matsutani S, Saisho H et al (2004) Different behaviors of microbubble in the liver: time-related quantitative analysis of two ultrasound contrast agents, Levovist and Definity. Ultrasound Med Biol 30:1035-1040

Matsuda Y, Yabuuchi I, Ito T (1998) Properties of gas (CO2) microbubbles made by hand agitation and it's contrast enhancing effect. Nippon Rinsho 56:866-870

Mattrey RF, Aguirre D (2003) Advances in contrast media research. Acad Radiol 10:1450-1460

Mattrey RF, Pelura TJ (1997) Perfluorocarbon-based ultrasound contrast agents. In: Goldberg BB (ed) Ultrasound contrast agents. Dunitz, London, pp 83-99

Mattrey RF, Scheible FW, Gosink BB et al (1982) Perfluorooctyl bromide: a liver/spleen-specific and tumour-imaging ultrasound contrast material. Radiology 145:759-762

Mattrey RF, Wrigley R, Steinbach GC et al (1994) Gas emulsions as ultrasound contrast agents. Preliminary results in rabbits and dogs. Invest Radiol 29 [Suppl 2]:S139-S141

Meuwl JY, Correas JM, Bleuzen A, Tranquart F (2003) Detection modes of ultrasound contrast agents. J Radiol 84:2013-2024

Morel DR, Schwieger I, Hohn L et al (2000) Human pharmacokinetics and safety evaluation of SonoVue™, a new contrast agent for ultrasound imaging. Invest Radiol 35:80-85

Perkins AC, Frier M, Hindle AJ et al (1997) Human biodistribution of an ultrasound contrast agent (Quantison) by radiolabelling and gamma scintigraphy. Br J Radiol 70:603-611

Quaia E, Blomley MJK, Patel S et al (2002) Initial observations on the effect of irradiation on the liver-specific uptake of Levovist. Eur J Radiol 41:192-199

Rott HD (1999) Safety of ultrasonic contrast agents. European Committee for Medical Ultrasound Safety. Eur J Ultrasound 9:195-197

Schneider M, Arditi M, Barrau MB et al (1995) BR1 a new ultrasonographic contrast agent based on sulphur hexafluoride-filled microbubbles. Invest Radiol 30:451-457

Schneider M, Broillet A, Bussat P et al (1997) Gray-scale liver enhancement in VX2 tumor bearing rabbits using BR14, a new ultrasonographic contrast agent. Invest Radiol 32:410-417

Schutt EG, Klein DH, Mattrey RM, Riess JG (2003) Injectable microbubbles as contrast agents for diagnostic ultrasound imaging: the key role of perfluorochemicals. Angew Chem Int Ed Engl 42:3218-3235

Shen CC, Li PC (2003) Pulse-inversion-based fundamental imaging for contrast detection. IEEE Trans Ultrason Ferroelectr Freq Control 50:1124-1133

Unger E, Fritz T, McCreery T et al (1997) Lyposomes as myocardial perfusion ultrasound contrast agents. In: Goldberg BB (ed) Ultrasound contrast agents. Dunitz, London, pp 57-74

Walday P, Tolleshaug H, Gjoen T et al (1994) Biodistributions of air-filled albumin microspheres in rats and pigs. Biochem J 199:437-443

Wheatley MA (2001) Composition of contrast microbubbles: basic chemistry of encapsulated and surfactant-coated bubbles. In: Goldberg B, Raichlen JS, Forsberg F (eds) Ultrasound contrast agents: basic principles and clinical applications. Dunitz, London, pp 3-11

2 Physical Basis and Principles of Action of Microbubble-based Contrast Agents

Emilio Quaia

CONTENTS

2.1 Introduction 15
2.2 Microbubble Persistence in the Bloodstream 15
2.2.1 Diffusibility of the Filling Gas 15
2.2.2 Surface Tension 16
2.2.3 Osmotic Pressure of the Filling Gas 16
2.2.4 Diffusion and Ostwald Coefficients 16
2.2.5 Nature of the Peripheral Capsule 16
2.3 Physical Basis and Principles of Action 17
2.3.1 Resonant Frequency 17
2.3.2 The Fundamental Equation of Microbubble Backscattering: Rayleigh–Plesset 19
2.3.3 Scattering Cross Section – Echogenicity of Microbubbles 20
2.3.4 US Beam Attenuation and Microbubble Size Distribution 22
2.3.5 Scattering to Attenuation Ratio 23
2.3.6 Acoustic Power of Insonation 23
2.4 Artefacts from Microbubble-Based Agents 25
2.4.1 Microbubble Artefacts with Doppler 25
2.4.2 Microbubble Artefacts with Contrast-Specific Modes 28
References 29

2.1 Introduction

Microbubble-based contrast agents consist of microbubbles of air or other gases, encapsulated by a shell of different composition and with a diameter of approximately 2–6 µm. The high difference in acoustic impedance between the gas in the microbubble and the surrounding tissue in vivo makes microbubbles highly reflective resulting in the enhanced acoustic backscattering from blood by up to 27 dB in both colour and spectral Doppler modes (Forsberg et al. 1999).

The oscillation of the microbubble under US beam is governed by parameters such as resonance frequency, pulse repetition frequency, acoustic power, the filling gas, damping coefficients and shell prop-

---

E. Quaia, MD
Assistant Professor of Radiology, Department of Radiology, Cattinara Hospital, University of Trieste, Strada di Fiume 447, 34149 Trieste, Italy

erties. Besides the other factors, the local acoustic power is the principal parameter affecting microbubbles behaviour (Powers et al. 1997; Correas et al. 2001). At low acoustic power, the microbubbles destruction from the US beam is minimized and microbubbles oscillate synchronously with the incident US and emit non-linear echoes. With increasing acoustic power of the insonating US beam, signals returning from microbubbles are increased by several orders of magnitude due to interactions between the insonating beam and the microbubbles, which include fundamental scattering, harmonic resonance and microbubble destruction.

2.2 Microbubble Persistence in the Bloodstream

To act as effective contrast agents in the peripheral circulation, microbubbles have to persist in the bloodstream. Various chemical strategies have been adopted to produce stabilized gas microbubbles in the peripheral circulation and the different compositions have an important influence upon the performance of the resulting agent.

2.2.1 Diffusibility of the Filling Gas

The first factor which determines the persistence of microbubbles in the peripheral circle is the diffusibility of the filling gas throughout the peripheral shell. The diffusibility, expressed by the diffusion coefficient, and the solubility of the filling gas in the blood, strongly affect microbubble persistence in the circle, according to the following equation:

$$T = \frac{\rho R^2}{2 D C_s} \quad (1)$$

where T = microbubble persistence in the blood, ρ = density of the gas, R = initial radius of the microbubble, D = diffusion coefficient of the gas in the substance of the shell, C_s = saturation coefficient of exchange of gas between aqueous and gaseous phases, which is higher in gas with increased solubility in the blood.

2.2.2
Surface Tension

Equation 1 is an effective approximation of microbubble persistence in the bloodstream. However, surface tension is another important mechanism responsible for the disappearance of the filling microbubble gas in a gas saturated liquid. The microbubble shell contains surface-active molecules, namely phospholipids, which act as a surfactant reducing the surface tension. The surfactant layer exerts a counterpressure against the tendency of surface tension and other forces to cause gas diffusion from a microbubble. The relation of the surface tension with microbubble dissolution was shown by Frinking (1999):

$$\frac{dR}{dt} = D \times L \left(\frac{\frac{C_i}{C_s} - 1 - \frac{2S_T}{Rp_0}}{1 + \frac{4S_T}{3Rp_0}} \right) \left(\frac{1}{R} + \frac{1}{\sqrt{\pi Dt}} \right) \quad (2)$$

where $\left(\frac{dR}{dt}\right)$ = variation of microbubble radius (R), with time (t) which is related to microbubble disappearance from the peripheral circle; D = diffusion coefficient of the gas; L = Ostwald coefficient which corresponds to the ratio of the amount of gas dissolved in the surrounding liquid and in the gas phase per unit volume; C_i/C_s = ratio of the dissolved gas concentration to the saturation concentration; S_T = surface tension; p_0 = ambient pressure. In Eq. 2 the surface tension is shown to strongly affect the dissolution of microbubbles and the higher the surface tension, the lower the microbubble persistence.

2.2.3
Osmotic Pressure of the Filling Gas

Kabalnov et al. (1998) showed that the stability of a microbubble in the peripheral circle is related to the osmotic pressure of the filling gas which counters the sum of the surface tension and blood arterial pressure:

$$(C_G + C_A) K \times T = \frac{2S_T}{R} + p_b + p_{atm} \quad (3)$$

where C_G and C_A = concentration of the filling gas ($_G$) and air ($_A$), K = gas constant, T = absolute temperature, S_T = surface tension, R = bubbles radius, p_b = systemic blood pressure, p_{atm} = atmospheric pressure (101 kPa). The limited solubility in blood determines an elevated vapour concentration in the microbubble relative to the surrounding blood and establishes an osmotic gradient that oppose the gas diffusion out of the microbubble. After the initial size adjustment due to the effect of body temperature, the microbubbles will either swell or shrink depending on the partial pressure of the air in the bubble, followed by a period of slow diffusion of gas into the bloodstream (Forsberg and Tao Shi 2001).

2.2.4
Diffusion and Ostwald Coefficients

Diffusion and Ostwald coefficients also strongly determine the rate of decrease of the bubble radius, which is a direct measure for the disappearance rate of the microbubble:

$$-\frac{d}{dt}(C_G R^3) = 3RD_G L_G C_G \quad (4)$$

$$-\frac{d}{dt}(C_A R^3) = 3RD_A L_A \left(C_A - \frac{p_{atm}}{KT} \right) \quad (5)$$

where C_G and C_A = concentration of the filling gas ($_G$) and air ($_A$), R = bubbles radius, D_G, D_a and L_G, L_a = diffusion and Ostwald coefficients respectively for the filling gas ($_G$) and the air ($_A$), p_{atm} = atmospheric pressure (101 kPa), K = gas constant and T = absolute temperature. From Eqs. 4 and 5 it can be derived that the diffusion and Ostwald coefficients determine the rate of decrease of the bubble radius, which is a direct measure for the disappearance rate of the microbubble. Thus, microbubbles filled with gases having lower diffusion and/or the Ostwald coefficient will persist longer in the bloodstream (Fig. 2.1) (Correas et al. 1997). This result was reached with the introduction of new generation of microbubble-based agents.

2.2.5
Nature of the Peripheral Capsule

The nature of the encapsulating shell is the last fundamental factor which affects microbubble persistence in the bloodstream. Of course, the more

Physical Basis and Principles of Action of Microbubble-based Contrast Agents

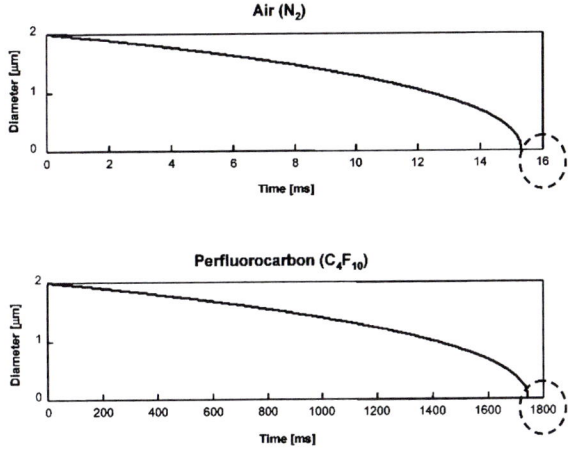

Fig. 2.1a,b. Difference of microbubble persistence in the bloodstream according to the filling gas: air (a) or perfluorocarbon gas (b), respectively. The microbubbles are completely dissolved when the diameter is equal to 0 and this happens after 16 ms for air (a) and 1800 ms for perfluorocarbon gas (b). (Images courtesy of Peter JA Frinking, Bracco Research, Geneva, Switzerland)

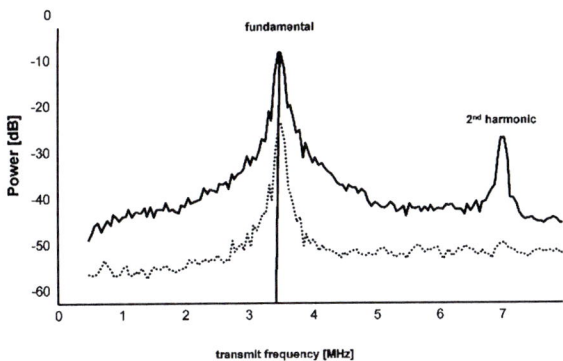

Fig. 2.2. Power spectral density of SonoVue for low (*broken line*) and high (*solid line*) acoustic power. The power of the backscattered signal presents a peak at the fundamental (resonant) frequency. (Image courtesy of Peter JA Frinking, Bracco Research, Geneva, Switzerland)

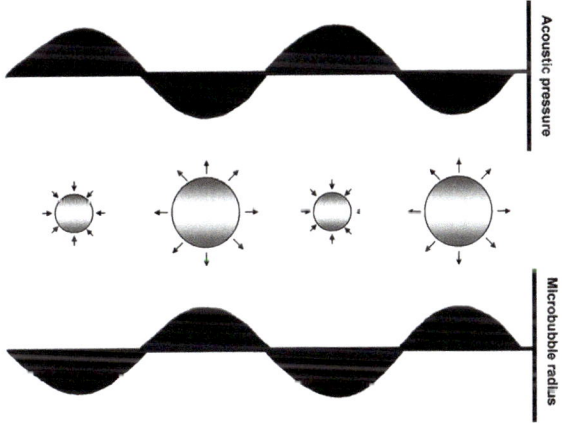

Fig. 2.3. Microbubble shows linear behaviour at very low acoustic power insonation. Microbubble radius presents a degree of compression at positive acoustic pressure which is equal to the degree of expansion at negative acoustic pressure.

stable the peripheral shell or the lower its solubility in water, the longer the microbubble persistence and echo-enhancing effect. Galactose-covered microbubbles present a low persistence for the high solubility of the sugar in the water. New generation microbubble-based agents present an albumin or phospholipids shell which present low solubility in water, further improving microbubble persistence in the bloodstream and the effect of scattering.

2.3
Physical Basis and Principles of Action

2.3.1
Resonant Frequency

The first theoretical description of free microbubble response to pressure was developed by RAYLEIGH (1917). Encapsulation of microbubbles affects their ability to oscillate, due to the presence of viscoelastic damping effects determined by the shell which influences the microbubble acoustic properties (DE JONG et al 1992, 1994; DE JONG and HOFF 1994; FRINKING and DE JONG 1999). To produce effective backscattering microbubbles have to be insonated by their characteristic resonant frequency (Fig. 2.2) and the exposure to US at their resonant frequency forces microbubbles to contract and expand their diameter several-fold. At low acoustic power microbubbles produce a US signal with the same frequency as the sound that excited them (Fig. 2.3). By increasing the acoustic power of insonation microbubbles exhibit non-linear vibrations (Fig. 2.4) at their resonant frequency (f_0) generating signals at f_0, harmonics ($2f_0$, $3f_0$, $4f_0$, etc.) and subharmonics ($f_0/2$, $f_0/3$, etc.) (Fig. 2.5) (FORSBERG et al. 1996; SHANKAR et al. 1998). At further higher acoustic power the expansion eventually disrupts the microbubbles shell generating a wide-band harmonic signal similar to a burst.

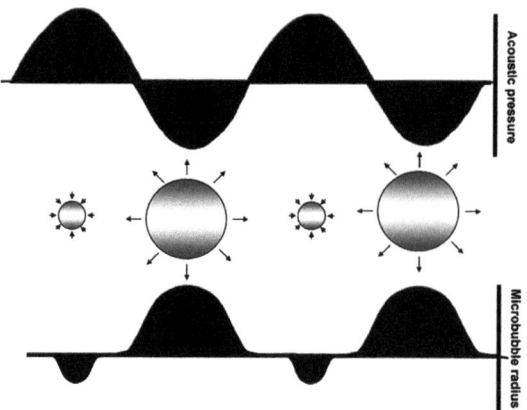

Fig. 2.4. Microbubble shows nonlinear behaviour if the acoustic power of insonation is progressively increased at the resonant frequency. With non-linear oscillation, the duration and degree of microbubble expansion is greater than its compression phase. This non-linear response to the insonation determines the production of harmonic frequencies.

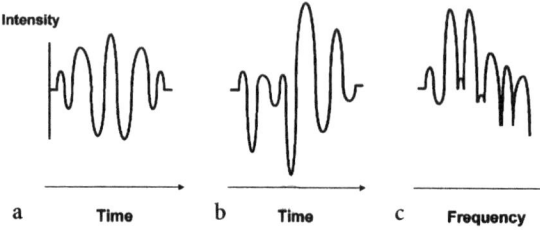

Fig. 2.5a–c. Microbubble non-linear behaviour. The transmitted acoustic wave (a) presents a definite periodic shape. The echo produced by microbubble resonance (b) presents an irregular shape in the time domain which becomes more definite in the frequency time (c) after Fourier transformation revealing multiple harmonic and subharmonic frequency components.

According to ANDERSON and HAMPTON (1980) the resonant – fundamental – frequency (f_0) is inversely related to the microbubble diameter and it may be expressed as:

$$f_0 \approx \frac{1}{2\pi R} \sqrt{\frac{3\gamma p_0}{\rho_0}} \qquad (6)$$

where R = microbubble diameter; γ = the ideal adiabatic constant of gas; p_0 = ambient fluid pressure; ρ_0 = density of the surrounding medium. To derive Eq. 6 the damping caused by the surrounding medium is assumed negligible, as there are no effects due to bubble surface tension or thermal conductivity.

Considering the same model employed for the backscattering of an air-filled microbubble surrounded by a thin elastic shell, and taking into account the increased restoring force due to shell elasticity, a further equation was developed by DE JONG et al. (1992):

$$f_0 \approx \frac{1}{2\pi r} \sqrt{\frac{3\gamma}{\rho}\left(P_0 + \frac{\pi}{3\gamma}\frac{S_e}{r}\right)} \qquad (7)$$

where S_e is the shell elasticity parameter which is defined as:

$$S_e = 8\pi \frac{R_o - R_i}{1-\nu} E \qquad (8)$$

where R_i and R_o = inner (i) and the outer (o) diameter of the microbubble (the difference $R_o - R_i$ is the thickness of the shell), ν is the Poisson's ratio which describes the ratio of transverse contraction strain to longitudinal extension strain in the direction of stretching acoustic pressure (tensile deformation is considered positive and compressive deformation is considered negative) and E is the modulus of Young – modulus of elasticity in tension – which describes the stiffness of a microbubble.

2.3.1.1
Practical Application

According to Eq. 7 the higher the shell elasticity due to encapsulation, the higher the resonant frequency, at equivalent microbubble radius. Moreover, the lower the shell elasticity due to encapsulation, the lower the generation of harmonics, due to the damping provided by the shell viscosity which produces a notable decrease in the pulsation amplitude. So, for a stiff and thick shell the stability in the peripheral blood is higher if compared with a flexible and thin shell, but production of harmonics is lower. In practical terms, for any given US power and frequency, less acoustic signal can be expected from microbubbles with thick, stiff shells. Since microbubbles with thick and stiff shells present an increased resistance to the US acoustic power of insonation, the produced acoustical backscattering signal may be improved simply by increasing the acoustic power of insonation.

Moreover, according to Eq. 7, the ideal resonant frequency for a microbubble is inversely related to the square of its radius (DE JONG et al. 1996; FRINKING and DE JONG 1999). The larger the microbubble radius, the lower the resonant frequency (Fig. 2.6), and the resonant frequency of a microbubble with a diameter of a few micrometres is comprised in the low MHz frequency range, which is employed

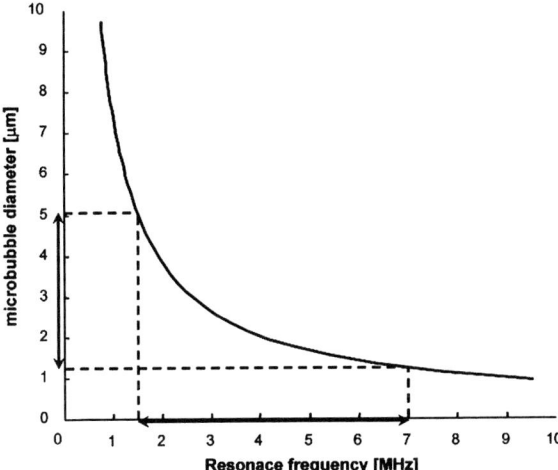

Fig. 2.6. Free air microbubble. Inverse hyperbolic relation between the resonance frequency and the microbubble diameter. (Image courtesy of Peter JA Frinking, Bracco Research, Geneva, Switzerland)

in abdominal US. Specifically, the resonant frequency for phospholipid-coated microbubbles with a diameters of 1–5 µm is approximately 4–0.6 MHz (Dayton and Ferrara 2002).

2.3.2
The Fundamental Equation of Microbubble Backscattering: Rayleigh–Plesset

The Rayleigh, Plesset, Noltingk, Neppiras, Poritsky equation, also known as the RPNNP equation and which was further developed by Church (1995), considers a free microbubble gas-filled model and describes both the linear and the non-linear characteristics of a shell-encapsulated microbubble.

In this model, the microbubble is considered coated by a continuous layer of incompressible solid elastic material, with a spherically symmetric motion, and surrounded by an incompressible liquid which presents infinite extent and a constant viscosity according to Newton's law. A Newtonian fluid is a fluid in which the shear stress – the ratio of force up to the area subjected to the force – is proportional to viscosity and velocity gradient (Chatterjee and Sarkar 2003). The rheological parameters (surface tension and viscosity) for microbubble-based agents may be calculated. The wavelength of the US field is assumed to be much larger than the microbubble diameter, and only the motion of the bubble surface is of interest. It is assumed that the vapour pressure remains constant during the compression and expansion phase, and that there is no rectified diffusion during the short period of exposure to US. The gas in the bubble is assumed to be ideal and compressed and expanded according to the ideal gas law with the polytropic exponent (Γ) remaining constant during vibration (Frinking 1999).

2.3.2.1
Motion of the microbubble wall

The first parameter to be considered in the backscattering is the motion of the microbubble wall (Frinking 1999):

$$\rho R R^{\cdot\cdot} + \frac{3}{2}\rho R^{\cdot 2} = p_L - p_0 \rho R^{\cdot 2} = p_L - p_\infty \qquad (9)$$

where ρ = density of the surrounding liquid medium (= 998 kg/m³); R = instantaneous microbubble radius; R˙ = first time derivative of the radius (the velocity of the microbubble wall); R¨ = second time derivative of the radius (the acceleration of the microbubble wall); p_L = liquid pressure at the microbubble wall; p_∞ = liquid pressure at infinity.

The assumption is that presence of the microbubble shell completely dominates the motion of the microbubble wall. Therefore, the microbubbles are considered to be elastic particles, which have an effective bulk modulus, K_{eff}, describing the elasticity of the shell, and a friction parameter describing the viscosity of the shell.

2.3.2.2
Bulk Modulus ≈ Elasticity of the Shell

The effective bulk modulus describes the elasticity of the shell. For a spherical volume V deformed by a quasi-static pressure change, ΔP determines the volume change of the microbubble and it is uniform over the microbubble surface. The volume strain (deformation) corresponds to $-\Delta V/V$, where V is the initial volume and ΔV is the change in volume, while the volume stress (ΔP) corresponds to the ratio of the magnitude of the normal force to the area. The effective bulk modulus, K_{eff} (Frinking and de Jong 1999), is given by the ratio of the volume stress to the volume strain:

$$K_{eff} = -V\frac{\Delta P}{\Delta V} \qquad (10)$$

Since the volume is spherical, symmetric and defined by the radius, the volume strain can be written as:

$$\frac{\Delta V}{V} = \left(\frac{R}{R_0}\right)^3 - 1 \quad (11)$$

where R_0 is the initial microbubble radius. Combining Eqs. 10 and 11 gives:

$$\Delta P = -K_{eff}\left[\left(\frac{R}{R_0}\right)^3 - 1\right] \quad (12)$$

2.3.2.3
Friction Damping ≈ Viscosity of the Shell

The friction damping parameter describes the viscosity of the shell. Since the pressure change ΔP, determining the volume change of the microbubble, can be split into three parts: (1) the liquid pressure at the bubble wall (p_L); (2) the damping pressure caused by friction damping of the system bubble – liquid (p_d), and (3) the hydrostatic pressure (p_0), it may be expressed as:

$$\Delta P = p_L + p_d - p_0 \quad (13)$$

Substitution of Eqs. 12 and 13 into Eq. 9, and using the expanded expression for p_∞ ($p_\infty = p_0 + P_{(t)}$; where p_0 = hydrostatic pressure; $P_{(t)}$ = time-varying applied acoustic pressure) yields:

$$\rho R R^{..} + \frac{3}{2}\rho R^{.2} = -K_{eff}\left[\left(\frac{R}{R_0}\right)^3 - 1\right] - p_d - P_{(t)} \quad (14)$$

By equating the damping pressure, multiplied by the bubble surface, to the damping force, an expression for p_d can be derived from the equation of motion of a damped forced oscillator:

$$4\pi R^2 p_d = \beta R^{.} \quad (15)$$

where β is the mechanical resistance, R = instantaneous microbubble radius; $R^{.}$ = first time derivative of the radius (the velocity of the microbubble wall).

According to the expression of MEDWIN (1977) for the total viscous and friction damping coefficient, $\delta_{tot} = \beta/\omega m$, where ω = insonating frequency of the applied acoustic field and m = effective microbubble mass [$(3/4)\pi R^3 \rho$], the damping pressure can be written as:

$$p_d = \delta_{tot}\rho\omega R R^{.} \quad (16)$$

where $\delta_{tot} = \delta_{rad} + \delta_{vis} + \delta_{th} + \delta_{fr}$, and δ_{rad} = damping coefficient due to reradiation; δ_{vis} = damping coefficient due to the viscosity of the surrounding medium; δ_{th} = damping coefficient due to heat conduction (MEDWIN 1977) and δ_{fr} = damping due to internal friction or viscosity of the shell (HOFF 1996).

Including friction damping, the final expression for the Rayleigh–Plesset theory is:

$$\rho R R^{..} + \frac{3}{2}\rho R^{.2} = p_{go}\left(\frac{R_0}{R}\right)^{3\Gamma} + p_v - p_0 - \frac{2S_T}{R} - \delta_{tot}\omega\rho R R^{.} - P_{(t)} \quad (17)$$

or

$$\rho R R^{..} + \frac{3}{2}\rho R^{.2} = -K_{eff}\left[\left(\frac{R_0}{R}\right)^3 - 1\right] - \delta_{tot}\rho\omega R R^{.} - P_{(t)} \quad (18)$$

or

$$\rho R R^{..} + \frac{3}{2}\rho R^{.2} = p_{go} - p_0 - \frac{2S_T}{R} - \frac{4\eta}{R}R^{.} \quad (19)$$

or

$$\rho R R^{..} + \frac{3}{2}\rho R^{.2} = p_{go}\left(\frac{R_0}{R}\right)^{3\Gamma} - \frac{2S_T}{R} - \frac{4\eta R^{.}}{R} - p_0 + P_{(t)}\sin\omega t \quad (20)$$

where R = instantaneous microbubble radius; $R^{.}$ = first time derivative of the radius (the velocity of the microbubble wall); $R^{..}$ = second time derivative of the radius (the acceleration of the microbubble wall); p_{go} = initial internal gas pressure in the microbubble (= [$C_A + C_G$] R T; where C_A and C_G = concentration of the filling air and gas respectively and T = absolute temperature); R_0 = initial microbubble radius; Γ = polytropic exponent of the gas; p_v = vapour pressure; p_0 = ambient hydrostatic pressure; S_T = surface tension; δ_{tot} = total damping constant (CHURCH 1995); ω = angular frequency of the applied acoustic field; ρ = density of the surrounding medium; $P_{(t)}$ = time-varying applied acoustic pressure; η = shear viscosity of liquid; ω = driving frequency; t = time.

These differential equations predict that the surface shell supports a strain that counters the surface tension and thereby stabilizes the microbubble against dissolution.

2.3.3
Scattering Cross Section – Echogenicity of Microbubbles

The scattering cross-section, σ, is used as the parameter defining the acoustical behaviour of the microbubble and is defined as the quotient of the acoustic power scattered in all directions per unit incident acoustic intensity. The scattered US intensity (I_s) is a function of the incident intensity I_0, the distance between the receiving transducer and the scatterer z, and the scattering cross-section of the scatterer σ according to:

$$I_s = \frac{I_0 \sigma}{4\pi z^2} \qquad (21)$$

The scattering cross-section is directly related to the scattered acoustic power and to microbubble radius (Fig. 2.7) and inversely related to the applied pressure.

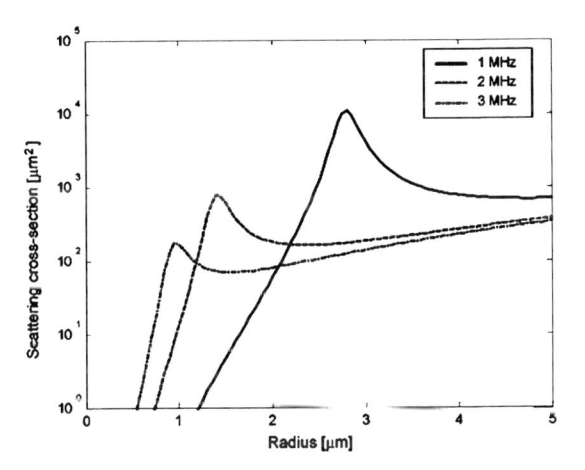

Fig. 2.7. Scattering cross section related to microbubble diameter for an encapsulated air-filled microbubble according to different frequencies of insonation. (Image courtesy of Peter JA Frinking, Bracco Research, Geneva, Switzerland)

The general expression for the scattering cross section in the frequency domain including higher harmonics is:

$$\sigma(R, \omega) = 4\pi R_0^2 \frac{\Omega^4}{(1-\Omega)^2 + (\Omega\delta)^2} \qquad (22)$$

where R = microbubble radius, R_0 = initial microbubble radius, ω = insonating frequency, $\Omega = \omega/f_0$ with f_0 = resonance frequency, δ = damping constant.

Equation 22, may be further developed as:

$$\sigma = \frac{4\pi R_0^2}{\left[\left(\frac{f_0}{f}\right)^2 - 1\right]^2 + \left(\frac{f_0}{f}\right)^4 \delta^2} \qquad (23)$$

$$\sigma = \frac{4\pi}{9} k^4 R^6 \left[\left(\frac{k_s - k}{k}\right)^2 + \frac{1}{3}\left(\frac{3(\rho_s - \rho)}{2\rho_s + \rho}\right)^2\right] \qquad (24)$$

where δ = damping constant, ρ = density respectively of the scatterer (subscript s, microbubble) and the surrounding medium (tissue or plasma), and k = adiabatic compressibility. The k and ρ are also related to the speed of sound ($c = 1 / \sqrt{\rho k}$). Consequently, the scattering cross section is strongly dependent from frequency both for free air (Fig. 2.8) and encapsulated microbubbles (Fig. 2.9) and from the difference in density between the microbubble and the surrounding medium.

2.3.3.1
Practical Applications

At the resonant frequency, the scattering cross section of a microbubble is no longer simply dependent on its size, and can reach peak (Fig. 2.8, 2.9) values a thousand times higher compared to values at off-resonance frequencies (DE JONG et al. 1996). Since the scattering cross section is strongly dependent on the ratio between the insonating frequency and the resonant frequency (Eq. 23), at frequency below resonance most of the scattering occurs at 180° relative to the incident wave, with an angular distribution pattern depending on the scatterer shape and the contrast in the acoustic properties between the particle and the surrounding medium (COUSSIOS et al. 2004).

The compressibility (k value, see Eq. 24) of air is 7.65×10^{-6} m²/N and the compressibility of water is 4.5×10^{-11} m²/N, similarly to tissue and plasma, while

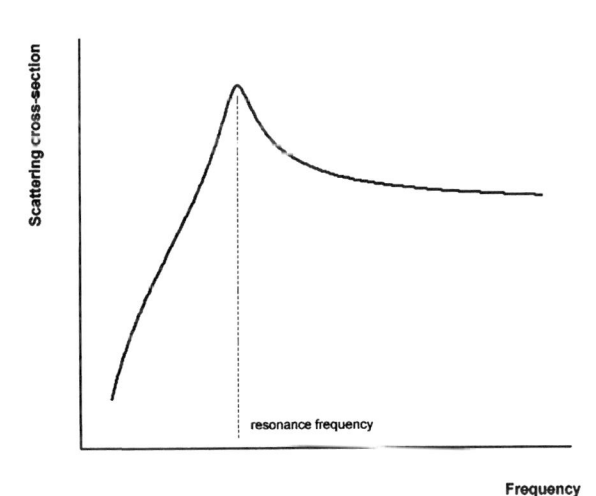

Fig. 2.8. Scattering cross section related to the insonating frequency for free-air microbubble. Scattering cross section abruptly increases at the resonance frequency of the microbubble. (Image courtesy of Peter JA Frinking, Bracco Research, Geneva, Switzerland)

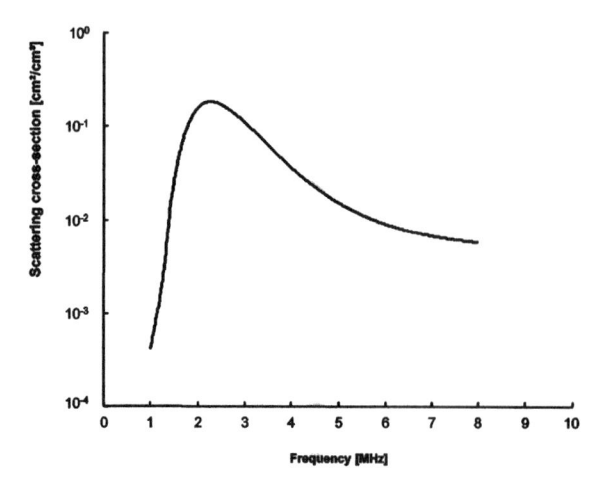

Fig. 2.9. Scattering cross section related to the insonating frequency for encapsulated air-filled microbubble. The lower the shell elasticity due to encapsulation, the higher the resonant frequency and the lower the scattering cross section and generation of harmonics. (Image courtesy of Peter JA Frinking, Bracco Research, Geneva, Switzerland)

the compressibility of a coated microbubble-based agent falls within this range (5×10^{-7} m^2/N in the case of Albunex). This high difference in compressibility, and so in impedance, results in a very high echogenicity which increases the sensitivity of US equipment to microbubbles (DAYTON and FERRARA 2002).

Scattering cross-section equations may be simplified to:

$$\sigma = R_0^6 f_0^4 [\approx Z] \tag{25}$$

known as Born approximation, where R_0 is the initial microbubble radius, f_0 is the resonance frequency and Z is the difference in acoustic impedance (ratio of acoustic pressure to sound flow) between the surrounding medium and the microbubble. Encapsulation drastically reduces the influence of resonance frequency on scattering cross section since the lower the shell elasticity due to encapsulation, the higher the resonant frequency (CHATTERJEE and SARKAR 2003). Moreover, since Eq. 22 shows that the scattering cross section is inversely related to the damping constant, the encapsulation of microbubbles with a thick and stiff shell produces a lower scattering cross section also for the viscoelastic properties of the surrounding shell.

2.3.4
US Beam Attenuation and Microbubble Size Distribution

The US weakening results from *scattering* and *absorption*. The combined effect of scattering and attenuation depend on microbubble concentration (Fig. 2.10). Scattering is the prevalent phenomenon with low microbubble concentrations while the attenuation, caused by multiple scattering, dominates when the microbubble concentration increases.

$$a_{(f)} = \int_{R\min}^{R\max} n(r)\sigma(r)\,dr \tag{26}$$

where a(f) = US frequency-dependent attenuation coefficient expressed in nepers[Np]/length and nepers is a dimensionless quantity, R_{max} and R_{min} = minimum and maximum microbubble radii, n(r) = microbubble concentration and σ = scattering cross-section.

Equation 26 may be employed to calculate the microbubble size distribution which is in agreement

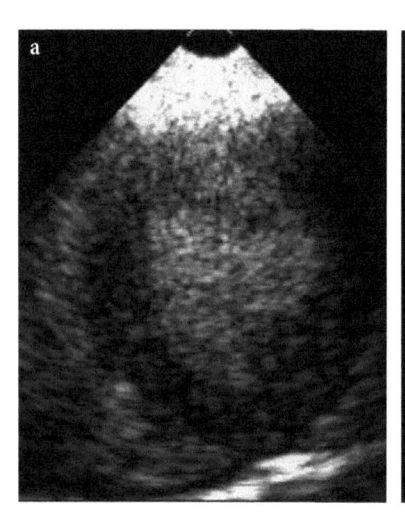

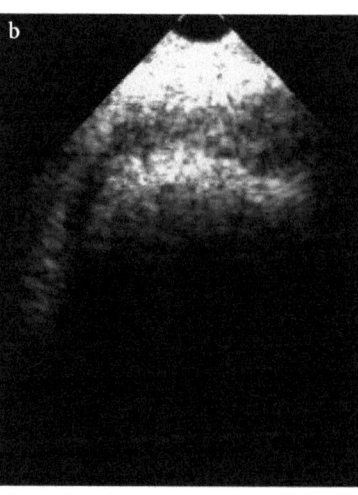

Fig. 2.10a,b. US attenuation determined by a microbubble-based agent (**a**). The attenuation expressed by the posterior acoustic shadowing increases by increasing microbubble concentration (**b**). (Images courtesy of Peter JA Frinking, Bracco Research, Geneva, Switzerland)

with values measured with optical methods. Microbubble-based agents size distribution is normal-shaped (Fig. 2.11) and the standard deviation is larger for first generation agents and lower for new generation agents which present a more uniform microbubble diameter.

2.3.5
Scattering to Attenuation Ratio

In a suspension of microbubbles each microbubble has to be considered as an element which absorbs and scatters US at the same time. The total energy loss or attenuation for an acoustical beam travelling through a screen of microbubbles is called the extinction coefficient, $\mu_e(\omega)$, and is given by:

$$\mu_e(\omega) = \mu_a(\omega) + \mu_s(\omega) \tag{27}$$

where $\mu_a(\omega)$ is the absorption coefficient and $\mu_s(\omega)$ is the scattering coefficient.

The scattering to attenuation ratio (STAR) is a measure of the acoustical effectiveness of the contrast agent. The STAR is defined as:

$$STAR(\omega) = \frac{\mu_s(\omega)}{\mu_e(\omega)} \tag{28}$$

and substituting Eq. 28 into Eq. 27 gives:

$$STAR(\omega) = \frac{\mu_s(\omega)}{\mu_a(\omega) + \mu_s(\omega)} \tag{29}$$

where $\mu_s(\omega)$ represents the part of the energy that is scattered away omnidirectionally by the microbubbles, while $\mu_a(\omega)$ represents the part of the energy that is absorbed by the microbubbles.

Therefore, the lower the absorption of the incoming plane US wave, the higher the STAR. A maximum value of STAR = 1 is obtained when there is no absorption. However, this index is only valid for low acoustic pressures and at high acoustic pressures non-linear transient effects appear.

2.3.5.1
Practical Application

The attenuation of the acoustical beam travelling through a screen of microbubbles can cause shadowing of underlying biological structures and is not considered to be a useful parameter. An effective contrast agent, therefore, is defined by good scattering properties and low attenuation. For these reasons, the higher the STAR, the more effective the contrast agent. DE JONG and HOFF (1993) and DE JONG et al. (1994) showed a non-linear relation between the increase in the acoustic pressure of insonation and the produced backscattering and attenuation. Some experimental evidence (COUSSIOS et al. 2004) suggests that liposomes present a higher scattering to attenuation ratio than albumin-coated microbubbles and could be more efficient as contrast agents.

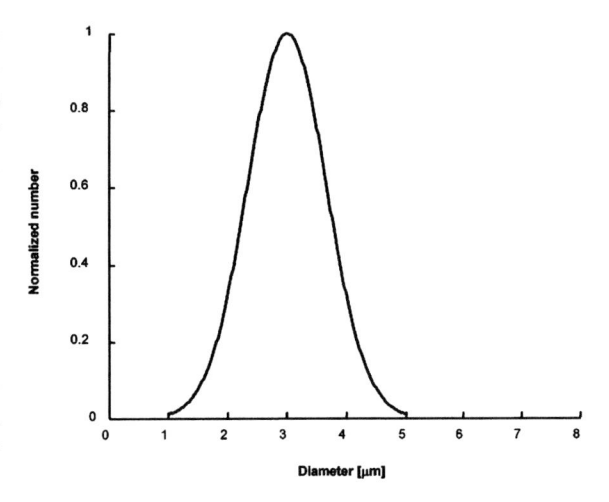

Fig. 2.11. Microbubbles diameter normal distribution. The mean diameter is 3 µm (Courtesy of Peter JA Frinking, Bracco Research, Geneva, Switzerland)

2.3.6
Acoustic Power of Insonation

The probability for a single US pulse to destroy a microbubble (Fig. 2.12) increases for high acoustic power amplitudes, long US pulse lengths and low frequencies according to the following equation:

$$E_{acoustic} = \int_0^k (P_0 \sin 2\pi f t)^2 \, dt = KP_0^2 \frac{1}{f} \approx K(MI)^2 \tag{30}$$

where $E_{acoustic}$ = acoustic power of insonation (W_0), P_0 = acoustic pressure amplitude, f = frequency, t = time, K = number of cycles per burst which determines the US pulse length, MI = mechanical index.

The acoustic power of insonation is usually considered related to the employed MI which measures the potential for mechanical damage to tissues exposed to intense US pulses.

$$MI = \frac{P-}{\sqrt{f}} \tag{31}$$

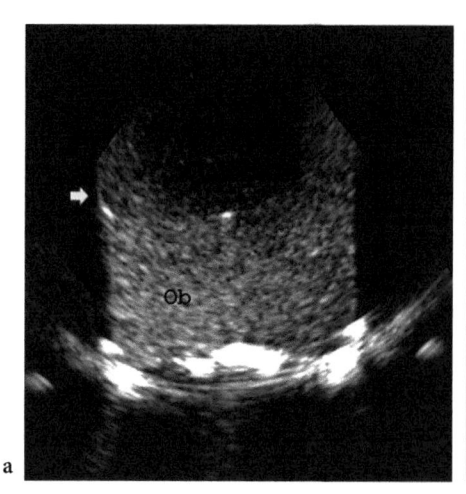

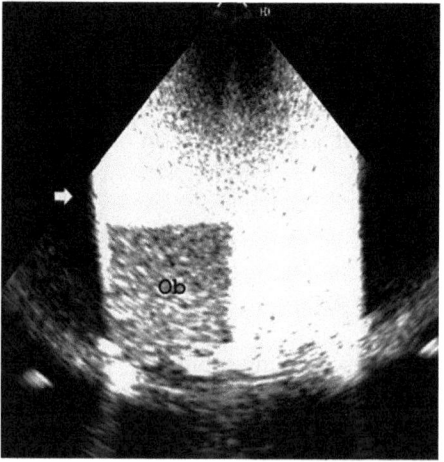

Fig. 2.12a,b. Microbubble rupture shown in a tissue-simulating model. Microbubbles are suspended in a water bath containing a reference echoic object similar to tissues (*Ob*). At low acoustic power insonation (**a**) there is evidence of microbubble resonance with production of low intensity echoes (*arrow*). At high acoustic power insonation (**b**) there is evidence of microbubble destruction. The flash is produced by microbubble destruction (*arrow*) which produces a broadband frequency signal (Courtesy of Peter JA Frinking, Bracco Research, Geneva, Switzerland)

with the peak negative acoustic pressure (P–) in megapascals (MPa; 1 Pa = 1 Newton/m^2), and the frequency in MHz. In clinical practice, the range for MI varies from 0.05 to 1.9. The lower the frequency of US, the greater its MI and therefore its destructive properties. However, the MI is an unreliable predictor of microbubble destruction, since at the same MI value different values of acoustic powers of insonation may be measured in different US systems (MERRITT et al. 2000).

2.3.6.1
High Acoustic Power

High acoustic power (Wo = peak negative pressure; 0.8–2.5 MPa) of insonation alters stabilized microbubbles and increases both the likelihood and rate of microbubble destruction (SHI et al. 2000). High acoustic power insonation induces changes of microbubble-based agents corresponding to fragmentation, coalescence, sonic cracking, jetting and to destruction of microbubbles (DAYTON et al. 1999; DE JONG et al. 1999; POSTEMA et al. 2004).

Fragmentation is the fission of a bubble into smaller microbubbles (POSTEMA et al. 2002, 2004) which was first visualized with high-speed cameras (POSTEMA et al. 2001, 2004). Fragmentation occurs around peak microbubble contraction (CHOMAS et al. 2001), when the bubble collapse is driven by inertial forces because the inward acceleration continues to increase as the bubble approaches its minimus radius, and suddenly changes sign as the bubble begins a rebound (POSTEMA et al. 2004).

Coalescence is the fusion of two or more microbubbles. As adjacent microbubbles expand, the pressure in the film between them increases, resulting in a deformation of the bubble surfaces. This thinning continues until a critical thickness around 0.1 μm, at which Van der Waals attractive forces results in capsule rupture and the coalescence of the bubbles (POSTEMA et al. 2004). Sonic cracking is the US-induced formation of a shell defect causing gas to escape from microbubbles (POSTEMA et al. 2004), and it was observed with rigid-shell microbubbles (POSTEMA et al. 2002). Jetting corresponds to asymmetric microbubble collapse, which causes the velocity of the upper bubble wall to exceed the velocity of the lower wall. For this phenomenon the fluid above the bubble is accelerated and focused during collapse, leading to the formation of a high-speed liquid jet (POSTEMA et al. 2004).

US energy-mediated destruction, expressed as disappearance time, of microbubbles is directly related to US intensity, duration and frequency (WALKER et al. 1997). Microbubble destruction produces the emission of a broadband frequency (Fig. 2.12) that includes both sub- and higher harmonics. The resulting fragments differ in their echo spectra and may be differentiated from the original microbubble-based contrast agent and subtraction contrast-specific modes, processing the echoes obtained before and after microbubble destruction (DAYTON and FERRARA 2002), improve microbubble detection.

When the applied acoustic power exceeds a specific threshold, the scattering level increases abruptly for a few seconds producing an increased echogenicity in conventional US and a coloured mosaic map at colour Doppler (FRINKING 1999). The effect is most effective when the US wave hits the microbubble for the first time. This particular transient response, known also as stimulated acoustic emission or flash echo imaging, may be considered as a signature of each contrast agent and was particularly observed in some contrast agents such as Sonavist (Schering AG, Germany) and Quantison (Quadrant, UK).

2.3.6.2
Low Acoustic Power

Low acoustic power (Wo = peak negative pressure 100–600 kPa) is used to produce the non-linear harmonic response of microbubbles. Below an acoustic power threshold, microbubbles act as stable linear or non-linear scatterers depending on the applied acoustic power. With non-linear oscillation, the duration and degree of microbubble expansion is greater than its compression phase. Non-linear oscillations of microbubble-based contrast agents generate significant scattered echoes at harmonic multiples of the transmitted frequency (Fig. 2.12). These harmonic echoes may be differentiated from tissue echoes from their spectral characteristic, containing prevalently echoes at double frequency, from the lower acoustic power and from their phase. The more recently introduced contrast-specific modes employ pulse trains with multiple frequencies, amplitudes and phases which increase significantly the sensitivity to the harmonic signal produced by microbubbles (Chap. 4).

2.4
Artefacts from Microbubble-Based Agents

2.4.1
Microbubble Artefacts with Doppler

Most microbubble-specific artefacts are found with colour and power Doppler modes because the settings of US equipment become inappropriate following a strong increase of the backscattered signals (Fig. 2.13) and need to be recognized to avoid interpretative errors (FORSBERG et al. 1994).

2.4.1.1
High-Intensity Transient Signals

This artefact is determined by microbubble collapse or by aggregates of macrobubbles producing sharp spikes on the Doppler spectral tracing, heard as crackling on the audio output (Figs. 2.14, 2.15). These spikes are easily recognized since they cover the entire frequency spectrum. This artefact may also be detected with colour and power Doppler imaging appearing as colour pixels of higher intensity within the more uniform signal of the vessel.

2.4.1.2
Pseudoacceleration of the Systolic Peak Velocity

An increase in the systolic peak velocity of up to 50% can be found at peak enhancement. This artefact is probably the result of signals that were too weak to be detected before microbubble injection and it may be almost completely cancelled by reducing the Doppler gain or by employing slow infusion of microbubbles. The increase in systolic peak velocity may produce error in grading stenotic lesions of the vessels.

2.4.1.3
Clutter

Clutter may be defined as unwanted strong echoes produced by stationary or slow moving tissues. The flow signals, registered at Doppler, are disturbed by clutter signals produced by muscular tissue and vessel walls which can be much stronger than the blood signals even after the injection of a microbubble-based contrast agent. These signals are also produced by the relative movement

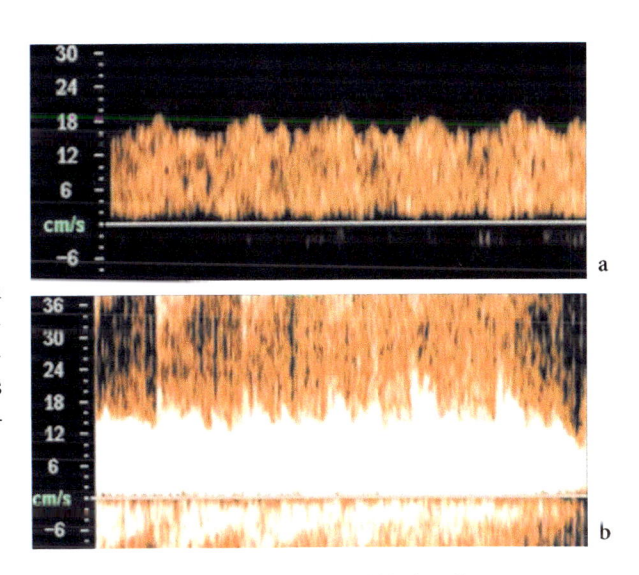

Fig. 2.13a,b. Artefacts from microbubble-based agents. Doppler signal before microbubble injection (a). Excessive amplifications of Doppler signal after microbubble injection (b)

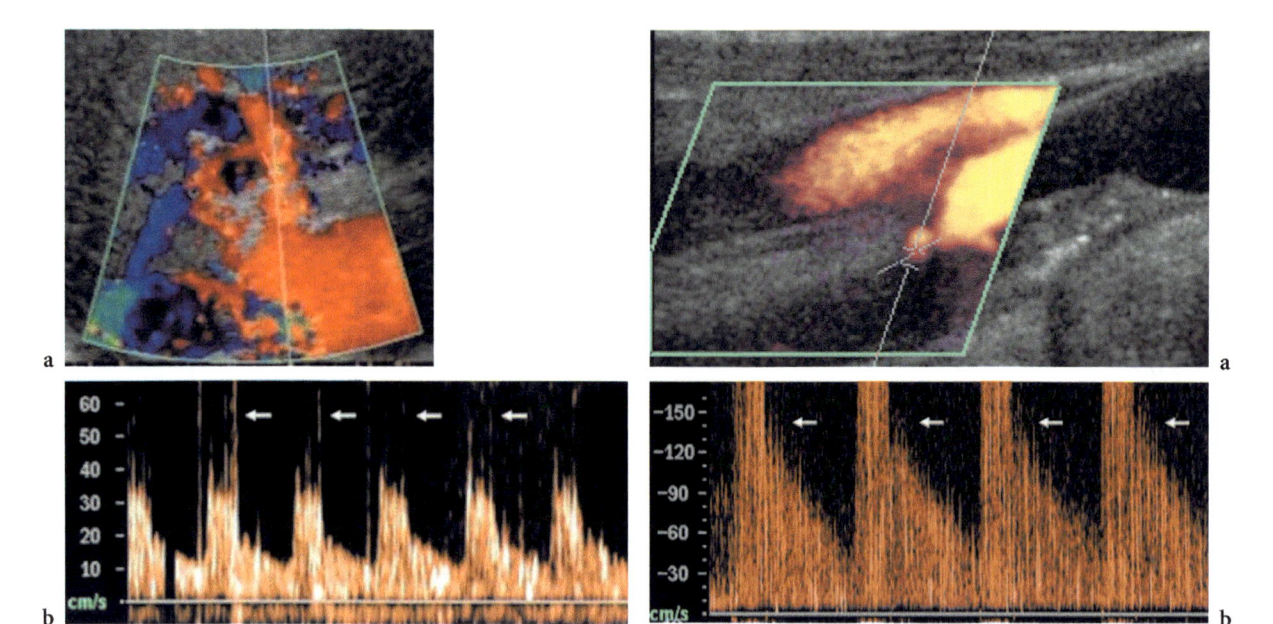

Fig. 2.14a,b. Artefacts from microbubble-based agents. Spikes (*arrows*) due to macrobubble presence in the bloodstream. Colour Doppler and Doppler interrogation of the hepatic artery (**a**) after microbubble injection. In the Doppler spectra (**b**) different spikes, covering the entire frequency spectrum, are evident due to macrobubble aggregates

Fig. 2.15a,b. Artefacts from microbubble-based agents. Spikes (*arrows*) due to macrobubble presence in the bloodstream. Colour Doppler and Doppler interrogation of the internal carotid artery (**a**) after microbubble injection. In the Doppler spectra (**b**) different spikes are evident due to macrobubble aggregates or microbubbles collapse

between the US probe and the unwanted tissue targets due to the cardiac beating, patient breathing and the operator moving while keeping the probe. Clutter may be reduced by using specific filters, harmonic power Doppler (Chap. 4) or by contrast-specific modes as three stage multi-pulse contrast agent detection (FRINKING et al. 1998; KIRKHORN et al. 2001). The principle of this multi-pulse technique is that the scattering properties are modified if microbubbles are insonated at high acoustic power while remaining unchanged at low acoustic power. The first stage of the pulsing sequence is to use low acoustic power pulses to obtain high resolution reference images without altering the agents; the second stage is to use high acoustic power, called the release burst, to modify the agent; and the third stage is to detect the changes using low acoustic power.

2.4.1.4
Blooming Artefact

In Doppler tracing only the mean frequency shift is displayed, while the Doppler signal intensity is increased after microbubble injection since the increase in backscattering echo-signal intensity determines the appearance also of the lowest velocities that were too weak to be registered before microbubble injection. When colour or power Doppler is turned on the overload of the Doppler signal registration apparatus is determined by the strong signals and multiple re-reflections between adjacent microbubbles. Such artefact (Figs. 2.16, 2.17) can be limited by reducing the colour gain and persistence and the MI or by increasing the wall filter and the pulse repetition frequency, resulting in a decreased sensitivity of the system. The slow infusion of microbubbles limits this artefact because of a decrease in the peak signal intensity. Dedicated US contrast-specific modes were introduced principally to avoid this artefact.

2.4.1.5
Jail Bar Artefact

The jail bar artefact (Fig. 2.18) is prevalently observed with power Doppler mode. It is determined by an error in image interpolation when the management of the backscattering signal intensity from the US system approaches saturation. Since each frame is reconstructed from an interpolation mathematical procedure of the image view lines, the saturation of signal determines a lack of colour along the interpolating view.

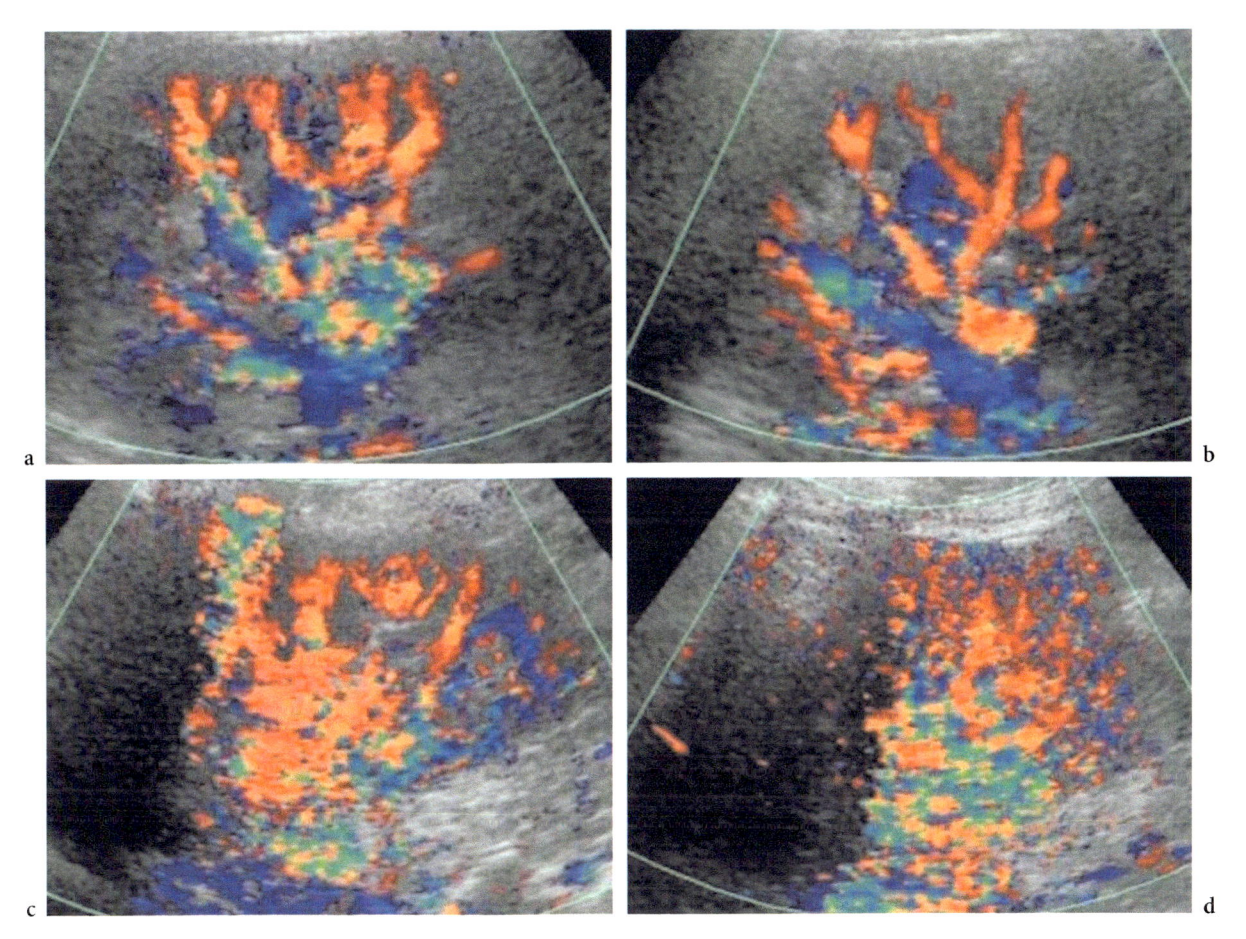

Physical Basis and Principles of Action of Microbubble-based Contrast Agents

Fig. 2.16a–d. Artefacts from microbubble-based agents. Blooming artefact consisting in the presence of colour signal outside the vessels. Baseline colour Doppler US (**a,b**) of the right kidney. The renal parenchymal vessels are identified. After microbubble-based agents injection (**c,d**) colour signal becomes diffuse and identified outside the renal vessels

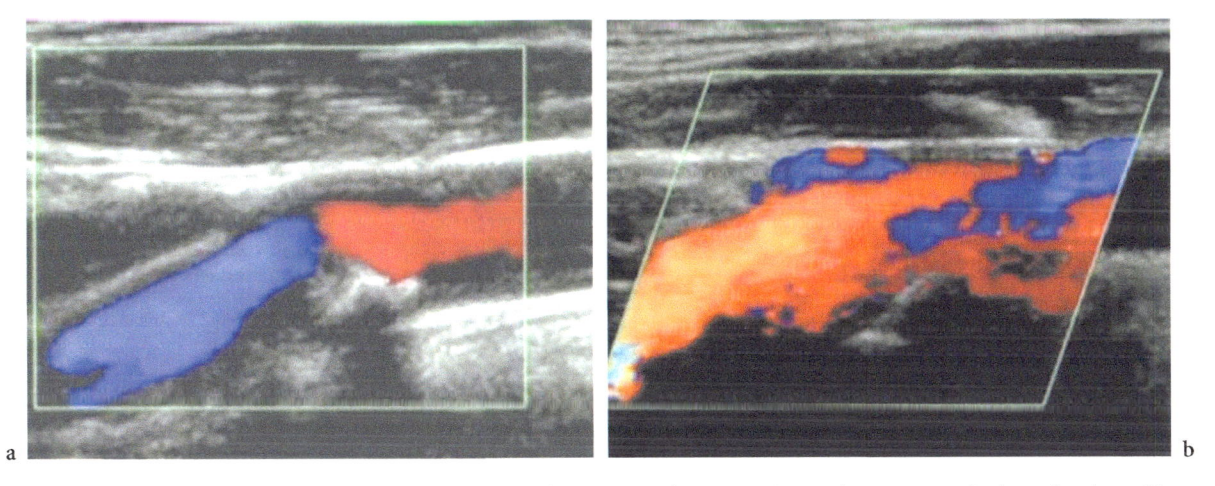

Fig. 2.17a,b. Artefacts from microbubble-based agents. Blooming artefact consisting in the presence of colour signal outside the vessels. Baseline colour Doppler US (**a**) of the right carotid bulb. After microbubble-based agents injection (**b**) colour signal becomes diffuse and identified outside the carotids

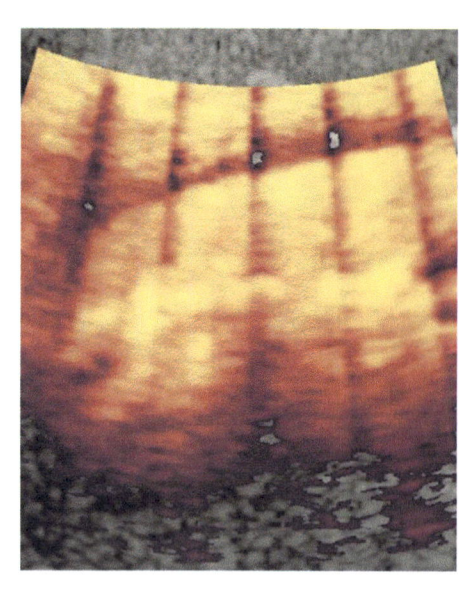

Fig. 2.18. Artefacts from microbubble-based agents. Jail-bar artefact consisting in the presence of black vertical signals void throughout the image

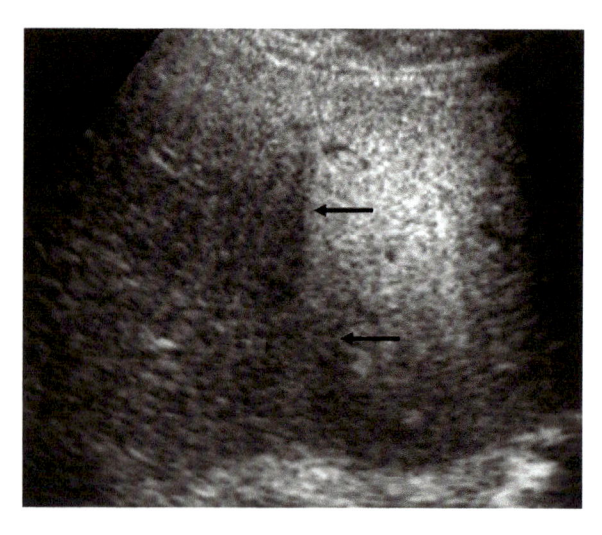

Fig. 2.19. Artefacts from microbubble-based agents (*arrows*). Artefact arising from the second scan in the same region of the liver. The areas of the liver where microbubbles were previously destroyed (*arrows*) appear as hypoechoic if compared to the adjacent areas of the liver not previously scanned

2.4.2
Microbubble Artefacts with Contrast-Specific Modes

2.4.2.1
Attenuation of the Sound Beam

This artefact is produced when the sound beam travels through high concentrations of microbubble-based agents (JAKOBSEN and CORREAS 2001). This artefact is frequently observed in the heart, and sometimes also observed in the liver.

2.4.2.2
Artefact from Multiple Insonations

This artefact results from different scans performed orthogonally which causes microbubble disruption, e.g. when the right liver lobe is scanned at a transverse insonating plane after initial longitudinal sweep through the left lobe and part of the right lobe (Figs. 2.19, 2.20) (HARVEY et al. 2000). Another artefact consisting in vertical signal void may be determined by small tissue movement between the two out-of-phase pulses in pulse inversion mode (Fig. 2.21) and may be eliminated by power pulse inversion mode which works as a multi-pulse technique by considering as linear the tissue movement between the different pulses and by summing the resulting phase shift.

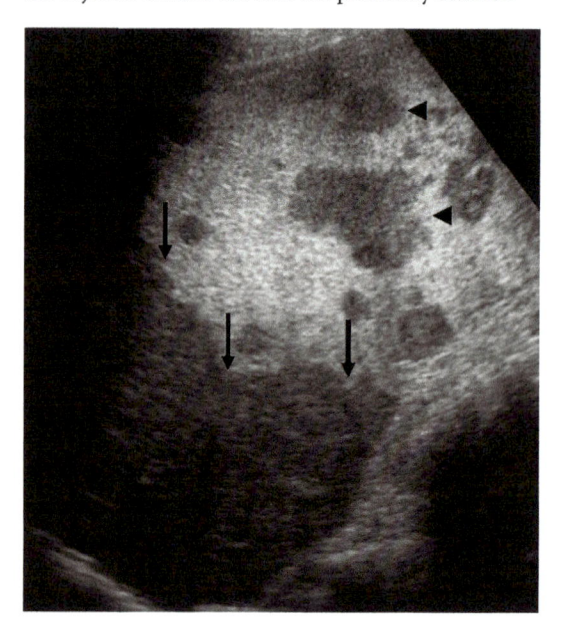

Fig. 2.20. Microbubble artefacts. Artefact (*arrows*) arising from the second scan in the same region of the liver. The areas of the liver where microbubbles were previously destroyed appear as hypoechoic compared to the adjacent areas of the liver not previously scanned. Some liver metastases are also evident (*arrowheads*)

2.4.2.3
Artefact from Heterogeneous Rate of Microbubble Rupture

Destructive mode presents some technical disadvantages. To produce a uniform microbubble rup-

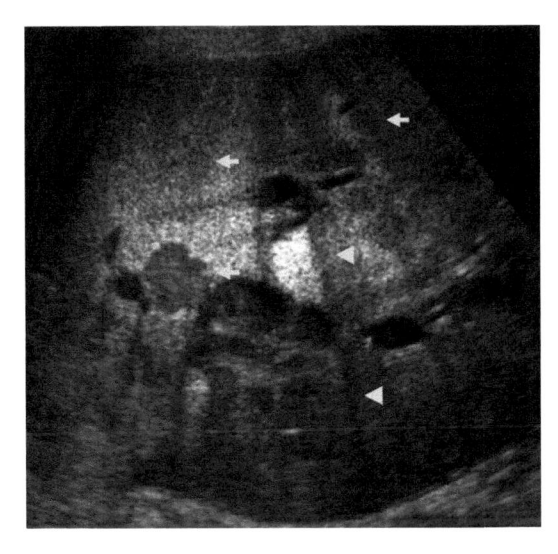

Fig. 2.21. Artefacts from microbubble-based agents. Pulse inversion mode. Artefacts arising from stationary tissue movement (*arrowheads*) between the first and the second out-of-phase pulse which determines the cancellation of the signal. Liver metastases (*arrows*) are also identified

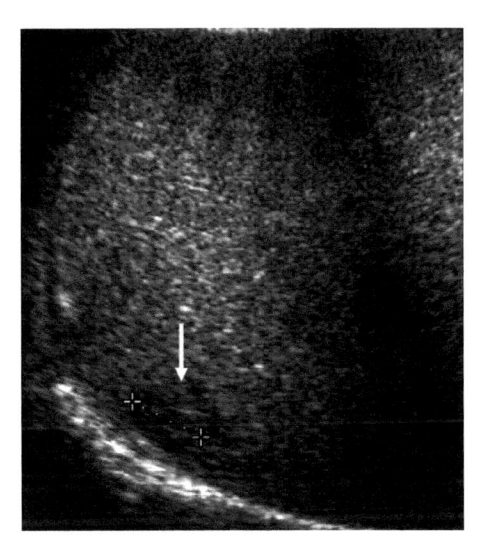

Fig. 2.22. Artefacts from microbubble-based agents. Pulse inversion mode. Artefact arising from heterogeneous microbubble rupture throughout the liver parenchyma which simulate one focal liver lesion (*arrow*) adjacent to the diaphragm

ture on liver parenchyma, which is necessary to produce a wideband frequency signal, rapid and uniform sweeps are necessary. The largest amount of microbubbles entrapped in liver sinusoids are destroyed after one single high MI sweep, so there is no possibility to analyze focal liver lesions with US acoustic windows other than transabdominal, such as an intercostal view. Scanning irregularities determined by a not completely uniform sweep or liver movements during emission of the two out phase pulses or to the heterogeneous distribution of acoustic power produce artefacts simulating focal liver lesions (Fig. 2.22). In order to reduce bubble destruction and to prolong bubble permanence, the lowest real time frame rate (7–9 Hz) has to be employed. However, a low frame rate increases US artefacts related to motion and to bubble rupture heterogeneously, which can simulate focal liver defects producing focal positive findings misinterpreted as metastases.

References

Anderson AL, Hampton LD (1980) Acoustics of gas-bearing sediments. Background. J Acoust Soc Am 67:1865-1889
Bauer A, Blomley MJK, Leen E, Cosgrove D, Schlief R (1999) Liver-specific imaging with SHU 563 A: diagnostic potential of a new class of ultrasound contrast media. Eur Radiol 9 [Suppl 3]:S349-S352
Chatterjee D, Sarkar K (2003) A Newtonian rheological model for the interface of microbubble contrast agents. Ultrasound Med Biol 29:1749-1757
Chomas JE, Dayton P, May D, Ferrara K (2001) Threshold of fragmentation for ultrasonic contrast. J Biomed Opt 6:141-150
Church CC (1995) The effect of an elastic solid surface layer on the radial pulsation of gas bubbles. J Acoust Soc Am 97:1510-1521
Correas JM, Kessler D, Worah D, Quay SC (1997) The first phase shift ultrasound contrast agent: EchoGen. In: Goldberg BB (ed) Ultrasound contrast agents. Dunitz, London, pp 83-99
Correas JM, Burns PN, Lai X, Qi X (2000) Infusion versus Bolus of an ultrasound contrast agent: in vivo dose-response measurements of BR1. Invest Radiol 35:72-79
Correas JM, Bridal L, Lesavre A et al (2001) Ultrasound contrast agents: properties, principles of action, tolerance, and artifacts. Eur Radiol 11:1316-1328
Coussios CC, Holland CK, Jakubowska L et al (2004) In vitro characterization of liposomes and Optison by acoustic scattering at 3.5 MHz. Ultrasound Med Biol 30:181-190
Dayton PA, Ferrara KW (2002) Targeted imaging using ultrasound. J Magn Res Imaging 16:362-377
De Jong N, Hoff L (1993) Ultrasound scattering properties of Albunex® microspheres. Ultrasonics 31:175-181
De Jong N, Hoff L, Skotland T, Bom N (1992) Absorption and scatter of encapsulated gas filled microspheres: theoretical considerations and some measurements. Ultrasonics 30:95-103
De Jong N, Cornet R, Lancée CT (1994a) Higher harmonics of vibrating gas filled microbubbles, part one: simulations. Ultrasonics 32:447-453
De Jong N, Cornet R, Lancée CT (1994b) Higher harmonics of vibrating gas filled microbubbles, part two: measurements. Ultrasonics 32:455-459

De Jong N, Frinking P, ten Cate F, van der Wouw P (1996) Characteristics of contrast agents and 2D imaging. IEEE ultrasonics symposium, pp 1449-1458

De Jong N, Frinking PJ, Bouakaz A et al (1999) Optical imaging of contrast agent microbubbles in an ultrasound field with a 100-MHz camera. Ultrasound Med Biol 26:487-492

Fisher NG, Christiansen JP, Leong-Poi H et al (2002) Myocardial and microcirculatory kinetics of BR14, a novel third-generation intravenous ultrasound contrast agent. J Am Coll Cardiol 39:530-537

Forsberg F, Tao Shi W (2001) Physics of contrast microbubbles. In: Goldberg B, Raichlen JS, Forsberg F (eds) Ultrasound contrast agents: basic principles and clinical applications. Dunitz, London, pp 15-23

Forsberg F, Basude R, Liu JB et al (1999) Effect of filling gasses on the backscatterer from contrast microbubble: theory and in vivo measurements. Ultrasound Med Biol 25:1203-1211

Frinking PJA, Céspedes EI, de Jong N (1998) Multi-pulse ultrasound contrast imaging based on a decorrelation detection strategy. Proc IEEE Ultras Symp 2:1787-1790

Frinking PJA (1999) Ultrasound contrast agents: acoustic characterization and diagnostic imaging. Optima Grafische Communicatie, Rotterdam, pp 33-37

Frinking PJA, de Jong N (1999) Scattering properties of encapsulated gas bubbles at high ultrasound pressures. J Acoust Soc Am 105:1989-1996

Forsberg F, Goldberg BB, Liu JB (1996) On the feasibility of real time in vivo harmonic imaging with proteinaceous microspheres. J Ultrasound Med 15:853-860

Gorce JM, Arditi M, Schneider M (2000) Influence of bubble size distribution on the echogenicity of ultrasound contrast agents: a study of SonoVue. Invest Radiol 35:661-671

Gramiak R, Shah PM (1968) Echocardiography of the aortic root. Invest Radiol 3:356-366

Harvey CJ, Blomley MJ, Eckersley RJ et al (2000) Hepatic malignancies: improved detection with pulse inversion US in late phase of enhancement with SH U 508 A - early experience. Radiology 216:903-908

Harvey CJ, Blomley MJK, Eckersley RJ, Cosgrove DO (2001) Developments in ultrasound contrast media. Eur Radiol 11:675-689

Hauff P, Fritsch T, Reinhardt M et al (1997) Delineation of experimental liver tumors in rabbits by a new ultrasound contrast agent and stimulated acoustic emission. Invest Radiol 32:94-99

Hoff L (1996) Acoustic properties of ultrasonic contrast agents. Ultrasonics 34:591-593

Jakobsen JA, Correas JM (2001) Ultrasound contrast agents and their use in urogenital radiology: status and prospects. Eur Radiol 11:2082-2091

Kabalnov A, Klein D, Pelura T et al (1998a) Dissolution of multicomponent microbubble in the blood stream 1. Theory. Ultrasound Med Biol 24:739-749

Kabalnov A, Bradley JA, Flam S et al (1998b) Dissolution of multicomponent microbubble in the blood stream 2. Experiment. Ultrasound Med Biol 24:751-760

Kono Y, Steinbach GC, Peterson T et al (2002) Mechanism of parenchymal enhancement of the liver with a microbubble-based US contrast medium: an intravital microscopy study in rats. Radiology 224:253-257

Lindner JR, Dayton PA, Coggins MP et al (2000) Noninvasive imaging of inflammation by ultrasound detection of phagocytosed microbubbles. Circulation 102:531-538

Marelli C (1999) Preliminary experience with NC100100, a new ultrasound contrast agent for intravenous injection. Eur Radiol 9 [Suppl 3]:S343-S346

Medwin H (1977) Counting bubbles acoustically: a review. Ultrasonics 1:7-13

Merritt CR, Forsberg F, Shi WT et al (2000) The mechanical index: an inappropriate and misleading indicator for desctruction of ultrasound microbubble contrast agents. Radiology 217:395

Meuwl JY, Correas JM, Bleuzen A, Tranquart F (2003) Detection modes of ultrasound contrast agents. J Radiol 84:2013-2024

Morel DR, Schwieger I, Hohn L et al (2000) Human pharmacokinetics and safety evaluation of SonoVue™, a new contrast agent for ultrasound imaging. Invest Radiol 35:80-85

Powers JE, Burns PN, Souquet J (1997) Imaging instrumentation for ultrasound contrast agents. In: Nanda NCSR, Goldberg BB (eds) Advances in echo imaging using contrast enhancement. Kluwer, Dordrecht, pp 137-170

Postema M, Bouakaz A, Chin CT, de Jong N (2001) Real-time optical imaging of individual microbubbles in an ultrasonic field. Proc IEEE Ultras Symp 1679-1682

Postema M, Bouakaz A, Chin CT, de Jong N (2002) Optically observed microbubble coalescence and collapse. Proc IEEE Ultras Symp 1900-1903

Postema M, van Wamel A, Lancée CT, de Jong N (2004) Ultrasound-induced encapsulated microbubble phenomena. Ultrasound Med Biol 30:827-840

Quaia E, Blomley MJK, Patel S et al (2002) Initial observations on the effect of irradiation on the liver-specific uptake of Levovist. Eur J Radiol 41:192-199

Rayleigh (1917) On the pressure developed in a liquid during the collapse of a spherical cavity. Philos Mag 34:94-98

Schneider M, Arditi M, Barrau MB et al (1995) BR1: a new ultrasonographic contrast agent based on sulphur hexafluoride-filled microbubbles. Invest Radiol 30:451-457

Schneider M, Broillet A, Bussat P et al (1997) Gray-scale liver enhancement in VX2 tumor bearing rabbits using BR14, a new ultrasonographic contrast agent. Invest Radiol 32:410-417

Shankar PM, Krishna PD, Newhouse VL (1998) Advantages of subharmonic over second harmonic backscatterer for contrast-to-tissue echo enhancement. Ultrasound Med Biol 24:395-399

Shen CC, Li PC (2003) Pulse-inversion-based fundamental imaging for contrast detection. IEEE Trans Ultrason Ferroelectr Freq Control 50:1124-1133

Shi WT, Forsberg F, Tornes A et al (2000) Destruction of contrast microbubbles and the association with inertial cavitation. Ultrasound Med Biol 26:1009-1019

Takeuchi H, Ohmori K, Kondo I (2004) Interaction with leukocytes: phospholipid-stabilized versus albumin-shell microbubbles. Radiology 230:735-742

Walker KW, Pantely GA, Sahn DJ (1997) Ultrasound-mediated destruction of contrast agents. Effect of ultrasound intensity, exposure, and frequency. Invest Radiol 32:728-734

3 Characterization and Design of Microbubble-Based Contrast Agents Suitable for Diagnostic Imaging

Eleanor Stride

CONTENTS

3.1 Introduction *31*
3.1.1 Contrast Agent Design *31*
3.1.2 Aims and Requirements *32*
3.2 Modelling and Analysis *33*
3.2.1 Derivation of a General Model *33*
3.2.2 Sensitivity Analysis *34*
3.2.3 Results and Implications *35*
3.3 Design and Engineering *37*
3.3.1 The Encapsulating Shell *37*
3.3.1.1 Improving the Shell Model *37*
3.3.1.2 Designing the Shell *38*
3.3.2 The Insonating Field *39*
3.3.2.1 Influence of the Field Parameters *39*
3.3.2.2 Influence of the Surrounding Fluid *40*
3.3.3 The Filling Gas *40*
3.4 Concluding Remarks *41*
References *41*

3.1 Introduction

The benefits of coated microbubble-based contrast agents in ultrasound (US) image enhancement have been clearly demonstrated since the development of the first commercial agents in the 1970s. More recently, their potential use in therapeutic applications such as targeted drug delivery has also become an active area of research. However, existing theoretical descriptions of coated microbubble are inadequate in several respects and despite considerable investigation, coated microbubbles behaviour is by no means fully understood. There is consequently substantial scope for improving the effectiveness of contrast agents, and despite a lack of definite evidence for harmful effects, there inevitably remain some concerns as to their safety.

The aim of this chapter is to discuss the deficiencies in coated microbubble characterisation and examine how these may be addressed in order to improve contrast agent design.

3.1.1 Contrast Agent Design

The first step in any design process is to define the requirements for a particular application. In the case of diagnostic imaging, the aim is to obtain a satisfactory image of the region of interest, quickly, safely and, if possible, economically. In terms of equipment costs and portability, scanning time and patient risk, US is superior to alternative imaging techniques such as CT and MR imaging. In terms of image quality, however, it is generally inferior, and the requirement for a contrast agent is to lessen this disadvantage by increasing the reflectivity of a particular feature compared with that of the surrounding tissue.

Gas microbubbles are effective contrast agents because their presence vastly increases the difference in acoustic impedance between the normally liquid filled blood vessels and the neighbouring solid or semi solid tissue. There is, in addition, a fortuitous coincidence between the frequency range over which coated microbubbles resonate and that which is used in diagnostic imaging, and under the right conditions, coated microbubbles will exhibit significantly non-linear behaviour. This can be exploited very effectively for imaging, as will be described below. Thus, whilst the discovery of microbubble contrast agents was in fact accidental (Gramiak and Shah 1968), in design terms, they represent an ideal choice for US contrast enhancement.

In therapeutic applications the aim is to target treatment, be it a drug or a physical effect such as heating, to a specific region of the body in order to minimise unwanted side effects. There is a wider range of factors to consider in assessing the optimality of microbubbles for this purpose than for

E. Stride, PhD
Department of Mechanical Engineering, University College London, Torrington Place, London, WC1E 7JE, UK

contrast enhancement. For example, in addition to ensuring the survival of the microbubbles in vivo, the microbubble coating may be required to act as an anchor site for certain species according to the type of therapy to be delivered and/or the target area.

There may also be differing requirements regarding the shape of coated microbubbles. Spheres have a low ratio of surface area to volume, whereas to increase the probability of a particle adhering to a target, a large surface area is desirable. Notwithstanding the question of optimality, however, coated microbubbles are undoubtedly an effective means of delivering therapy, particularly if there is an additional requirement for imaging, for example to trace the passage of the coated microbubbles to the target site. They can also be destroyed using US, which enables treatment to be delivered directly to the target site.

3.1.2
Aims and Requirements

Having established the suitability of microbubbles for diagnostic and therapeutic applications in a general sense, the design of the coated microbubbles themselves must now be examined more closely to identify areas for improvement. The precise requirements will naturally vary according to the application and, for the purposes of illustration, the following discussion will therefore concentrate upon coated microbubble design for image enhancement. The procedure may easily be adapted for therapeutic applications however.

The three main requirements for an US contrast agent are:
- Detectability – Coated microbubbles should produce as large a contrast effect as possible for a given dose.
- Longevity – Coated microbubble survival times should be sufficient to enable imaging of the required region.
- Safety – Coated microbubbles should pose no risk to the patient.

For existing contrast agents these are conflicting requirements. In order to achieve a large contrast effect, and thereby minimise the dose required, the scattered signal from the coated microbubbles must be distinct from that generated by tissue. At present, the most effective way of obtaining a distinctive signal is to use a high acoustic power of insonation (high mechanical index, MI). This not only increases the amplitude of the signal and the proportion of coated microbubbles excited, but also causes the microbubbles to behave non-linearly. In theory, the non-linear components in the overall scattered signal will be due primarily to this behaviour. Thus, by using an appropriate imaging technique such as pulse inversion (Chap. 4), which isolates these components, much of the noise from the surrounding tissue can be eliminated. However, using a high acoustic power also increases the likelihood of coated microbubble destruction. This may be desirable for certain types of imaging, but it requires larger and/or more frequent doses to be administered and is clearly unacceptable if, for example, drug carrying coated microbubbles are being imaged away from the target site. Moreover, at high acoustic power the potential for harmful bio-effects is necessarily increased, and the effects of non-linear propagation through the surrounding tissue will become noticeable, thus limiting the maximum microbubble/tissue signal ratio that may be achieved.

The possibility of designing coated microbubbles in order to overcome this problem is discussed in Sect. 3.2. There are some further requirements to consider first however. These are general to all applications.

An ideal coated microbubble should:
- Respond predictably and reproducibly
- Have a well defined destruction threshold
- Locate preferentially in the area required
- Be economical to produce
- Be convenient to administer
- Eventually disintegrate or be eliminated from the body

The reproducibility of coated microbubble response, the ease with which coated microbubbles can be administered and their cost, will be determined primarily by the manufacturing process. It should perhaps be noted at this point that the main disadvantage of ultrasound contrast agents is the fact that the need to administer them increases the time, skill and resources required for performing a scan. Since this must be offset against the benefits of contrast agents, it is important that manufacturing requirements are considered in the design process.

As indicated above, the ability of coated microbubbles to "locate preferentially", whether for imaging or treatment, is related primarily to their surface chemistry, as is their ability to disintegrate and/or be eliminated from the body. These properties will be discussed further in Sect. 3.3. To predict either the acoustic response or the destruction threshold of a coated microbubble, an accurate model is required. This is also the principle requirement for determining the most important factors on which to concentrate for design. The development of a suitable model is the subject of the next section.

3.2
Modelling and Analysis

3.2.1
Derivation of a General Model

A number of models describing the response of a single, coated gas microbubble to an imposed US field have been developed (Fox and HERZFELD 1954; GLAZMAN 1983; LORD et al. 1990; DE JONG et al. 1992; CHURCH 1995; KHISMATULLIN and NADIM 2002; MORGAN et al. 1999). They vary in terms of their complexity but, regardless of the rigour with which they were originally derived, they can be shown to be mathematically equivalent. In the absence of reliable experimental data it is not possible to assess their relative worth. The following discussion will therefore be based on a generalised model, of which the models mentioned above represent specific forms.

A spherical volume of gas enclosed by a stabilising outer layer and suspended in a volume of liquid is considered (Fig. 3.1). The notation used is defined in Table 3.1. The validity of the assumptions underlying the model will be assessed subsequently. For the present, spherical symmetry is assumed and conservation of momentum in spherical polar coordinates yields:

$$\rho\left(\frac{\partial u}{\partial t}+u\frac{\partial u}{\partial r}\right)+\frac{\partial p}{\partial r}=\frac{\partial T_{rr}}{\partial r}+\frac{2T_{rr}-T_{\theta\theta}-T_{\phi\phi}}{r} \quad (3.1)$$

Similarly, from conservation of mass:

$$\frac{\partial \rho}{\partial t}+\rho\frac{\partial u}{\partial t}+u\frac{\partial \rho}{\partial r}+\frac{2\rho u}{r}=0 \quad (3.2)$$

Table 3.1. Notation

Symbol	Definition	Subscript	Definition
u	radial velocity	r	radial
t	time	G	gas
p	pressure	S	shell
T	stress	L	liquid
r	radial coordinate	1	inner surface
R	radius	2	outer surface
$\dot{R}$	radial velocity	∞	conditions at infinity
$\ddot{R}$	radial acceleration	o	initial conditions
f	factor	v	viscous
V	volume	s	stiffness
G	shear modulus	rad	radiation
M	strain time derivative	th	thermal
d	thickness	A	acoustic
k	constant	e	equilibrium conditions
		max	maximum
δ	damping factor	min	minimum
σ	surface tension	θ	latitudinal
ω	frequency	ϕ	longitudinal
μ	viscosity		
κ	polytropic constant		
ψ	material function		
τ	time variable		
α	material constant		
Γ	concentration		
χ	elasticity parameter		
ρ	density		

Integrating Eq. 3.1 over three regimes for the gas, shell and surrounding fluid gives:

$$\int_{0}^{R_{1}}\left[\rho_{G}\left(\frac{\partial u}{\partial t}+u\frac{\partial u}{\partial r}\right)+\frac{\partial p}{\partial r}-\frac{\partial T_{G,rr}}{\partial r}-\frac{2T_{G,rr}-T_{G,\theta\theta}-T_{G,\phi\phi}}{r}\right]dr$$
$$+\int_{R_{1}}^{R_{2}}\left[\rho_{S}\left(\frac{\partial u}{\partial t}+u\frac{\partial u}{\partial r}\right)+\frac{\partial p}{\partial r}-\frac{\partial T_{S,rr}}{\partial r}-\frac{2T_{S,rr}-T_{S,\theta\theta}-T_{S,\phi\phi}}{r}\right]dr \quad (3.3)$$
$$+\int_{R_{2}}^{\infty}\left[\rho_{L}\left(\frac{\partial u}{\partial t}+u\frac{\partial u}{\partial r}\right)+\frac{\partial p}{\partial r}-\frac{\partial T_{L,rr}}{\partial r}-\frac{2T_{L,rr}-T_{L,\theta\theta}-T_{L,\phi\phi}}{r}\right]dr=0$$

The density, elasticity and viscosity of the filling gas will be considerably smaller than those of the solid shell or surrounding fluid, particularly at the low insonation pressures which are of most interest in this discussion. The first integral may therefore be neglected. If the surrounding fluid is considered to be infinite, i.e. the presence of boundaries such blood vessel walls and other coated microbubbles is ignored, there is no need to modify the third integral.

If the presence of other coated microbubbles in the fluid is ignored, then, at the relevant frequencies and radial amplitudes, the speed of the coated microbubble wall (≈ 5 m/s) will be much smaller than the speed of sound in either the shell or the surrounding fluid (≈ 1500 m/s). ρ_s and ρ_L may therefore be treated as constants and hence from Eq. 3.2:

$$u(r,t)=\frac{R_{1}^{2}(t)\dot{R}_{1}(t)}{r^{2}} \quad (3.4)$$

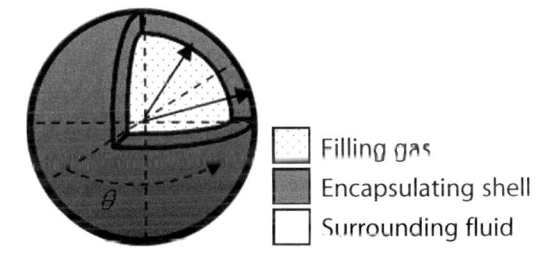

Fig. 3.1. The coated microbubble system considered

From conservation of radial stress on either side of the shell:

$$p_G(R_1,t) = p_S(R_1,t) - T_{S,rr}(R_1,t) + \frac{2\sigma_1}{R_1} \quad (3.5)$$

$$p_S(R_2,t) - T_{S,rr}(R_2,t) = p_L(R_2,t) - T_{L,rr}(R_2,t) + \frac{2\sigma_2}{R_2} \quad (3.6)$$

Surface tension has been treated as a constant in Eqs. 3.5 and 3.6 since, as will be shown in Sect. 3.3, the elastic effect due to variation in the concentration of surface molecules can be included in the definition of $T_{s,rr}(R_{1or2}, t)$. It has also been assumed that the vapour pressure inside the coated microbubble will be negligible.

Substituting into Eqs. 3.4–3.6 gives:

$$\rho_S\left(R_1\ddot{R}_1 - R_1\ddot{R}_1\frac{R_1}{R_2} + \frac{3}{2}\dot{R}_1^2 - \left(\frac{4R_2^3 - R_1^3}{2R_2^3}\right)\frac{\dot{R}_1^2 R_1}{R_2}\right) + \rho_L\left(\left(\frac{4R_2^3 - R_1^3}{2R_2^3}\right)\frac{\dot{R}_1^2 R_1}{R_2} + R_1\ddot{R}_1\frac{R_1}{R_2}\right)$$
$$= \left(p_G - p_\infty(t) - \frac{2\sigma_1}{R_1} - \frac{2\sigma_2}{R_2} + \int_{R_1}^{R_2}\left[\frac{2T_{S,rr} - T_{S,\theta\theta} - T_{S,\phi\phi}}{r}\right]dr + \int_{R_2}^{\infty}\left[\frac{2T_{L,rr} - T_{L,\theta\theta} - T_{L,\phi\phi}}{r}\right]dr\right)$$

This may be rewritten as:

$$R_1\ddot{R}_1\left(1 + \left(\frac{\rho_L - \rho_S}{\rho_S}\right)\frac{R_1}{R_2}\right) + \dot{R}_1^2\left(\frac{3}{2} + \left(\frac{\rho_L - \rho_S}{\rho_S}\right)\left(\frac{4R_2^3 - R_1^3}{2R_2^3}\right)\frac{R_1}{R_2}\right)$$
$$= \frac{1}{\rho_S}\left(p_G - p_\infty(t) - \frac{2\sigma_1}{R_1} - \frac{2\sigma_2}{R_2} + f_{Ls} + f_{Ss} + f_{Lv} + f_{Sv} + f_{\delta rad} + f_{\delta th}\right) \quad (3.7)$$

f_{Sv}, f_{Ss}, f_{Lv} and f_{Ls} correspond to the integrals for stress in the shell and fluid. The two additional factors, $f_{\delta rad}$ and $f_{\delta th}$, represent respectively the damping of coated microbubbles oscillations due to the reradiation of the sound field and that due to conduction from the filling gas to the surroundings. The rigorous derivation of these last two terms will be discussed later. In its present form Eq. 3.7 represents a generalised model for coated microbubble behaviour. The existing models differ only in the way in which the last six terms are defined.

3.2.2
Sensitivity Analysis

Before seeking to define f_{Sv}, f_{Ss}, f_{Lv}, f_{Ls}, $f_{\delta rad}$, $f_{\delta th}$, p_G and p_∞, it is desirable to identify which factors are the most significant in controlling coated microbubble behaviour, and hence which areas are the most important for modelling and design. It is therefore necessary to make some preliminary simplifying assumptions from which initial definitions of the above terms can be derived.

Firstly, if the assumption that the surrounding fluid is incompressible is retained for the present, then $f_{\delta rad} = 0$. If it also assumed that the fluid is purely Newtonian then:

$$f_{Ls} = 0 \quad \text{and} \quad 2T_{\theta\theta} = 2T_{\phi\phi} = -T_{rr} = T_{L,rr} = 2\mu_l\frac{\partial u}{\partial r}$$

and hence

$$f_{Lv} = 3\int_{R_2}^{\infty}\frac{T_{L,rr}}{r}dr = -4\mu_l\frac{R_1^2\dot{R}_1}{R_2^3}$$

Similarly, if the shell is assumed to be a homogeneous, linear viscoelastic solid layer having finite thickness, then for small strain:

$$f_{Ss} = \frac{-4G_S(R_1 - R_{1e})(R_2^3 - R_1^3)}{R_2^3 R_1} \quad \text{and,} \quad f_{Sv} = -4\mu_S\dot{R}_1\left(\frac{R_2^3 - R_1^3}{R_2^3 R_1}\right)$$

For these conditions it is justifiable to assume that gas behaviour will be polytropic and since coated microbubbles are unlikely to be perfectly gas-tight, the gas pressure at equilibrium may be taken to be equal to the ambient pressure p_o.

Thus $\quad p_G(R_1,t) = p_o\left(\frac{R_{o1}}{R_1}\right)^{3\kappa} \quad$ and $\quad f_{\delta th} = 0$.

The maximum coated microbubble diameter is restricted by the size of the smallest human blood vessels to approximately 8 μm. For the range of frequencies used in diagnostic imaging (1–10 MHz) this will be at least an order of magnitude smaller than the wavelength of the incident sound field. In the absence of any other coated microbubbles or neighbouring boundaries therefore, the incident pressure may be considered to be uniform over the surface of the coated microbubble. At low acoustic power of insonation, distortion due to non-linear propagation will be small and, for the purposes of this preliminary analysis, the incident field may be modelled as a simple sinusoid $p_\infty(t) = p_o + p_A\sin(\omega t)$.

Substituting from the above into Eq. 3.7 gives:

$$R_1\ddot{R}_1\left(1 + \left(\frac{\rho_L - \rho_S}{\rho_S}\right)\frac{R_1}{R_2}\right) + \dot{R}_1^2\left(\frac{3}{2} + \left(\frac{\rho_L - \rho_S}{\rho_S}\right)\left(\frac{4R_2^3 - R_1^3}{2R_2^3}\right)\frac{R_1}{R_2}\right)$$
$$= \frac{1}{\rho_S}\left(p_o\left(\frac{R_{o1}}{R_1}\right)^{3\kappa} - p_o - p_A\sin(\omega t) - \frac{2\sigma_1}{R_1} - \frac{2\sigma_2}{R_2} - \frac{4\dot{R}_1 R_1^2 \mu_L}{R_2^3} - \frac{4\dot{R}_1 V_S \mu_S}{R_2^3 R_1} - \frac{4V_S G_S}{R_2^3 R_1}\left(1 - \frac{R_{1e}}{R_1}\right)\right)$$
(3.8)

This is equivalent to the form derived by Church (1995).

To determine the factors having the most significant effect upon coated microbubble behaviour, Eq. 3.8 may be rearranged once again in terms of wall acceleration $\ddot{R}_1$, and broken down into seven components representing: the filling gas pressure (PF), the inertia of the shell and surrounding fluid (IF), the incident pressure (AF), surface tension (SF), fluid viscosity (L_vF), shell viscosity (S_vF), and shell stiffness (S_sF).

$$\ddot{R}_1 = PF + IF + AF + TF + L_vF + S_vF + S_sF$$

$$\ddot{R}_1 = \underbrace{\frac{P_o}{A}\left(\frac{R_{o1}}{R_1}\right)^3}_{PF} - \underbrace{\frac{\rho_s \dot{R}_1^2}{A}\left(\frac{3}{2} + \left(\frac{\rho_L - \rho_s}{\rho_s}\right)\left(\frac{4R_2^3 - R_1^3}{2R_2^3}\right)\frac{R_1}{R_2}\right)}_{IF} - \underbrace{\frac{p_o + p_A Sin(\omega t)}{A}}_{AF}$$

$$- \underbrace{\frac{2}{A}\left(\frac{\sigma_1}{R_1} + \frac{\sigma_2}{R_2}\right)}_{TF} - \underbrace{\frac{4\dot{R}_1 V_s \mu_S}{AR_1R_2^3}}_{L_vF} - \underbrace{\frac{4\dot{R}_1 R_1^2 \mu_L}{AR_2^3}}_{S_vF} - \underbrace{\frac{4V_S G_S}{AR_2^3}\left(1 - \frac{R_{1e}}{R_1}\right)}_{S_sF}$$

$$A = \rho_s R_1\left(1 + \left(\frac{\rho_L - \rho_s}{\rho_s}\right)\frac{R_1}{R_2}\right) \quad (3.9)$$

This type of analysis is similar to that carried out by FLYNN (1964) to investigate the nature of free bubble cavitation behaviour.

Equation 3.9 may either be solved numerically or else linearised to enable an analytical solution. Since ultimately it is the non-linear behaviour of coated microbubbles which is of interest for design, a numerical approach is preferable. The size of the acceleration factors may then be compared and their relative importance determined. This type of analysis also enables the sensitivity of coated microbubble behaviour to variation in the model parameters to be assessed as shown in the next section.

3.2.3
Results and Implications

Figure 3.2 shows plots of the acceleration factors for a coated microbubble and a free microbubble of the same size exposed to the same insonation conditions. These were obtained for the parameters shown in Table 3.2 according to the procedure described in STRIDE and SAFFARI (2003). The shell parameters were selected to be of the same order of magnitude as those obtained for commercial contrast agents (DE JONG et al. 1992; GORCE et al. 2000). For reasons that will be explained subsequently, the fluid parameters used were those of plasma and it was assumed that the gas would behave ideally and isothermally. A variety of insonation frequencies were used, corresponding to resonant, sub-resonant and super-resonant regimes. Figure 3.2 shows the case for 3 MHz at which the radial amplitude was maximised. The relative magnitude of the different components of Eq. 3.9 was similar at all frequencies however. The insonation pressure was varied within the range of pressures (0.05–0.1 MPa) at which it would be reasonable to expect a coated microbubble to remain intact (STRIDE and SAFFARI 2003) and for which Eq. 3.9 would be valid.

Table 3.2. Simulation parameter values

	Parameter	Symbol	Value	Unit
Gas (air) CENGEL and BOLES (1989)	Polytropic constant	κ	1.0	
Shell (Albunex) CHURCH (1995)	Ambient pressure	p_o	0.1	MPa
	Shear modulus	G_s	88.8	MPa
	Density	ρ_s	1100	Kgm^{-3}
	Viscosity	μ_s	1.77	Pas
	Inner radius	R_1	3.635	μm
	Thickness	d_e	15	nm
	Inner surface tension	σ_1	0.04	Nm^{-1}
	Outer surface tension	σ_2	0.005	Nm^{-1}
Liquid (plasma) DUCK (1990)	Density	ρ_l	1030	Kgm^{-3}
	Viscosity	μ_l	0.0015	Pas

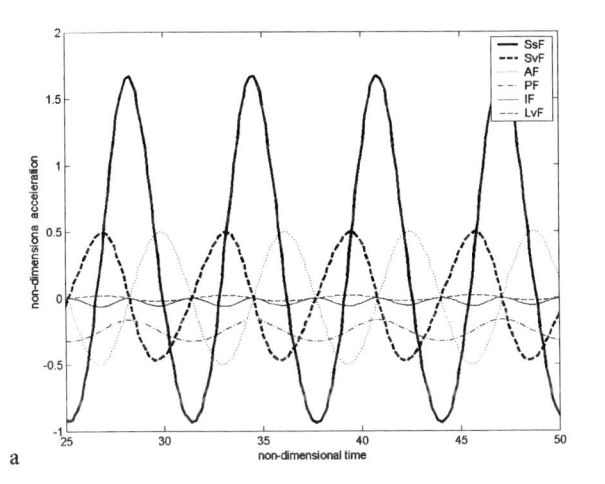

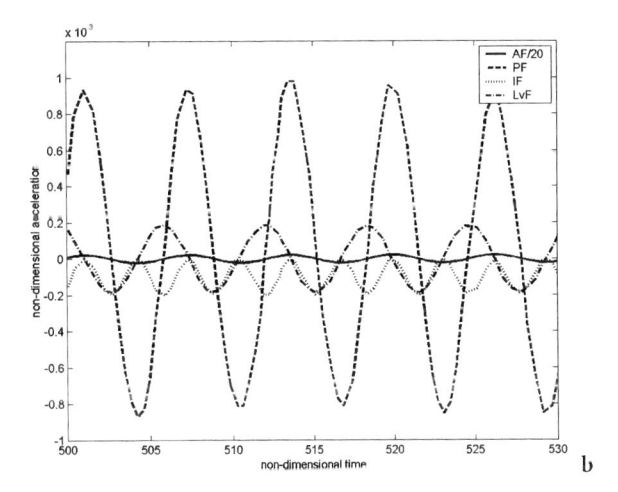

Fig. 3.2a,b. Acceleration factors for (a) an Albunex-coated microbubble and (b) a free bubble insonified at 3 MHz and 50 kPa. Factors IF and L$_v$F have been omitted in (a) and (b), respectively, as they have negligible amplitude.

A comparison of Fig. 3.2a and Fig. 3.2b indicates that the factors controlling the behaviour of a coated microbubble may differ considerably from those controlling the behaviour of a free bubble. Whilst the latter is primarily determined by either pressure or inertia, microbubble response is dominated by the stiffness and viscosity of the encapsulating shell. This finding has a number of implications. For example, it calls into question the validity of relating results obtained from work on free bubbles to coated microbubbles. This is particularly relevant for the assessment of contrast agent safety, which has in many cases been based on results derived from free bubble models (Nyborg 2001). For the purposes of design, the main conclusion is the importance of the shell as an area requiring accurate modelling and offering opportunities for modifying coated microbubble response. Similarly, the relatively large amplitude of the incident pressure factor indicates that the sound field should also be a focus for modelling and design.

Figure 3.3 indicates the sensitivity of coated microbubble radial acceleration to a change of ±20% in each of the variables shown in Table 3.2. The results suggest that, as might be expected, coated microbubble response is most sensitive to changes in the shell and sound field parameters (G_s, m_s, d_s, f, p_A). This reinforces the finding from Fig. 3.2 that these factors are the most significant in terms of coated microbubble design.

Before the modelling and/or design of the shell and sound field can be considered further, the validity of the sensitivity analysis itself must be examined. The results of the analysis present something of a paradox: the aim of the sensitivity analysis is to determine which parts of the model it is most important to improve. In order to perform the analysis however, a model is required which, by implication, must be inferior. It is therefore necessary to re-examine the assumptions made above and determine under which circumstances the sensitivity analysis could be invalidated.

The first point to examine is the model of the filling gas. Potentially, a different model could increase the relative amplitude of PF in Eq. 3.9. However, at the small amplitudes of oscillation considered, the temperatures and pressures inside the coated microbubble would be, respectively, high and low compared with the critical values for the gas, and deviation from ideal gas behaviour would be expected to be minimal. Secondly, if the stiffness and viscosity of the shell were much lower than those given in Table 3.2, or if the shell was damaged so that its influence were lessened, then coated microbubble behaviour would be expected to be closer to that of a free bubble. At present, however, it is only shells having a strong influence upon coated microbubble behaviour at non-destructive insonation pressures that are of interest for the purposes of design.

The justification for ignoring fluid compressibility has already been given. An additional term taking account of the elasticity of the surrounding fluid could be included in Eq. 3.8. However, for fluids such as plasma, and indeed for whole blood, the size of this term is so small compared with the shell elasticity that its influence upon coated microbubble dynamics is negligible (Stride and Saffari 2004). For coated microbubbles enclosed in narrow blood vessels and/or other types of denser, stiffer tissue, the non-Newtonian behaviour of the surroundings may be more significant and require careful modelling (Allen and Roy 2000). The validity of the sensitivity analysis is therefore restricted to the behaviour of coated microbubbles in relatively large blood vessels. Fortunately, for the application of diagnostic imaging, this is frequently a reasonable assumption.

A similar analysis could be carried out for different coated microbubble applications again by examining the equations describing the relevant physical processes and identifying the controlling factors. In the case of coated microbubble acoustic response, the most important factors were found to be the encapsulating shell and the sound field. For controlling the long term stability of coated microbubbles on the other hand, the diffusivity of the gas is likely to be important as well as the permeability and solubility of the shell. Some of these considerations will be discussed again later. The next section considers modelling and engineering coated microbubbles to control and improve their acoustic response.

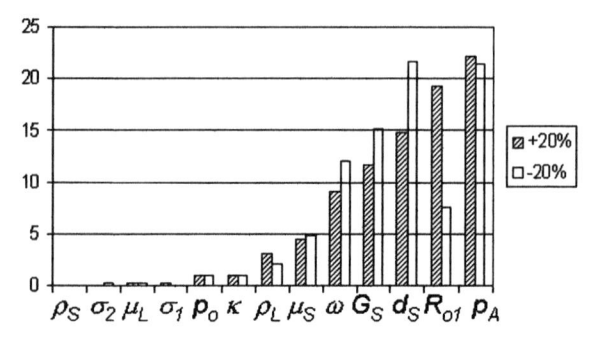

Fig. 3.3. The sensitivity of coated microbubble wall radial acceleration to variations of ±20% in each of the model parameters shown in Table 3.2 for insonation at 1 MHz and 50 kPa

3.3
Design and Engineering

There are two types of variables involved in the design and engineering of coated microbubbles. Firstly, there are those which, within limits, can be controlled, such as the shell, the gas and the sound field. Secondly, there are those, such as the surrounding fluid, which cannot be controlled but whose influence upon coated microbubble behaviour must be considered since it may affect the design requirements.

3.3.1
The Encapsulating Shell

The conclusion from the preceding analysis was that the main determinant of response is the encapsulating shell. It is therefore important that its behaviour should be modelled correctly, not only to enable coated microbubble response to be accurately predicted, but also to indicate the most effective means of engineering the shell to achieve a particular response. To do this, the assumptions underlying the modelling of the shell must be reviewed to determine their validity.

3.3.1.1
Improving the Shell Model

It was assumed above that coated microbubble behaviour would be spherically symmetric. On the basis of optical studies by POSTEMA et al. (2003) this assumption would appear to be incorrect. In terms of coated microbubble acoustic response, however, the effect of asymmetric behaviour would be expected to be relatively small. The decay rate for the pressure wave generated by aspherical oscillations will be very rapid compared with that for the wave due to radial pulsations (LEIGHTON 1994). For the purposes of this study therefore, it is justifiable to retain the assumption of sphericity and thereby confine the analysis to one dimension.

It was also assumed in deriving Eq. 3.8 that the shell was of finite thickness and consisted of a homogeneous, linear viscoelastic solid. This too may be seen to be invalid. A simple linear model is inappropriate if decisions regarding the optimum shell material are to be made. A fairly wide range of materials has been used for coating microbubbles, from palmitic acid to cyanoacrylate. Thus, even if it is justifiable to regard some materials as behaving linearly at low amplitudes of oscillation, this may not be the case in general. Moreover, some shell materials are far more fluid in nature than others and it may be more appropriate to consider them as liquids or as two-dimensional layers, i.e. having negligible thickness, than as solid shells.

Considering firstly non-linear viscoelastic behaviour: it cannot be assumed in this case that the trace of the stress tensor **T** in Eq. 3.3 will be zero and the shell functions will therefore be of the form

$$f_{Ss} + f_{Sv} = 2\int_{R_1}^{R_2} \frac{T_{S,rr} - T_{S,\theta\theta}}{r} dr$$

Again spherical symmetry has been assumed so that $T_{\phi\phi} = T_{\theta\theta}$.

There are several models available for describing this type of material. One of the most general is that due to GREEN and RIVLIN (1957).

$$\mathbf{T}(t) = \int_{-\infty}^{t} \{\mathbf{I}\psi_1 tr(\mathbf{M}_1) + \psi_2 \mathbf{M}_1\} d\tau_1$$
$$+ \int_{-\infty}^{t}\int_{-\infty}^{t} \{\mathbf{I}\psi_3 tr(\mathbf{M}_1)tr(\mathbf{M}_2) + \mathbf{I}\psi_4 tr(\mathbf{M}_1\mathbf{M}_2) + \mathbf{I}\psi_5 tr(\mathbf{M}_2) + \psi_6 \mathbf{M}_1\mathbf{M}_2\} d\tau_1 d\tau_2 + \ldots$$

(3.10)

where $\tau_{1,2}$ are time variables of integration, **I** is the identity matrix and $\mathbf{M}_{1,2}$ are the time derivatives of the strain tensor with respect to $\tau_{1,2}$, etc. Functions $\psi_{1,2}$, etc. must be determined experimentally for a particular material. Incorporating Eq. 3.10 into Eq. 3.7 generates a system of differential equations which can be solved numerically. This form of Eq. 3.7 is also suitable for modelling large amplitude deformations.

The next case to consider is that of a surfactant layer. It has already been shown that there may be a significant difference between the behaviour of a free bubble and an encapsulated microbubble (Fig. 3.2). The nature of a surfactant coated microbubble is currently unclear in this respect. According to the results obtained by GORCE et al. (2000) the shell parameters for phospholipid monolayers are of the same order of magnitude as those obtained for albumin shells. However, results reported by POSTEMA et al. (2003) suggest that phospholipids-coated microbubbles behaviour is closer to that of a free bubble. Further controlled experiments are required to resolve this discrepancy.

It is undoubtedly true, however, that the material microstructure is different for surfactants and polymers. A phospholipid monolayer for example, consists of a single layer of molecules bound together by secondary (Van de Waals) bonds. These are continuously broken and reformed, with the result that the molecules can "slip" over each other, allowing the layer to deform without wrinkling. Polymers such as serum albumin, on the other hand, consist of much larger intertwined molecular chains which may be cross-linked by covalent bonds. This prevents continuous deformation so that the shell is more likely to buckle and/or rupture. In both cases, resistance to tension and compression is due to intermolecular forces opposing the movement of molecules from their equilibrium positions. However, given the monomolecular thickness of the surfactant layer, it may be more appropriate to treat this resistance as a variation in surface tension of a single interface, rather than as the elasticity of a finite solid layer as is appropriate for thicker polymer shells.

The boundary condition (Eq. 3.5) for a single interface with a surfactant layer may be expressed as:

$$p_G(R,t) = p_L(R,t) - T_{L,rr}(R,t) + \frac{2\sigma}{R} + \frac{\partial \sigma}{\partial R} + \frac{1}{R^3}\frac{\partial \alpha}{\partial R} - \frac{\alpha}{R^4}$$

where σ is surface tension and α is a parameter relating to repulsion between molecules.
The corresponding form of Eq. 3.7 is:

$$\rho_L\left(R\ddot{R} - R\ddot{R}_1 + \frac{3}{2}\dot{R}_1^2\right)$$
$$= \left(p_G(R,t) - p_\infty(t) - \frac{2\sigma}{R} - \frac{\partial\sigma}{\partial R} - \frac{1}{R^3}\frac{\partial\alpha}{\partial R} + \frac{\alpha}{R^4} - \frac{4\mu_L \dot{R}}{R}\right)$$

The variation in surface tension depends upon the variation in surface concentration of the surfactant Γ.

$$\frac{\partial \sigma}{\partial R} = \frac{\partial \sigma}{\partial \Gamma}\frac{\dot{\Gamma}}{\dot{R}} = \frac{-\chi}{\Gamma_o}\frac{\dot{\Gamma}}{\dot{R}} = \frac{2R_o^2 \chi}{R^3} \quad \text{since} \quad 4\pi R^2 \Gamma = 4\pi R_o^2 \Gamma_o$$

so

$$\dot{\Gamma} = \frac{\partial}{\partial t}\left(\frac{R_o^2 \Gamma_o}{R^2}\right) = \frac{-2R_o^2 \Gamma_o \dot{R}}{R^3} \quad \text{where } \chi \text{ is defined as } -\frac{\partial \sigma}{\partial \Gamma}\Gamma_o$$

thus

$$\rho_L\left(R\ddot{R} + \frac{3}{2}\dot{R}_1^2\right) = \left(p_G(R,t) - p_\infty(t) - \frac{2\sigma}{R} - \frac{2\chi R_o^2}{R^3} - \frac{1}{R^3}\frac{\partial \alpha}{\partial R} + \frac{\alpha}{R^4} - \frac{4\mu_L \dot{R}}{R}\right)$$
(3.11)

Equation 3.11 is similar in form to those derived for the radial oscillations of ocean bubbles with organic film coatings (e.g. Glazman 1983). More advanced descriptions of the monolayer than the simple treatment expressed by Eq. 3.11 are available. For example, additional terms accounting for viscous dissipation in the surfactant layer may be included together with terms having a higher order dependence upon R^{-2} (Israelachvili 1991). The difficulty, however, is obtaining reliable experimental data from which the model parameters may be derived. For example, direct measurements of χ have been made for a variety of liquid-condensed and solid-state films (e.g. Joly 1972), but there is no data available for χ or α at frequencies in the MHz range. Predictions from molecular modelling are at present inadequate, and as mentioned earlier, in the absence of this data, Eqs. 3.8 and 3.11 are of equivalent value.

From Eq. 3.11 $\quad f_{Ss} = \frac{1}{R^3}\left(\frac{\alpha}{R} - 2\chi R_o^2 - \frac{\partial \alpha}{\partial R}\right) = \frac{1}{R^3}\left(\frac{k_1}{R} - k_2\right)$

From Eq. 3.8 $\quad f_{Ss} = \frac{-4G_S(R_1 - R_{1e})(R_2^3 - R_1^3)}{R_2^3 R_1}$

In the limit of negligible shell thickness this reduces to:

$$f_{Ss} = \frac{1}{R^3}\left(12G_S R_o^2 d_o \frac{R_e}{R} - 12G_S R_o^2 d_o\right) = \frac{1}{R^3}\left(\frac{k_1}{R} - k_2\right)$$

In spite of its potential for describing complex material behaviour Eq. 3.10 is also of limited value until functions $E_{1,2}$, etc. can be specified on the basis of reliable experimental data.

In order to improve the overall understanding of coated microbubble behaviour this lack of material data needs to be addressed. For coated microbubble design, however, it is a comparatively minor obstacle. The aim of the design process is to establish the optimum characteristics for a product and determine how these may be achieved. The absence of data for existing coated microbubbles is thus relatively insignificant, as demonstrated in the following section.

3.3.1.2
Designing the Shell

In order to meet the requirements for the ideal coated microbubble set out in Sect. 3.1.2, an improvement in coated microbubble detectability at low insonation pressures is needed. The most obvious means of achieving this would be to increase the harmonic content of the signal radiated by the microbubbles. The presence of harmonics in the coated microbubble signal is due to the fact that, for equal peak positive and negative insonation pressures, the amplitude of coated microbubble oscillations will be greater during expansion than during compression ($|R_{max}| > |R_{min}|$). Therefore, if the ratio $R_{max}:R_{min}$ could be increased, the harmonic content and hence microbubble detectability could be enhanced. It is clear from the previous discussion that the most effective way of modifying coated microbubble response is likely to lie with the encapsulating shell.

Both the structure and the material of the shell may be modified and there are a number of possible approaches. For example, the shell material may be selected or engineered so that the shear modulus G_s is smaller in tension than in compression. It would be inappropriate in an article of this length to include the rigorous modelling of this behaviour, and again such a demonstration would be of limited value given the lack of specific material data. The principle, however, can be demonstrated effectively using a much simpler model, of the type derived by Hoff et al. (2000), etc. for a shell of negligible thickness.

$$\rho_L\left(R\ddot{R} + \frac{3}{2}\dot{R}_1^2\right)$$
$$= \left(p_o\left(\frac{R_o}{R}\right)^{3\kappa} - p_o - p_A\sin(\omega t) - \frac{2\sigma}{R} - \frac{12G_s R_o^2 d_o}{R^3}\left(1 - \frac{R_e}{R}\right) - \frac{12\mu_s R_o^2 d_o \dot{R}}{R^4} - \frac{4\mu_L \dot{R}}{R}\right)$$

with G_S defined by $G_S(R_1) = \begin{cases} G_{Si}, R_1 \geq R_{e1} \\ G_{Sii}, R_1 < R_{e1} \end{cases}$

The frequency spectra for the pressure radiated by coated microbubbles having $G_{sii} = G_{si}$ and $G_{sii} = x\, G_{si}$ under identical insonation conditions is shown in Fig. 3.4 for various values of x. As may be seen, there is a distinct enhancement in the harmonic content when $x > 1$. There are a number of materials which naturally display this behaviour. The response of TiNi crystals, for example, has long been recognised as being asymmetric in tension and compression (Gall et al. 1999). Clearly this type of material is unsuitable for coating microbubbles, but similar behaviour has also been demonstrated for materials such as cartilage (Provenzano et al. 2002) and other natural polymers. The reported tensile and compressive moduli are derived from relatively large samples and may relate to material structure on a scale which is large compared with the thickness of a microbubble coating. However, it may be possible to imitate these structures on a much smaller scale. The inclusion of cholesterol molecules in a cell membrane for example has been shown to produce a highly non-linear increase in its resistance to deformation (Boal 2002). Since the coatings of phospholipid-coated microbubbles are very similar in composition to cell membranes, it is perfectly feasible that they could be similarly engineered.

There are alternative means by which enhanced non-linear behaviour may be achieved. The shell may be constructed so that it will buckle in compression, for example by varying its thickness over the coated microbubble surface. This will have a similar effect to increasing the ratio of compressive to tensile modulus, since a buckled shell will not compress to the same degree as one which remains smooth. Similarly, it is easy to envisage various ways in which the shell structure may be designed to alter its relative resistance to tension and compression that would be easily within the capabilities of available manufacturing methods.

3.3.2
The Insonating Field

As indicated in Figs. 3.3 and 3.4, variation in the US field parameters will have a strong impact on coated microbubble behaviour (Simpson et al. 1999; Uhlendorf and Hoffmann 1994). It will also affect the quality of the scan image directly, in terms of resolution, etc. Both the nature of the input waveform and its propagation through the microbubbles' surroundings must be taken into account.

3.3.2.1
Influence of the Field Parameters

Provided the thickness and viscosity of the encapsulating shell is not too great compared with their diameter, coated microbubbles will resonate at a specific frequency. The most appropriate range of frequencies for a given application will thus depend strongly upon the size distribution of the coated microbubble population, and either the incident spectrum must be selected accordingly or it may be desirable to control the size of the coated microbubbles to enable a particular frequency range to be used, e.g. to achieve a particular level of resolution.

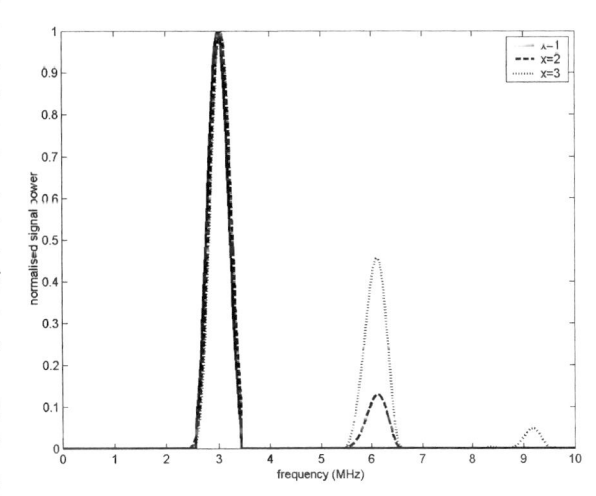

Fig. 3.4. Frequency spectra for the pressure radiated by coated microbubbles insonated at 3 MHz and 50 kPa with shells of varying degrees of non-linearity

Resonance, however, is not the only consideration in the selection of the insonation frequency. A number of methods have been investigated with the aim of improving image quality by manipulation of the input spectrum. One of the most common is to use a combination of two frequencies in order to generate an enhanced response at the difference frequency. Various different versions of this technique have been developed (Wyzalkowski and Szeri 2003). The use of coded excitation ("chirps") has also been examined (Borsboom et al. 2003). The imaging strategies which have been developed to take advantage of these techniques will be reviewed in subsequent chapters.

The amplitude of the incident field is also a significant factor. As mentioned earlier, it will determine the degree of non-linear behaviour exhibited by existing coated microbubbles and is clearly important in terms of coated microbubble destruction. It is also likely to be a factor in determining the fraction of a coated microbubble population activated by the incident field. The maximum and minimum pressures which may be used for an ultrasound scan are limited by considerations of patient safety and signal attenuation respectively. The aim in improving coated microbubble design is to minimise the insonation pressure required to obtain the desired image quality.

3.3.2.2
Influence of the Surrounding Fluid

Between transmission and detection, the incident and scattered fields must propagate through the surrounding tissue and will inevitably be modified to some extent in the process. Whilst it has been assumed that the effects of compressibility will be small in terms of coated microbubble dynamics, they may have a greater impact on the propagation of the sound field. During compression, the local density of the tissue is increased slightly and so too therefore is the speed at which the wave travels through it. The reverse occurs during rarefaction, with the result that the shape of the wave or pulse, in the case of imaging, will be distorted. This distortion corresponds to an increase in the harmonic content of the frequency spectrum and will affect both the response of the coated microbubbles and the degree to which the pulse is attenuated. Thus, to achieve a particular coated microbubble response and signal amplitude, this effect must be taken into account.

The compressibility of the surrounding fluid must also be included when a population rather than a single coated microbubble is considered.

For the reasons given in Sect. 3.2.1, acoustic radiation damping is a small effect for a single coated microbubble at low insonation power, particularly if the viscosity of the shell is relatively large and thus forms the main contribution to the overall damping. In a coated microbubble population, however, the presence of the other coated microbubbles can increase the effective compressibility of the surroundings considerably, and also introduces the problem of multiple scattering between microbubbles. At sufficiently low concentrations it is still reasonable to neglect acoustic damping and predict the overall acoustic signal by linear summation of single coated microbubble responses, assuming that the activated proportion of the population is known. At higher concentrations, however, and importantly in the range corresponding to coated microbubble injections, it has been shown experimentally that linear summation fails to accurately predict acoustic response (Marsh et al. 1997).

3.3.3
The Filling Gas

It was assumed in deriving Eq. 3.8 that the filling gas would behave polytropically, on the basis that the pressure inside the coated encapsulating at low amplitudes of oscillation would be relatively low compared with the critical pressure for the gas. This assumption is valid for air and many other gases (Cengel and Boles 1989), although it should not be made automatically for every gas. It was also assumed that the gas behaviour would be isothermal ($\kappa=1$). Given the high specific heat capacity of plasma and the small size of the coated microbubble, it is reasonable to assume that the surrounding fluid will behave as a heat sink and that the temperature gradient within the coated microbubble will be very small at low insonation pressures (Neppiras 1980). Moreover, it was determined subsequently that microbubble response was relatively insensitive to the value of κ (Fig. 3.3).

The choice of filling gas will also affect the long term stability of the coated microbubble. If the shell is gas permeable and/or soluble, then the rate at which the coated microbubble dissolves will depend upon the solubility of the gas as well as the durability of the shell. Clearly, any shrinkage of the coated microbubbles due to dissolution will affect their acoustic response and this may be important for some applications. In addition there may be some safety issues relating to very low solubility gases. If free bubbles are able to persist after the microbubble shells have degraded they could potentially coalesce to form a relatively large bubble capable of causing an embolism. Finally, the possibility of chemical interaction between the filling gas and the shell material or any therapeutic compounds may need to be considered.

3.4
Concluding Remarks

Advances in imaging technology, and more recently in therapeutic applications, such as drug delivery, have greatly increased the range of potential benefits offered by ultrasound contrast agents. Hence, the need to develop agents for specific tasks has also increased. The aim of this chapter has been to present an overview of how contrast agents may be designed in order to improve their suitability for particular applications. It has been shown that analytical techniques may be applied to identify the most important factors for modelling and design, and that this knowledge may be employed to modify coated microbubbles behaviour.

There are still some areas of uncertainty. The characterisation of existing agents is currently unsatisfactory and there is undoubtedly scope for improvement in the modelling of contrast agent behaviour in vivo. Even using existing knowledge, however, there are considerable advantages to be gained through coated microbubble design. In the example given, it was shown how the material and/or structure of the encapsulating shell could be selected in order to enhance the non-linearity of coated microbubble oscillations at low insonation pressures. Similar improvements may be achieved by appropriate selection of the filling gas to control coated microbubble longevity, and coated microbubble structure may be modified to improve targeting. More and more benefits will be realised as the deficiencies in the existing theory are addressed.

References

Allen J, Roy R (2000) Dynamics of gas bubbles in viscoelastic fluids II. Non-linear viscoelasticity. J Acoust Soc Am 108:1640-1650
Boal D (2002) Mechanics of the cell, 1st edn. Cambridge University Press, Cambridge
Borsboom J, Chin C, de Jong N (2003) Non-linear coded excitation method for ultrasound contrast imaging. Ultrasound Med Biol 29:285-292
Cengel Y, Boles M (1989) Thermodynamics: an engineering approach. Ultrasound Med Biol 29:1749:1757
Church C (1995) The effects of an elastic solid surface layer on the radial pulsations of gas bubbles. J Acoust Soc Am 97:1510-1520
De Jong N, Hoff L, Skotland T, Bom N (1992) Absorption and scatter of encapsulated gas filled microspheres: theoretical considerations and some measurements. Ultrasonics 30:95-103
Duck F (1990) Physical properties of tissue: a comprehensive reference book, 1st edn. Academic, London
Flynn H (1964) Physics of acoustic cavitation in liquids. In: Mason W (ed) Physical acoustics 1B. Academic, London
Fox F, Herzfeld J (1954) Gas bubbles with organic skin as cavitation nuclei. J Acoust Soc Am 26:984-989
Gall K, Sehitoglu H, Chumlyakov Y, Kireeva I (1999) Tension compression asymmetry of the stress-strain response in aged single crystal and polycrystalline NiTi. Acta Mater 47:1203-1217
Glazman R (1983) Effects of adsorbed films on gas bubble radial oscillations. J Acoust Soc Am 74:980-986
Gorce J, Arditi M, Schneider M (2000) Influence of bubble size distribution on the echogenicity of ultrasound contrast agents: a study of SonoVue. Invest Radiol 35:661-671
Gramiak R, Shah PM (1968) Echocardiography of the aortic root. Invest Radiol 3:356-366
Green E, Rivlin R (1957) The mechanics of non-linear materials with memory. Arch Rational Mech Anal 1:1-21
Hoff L, Sontum P, Hovem J (2000) Oscillations of polymeric microbubbles: Effect of the encapsulating shell. J Acoust Soc Am 107:2272-2280.
Israelachvili J (1991) Intermolecular and surface forces, 2nd edn. Academic, London
Joly M (1972) Rheological properties of monomolecular films, part II. Experimental results, theoretical interpretation and applications. In: Matijevic E (ed) Surface colloid science. Wiley, New York, pp 79-194
Khismatullin D, Nadim A (2002) Radial oscillations of encapsulated microbubbles in viscoelastic liquids. Phys Fluids 14:3534-3557
Leighton T (1994) The acoustic bubble, 1st edn. Academic, London
Lord W, Ludwig R, You Z (1990) Developments in ultrasonic modelling with finite element analysis. J Non Destruct Eval 9:129-139
Marsh J, Hall C, Hughes M (1997) Broadband through-transmission signal loss measurements of Albunex® suspensions at concentrations approaching in vivo doses. J Acoust Soc Am 101:115-1161
Morgan K, Allen J, Chomas J, Dayton P, Ferrara K (1999) Experimental and theoretical analysis of individual contrast agent behavior. IEEE Proc Ultrason Symp 2:1685-1688
Neppiras E (1980) Acoustic cavitation. Phys Rep (Phys Lett) 61:159-251
Nyborg W (2001) Biological effects of ultrasound: development of safety guidelines, part II. General review. Ultrasound Med Biol 27:301-333
Postema M, Bouakaz A, Chin C, de Jong N (2003) Simulations and measurements of optical images of insonified ultrasound contrast microbubbles. IEEE Trans Ultrason Ferr Freq Cont 50:523-535
Provenzano P, Lakes R, Corr D, Vanderby R Jr (2002) Application of non-linear viscoelastic models to describe ligament behaviour. Biomech Mod Mechanobiol 1:45-57

Simpson DH, Chin C, Burns P (1999) Pulse inversion Doppler: a new method for detecting non-linear echoes from microbubble contrast agents. IEEE Trans Ultrason Ferr Freq Cont 46:372-382

Stride E, Saffari N (2003) The destruction of microbubble ultrasound contrast agents. Ultrasound Med Biol 29:563-573

Stride E, Saffari N (2004) Theoretical and experimental investigation of the behaviour of ultrasound contrast agent particles in whole blood. Ultrasound Med Biol 30(11):1495-1509

Uhlendorf V, Hoffmann C (1994) Non-linear acoustic response of coated microbubbles in diagnostic ultrasound. Proc IEEE Symp Ultrason 2:1559-1562

Wyzalkowski M, Szeri A (2003) Optimization of acoustic scattering from dual frequency driven microbubbles at the difference frequency. J Acoust Soc Am 113:3073-3079

4 Contrast-Specific Imaging Techniques: Technical Perspective

THOMAS ANTHONY WHITTINGHAM

CONTENTS

4.1	Introduction	43
4.2	Non-linearity and Harmonic Generation	44
4.2.1	Harmonics	44
4.2.2	Non-linear Scattering by Microbubbles	45
4.2.3	Non-linear Propagation in Tissue	47
4.3	Early Methods of Microbubble-Based Agent Visualisation	47
4.3.1	Conventional B-Mode	47
4.3.2	Conventional Spectral Doppler	48
4.3.3	Conventional Colour Doppler	48
4.3.4	Harmonic B-Mode Imaging by High-Pass Filtering	49
4.3.5	Harmonic Colour Flow Imaging by High Pass Filtering	50
4.3.6	Harmonic Power Doppler Imaging by High-Pass Filtering	50
4.3.7	Intermittent Imaging in B-Mode	50
4.3.8	Intermittent Colour Flow Imaging	51
4.3.9	Intermittent Power Doppler Imaging	52
4.3.10	The Need for Further Improvements	52
4.4	Low-MI Techniques	53
4.4.1	Pulse Inversion with Two Transmissions	53
4.4.2	Pulse Inversion on Alternate Scan Lines	54
4.4.3	Pulse Inversion with Three Transmissions	55
4.4.4	Harmonic Detection by Coded Excitation	56
4.4.5	Amplitude Modulation (Power Modulation)	57
4.4.6	Combined Amplitude Modulation and Pulse Inversion/Phase Shift. Contrast Pulse Sequence (CPS) Imaging	59
4.4.7	Developments in Low-MI Doppler Imaging	63
4.5	High-MI Techniques	65
4.5.1	Development in High-MI Doppler Imaging	66
4.5.2	Pulse Subtraction	67
4.5.3	1.5 Harmonic Imaging (1.5 HI)	67
4.6	Techniques for Imaging Perfusion and Flow in Very Small Vessels	68
4.7	Techniques in Development	69
4.7.1	Subharmonic Imaging	69
4.7.2	Release Burst Imaging	69
	References	70

T. A. WHITTINGHAM, PhD
Regional Medical Physics Department, Newcastle General Hospital, Westgate Road, Newcastle Upon Tyne, NE4 6BE, UK

4.1 Introduction

This chapter discusses the technical principles behind a range of contrast-specific techniques. New techniques are constantly being developed to take advantage of the properties of new microbubble-based ultrasound (US) contrast agents and the range discussed here is by no means exhaustive.

The discussion is primarily concerned with techniques for discriminating microbubble-based contrast agents from tissue. However, some techniques are so successful at suppressing tissue echoes that, by themselves they would be difficult to use, since the user would have no tissue landmarks to navigate by. Most commercial contrast-specific imaging modes, therefore, combine contrast agent imaging with a tissue visualising B-mode method. Details are not given of how conventional B-mode images are obtained and integrated with the contrast agent image. They can use one or more of the pulses that are transmitted to image the contrast agent, or use separate transmissions. The B-mode processing can be carried out in a completely separate channel, or be little more than a separate final stage in an otherwise common processing chain. Some systems offer the user the choice of separately displaying a contrast image, a tissue image or a combination of both.

Manufacturers often use very similar techniques to each other, but this is not apparent in their marketing literature. Even though a technique is mentioned here in association with a selection of trade names, it may be also associated with other trade names used by other manufacturers. The omission of any particular trade name is not due to any bias; those mentioned are simply examples with published descriptions known to the author.

4.2
Non-linearity and Harmonic Generation

4.2.1
Harmonics

As the terms fundamental and harmonic are much used when discussing contrast agents, a brief explanation may be helpful. Only a continuous sine-wave can be characterised by a single frequency f (Fig. 4.1a). If a waveform is anything other than this pure mathematical concept there must be more than one frequency present, and it is necessary to talk about a spectrum of frequencies rather than a single frequency. The continuous but distorted waveform of Fig. 4.1b can be obtained by summing a number of suitably aligned sinusoidal waveforms at frequencies f, $2f$, $3f$, $4f$ etc., each with a different amplitude. Transmitting such a wave is entirely equivalent to transmitting this set of continuous sine-waves, which are known respectively as the fundamental or first harmonic, second harmonic, third harmonic, fourth harmonic etc., frequency components of the waveform.

Real transmitted pulses, of course, are neither purely sinusoidal nor continuous. A pulse consisting of N sinusoidal cycles has energy over a spectrum of frequencies, with a centre frequency f_c and a 3 dB bandwidth of f_c/N, as shown in Fig. 4.1c. In a real pulse, each cycle may be different in amplitude and duration to the others, and may not have a perfect sinusoidal shape. The spectrum of such a pulse consists of a number of harmonic spectra, with centre frequencies f_c, $2f_c$, $3f_c$, $4f_c$ etc., as shown in Fig. 4.1d. That centred on f_c is the fundamental spectrum of the pulse, that centred on $2f_c$ is the second harmonic spectrum etc., although it is common to simply talk about the fundamental or second harmonic fre-

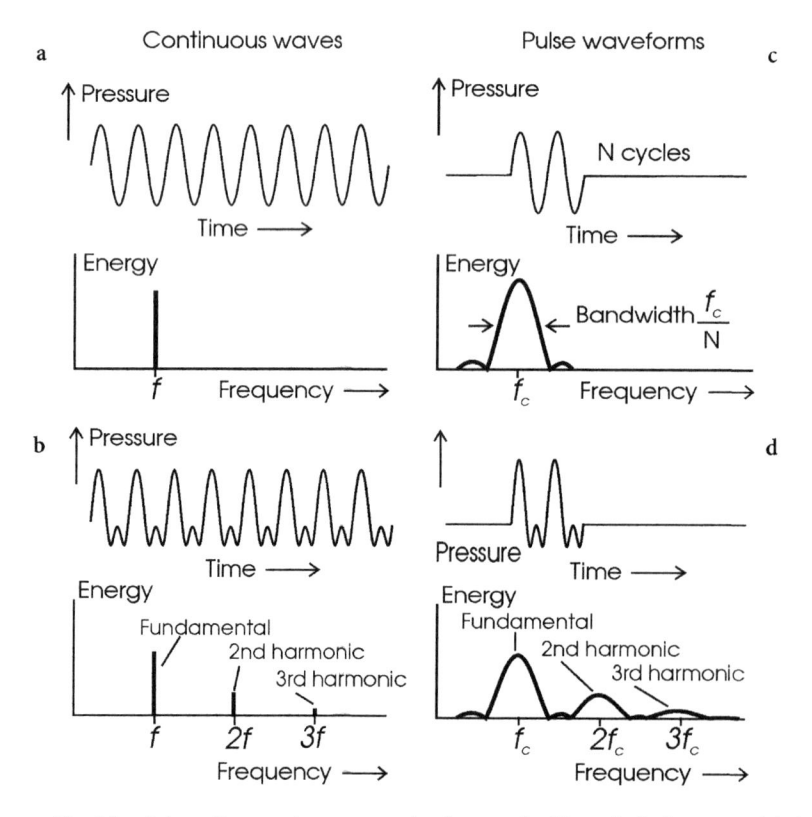

Fig. 4.1a–d. A continuous sine-wave can be characterised by a single frequency (a). A continuous but distorted waveform (b) can be obtained by summing a number of suitably aligned sinusoidal waveforms at frequencies f, $2f$, $3f$, $4f$ etc., each with a different amplitude. A pulse consisting of N sinusoidal cycles (c) has energy over a spectrum of frequencies, with a centre frequency f_c and a 3 dB bandwidth of f_c/N. In a real pulse, each cycle may be different in amplitude and duration to the others, and may not have a perfect sinusoidal shape. The spectrum of such a pulse (d) consists of a number of harmonic spectra, with centre frequencies f_c, $2f_c$, $3f_c$, $4f_c$, etc.

quency rather than the fundamental spectrum or the second harmonic spectrum. In practice, third and higher harmonics will contribute very little to the useable signal, as they are likely to be outside the frequency response of the transducer and will also be highly attenuated in tissue.

When seeking an understanding of the interaction of a real pulse with say a bubble, it is often very helpful to consider what would happen to the fundamental and the harmonic waves individually. An important example is in pulse inversion imaging (Sect. 4.4.1) which involves comparing the echoes produced by one pulse with those produced by a second pulse that is an inverted version of the first pulse. Figure 4.2 shows that distorted echoes scattered from a non-linear target (such as a microbubble) for the two pulses differ in that the fundamental and the odd harmonics are inverted in the echo from the inverted pulse. However, the second and other even harmonics are the same in the two echoes.

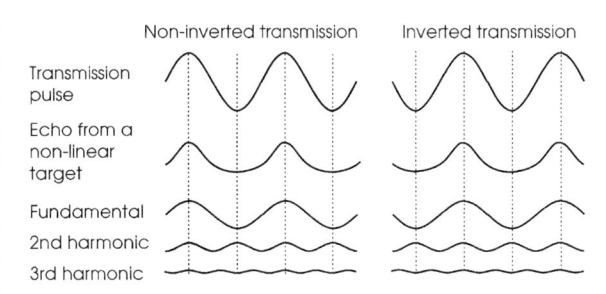

Fig. 4.2 If a transmission pulse is inverted the fundamental and odd harmonics of the echo from a non-linear target are inverted but the second harmonic component and other even harmonics are not.

4.2.2
Non-linear Scattering by Microbubbles

A linear reflector or scatterer is one that produces an echo whose amplitude is always the same fraction of the incident amplitude, whatever that amplitude might be. As this applies at every instant of the incident pulse, it follows that the waveform (amplitude versus time) of the echo pulse will be the same as that of the incident pulse. Scattering from tissue is considered to be linear. Scattering by a microbubble is also approximately linear if the incident pulse has a very low peak pressure amplitude (say below about 0.03 MPa). However, if the peak pressure amplitude of the incident pulse is increased, scattering by microbubbles becomes more and more non-linear – in other words the peak amplitude of the echo pulse is not in direct proportion to the peak amplitude of the incident pulse. This non-linearity results from the asymmetrical way that microbubbles expand and contract in a sound wave (Fig. 4.3). Bubbles compress less in response to a rise in pressure than they expand in response to a drop in pressure of the same magnitude. This is because the density, and hence the stiffness, of the gas in a bubble is increased during compression and reduced in expansion. Since the in and out movements of the bubble wall are asymmetric, the waveform of the echo is also asymmetric, with a peak amplitude that is not in proportion to the peak amplitude of the incident pulse.

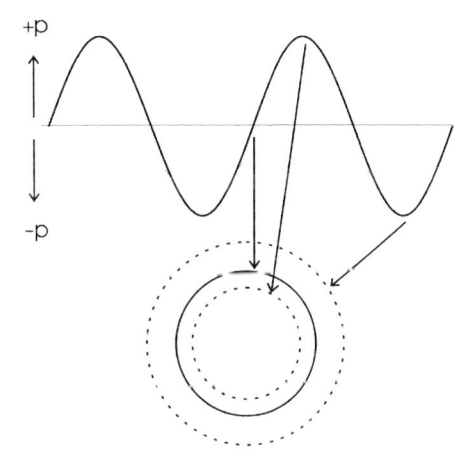

Fig. 4.3. Simplified model of the asymmetrical way that microbubbles expand and contract in a sound wave.

Curve s in Fig. 4.4 shows an idealised model of the relationship between the scattered echo waveform (E) and the incident sinusoidal waveform (I) for a non-linear scatterer such as a microbubble. The peak negative pressure of E is less than the peak positive pressure due to the non-linearity of curve s. Curve s can be expressed as the sum of a series of other curves, namely a straight line ($s_1 = k_1 p$), a quadratic function ($s_2 = k_2 p^2$), a cubic function ($s_3 = k_3 p^3$), etc. The first three of these curves are shown in the figure as s_1, s_2, s_3, and each of them defines an "order" of scattering. For a linear scatterer, S would be a straight line, such as s_1, and there would only be first-order scattering. Each of these different orders of scattering curves can be thought of as producing its own echo waveform, the sum of all of these being the actual echo waveform. That produced by first-order (linear) scattering is shown as e_1, that by second-order scattering is shown as e_2, and that as third-order scattering is shown as e_3. Higher-order scattering is omitted for clarity. Adding together e_1, e_2 and e_3 etc., forms the actual echo E.

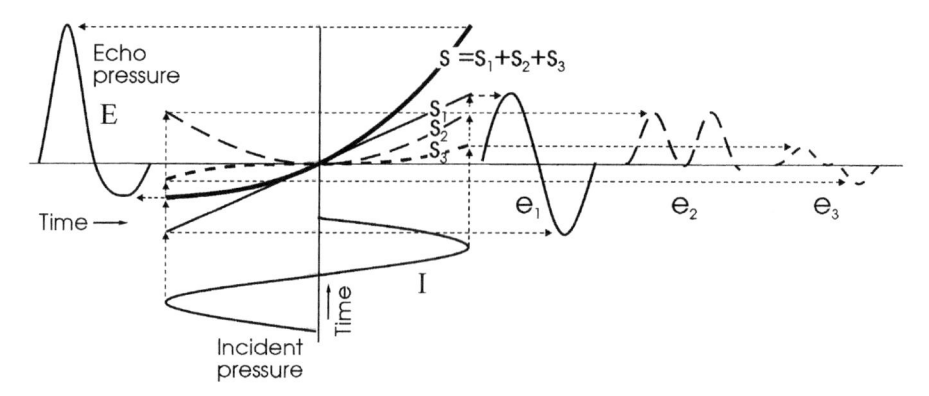

Fig. 4.4. Simplified model of the relationship (curve s) between an incident waveform I and the echo E scattered by a non-linear target such as a microbubble. Curve s can be considered as the sum of other curves (s_1, s_2, s_3...) of different orders: s_1 is a linear (first order) relationship, s_2 is a quadratic relationship (second order), and s_3 is a cubic relationship (third order). The echo E can be considered as the sum of the components (e_1, e_2, e_3...) contributed by each order.

It is important to distinguish between orders of scattering and harmonics. First-order scattering produces an amplitude-scaled replica of the incident pulse. Higher orders of scattering introduce harmonics of the various frequencies present in the incident pulse. In the example of Fig. 4.4, which shows one cycle of a single frequency incident wave, the first-order echo waveform e_1 contains only that (fundamental) frequency. The second-order echo waveform e_2 has none of the fundamental frequency, but consists of a component at twice the fundamental frequency (second harmonic) and a constant, which can be thought of as a zero frequency component. The third-order echo waveform e_3 consists of a component at three times the fundamental frequency (third harmonic) as well as a component at the fundamental frequency, as shown in Fig. 4.5. Although not shown, a fourth-order echo waveform would have both second- and fourth-order harmonics as well as a constant component.

The signal at the fundamental frequency, produced by third and other odd orders of scattering, is the basis of an important contrast detection method known as amplitude or power modulation, discussed in Sect. 4.4.5. This "non-linear fundamental" signal is distinct from the fundamental signal due to first-order scattering and is only present because of the non-linearity of the scattering process.

The amplitude of any particular frequency in the spectrum of echoes from microbubble is strongly dependent on the phenomenon of resonance. A microbubble will expand and contract most vigorously at one particular frequency, known as its natural resonance frequency, which is higher for smaller bubbles and stiffer shells. An injection of US contrast agent introduces microbubbles with a wide range of diameters so the centre frequency of the incident pulse is generally chosen to coincide with the mean resonant frequency of the microbubble population. However, it is likely that there will be some bubbles of the ideal size to resonate at most of the frequencies in the spectrum of the incident pulse.

Figure 4.6, adapted from AVERKIOU et al. (2003), shows the echo non-linearly scattered by a microbubble, for a typical incident pulse.

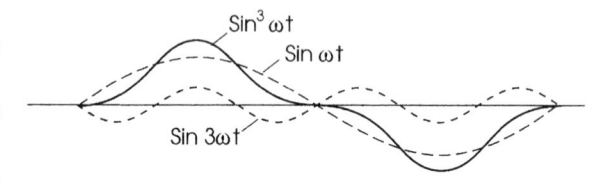

Fig. 4.5. The third order echo contribution e_3 in Fig. 4.4, in which pressure varies in proportion to the cube of a sine wave of frequency f. It is the sum of a fundamental component with a frequency f and a third harmonic component at frequency $3f$. (N.B. $\omega = 2\pi f$, t = time.)

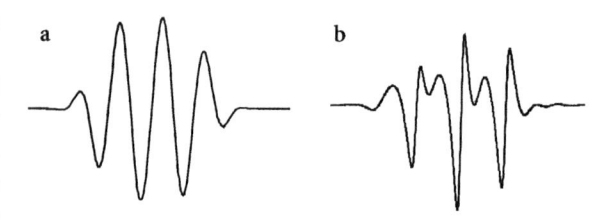

Fig. 4.6a,b. Typical incident pulse (**a**) and the echo (**b**) from a microbubble. From AVERKIOU et al. (2003).

4.2.3
Non-linear Propagation in Tissue

As a pulse propagates in tissue, as in most media, it becomes progressively distorted – a process known as non-linear propagation. This is a consequence of the fact that the peaks of a pressure wave are more compressed and therefore have a higher speed than the troughs. The peaks catch up with the troughs to an extent that increases with the pulse amplitude and distance travelled. The resulting waveform distortion may be negligible for low amplitude pulses but can be very obvious in the waveforms of large amplitude pulses. Consequently, since waveform distortion implies harmonic content, the echo reflected or scattered from a tissue interface will have some degree of second harmonic component, depending on the transmitted pulse amplitude and the position of the interface in the beam. There will also be weaker third and higher harmonics, but the transducer bandwidth is generally too small for these to be of practical interest.

This phenomenon is used to great advantage in the B-mode imaging technique known as tissue harmonic imaging. Here acoustic noise (clutter) due to reverberations, grating lobes and other side lobes, etc. is much reduced by restricting the display of echoes to those with a significant harmonic content – in other words echoes from targets close to the beam axis where transmitted pulses are stronger and more distorted.

It is important to note that the harmonic components in tissue echoes arise in a quite different way to that for microbubble echoes. In tissue, the scattering process is approximately linear; any distortion, and hence harmonics, in the echoes arises from the faithful mimicking of any distortion already in the waveform of the incident pulse. In the case of a microbubble, the harmonic components are generated at the moment of scattering – they do not depend on any pre-existing harmonic component in the incident pulse. In both cases, the magnitude of the harmonic content will be greater the larger the amplitude of the transmitted pulse.

In this chapter, the second harmonic component present in tissue echoes due to non-linear propagation of the transmitted pulse will be referred to simply as the "tissue harmonic". It is always present to some extent, increasingly so for higher transmitted amplitudes. It presents a particular challenge to those contrast agent visualising techniques that differentiate between microbubble echoes and tissue echoes on the basis of their second harmonic component (see Sects. 4.4.1–4.4.4 and 4.4.6–4.4.7).

4.3
Early Methods of Microbubble-Based Agent Visualisation

The reason for using US contrast agent microbubbles is that they scatter ultrasound much more strongly than do blood cells. The ratio of the power scattered by a microbubble to that scattered by a single blood cell has been estimated at about 10^{14}:1 (140 dB). This is due mainly to the large difference in acoustic impedance that exists between a gas and a liquid, but it is also due to the fact that bubbles of typical US contrast agent dimensions (around 3 μm diameter) exhibit resonance, i.e. oscillate particularly vigorously, at frequencies that are typical (around 3 MHz) of diagnostic US. In clinical use, of course, the concentration of microbubbles must be much less than that of blood cells, and so the actual increase in scattered power is much less than 140 dB. Nevertheless, even without any special instrumentation or processing, contrast agent microbubbles in practical concentrations can increase the echogenicity of the blood by about 20 dB.

4.3.1
Conventional B-Mode

Microbubble-based contrast agents gave some immediate benefits to B-mode imaging with conventional equipment, particularly in cardiology where, for example, the abundance of strongly scattering microbubbles in the left ventricle made it possible to delineate the wall of the chamber with much greater contrast and precision, allowing greatly improved estimates of ventricular volume and output.

However, efforts to use contrast agents to visualise blood vessels within tissue, such as the liver or myocardium, were less successful. The echo signal due to scattering from the many tiny interfaces within tissue was still much stronger, by as much as 20 dB, than that from within contrast-enhanced blood vessels. The echogenicity of blood vessels could be increased to a limited extent by increasing the concentration of microbubbles but, unfortunately, increasing the concentration also increased the attenuating affect of the US contrast agent itself, leading to shadowing of deeper regions. Also, although not appreciated at first, much of the signal was due to collapsing microbubbles (see Sect. 4.4.3) and these could not be replenished in the smaller vessels between real-time frames.

4.3.2
Conventional Spectral Doppler

Microbubble-based agents were also of benefit in spectral Doppler studies of blood flow. The increase of about 20 dB in echo strength that they produced allowed spectral Doppler techniques to detect and measure blood flow in vessels that would be otherwise too deep. This type of application is sometimes referred to as "Doppler rescue".

4.3.3
Conventional Colour Doppler

Colour Doppler imaging techniques, such as colour flow imaging (CFI) or power Doppler imaging (PDI), also benefited since the arrival and distribution of microbubbles, at least in the larger arteries, could be demonstrated more easily. In CFI a B-mode tissue image is overlaid with a colour map in which the colour of each pixel is determined by the mean Doppler shift for that location. There is no information about the strength (power) of the Doppler signal and all coloured pixels are shown at fixed brightness. In PDI, the colour intensity of each pixel of the colour overlay is proportional to the mean power of the Doppler signal at that location (irrespective of the Doppler shift), providing an indication of the number of moving blood cells there. No information about the Doppler shift is given, so the colour used is either fixed or only changes a little with signal strength (e.g. from dull orange for low strength to bright yellow for maximum strength). In both CFI and PDI, the increased signal to noise ratio provided by microbubbles was valuable in itself, but it could also be used to improve spatial resolution by permitting the use of higher frequencies.

A disadvantage of using CFI with contrast agent is that it is subject to "blooming" – this is the spreading of full brightness colour beyond the walls of the vessel to which it should ideally be confined. This leads to loss of spatial resolution, with blooming around adjacent vessels merging together and blooming from larger arteries obscuring signals from smaller ones. It is caused by the sensitivity being so high with microbubbles that the effective spatial dimensions of the transmitted pulse are increased. Without microbubbles, blood cells are normally unable to generate echoes above noise level unless the most intense, central part of the pulse is within the blood vessel, or only a small distance outside it. With US contrast agent present, microbubbles at the vessel wall are still able to produce detectable echoes when the centre of the pulse is some distance outside the vessel.

The problem with CFI in this regard is the "priority" algorithm used to decide whether a particular pixel displays grey-scale B-mode information or colour Doppler shift information. Without US contrast agent, Doppler signals are generally weak, so an algorithm is used that always shows the Doppler information, provided the Doppler signal has a strength above a specific threshold (which the user sets with the priority control). When US contrast agent is used, the increased strength of Doppler signals means this threshold is exceeded well beyond the vessel wall, resulting in many pixels outside the vessel being shown in a conspicuous colour appropriate to the Doppler shift, irrespective of whether the Doppler signal strength is only just above threshold or very high.

PDI is potentially the more attractive of the two modes for microbubble imaging since it shows the concentration of microbubbles directly. It suffers much less from blooming than does CFI since low strength Doppler signals from outside a vessel are shown at low brightness. It is also the most sensitive method for detecting moving blood. One reason for this is that it uses just one colour rather than many, helping the eye to better appreciate the dynamic range of signals. Another is that it gives a signal even when the beam is perpendicular to a vessel, due to the angular spread of the beam. Some of this high sensitivity can be traded for improved temporal resolution. Whereas it is normally necessary to interrogate each scan line about 10 times in order to obtain the Doppler information, the stronger signals from microbubbles means that sufficient sensitivity can be achieved with fewer transmission/reception sequences. A consequence of spending less time interrogating each scan line is poorer accuracy in the measurement of the Doppler frequency shifts, but this is of no concern in PDI.

The problem of using PDI with contrast agents, however, is that it suffers from "flash" artefact. Moving tissue produces much stronger Doppler signals than does even microbubble-enhanced blood. Since the brightness of each pixel in a PDI image is proportional to signal strength, this signal would swamp the weaker Doppler signals from blood, if it were not filtered out. A high-pass "clutter" (wall thump) filter is therefore incorporated into all Doppler equipment, taking advantage of the fact that Doppler signals from relatively slow moving tissue generally have a lower frequency than that from the blood. Such filters are reasonably effective when imaging flow in larger vessels because of the higher blood speeds, but, even then, movements of the probe or tissue that produce Doppler frequencies above the filter's cut-off frequency result in bright transient colour patches, known as "flash" artefacts. Unfortunately, the low frequency Doppler signals from the slow moving blood in the smaller vessels are rejected by the clutter filter along with the unwanted tissue signals.

This, together with poor replenishment of collapsed microbubbles between imaging frames, meant there was less success in using microbubbles to visualise flow in smaller vessels, such as in the liver or myocardium.

4.3.4
Harmonic B-Mode Imaging by High-Pass Filtering

Alternative / associated names: Contrast Harmonic Imaging (CHI), Narrow Band Harmonic Imaging, Dual Frequency Harmonic Imaging, Harmonic Greyscale Imaging.

A considerable improvement in contrast between blood and tissue was achieved by using a high-pass filter to suppress the fundamental component of the echoes but leave the second harmonic. This suppressed all the signal from tissue apart from the tissue harmonic component (see Sect. 4.2.3). The amplitude of the transmission pulses was chosen to be large enough to ensure a useful second harmonic signal from microbubbles, but not so large as to cause excessive bubble destruction or to generate a conspicuous second harmonic signal from tissue. Harmonic detection sacrificed some sensitivity since, for both microbubble and tissue echoes, most energy is in the suppressed fundamental frequency band. However, the second harmonic signal from microbubbles is much more than that from tissue, allowing vessels within tissue to show up brightly against a darker background. A further benefit of the improved contrast was an increase in the time for which the signal from an injected bolus of microbubbles could be detected.

It is necessary to lower the frequency of the transmitted pulse so that both it and the second harmonic spectrum can be accommodated within the frequency range of the transducer. Thus, a transducer with a frequency range from say 1.5 MHz to 4.5 MHz can be used to transmit a 2 MHz pulse and still have sufficient bandwidth to receive the second harmonic spectrum of the echoes, centred on 4 MHz. This requires a transducer with a bandwidth (3 MHz in this case) approximately equal to its centre frequency. Fortunately, transducer technology has advanced sufficiently to make this possible. There is some loss of efficiency due to either the transmission or reception centre frequency, or both, not being at the peak of the transducer frequency response curve, but this is more than offset by the greater echo strength due to the use of microbubbles. Some manufacturers arrange for transducers that are to be used for harmonic imaging to have their greatest efficiency at the second harmonic frequency.

The method has limitations, however. Firstly, any overlap between the spectrum of the transmitted pulse and second harmonic spectrum of the echoes should be as small as possible, if the filter is to separate them successfully. This means the bandwidth of both spectra should be less than half the bandwidth of the transducer (Fig. 4.7a). Since

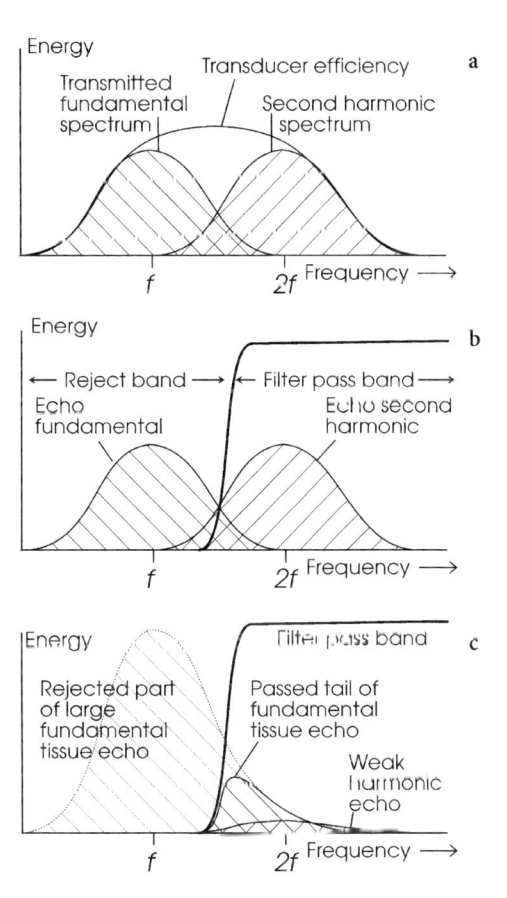

Fig. 4.7a–c. Harmonic B-mode imaging with a high-pass filter. The bandwidth of the transmitted pulse must be less than half the transducer bandwidth in order to reduce overlap with the second harmonic spectrum (**a**). Inevitably there is some overlap and the signal rejected by the filter contains part of the second harmonic spectrum, reducing the strength of the harmonic microbubble signal available for display. Also, the passed signal is contaminated by part of the fundamental spectrum, increasing tissue clutter (**b**). The high frequency tail of a strong tissue echo can overwhelm a weak harmonic signal (**c**).

axial resolution improves in proportion to echo bandwidth, it is twice as poor as that which can be achieved in conventional B-mode imaging, where the full transducer bandwidth is used to transmit and receive.

Secondly, as in practice there will always be some overlap, the signal rejected by the filter must contain part of the low frequency end of the second harmonic spectrum (Fig. 4.7b), reducing the strength of the harmonic microbubble signal available for display. Conversely, the signal passed by the filter will contains the high frequency tail of the fundamental spectrum from tissue. If the tissue signal is strong, or the microbubble signal is weak, this tail can overwhelm the peak of the second harmonic spectrum (Fig. 4.7c). This places a limit on the strength of blood echoes that can be detected.

Although the contrast between microbubbles and tissue was much improved by harmonic imaging, the tissue harmonic signal limited the improvement. Also, axial resolution and sensitivity remained poor. These limitations have largely been overcome in the more recent techniques for harmonic imaging, described later. However, these generally require that two or more pulses be transmitted down each scan line, so the filter method of harmonic imaging retains the advantage of a higher frame rate than is possible with the more recent methods.

4.3.5
Harmonic Colour Flow Imaging by High-Pass Filtering

Alternative / associated names: Harmonic Doppler Imaging

Using a high pass filter to remove the mainly fundamental tissue echoes brought similar improvements in contrast and imaging time to colour flow imaging (CFI). (It was, of course, necessary to detect the Doppler shifts relative to the second harmonic frequency). In particular, blood flow could be imaged in narrower vessels than before. The flash problem due to probe or tissue movement (see Sect. 4.3.3) was also very much reduced, since filtering out the fundamental spectrum suppresses echoes from all tissue, whether moving or not. The temporal resolution was poor because of the need to transmit several pulse down each line and spatial resolution remained poor in comparison to harmonic B-mode because of the long pulse length.

4.3.6
Harmonic Power Doppler Imaging by High-Pass Filtering

Alternative / associated names: Harmonic Power Doppler (HPD), Power Harmonic Imaging

The benefits of harmonic imaging were even more important for power Doppler imaging (PDI). By substantially reducing the serious flash artefact to which PDI is vulnerable, the advantages of PDI could be put to good use. These include its greater sensitivity than CFI and its smaller blooming artefact, as discussed in Sect. 4.3.3. Also, PDI is not concerned with Doppler shifts so aliasing is of no consequence. This means lower pulse repetition frequencies can be used, with the result that a slow moving microbubble will travel further between pulses. This in turn means a larger phase difference between the echoes from consecutive transmissions, increasing the probability of detection when only a few pulses are transmitted per line.

4.3.7
Intermittent Imaging in B-Mode

Alternative/associated names: Intermittent Second-Harmonic Gray-Scale (ISHGS), Transient Imaging, Interval Delay Imaging, Flash Echo Imaging, Triggered Imaging

As mentioned earlier (Sect. 4.3.1) the principal original application of microbubble-based agents was to opacify the left ventricle in order to better delineate the chamber wall. This worked well, as did visualisation of the major arteries in the liver, but efforts to visualise very small blood vessels in the abdomen or myocardium were much less successful. PORTER et al. (1995) found that microbubbles became visible in the myocardium when imaging was resumed after freezing the system, and proved that microbubbles were being destroyed by the scanning. In large vessels and the chambers of the heart, the blood is moving so rapidly that the imaged slice is replenished with microbubbles between frames. In the capillary bed, however, blood moves at only about 1 mm/s, so it can take several seconds to replenish the destroyed microbubbles in the imaged slice. Thus the bubbles were being continually destroyed by the real-time scanning. By using the ECG to trigger one image frame every two to four cardiac cycles, PORTER and XIE (1995) allowed time for microbubble replenishment in narrow vessels and were thus able to visualise microbubble-based agents in the myocardium itself.

The technique of intermittent imaging can also be used to visualise small vessels in the abdomen. ECG triggering is not necessary but the frame rate must be sufficiently low to allow replenishment of the tissue slice with microbubbles between frames. Again, the ability to monitor the scan plane in real time is lost. As an alternative to intermittent imaging of a fixed tissue slice, the probe can be swept sideways to view neighbouring slices of tissue, containing still-intact microbubbles.

The echoes produced by collapsing microbubbles contain a wide range of harmonics. This means harmonic B-mode imaging can be used to reduce tissue clutter signals. However, since the transmitted pulses have a large amplitude, there can be a high level of second harmonic component in the echoes from tissue. When using the technique to image perfusion in the myocardium, for example, the second harmonic microbubble signals may be only a few decibels above the tissue harmonic contrast signal (BECHER and BURNS 2000). In such cases, contrast between microbubbles and tissue can be increased by offline subtraction of a non-contrast-enhanced image of the same cross-section from the contrast-enhanced image.

4.3.8
Intermittent Colour Flow Imaging

Alternative / associated names: Pseudo-Doppler Imaging, Fundamental Imaging, Sono-scintigraphy, Stimulated Acoustic Emission Imaging (SAE)

It was also found that using large amplitude transmission pulses to deliberately destroy microbubbles provided a very sensitive way of visualising the distribution of microbubbles when in CFI mode, even when the blood was stationary (BLOMLEY et al. 1999). In this mode, the microbubbles shows as a random colour mosaic extending over a limited depth range close to focus of the transmitted ultrasound (Fig. 4.8). The effect quickly disappears over a few frames due to the destruction of the microbubbles. As microbubbles are destroyed, their attenuating effect no longer protects those at greater depths, so the deeper microbubbles then burst, generating their own colour signal. The appearance is that of a colour "veil" starting at the focal region (where the amplitude is greatest) and shifting down the screen. The technique was originally called stimulated acoustic emission as it was thought that the Doppler system was detecting the broad spectrum of ultrasonic energy generated by the bursting of microbubbles.

The technique is now more commonly referred to as loss of correlation (LOC) imaging in recognition of the difference between the way this signal is generated and the normal way Doppler systems work, which is by measuring the regular (correlated) changes in phase between consecutive echoes from a moving reflector. Colour Doppler imaging involves interrogating each scan line in the image with several transmission-reception sequences. Each line is divided into a number of sample volumes, one for each colour pixel, and after every transmission an echo signal for each of these is obtained by dividing up the echo sequence into corresponding time segments. For each sample volume, the mean Doppler frequency can be estimated from the average phase shift between echoes from consecutive transmissions. This is used to allocate the appropriate colour to the pixel, from a pre-defined scale of colour against Doppler frequency. When large amplitude pulses are used with microbubbles, many of the microbubbles in the beam collapse and release gas, which then dissolves, either immediately or over the course of the next few pulses, depending on the gas. This results in a substantial and largely random differences between the echoes from consecutive transmissions. The estimate of Doppler frequency, and hence the colour allocated to the pixel, is therefore random. It is different for every pixel and collapse event, resulting in the observed random colour mosaic.

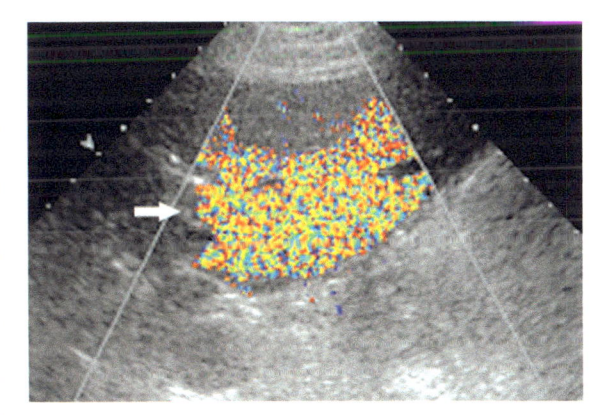

Fig. 4.8. Loss of Correlation (LOC) or stimulated acoustic emission (SAE) image, produced in colour flow imaging mode with large amplitude transmission pulses. The collapse of microbubbles produces changing echo signals that are interpreted as irregular Doppler signals, and displayed as a random colour mosaic.

In CFI, the need to interrogate each line of the colour box (the region of the image subject to Doppler imaging) several times means there is only time to interrogate a relatively small number of scan lines across the box. This means the colour pixels are wider than those in a B-mode image, and hence lateral resolution is poorer. The axial resolution is also poor because, in order to boost signal to noise ratio, pulse lengths used for Doppler are longer than those used for B-mode.

4.3.9
Intermittent Power Doppler Imaging

Alternative / associated names: Harmonic Power Doppler, Intermittent Harmonic Power Doppler, Colour Power Angio, Energy Imaging

The loss of correlation (LOC) signal described in the previous section can also be detected using power Doppler imaging (PDI). This replaces the multicolour mosaic seen in CFI with a narrow range of colours, the brightness indicating the local concentration of collapsing microbubbles (Fig. 4.9). In CFI, the accuracy of the estimates of Doppler frequency increase with the time spent interrogating each scan line. PDI does not display Doppler frequency information, so the fact that the microbubbles disappear after just one or two transmissions is of less consequence. Ultimately, an estimate of Doppler power can be obtained from just two transmissions per line. Suppression of tissue clutter is improved by detecting only second harmonic echo components and using the second harmonic frequency as the reference.

As with the all microbubble disrupting techniques, the method is not real-time and intermittent imaging must be used to view a fixed slice. It also suffers from poor axial resolution owing to the longer pulses used in Doppler imaging. Nevertheless, the technique is one of the most sensitive means of imaging microbubbles.

4.3.10
The Need for Further Improvements

Despite the improvements brought about by the filter method of harmonic imaging and the sensitivity of the LOC method, there remained a number of significant limitations. These included:

- The poor axial resolution in harmonic B-mode imaging due to the need to restrict the bandwidth of the transmitted pulse to less than half that of the transducer.
- The imperfect contrast between microbubbles and tissue in harmonic imaging when using a filter, due to the overlap between the fundamental spectrum and the second harmonic spectrum.
- The presence of a small but contrast limiting second harmonic component in the echoes from tissue, due to non-linear propagation of the transmitted pulse.
- Increased microbubble destruction, and hence an inability to image continuously in real-time if transmitted pulses of larger amplitude were used in an attempt to produce stronger second harmonic signals from microbubbles.
- Poor axial resolution with the otherwise sensitive Harmonic Power Doppler Imaging method based on microbubble destruction and LOC signals.

These problems have been addressed by two quite different approaches. One group of methods, commonly known as "low MI", seeks to minimise the incidence of microbubble destruction and the magnitude of tissue harmonic signal by transmitting pulses with low amplitudes and making use of the much greater non-linearity of scattering by microbubbles compared to that by tissues.

The other group of methods, commonly known as "high MI", uses larger pulse amplitudes (about 1 MPa), and make use of either the energy released

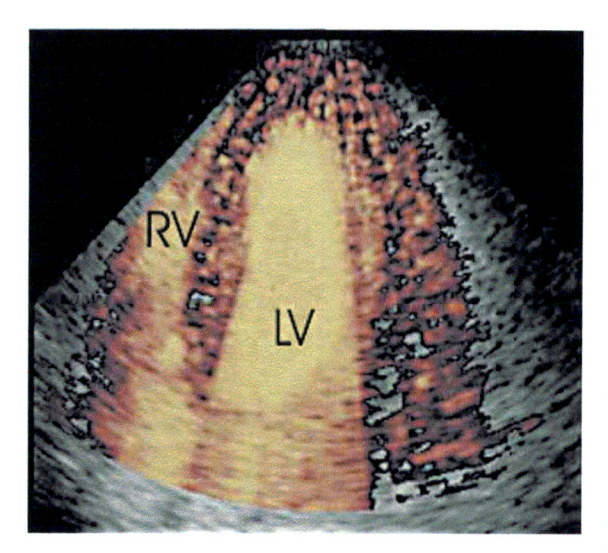

Fig. 4.9. Intermittent Harmonic Power Doppler image showing a four chamber view of a heart during continuous infusion of Levovist. Triggering every third cardiac cycle shows complete left ventricular (LV) and myocardial opacification. From KUNTZ-HEHNER et al (2002).

or the difference in the echo signals before and after the bubble destruction.

MI is actually a safety index, displayed on the screen of most modern ultrasound imaging machines, to indicate the potential for non-thermal bio-effects. It is defined as:

$$MI = p- / \sqrt{f_c}$$

where $p-$ is the largest peak negative (rarefactional) pressure that the transmitted pulse would achieve during its travel through a medium of specified attenuation coefficient (0.3 dB cm^{-1} MHz^{-1}) and f_c is the centre frequency of the pulse. The value displayed on the screen responds to changes of operating mode or any control settings that affect acoustic output. The theory behind the above formula for MI relates to the threshold for the production of inertial cavitation of free gas or vapour bubbles in water (HOLLAND and APFEL 1989; APFEL and HOLLAND 1991) so it cannot be assumed that MI will be a reliable quantitative indicator of the likelihood of the rupture of microbubbles with stabilising shells, as used in contrast agents. Nevertheless, it does provide a rough indication of this, at least for a given contrast agent, and it has the merit of being widely available on image screens.

The differences in shell strength and flexibility between microbubbles of different makes, and the uncertain relevance of MI to contrast microbubble destruction, mean there is no universally accepted boundary between "high" and "low" MI in regard to the potential for microbubble destruction. However, an MI of 1.0 would certainly be considered as high, while one of 0.1 would certainly be considered low in this regard, although values as low as 0.06 are used. Note that there is no known threshold below which bubble destruction does not occur; it is more a matter of probability.

4.4
Low-MI Techniques

As stated above, these methods use low amplitude pulses in ways that take advantage of the non-linear nature of scattering by microbubbles. Their evolution has gone hand in hand with the development of new types of microbubble-based agents with more flexible shells, able to expand and contract with larger amplitudes in a non-linear fashion. The new generation of microbubble-based agents also benefits from longer lifetimes, allowing observations over longer periods.

The principal advantage of low-MI techniques is that the microbubbles are not destroyed so readily, permitting continuous real-time imaging.

The principal disadvantage of low-MI techniques is that they have less sensitivity (dynamic range) than high-MI techniques. This is primarily due to the fact that low-MI techniques make use of the small differences between echoes from two or more separate transmissions, and the energy associated with this is only a small fraction of that in any individual echo.

Some low-MI techniques are based on the detection of the second harmonic signal from microbubbles, but avoid the limitations of earlier methods based on high-pass filtering (see Sects. 4.3.4–4.3.6). The newer methods of second harmonic detection use pulse inversion (Sects. 4.4.1–4.4.3) or coded transmissions and matched filters (Sect. 4.4.4). An alternative approach is to use amplitude modulation (Sect. 4.4.5) to detect the effects of non-linear scattering on the fundamental component of echoes. A third approach is contrast pulse sequence imaging (Sect. 4.4.6) which combines the first two.

Transmitted pulses with low intrinsic second harmonic content are desirable for the many microbubble imaging methods that are based on detecting the second harmonic component of microbubbles echoes. In general, the more abrupt the rise and fall of a pulse waveform, the greater the harmonic components. Transmitted pulses with a gently rising and falling bell-shaped (Gaussian) amplitude profile are therefore often used. It is also desirable that the input amplification stage of the receiver is very linear, in other words that the amplification factor (gain) is constant for all echoes whether large or small in amplitude. Any non-linearity will introduce distortion into the amplified waveforms and hence generate second harmonic components. Both sources of spurious second harmonic contamination will degrade the contrast between microbubble echoes and those from tissue.

4.4.1
Pulse Inversion with Two Transmissions

Alternative / associated names: Pulse Inversion (PI), Phase Inversion (PI), Pulse Subtraction (PS), Polarity Inversion (PI), Wideband Harmonic Imaging, Pulse Inversion Harmonic Imaging (PIHI), Pulse Inversion Contrast Harmonic Imaging (PICHI), Pulse Inversion Harmonics (PIH)

This very common technique involves interrogating each line twice. It avoids the filter method's limitations of poor axial resolution and imperfect separation of fundamental and second harmonic components, but at the expense of frame rate. Short (two to three cycle) pulses, as typically used in B-mode, are transmitted, with the waveform of the second pulse being the inverse of the first (Fig. 4.10). In other words, the positive half cycles in the first pulse are replaced by negative half cycles (with the same shape and magnitude) in the second pulse, and vice versa. The un-demodulated echo sequences produced by the two pulses are stored and added together. The resultant sum is used to determine the grey levels along the corresponding scan line on the display.

In the second echo sequence, linearly scattered echoes, such as those from tissue, will simply be inverted versions of those in the first echo sequence. Tissue echoes will therefore be cancelled when the two echo sequences are summed. If the scattering is non-linear, as is the case for microbubbles, the two sequences will not cancel on addition (Fig. 4.10).

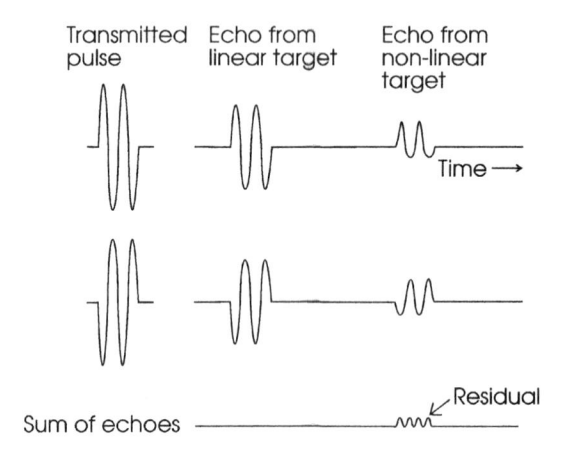

Fig. 4.10. Pulse inversion imaging involves summing echo sequences from a non-inverted and an inverted transmission pulse. Echoes from linear targets cancel whilst those from non-linear targets (microbubbles) form a residual signal, consisting of second and higher even harmonic signals.

An equivalent explanation may be given in terms of the effect of inverting the transmitted pulse on the fundamental and harmonic waveforms of an echo pulse. As illustrated in Fig. 4.2, inverting a transmitted pulse causes the fundamental waveform (and any odd order harmonics) of the echo to be inverted, but the second (and any even order harmonic) waveforms of the echo are not inverted. Thus, summing the two echo sequences cancels out the fundamental and the odd harmonics in the echoes but doubles the magnitude of the second and other even harmonics. The pulse inversion technique therefore provides a way of cancelling fundamental and odd harmonic components of echoes but preserving and amplifying second harmonic (and other even) components.

The advantage of the pulse inversion method over the filter method of harmonic detection (see Sect. 4.3.4) is that overlap between the fundamental and second harmonic spectra does not matter (Fig. 4.11). Hence, there is no need to restrict the

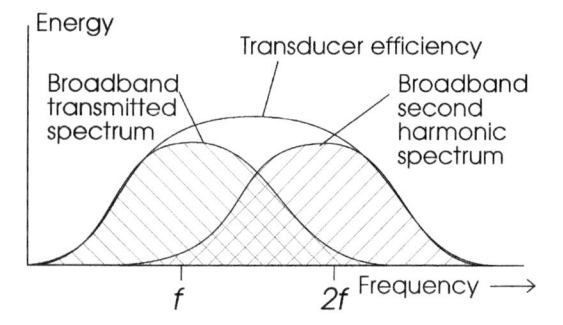

Fig. 4.11. The pulse inversion method of suppressing fundamentals signals does not depend on a high-pass filter. Overlap of the transmitted spectrum with the harmonic spectrum therefore does not matter, allowing the transmission spectrum to be broad and hence the axial resolution to be good.

transmission spectrum to the lower half of the transducer frequency range and so limit bandwidth. This allows short (large bandwidth) pulses to be used and hence good axial resolution to be achieved. The swamping of weak microbubble echoes by the high frequency tail of the fundamental spectrum of tissue echoes Fig. 4.7c) is eliminated. Similarly, the lower frequency tail of the harmonic spectrum is retained, increasing the strength of the harmonic signal. The disadvantage of the method, however, is a reduction in frame rate due to the need to interrogate each scan line twice.

Pulse inversion is also used in the B-mode tissue imaging method known as Tissue Harmonic Imaging (Sect. 4.2.3), which produces images with fewer acoustic noise artefacts and improved spatial resolution. In that application, transmission pulses with much greater amplitudes are used to ensure the deliberate generation of substantial tissue harmonic signals.

4.4.2
Pulse Inversion on Alternate Scan Lines

Alternative / associated names: Coherent Contrast Imaging (CCI)

The reduction in frame rate referred to above can be avoided by transmitting only one pulse per scan line, but inverting the transmitted pulse on alternate scan lines. The overlap between adjacent beams means that scatterers receive pulses of alternating polarity. Summing the echo sequences from adjacent lines therefore cancels out echoes from linear scatterers, as in the two-pulse method described in the previous section. The sum of the two echo sequences represents an average of the two contributing lines and is therefore displayed as a synthetic line situated midway between them. The avoidance of a frame rate penalty comes at the expense of a slightly imperfect cancellation of the fundamental, since not all points in a pair of overlapping beams experience matching but inverted versions of the same pulse waveform. This technique is well suited to machines which use parallel beam forming (see, for example, WHITTINGHAM 1997) as a time saving technique in normal B-scanning, since the necessary facilities for digitising storing and adding undemodulated echo sequences from adjacent scan lines already exist.

4.4.3
Pulse Inversion with Three Transmissions

Alternative / associated names: Power Pulse Inversion (PPI) Imaging, Power Pulse Inversion Contrast Harmonic (PPICH) Imaging

The tissue-contrast discrimination that can be achieved by pulse inversion as described in Sects. 4.4.1 or 4.4.2 is limited by any tissue movement between the two transmissions. Where there is tissue movement, the positions of the tissue interfaces in the second echo sequence will not match those in the first, and the cancellation of fundamental echo components will not be perfect. POWERS et al. (2000) have described how three interrogations of a line with alternately inverted pulses can greatly reduce the effect of tissue motion.

The processing amounts to forming an average of the first and third echo sequences (by adding them together and dividing by two) and adding this to the second echo sequence. If the tissue velocity is not too great, the difference in phase between echoes from the first and third pulses (less than a millisecond apart) will be small, say less than 30° or so. The average echo sequence will then be a close approximation to one with half the phase shift (Fig. 4.12), corresponding to what would have been returned if an imaginary pulse had been transmitted midway in time between these two real pulses. Assuming the tissue velocity to be constant, the positions of any tissue interface at this time would have been the same as when the second real pulse was transmitted. Consequently, the positions of any given tissue echo in the average echo sequence will match that in the real sequence from the second pulse (Fig. 4.13), overcoming the tissue motion problem. As for the two-pulse method, adding the average echo sequence from the two non-inverted pulses to the real sequence from the second (inverted) pulse will give cancellation of linear tissue echoes but not of microbubble echoes.

The method can be considered to be a three-pulse example of the contrast pulse sequence (CPS) technique discussed in Sect. 4.4.6.

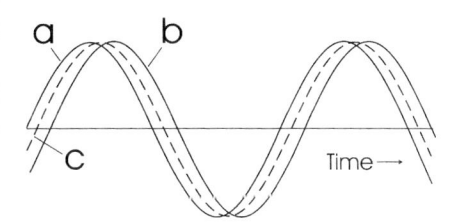

Figure 4.12. Pulse inversion with three transmissions. If the tissue velocity is not too great, the difference in phase between echoes from the first (*a*) and third (*b*) pulses (less than a millisecond apart) will be small, say less than 30° or so. The average echo sequence (*c*) will then be a close approximation to one with half the phase shift, corresponding to what would have been returned if an imaginary pulse had been transmitted midway in time between these two real pulses.

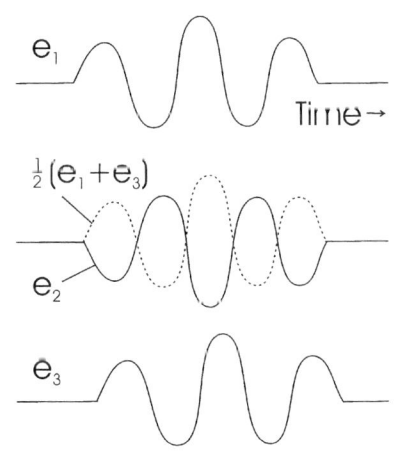

Fig. 4.13. Pulse inversion with three transmissions. Forming an average of the first echo sequence with the third echo sequence means that the echoes e_1 and e_3 from a given moving tissue interface form an average echo $½(e_1 + e_3)$ whose position is midway between e_1 and e_3 (Fig. 4.12). This average echo will be in the same position as, and therefore cancel, the real echo e_2 from the same interface in the echo sequence produced by the second (inverted) transmission pulse.

4.4.4
Harmonic Detection by Coded Excitation

Coded transmission pulses (coded excitation) were originally developed for B-mode tissue imaging, where they allowed signal to noise ratio to be improved without the need to exceed regulatory safety limits on pulse amplitudes. Rather than using larger amplitude pulses to increase the transmitted energy and hence achieve greater sensitivity, longer pulses are used. In contrast agent applications, the use of long coded pulses allows either sensitivity to be increased for a given transmission amplitude, or sensitivity to be maintained while using lower amplitude pulses in order to reduce tissue harmonic signals.

Within the long pulses are frequency or phase changes that act as a code. This code is present in genuine echoes but not in noise, so by using a special "matched" filter, designed to respond strongly to the transmitted code, the signal to noise ratio can be improved. This filter compresses the long coded echo pulses into short high amplitude ones, effectively using the energy distributed along the length of the pulse to build up a shorter pulse of greater amplitude. The use of long pulses does not lead to poorer axial resolution since the signals produced by the matched filter inherit the large bandwidth that the frequency or phase changes gives to the transmitted pulses. The signals from the matched filter, therefore, have similar lengths to those of conventional echoes. Note that it is bandwidth, not simply pulse length, that limits axial resolution.

4.4.4.1
Binary Coding

Alternative / associated names: Coded Contrast Agent Imaging, Coded Phase Inversion, Coded Harmonic Angio, Coded Octave Harmonic Imaging

One coded excitation technique involves transmitting pulses in the form of several "base pulses", each say two cycles long, strung together end to end. If an inverted base pulse represents "-1" and a non-inverted base pulse represents "1", a pulse consisting of four base pulses in which the fourth was inverted would carry the four digit code 1,1,1,–1. A code in which the digits are either 1 or –1 is known as a binary code. As echoes return, they are stepped past a reference replica of the coded transmission pulse and compared, one code digit at a time. When an echo code lines up perfectly with the reference code the output is high. A mismatch in position of just one digit will produce only a low output. Thus a high amplitude signal is produced that has a duration equal to just one base pulse. However, as the echo is stepped past the reference there are some positions where a partial degree of similarity occurs and smaller but significant outputs are produced. The output of the comparison process (filter) for each echo therefore consists not only of a large amplitude "main lobe" but also smaller "range lobes" which degrade range (axial) resolution. The solution to the problem is to transmit a second pulse, with a different carefully chosen code (technically, the codes of the two pulses form a "Golay pair"). The filter output for an echo from this transmission also has a high amplitude main lobe as well as range lobes, but, if the two codes are chosen appropriately, the range lobes produced by the second pulse will be inverted versions of those produced by the first pulse. Summing the two filter outputs causes the range lobes to cancel, leaving a short main lobe of double amplitude. Thus the method has high sensitivity and an axial resolution equal to that of one base pulse.

In the above description, transmission codes are chosen such that echoes with these codes will give strong short output signals after filtering. This is what is required for B-mode imaging. It is possible, however, to do the opposite and use codes that totally suppress echoes with the transmission codes. Such codes are used to eliminate the fundamental signal in microbubble-based agents applications. The key to preserving the second harmonic component of the echoes is to use coded transmission sequences in which one or more of the base pulses is shifted by a quarter of a cycle. If second harmonic components are present in an echo, this quarter cycle shift at the fundamental frequency will become a half cycle shift at the second harmonic frequency. This amounts to an inversion of that base pulse at the second harmonic frequency, but not at the fundamental frequency. Thus, the code of the second harmonic component of an echo will be modified from that transmitted, whereas the fundamental component will retain the code of the transmitted pulse. By careful choice of the transmission codes and filters, it can be arranged that the modified codes of the second harmonic component cause the second harmonic component to be selectively detected, whilst the un-modified codes cause the fundamental component to be cancelled out.

4.4.4.2
Chirp Coding

Alternative / associated names: Chirp Excitation, Chirp Coded Excitation

Another form of coded pulse with a large bandwidth is a "chirp", in which the frequency and amplitude are progressively varied over say twenty or thirty cycles. Ultrasonic chirps are transmitted by some bats in order to help them recognise their own echoes in the presence of noise. Chirps with a Gaussian (bell shaped) waveform are sometimes used in coded B-mode tissue imaging since this shape has been shown to produce only small range lobes and to propagate in a medium with frequency dependent attenuation, such as tissue, with minimum change in bandwidth. Chirp transmissions offer a frame rate advantage over binary coded excitation, as just described, since only one transmission is needed per line.

The matched filtering process involves comparing the echoes with a stored reference version of the transmitted chirp. With reference to Fig. 4.14, the comparison process consists of moving the echo waveform past the stored reference version in small time steps and, for each step, integrating the product of the two waveforms over time. When two waveforms of identical shape, albeit with different amplitudes, are well out of alignment in time the output of this process is low (a). As they become almost aligned the output becomes larger, reaching a maximum at perfect alignment (b) and then falling off again (c). The filter output is thus a short, large amplitude "compressed" pulse for every match between a genuine chirp echo and the reference chirp. The output is low, however, for non-chirp noise.

BORSBOOM et al. (2003, 2004) have shown that by using a reference chirp in which the frequencies are doubled (e.g. from 4–8 MHz for a transmitted chirp in which the sweep is from 2–4 MHz) the filter will extract and compress the second harmonic component of microbubble echoes, and achieve an improvement in signal to noise ratio of approximately 10 dB over that when using a conventional short pulse of the same bandwidth.

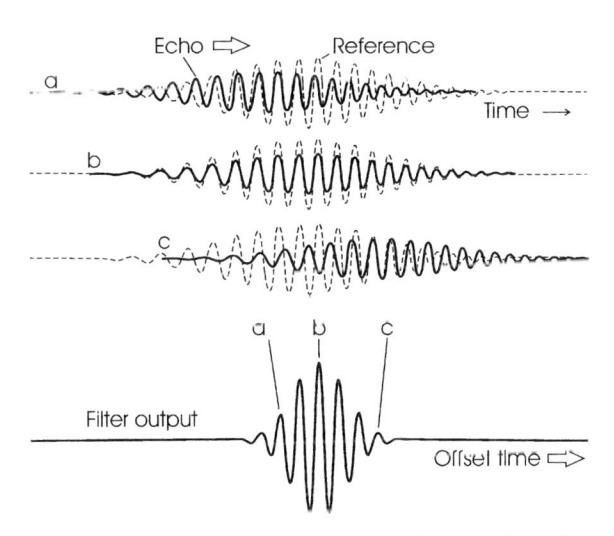

Fig. 4.14-c. Chirp detection in harmonic detection by coded excitation. The comparison process consists of moving the echo waveform past the stored reference version in small time steps and, for each step, integrating the product of the two waveforms over time. When two waveforms of identical shape, albeit with different amplitudes, are well out of alignment in time the output of this process is low (a). As they become almost aligned the output becomes larger, reaching a maximum at perfect alignment (b) and then falling off again (c). To detect the second harmonic, the start and finish frequencies in the reference chirp are doubled.

4.4.5
Amplitude Modulation (Power Modulation)

In this approach (BROCK-FISHER et al. 1996), the dependence of the amplitude of microbubble echoes on transmission pulse amplitude is utilised directly. The process is often called power modulation, although amplitude modulation is a more accurate description. Power can be high even if the amplitude is low, if the pulse repetition frequency or the pulse length is large.

At its simplest, the technique involves transmitting two pulses with different amplitudes (but otherwise identical waveforms) and storing the two resulting echo sequences. Assuming the typical case where the amplitude of the second pulse is twice that of the first, the first echo sequence is amplified by a factor of two before being subtracted from the second echo sequence. This results in the cancellation of the echoes from stationary tissue since, for linear scatterers, the second echo sequence will be identical to the first, apart from having twice the amplitude. This is not the case for a non-linear scatterer such as a microbubble, since the echoes produced by the two pulses will be distorted to different extents and the amplitudes of the second set of echoes will be less than twice those of the first. There is therefore a residual after subtraction, representing the "non-linear signal" from the microbubble. Importantly, this contains components at the fundamental frequency as well as at harmonics frequencies, as explained in Sect. 4.2.2 and shown in Fig. 4.5.

The ability of amplitude modulation techniques to make use of the fundamental component of microbubble echoes gives them more sensitivity than second harmonic detection methods, since:
- There is much more energy in the fundamental component of an echo than in any of its harmonic components
- The lower frequency of the fundamental echo component means it suffers much less attenuation in returning through tissue to the transducer than do the harmonic components
- The transducer efficiency is greater since its centre frequency can match that of the fundamental, whereas for second harmonic detection both the transmitted (fundamental) frequency and the second harmonic generally lie in the less efficient wings of the transducer's frequency response (but see Sect. 4.3.4)
- Second harmonic signals from tissue can be safely rejected without compromising the microbubble signals.

The simple two-pulse method just described has two limitations. Firstly, movement of tissue interfaces between transmissions will limit performance since the echoes from a given interface will not be in the same positions in their respective echo sequences when they are subtracted. Secondly, generating two pulses with one having precisely twice the amplitude of the other is not straightforward. Driving the transducer with electrical pulses of different peak to peak voltages presents challenges of precision and quality control if small but potentially important errors in pulse amplitudes are to be avoided. Using all the transducer elements in the transmitting aperture for one pulse, but only half for the other, introduces difficulties due to differences in the width, shape and/or position of the two beams. For example, if alternate elements in the array are used to generate the weaker beam, that beam will have more pronounced grating lobes.

Both problems can be solved by interrogating the scan line three times (HUNT et al. 2003). The same peak to peak voltage is applied to all the elements in the transmitting aperture, but only half the elements are used for the first pulse, while the remaining half are used for the third pulse (Fig. 4.15). All the elements are used for the second pulse. Processing consists of subtracting the second echo sequence from the sum of the first and third echo sequences.

Taken together, the elements and beam-forming delays used for the first and third transmissions are the same as used for the second transmission. Thus, the effective beam shape used to form the

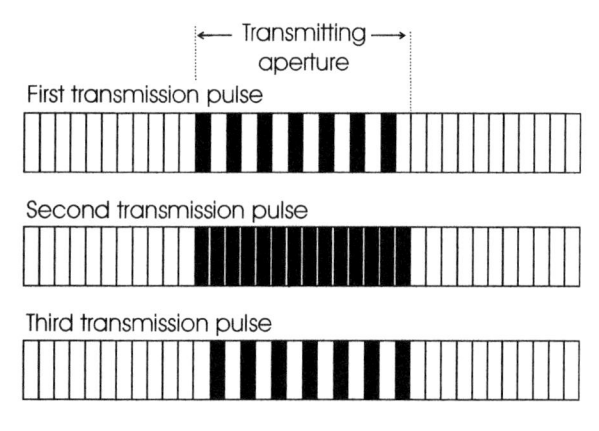

Fig. 4.15. Amplitude (power) modulation with three pulses. The same peak to peak voltage is applied to all the elements in the transmitting aperture, but only half the elements are used for the first pulse, while the remaining half are used for the third pulse. All the elements are used for the second pulse. Processing consists of subtracting the second echo sequence from the sum of the first and third echo sequences.

sum of the first and third echo sequences is identical to that used to form the second echo sequence. The fact that only half the elements are used for the first and third transmissions means that the pressure amplitudes generated by these in the focal zone are half those produced by the second transmission. For stationary linear scatterers, such as tissue interfaces, summing the echoes produced by the two half amplitude transmitted pulses gives the same result as would have been obtained by transmitting one full amplitude pulse. For non-linear scatterers, this sum will be slightly more than would have been obtained from one full amplitude pulse. Subtracting the second echo sequence from the sum of the first and third echo sequences will therefore give zero for tissue echoes but not for microbubble echoes.

The use of three pulses makes it possible to correct for uniform tissue movement in a similar way to that used for the three-pulse pulse inversion method (see Sect. 4.4.3). Provided the movements of tissue interfaces between the first and third pulses are much less than a wavelength, summing the echo sequences from the first and third pulses produces a double amplitude approximation to the echo sequence that would have been obtained for interfaces in the positions they had midway in time between the first and third transmissions (Fig. 4.16). If the speeds of all tissue interfaces are constant (albeit different for each scatterer) these positions will be the same as at the time of the second pulse. Subtraction of the second echo sequence from the sum of the first and third echo sequences therefore cancels tissue echoes but leaves a residual signal (at

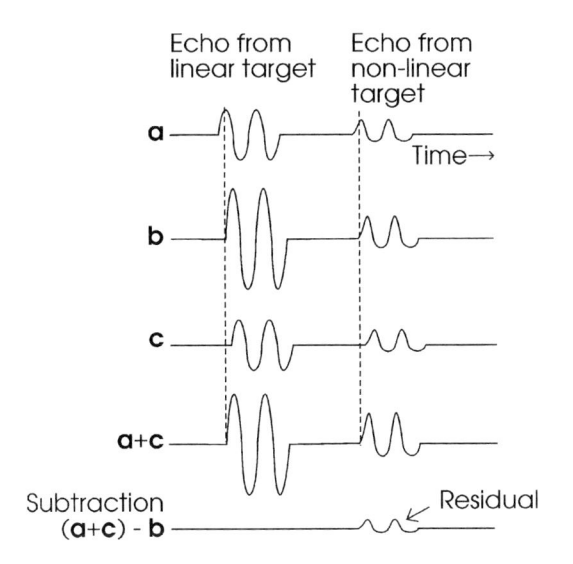

Fig. 4.16. Amplitude (power) modulation with three pulses. Echo sequences a and c are from half amplitude transmission pulses. Echo sequence b is from a full amplitude pulse transmitted midway in time between the first and third transmission. The linear target (tissue interface) is assumed to be moving whilst the non-linear target is stationary. The sum (a + c) has approximately double the amplitude of either a or c, with the tissue echo time-shifted to coincide in position with the tissue echo in sequence b. Subtracting b from (a + c) cancels echoes from stationary or slow moving linear targets but leaves a residual at the fundamental frequency for echoes from stationary or moving non-linear targets.

the fundamental frequency) for the microbubble echoes. Thus, the effects of slow steady motion are largely compensated for. Where the speed is changing with time, more pulses are needed, as discussed in Sect. 4.4.6.2. This method can be considered to be an example of a three-pulse CPS, as discussed next.

4.4.6
Combined Amplitude Modulation and Pulse Inversion/Phase Shift. Contrast Pulse Sequence (CPS) Imaging

Alternative / associated names: Power Modulated Pulse Inversion (PMPI), Cadence Imaging

Contrast pulse sequence (CPS) imaging is a general name for interrogating each scan lines a number of times with pulses having various amplitudes and phases. In practice, only two pulse amplitudes are usually involved, one being twice the other, and the change of phase between pulses is usually either 0° or 180° (i.e. pulse inversion). However, other phase shifts, such as 90° or 120° may be used (WILKENING et al. 2000). A processor first amplifies the echo sequence from each transmission by a particular weighting factor (for example ×2 or ×–1) and then sums all the weighted echo sequences. By suitable choice of transmission pulses and weighting factors it is possible to isolate or suppress the fundamental or any harmonic or combination of harmonics as required, with a controllable degree of sensitivity to motion.

Notation such as (½, –1, 1, –½) (–2, –1, 1, 2) is used to summarise the transmitted pulse amplitudes and their weighting factors (PHILLIPS 2001). In this example, the first set of numbers (½, –1, 1, –½) indicates that each line is interrogated four times, with the first and last transmitted pulses having amplitudes half that of the second and third pulses, and that the second and fourth transmitted pulses are inverted. The second set of numbers (–2, –1, 1, 2) indicates that the amplifier weighting factors for the first and last echo sequences are twice those for the second and third sequences and that the first two echo sequences are inverted before being summed. The pulse inversion and amplitude modulation techniques described previously may be considered as examples of this more general class of techniques. For example, the pulse inversion method using two pulses (Sect. 4.4.1) could be represented in CPS notation as (1, –1) (1, 1).

4.4.6.1
Selection or Suppression of Particular Fundamental and Harmonic Signals by CPS

A useful insight into how CPS is able to select particular harmonics can be gained by considering the echo from a non-linear scatterer as the sum of contributions from the different orders of scattering (see Sect. 4.2.2). Note that this is very much an idealised model of scattering as many other factors will be relevant in practice, including the occurrence of resonances at many different frequencies and differences in scattering characteristics in the wide range of bubble sizes involved. With reference to Fig. 4.4, where s(p) is the pressure amplitude of an echo from a microbubble and p is the pressure amplitude of the incident wave:

$$s(p) = k_1 p + k_2 p^2 + k_3 p^3 + \ldots \text{(higher orders)}$$

The coefficients k_1, k_2, k_3 etc. represent the relative strengths of the first-order (linear), second-order (quadratic) and third-order (cubic) scattering from the microbubble. Contributions of higher orders are likely to be smaller, so for clarity, the discussion will be limited to the first three orders.

Consider, as an example, the three-pulse amplitude modulation technique previously described (Sect. 4.4.5) which can be described by (½, 1, ½) (1,−1, 1). In the set of equations below, the three columns represent the first, second and third orders and the rows represents the weighted responses s(p) to each of the three transmitted pulses at the moment of peak transmitted amplitude. Summing the three orders (columns) independently shows that first-order (linear) echoes from tissue are suppressed and that second- and third-order scattering are enhanced. The third order contains the required non-linear fundamental signal from microbubbles (Fig. 4.5) while the second-order term shows that second harmonic microbubble echo components will also be preserved, albeit to a lesser degree.

Order:	1(linear)	2(quadratic)	3(cubic)
$1 \times s(½)$ =	$k_1 .½$	+ $k_2 .½^2$	+ $k_3 .½^3$
$-1 \times s(1)$ =	$-k_1 .1$	− $k_2 .1^2$	− $k_3 .1^3$
$1 \times s(½)$ =	$k_1 .½$	+ $k_2 .½^2$	+ $k_3 .½^3$
Sum =	0	− $k_2 .½$	− $k_3 .¾$

Another three-pulse sequence, marketed as Cadence CPS Imaging (Fig. 4.17) is (½, −1, ½) (1, 1, 1). Summing the three orders (below) shows that, although this achieves the same suppression of linear (first-order) tissue signals and selection of third-order (and hence non-linear fundamental) signals as the previous sequence, it generates three times the amount of second-order signal and hence a larger microbubble sensitivity, due to the greater second harmonic content:

Order:	1(linear)	2(quadratic)	3(cubic)
$1 \times s(½)$ =	$k_1 .½$	+ $k_2 .½^2$	+ $k_3 .½^3$
$1 \times s(-1)$ =	$k_1 .-1$	+ $k_2 .(-1)^2$	+ $k_3 .(-1)^3$
$1 \times s(½)$ =	$k_1 .½$	+ $k_2 .½^2$	+ $k_3 .½^3$
Sum =	0	+ $k_2 .1½$	− $k_3 .¾$

Although not involving amplitude modulation, the pulse-inversion method using three pulses (Sect. 4.4.3) could be described as the CPS (1, −1, 1) (1, 2, 1). The summation below shows that both first-order (linear) and third-order echo components are suppressed, leaving only second harmonic echo components:

Order:	1(linear)	2(quadratic)	3(cubic)
$1 \times s(1)$ =	$k_1 .1$	+ $k_2 .1^2$	+ $k_3 .1^3$
$2 \times s(-1)$ =	$2k_1 .-1$	+ $2k_2 .(-1)^2$	+ $2k_3 .(-1)^3$
$1 \times s(1)$ =	$k_1 .1$	+ $k_2 .1^2$	+ $k_3 .1^3$
Sum =	0	+ $k_2 .4$	+ 0

Longer sequences can give greater sensitivity, due to the summation of more echoes. For example, a similar summation for the five-pulse pulse inversion sequence (1, −1, 1, −1, 1) (1, 4, 6, 4, 1) gives a response with 16 times the amplitude (sum = 0 + $64k_2$ + 0) of the three-pulse sequence (sum = 0 + $4k_2$ + 0). Long sequences also allow greater control over

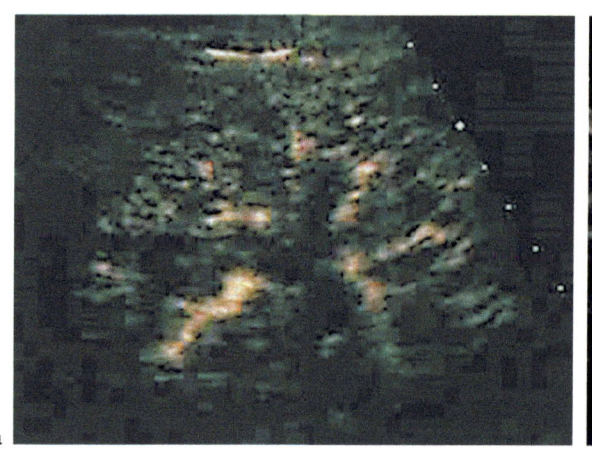

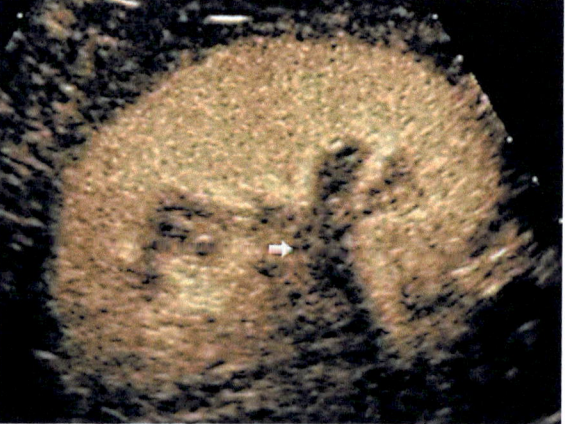

Fig. 4.17a,b. Cadence contrast pulse sequencing (CPS, Sequoia, Acuson-Siemens, USA). The microbubbles are depicted in a colour overlay over a B-mode image. Scan of the left kidney. **a** In the first seconds after microbubbles injection, the image is very dark because the background signal from the stationary tissues is completely suppressed. The only signal is produced by microbubbles which are arriving in the scanning plane. **b** After 45 s the renal parenchyma is completely filled by microbubbles. The renal sinus (*arrow*) is devoid of contrast enhancement, since microbubbles remain intravascular. The apparent slight signal in the renal sinus is due to the presence of renal parenchyma adjacent to the scanning plane (partial volume effect)

which harmonics are selected or suppressed. Consider the CPS (½, –1, 1, –½) (–2, –1, 1, 2):

Order:	1 (linear)	2 (quadratic)	3 (cubic)
$-2 \times s(½)$ =	$-2k_1 . ½$	$- 2k_2 . ½^2$	$- 2k_3 . ½^3$
$-1 \times s(-1)$ =	$-k_1 . -1$	$- k_2 . (-1)^2$	$- k_3 . (-1)^3$
$1 \times s(1)$ =	$k_1 . 1$	$+ k_2 . 1^2$	$+ k_3 . 1^3$
$2 \times s(-½)$ =	$2k_1 . -½$	$+ 2k_2 . (-½)^2$	$+ 2k_3 . (-½)^3$
Sum =	0	+ 0	$+ k_3 . 1½$

This CPS suppresses first-order and second-order scattering but gives a large response for third-order scattering, and hence for the non-linear fundamental signal from a microbubble. However, the greater time needed to transmit longer sequences means poorer temporal resolution. Further examples of CPS have been discussed by PHILLIPS (2001).

As in the power modulation method (Sect. 4.4.5), just half the elements in the transmitting aperture are fired for the half amplitude pulses, and all are fired for the full amplitude pulses (KRISHNAN et al. 2003).

4.4.6.2
Tolerance of Tissue Motion with CPS

The cancellation of first-order (linear) signals from tissue becomes less successful when the scattering and reflecting tissue interfaces move between transmissions, since the position of tissue echoes will be different in consecutive echo sequences. Fortunately, the CPS process can be made to fulfil another role – that of a filter to suppress the first-order clutter signals generated by moving tissue. How this works can be explained in engineering terms by considering each transmission as providing one sample of the echo signal from the moving target (tissue interface), and the weighting factors as coefficients of a digital filter that combines these samples. The more coefficients, the better the suppression of the sampled signal and the larger the range of target speeds over which suppression is effective. However, a more conceptual explanation is possible, as follows.

Let the echo sequence produced by the first transmission pulse be represented by a, and those from the other transmissions be represented by b, c, d, e ...etc., respectively. Consider the CPS processing as forming the weighted sum $w_1 a + w_2 b + w_3 c + w_4 d + w_5 e$ ...etc. Note that, for first-order (linear) scattering, a negative weight can be achieved by inverting either the transmission pulse or the echo sequence. Thus, the three-pulse pulse inversion method (1, –1, 1) (1, 2, 1) discussed in Sect. 4.4.3, and the three-pulse amplitude modulation method (½, 1, ½) (1, –1, 1) discussed in Sect. 4.4.5, both have the same overall relative weightings of $w_1 = \times 1$, $w_2 = \times -2$ and $w_3 = \times 1$. They can both be considered as forming the weighted sum $a -2b +c$, which is zero for linear echoes from stationary or slow steadily moving tissue.

In the case of the basic pulse inversion method discussed in Sect. 4.4.1, there are just two echo sequences, a and b, and cancellation of first-order signals is achieved by forming $a-b$. The three-pulse methods considered in the previous section are able to compensate for tissue movement at slow constant speed (albeit with the various interfaces moving at different speeds), by forming an "average" echo sequence $½(a +c)$ that corresponds to that which would have been obtained when the tissue interfaces were at the same positions as they were for the middle echo sequence b. Cancellation of the linear tissue signals can then be achieved by subtracting b from $½(a +c)$. In relative terms this is the same as forming the weighted sum $a -2b +c$.

If the speed of a tissue scatterer changes between the first and third interrogations, the positions of its echo in the average echo sequence $½(a +c)$ will not correspond exactly to that for echo sequence b. However, provided the acceleration is constant, the problem can be overcome by using four interrogations per line, generating echo sequences a, b, c and d. If the first three echo sequences a, b and c were used by themselves, the changing speed would mean $a -2b +c$ would not be quite zero. Similarly, if the last three echo sequences b, c, and d were used by themselves, the sum $b -2c +d$ would differ from zero by approximately the same error. By forming both these weighted sums and subtracting one from the other, the two errors will cancel and a zero result will be produced for tissue echoes. This means forming the weighted sum $(a -2b +c) - (b -2c +d) = a -3b +3c -d$. Thus CPS sequences such as (1, –1, 1, 1) (1, 3, 3, 1) or (1, 1, 1, 1) (1, –3, 3, –1) would extend compensation for slow tissue movement to include constant acceleration.

The argument can be extended to longer pulse sequences. Using five pulses, producing echo sequences a, b, c, d and e, it can be shown that the weighted sum $a -4b +6c -4d +e$ allows suppression of fundamental signals from tissue with uniformly changing acceleration. Examples of CPS with these overall relative weightings include the extended pulse inversion sequence (1, –1, 1, –1, 1) (1, 4, 6, 4, 1) mentioned in the previous section and the extended phase and amplitude modulation sequence (½, -1, ½, -1, ½) (1, 2, 6, 2, 1).

Figure 4.18, adapted from Thomas et al. (2002), shows that the suppression of first-order echoes by the latter five-pulse sequence (½, -1, ½, -1, ½) (1, 2, 6, 2, 1) is more than 20 dB better than that of the three-pulse version (½, -1, ½) (1, 1, 1) mentioned in the previous section. Note that the speed axis of this diagram is calibrated on the basis of a transmitted centre frequency of 3.85 MHz and an interval of 200 μs between pulses. The velocities marked would need to be increased in inverse proportion for smaller times between pulses, or lower frequencies.

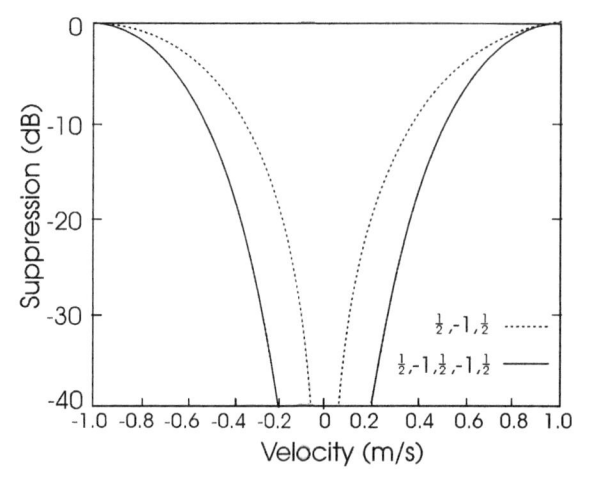

Fig. 4.18. Using a longer pulse sequence allows better suppression of signals from moving tissue. The transmission sequence (½, -1, ½, -1, ½) exhibits more than 20 dB better suppression than (½, -1, ½). The assumed frequency is 3.85 MHz and the interval between pulses is 200 μs. Adapted from THOMAS et al. (2002).

4.4.6.3
Dual Processing/Interleaving

Alternative / associated names: Convergent CPS

It is possible to make one transmission pulse sequence serve more than one purpose (Phillips et al. 2003). For example, echoes from the transmission sequence (1,-1,1,-1,1) might be summed with weights (1, 4, 6, 4, 1), allowing second harmonic signals to be detected with high sensitivity and good compensation for tissue movement, as mentioned in the previous section. Slow moving or stationary microbubbles in narrow vessels would be detected this way. Simultaneously and separately, the same echoes might be summed using weights (1, 0, -2, 0, 1). Since only the first, third and fifth pulses contribute to the output, this is equivalent to the CPS (1,1,1) (1,-2,1) at half the pulse repetition frequency. This CPS will cancel out echoes of all orders from stationary or slow moving scatterers, including both tissue interfaces and stable microbubbles. However, it will give a residual signal in response to echoes from changing or rapidly or irregularly moving microbubbles in heart chambers or large blood vessels. In this regard the reduced effective pulse repetition rate gives more time for bubble movement between consecutive pulses and so increases the likelihood of detection.

Thus, the two summation processes allow echoes from microbubbles in narrow vessels and those from microbubbles in larger vessels to be displayed separately, or together as different colour overlays, as desired. This can be of value, for example, in observing flow in the myocardium without the distraction of an extensive bright image of contrast in an adjacent heart chamber, or in observing arteries in the liver without losing them against a background of US contrast agents in the micro-circulation. Of course, another processing channel can simultaneously use one or more of the pulses in each sequence to produce B-mode echoes, providing a background image for the microbubble echo overlays.

Dual processing can be shared between two or more lines to further lower the effective pulse repetition frequency for movement detection. During gaps left in the sequence of pulses transmitted down one line, pulses can be transmitted down one or more neighbouring lines. In Fig. 4.19, two pairs of pulses separated by a longer gap are transmitted along each scan line. The long (1200 μs) spacing of the two pairs allows detection of slow moving microbubbles, whilst the short (200 μs) interval between pulses in a pair permits suppression of tissue movement. When more than one line is involved like this it is known as "interleaving".

Dual processing can also help to overcome limitations on CPS performance caused by reverberations. Reverberations are duplicate tissue echoes caused by multiple reflections between strongly

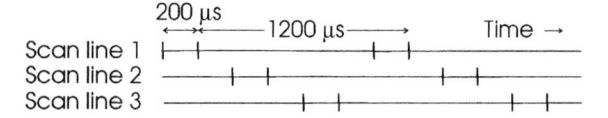

Fig. 4.19. Contrast Pulse Sequencing. An example of "interleaving" over three scan lines. Two pairs of pulses, separated by a longer gap, are transmitted along scan line 1. Similar sequences are transmitted along lines 2 and 3, interleaved with that of line 1, so that no time is wasted.

reflecting interfaces. Echoes from the second and subsequent pulses in a transmission sequence might contain reverberations produced by the preceding pulse in the sequence. However, there will be no such reverberations mixed in with echoes produced by the first pulse. This will upset the comparison of echoes from the different pulses. With dual processing, a pulse used for one process can act as a reverberation-generating pulse for the first pulse used in a second process. For example, the transmitted sequence (1, 1, –1, 1, 1) might be summed with weights (0, 1, 2, 1, 0) to detect echoes from microbubbles by pulse inversion (Sect. 4.4.3), and with weights (1, 0, 0, 0, –1) to detect irregularly moving or collapsing microbubbles. The first pulse in the sequence acts as a reverberation-generating pulse for the (0, 1, 2, 1, 0) processing. Additionally, it is possible to incorporate a "dummy" pulse at the beginning of a sequence. Apart from the reverberations this contributes to the echoes from the first active pulse, echoes from this pulse are disregarded.

4.4.7
Developments in Low-MI Doppler Imaging

4.4.7.1
Improvements in Spatial and Temporal Resolution

The spatial (axial/range) resolution of Doppler imaging methods have been dramatically improved by using short (broadband) pulses. A problem with using broadband pulses is that both the centre frequency and the bandwidth of echoes decrease with increasing scatterer depth, due the progressive loss of the higher frequencies in the spectra of the transmitted pulse and echoes as they propagate through tissue. In any Doppler method this would lead to a reduction in sensitivity with depth, due to the reference frequency f_m used for producing the Doppler signal becoming increasingly mismatched to the actual centre frequency of deeper echoes. Similarly, the centre frequency and bandwidth of the noise-limiting receiver filter become increasingly mismatched to those of the deeper echoes. A solution is to progressively lower f_m and the centre frequency and bandwidth of the noise-limiting band-pass filter in the receiving system with time after transmission to constantly match the changes in the echoes with depth.

An inconvenient consequence of changing f_m with depth in a CFI system is that the blood velocity associated with a given Doppler shift (given by the Doppler equation) changes at the same time. This means there is no single value of velocity that can be shown on screen as corresponding to the limits of the colour bar displayed beside the image. A way of dealing with this (SHIKI and MINE 2002a) is to show two velocity values at the ends of the colour bar, one for the top of the region of interest (colour box) and one for the bottom.

Another reason for varying the filter pass band with depth is to pass either the fundamental or second harmonic frequency bands, or both, as required. For example, near the surface, where sensitivity is not a problem, the fundamental can be suppressed to help clutter reduction, whereas at depth the fundamental may be needed to improve sensitivity.

Temporal resolution in power Doppler imaging has been improved by reducing the number of transmissions per line, bringing obvious benefits to cardiac applications. An even greater improvement in frame rate can be achieved by "parallel beam-forming" in reception. This involves transmitting a beam that is wide enough to include several (e.g. four) receiving beams, and have the echoes along each of these processed simultaneously. Without microbubble-based agents, parallel beam forming with a phased array probe can cause problems in complying with safety regulations, since the dilution of the transmitted power over a number of beams, emanating in a fan-like way from the centre of the probe face, means the temporal-average intensity near the probe must be high. With microbubble-based agents, this difficulty is avoided since low amplitude pulses are transmitted, taking advantage of the greater scattering ability of microbubbles.

4.4.7.2
Pulse Inversion Doppler (PID)

HOPE SIMPSON et al. (1999) have described a technique, which they named Pulse Inversion Doppler, that combines the improved spatial (axial/range) resolution and clutter rejection benefits of the pulse inversion method of harmonic detection with the flow indicating ability of Doppler imaging. In common with the latter, each scan line is interrogated by transmitting pulses along, and receiving from, each scan line several times, but it differs in that the transmitted pulses are as short as normal B-mode pulses and that alternate pulses are inverted. The use of microbubble-based agents permits operation at high frame rates, since the relatively large signals from microbubbles gives sufficient signal to noise ratio with only four or fewer transmission/receive sequences along each scan line.

Before explaining how PID works, it is useful to recall that Doppler systems generally measure the Doppler frequency shift as the rate at which the returning echoes come in and out of phase with a reference signal having the same frequency as the transmitted wave. For a reflector moving toward the probe at constant speed, the phase difference between the echoes and the reference signal will change between pulses due to the steadily reducing range. If the reflector advances by (say) one hundredth of a wavelength (λ) between pulses, it will take 100 pulses for this difference in phase to complete a cycle from say 0°–360°. This cycle will take a time of 100 T_P seconds, where T_P is the time between transmissions, and will therefore repeat 1 / 100 T_p times per second. As stated at the start of this paragraph, this repetition rate is the Doppler frequency shift f_D, whilst $1/T_P$ is the pulse repetition frequency prf. Thus, for this moving reflector, $f_D = prf / 100$. In general, if a reflector advances towards the probe by a distance λ/N between pulses, it will produce a Doppler shift of prf / N.

In the case of a sequence of alternately inverted pulses, even echoes from a stationary reflector would have an apparent phase change of half a wavelength between successive echoes. This would therefore be interpreted as a Doppler shift of $prf / 2$. Echoes from a reflector moving towards the probe at the same velocity as above would have an apparent Doppler shift of $prf / 2$ due to the alternating pulse inversion, and a further genuine Doppler shift of $prf / 100$ due to the reflector's movement. Thus the effect of transmitting alternately inverted pulses is to shift Doppler frequencies by $prf / 2$, as shown in Fig. 4.20.

However, since inverting the transmitted pulse does not invert the second harmonic component of the echoes (Fig. 4.2), as far as the second harmonic frequency component is concerned, the echoes from successive transmissions will all have the same polarity. Thus the Doppler spectrum is divided into two bands – one centred on $prf / 2$ containing only Doppler signals from fundamental components of echoes, and one centred on zero frequency, as normal, containing only Doppler signals from second harmonic components. This means that Doppler clutter from tissue, which is nearly all from fundamental echo signals at the low transmission amplitudes used, can be removed by filtering out the Doppler spectrum centred on $prf / 2$. This can be achieved with a low-pass filter that blocks all Doppler frequencies above $prf / 4$. Note that this is half the Nyquist limit for the onset of aliasing when using conventional Doppler. Strictly, the Doppler spectrum centred on $prf / 2$ will also contain Doppler signals due to odd harmonics as well as the fundamental, and the Doppler spectrum centred on zero frequency will contain Doppler signals due to all even harmonics, but only the second harmonic is likely to be within the transducer frequency response.

If any microbubbles move so fast as to produce a conventional Doppler shift of more than $prf / 4$, their second harmonic Doppler signals will overlap those in the fundamental Doppler spectrum and be blocked along with the fundamental clutter. This is not likely for blood in narrow vessels. Conversely, tissue or probe movements producing Doppler shifts above $prf / 4$ will extend into the low frequency pass band of the filter and manifest themselves as flash artefact.

One practical implementation (SATO 2004) involves transmitting four pulses, alternately inverted, along each scan line. The echoes from the first three are summed with weights (1, 2, 1) to give one fundamental-free signal (see Sect. 4.4.3), and the echoes from the last three are summed the same way to give a second fundamental-free signal. The phase difference between these two principally second harmonic signals gives a velocity estimate and the root mean square magnitude of all four echoes gives a power estimate. As already mentioned (see Sect. 4.3.3), a disadvantage of using only a few transmission/receive sequences for each scan line is that the accuracy of Doppler frequency measurement is much less than in conventional colour

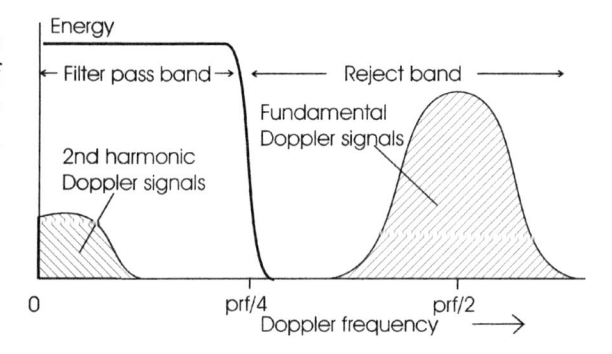

Fig. 4.20. Pulse Inversion Doppler. Doppler signals from fundamental echo components are shifted to a band centred at prf/2; even stationary targets will appear to have a Doppler shift of prf/2. Doppler signals from second harmonic echo components are not given this shift. A low-pass filter with a cut-off frequency at prf/4 will therefore suppress Doppler clutter from stationary or moving tissue but leave Doppler signals from second harmonic signals, such as from moving microbubbles (and moving tissue if tissue harmonics are present).

flow imaging. However, it is still possible to determine whether the Doppler frequency is positive (flow towards the probe), negative, or close to zero. In this method, a signal proportional to the power in the harmonic Doppler signal can be displayed in (say) red if flow is towards the probe, in blue if away from the probe and in green if slow moving or stationary. A grey background B-mode image of tissue can be added using the combined magnitudes of the echoes before separation into harmonic and fundamental components by the filter. The result is similar to conventional directional power Doppler, only having the advantages of good axial resolution and discrimination of stationary from moving microbubble-based agents. Vascular Recognition Imaging is a commercial technique which makes use of this approach (Fig. 4.21).

4.5
High-MI Techniques

High-MI methods achieve higher sensitivity than low-MI methods by using transmitted pulses with sufficient amplitude to vigorously excite or destroy some or all the microbubbles in the beam, and either using the energy released or making use of the difference in the echo signals before and after microbubble destruction. They are the only option for those contrast agents (e.g. Levovist) whose microbubbles are not flexible enough to give a useful nonlinear signal when insonated by low-MI pulses.

Where transmitted pulse amplitudes are sufficient to cause rapid destruction of the microbubble population, real-time scanning is not possible for small vessels, since the images disappear with the

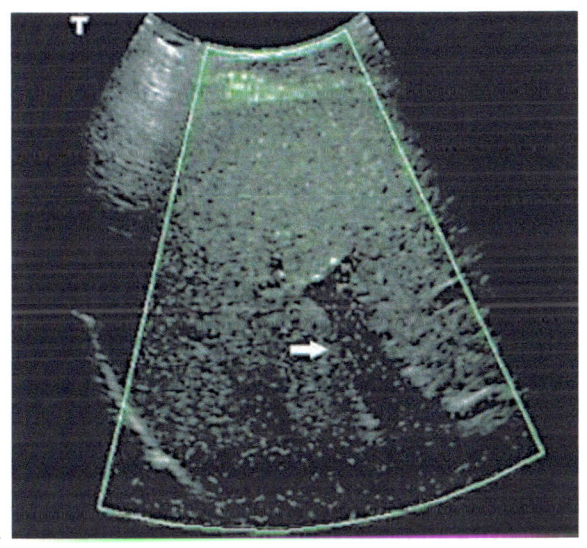

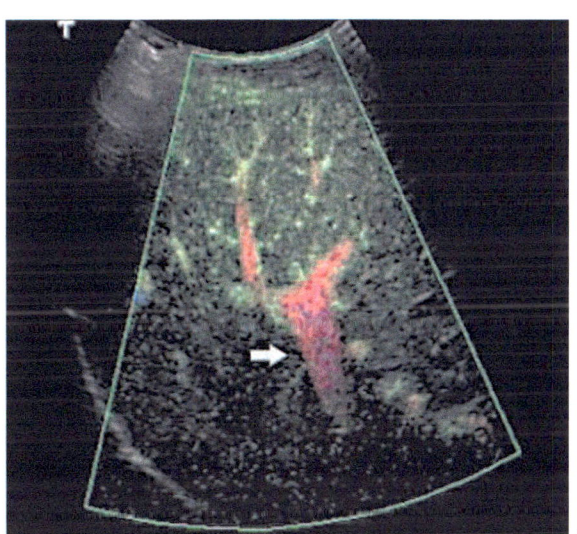

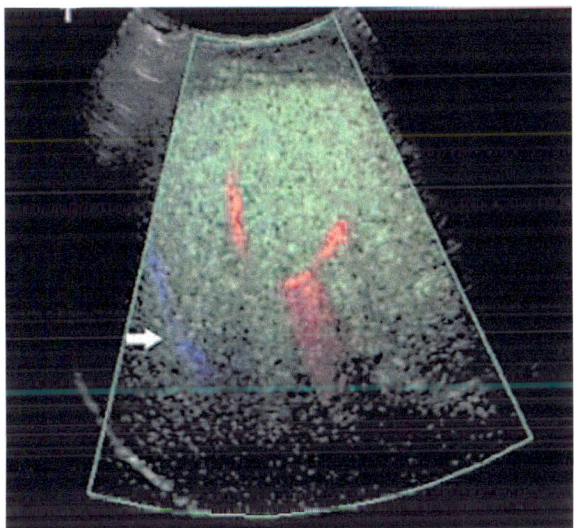

Fig. 4.21a–c. Vascular recognition imaging (VRI), Aplio, Toshiba, Japan. In this mode, stationary or slow moving microbubbles are depicted in a green colour, microbubbles moving toward the transducer are depicted in red, while microbubble moving away from the transducer are depicted in blue. Scan of the right lobe of the liver. **a** Before microbubble arrival no signal is revealed in the portal vein (*arrow*). **b** In the first seconds after microbubble arrival the portal vein is depicted in red, since it presents a flow toward the transducer. **c** From 45–70 s after microbubble injection the liver is homogeneously enhanced due to stationary microbubbles pooling in the liver sinusoids, which are represented in green. A larger vessel with flow away from the transducer (*arrow*) is represented in blue

microbubbles and there is insufficient time for replenishment between frames. However, as mentioned earlier (see Sect. 4.3.7), intermittent imaging can be used or the probe can be swept sideways over the patient's skin while recording the images. The distribution of microbubbles before its destruction can then be assessed by reviewing the recording frame by frame. This sweep may be repeated after a pause of several seconds during which microbubbles are replenished by fresh blood flowing into the region.

If pulse amplitudes are large enough to cause vigorous irregular oscillations in the microbubbles, but only a slow rate of microbubble destruction, real-time imaging of narrower vessels is possible at a few frames per second.

4.5.1
Development in High-MI Doppler Imaging

Alternative / associated names: Advanced Dynamic Flow, Contrast Burst Imaging (CBI)

Harmonic Power Doppler imaging (Sect. 4.3.9) can be used with Levovist. Since it is based on loss of correlation signals (LOC) from vigorously oscillating or collapsing microbubbles, it can detect even stationary or very slow moving microbubbles. However, it suffers from poor spatial resolution. More recent developments in this LOC technique use short (broadband) high amplitude pulses in order to improve spatial resolution. In general, the number of pulses transmitted down each scan line has also been reduced to improve temporal resolution – as is desirable for cardiac applications, for example.

The bandwidth of Doppler LOC signals (see Sect. 4.3.8) due to collapsing or irregularly oscillating microbubbles is large. As usual, a high-pass filter removes most of the clutter signal from tissue, as well as the low frequency part of the broad LOC Doppler spectrum. However, because of its large bandwidth, most of the Doppler spectrum is passed. The clutter filter performance is improved by using a high pulse repetition frequency (prf). In normal Doppler applications where low blood speeds are measured, a high prf cannot be used since the distance moved by the blood (or a microbubble) between transmissions would be too small to produce a measurable phase difference between consecutive echoes. In LOC techniques, blood speeds are not measured, so a high prf can be used. Tissue clutter filters work by cancelling out echoes that do not change much between transmissions. A high prf means greater tolerance of tissue movement since there is less phase shift between consecutive tissue echoes. The high prf also improves frame rate.

One example, marketed as Contrast Burst Imaging (CBI), uses typically six large amplitude short pulses per line to image perfusion in tissues where high sensitivity is wanted, for example in trans-cranial brain studies (MEVES et al. 2002).

Another example, marketed as Advanced Dynamic Flow (ADF), uses fewer (2–4) pulse transmissions per line (SATO 2003). A version described by SATO et al. (2003) uses slightly lower pulse amplitudes. This reduces the rate of bubble destruction, allowing real-time imaging, albeit at low frame rates (4–5 frames/s). Both Doppler power and B-mode signals are displayed in grey-scale, the moment to moment variations and pulsatility of the blood signals helping them to stand out from the tissue B-mode signals. The algorithm used to determine whether a particular pixel displays B-mode or Doppler power information is an important part of this technique. According to the algorithm used in conventional Power Doppler Imaging, a particular pixel will display a colour with a brightness proportional to the Doppler power for that pixel if this exceeds a threshold value (which the user sets with the colour priority control). Otherwise it displays a grey level proportional to the B-mode echo amplitude for that pixel. This algorithm works well in non-US contrast agent imaging, where Doppler signals are often weak, since it allows Doppler signals with sufficient strength to be displayed irrespective of tissue signal strength. When the threshold algorithm is used with US contrast agents, however, the greater strength of the Doppler signals from microbubbles means the threshold is too easily exceeded, resulting in blooming (see Sect. 4.3.3). In the ADF algorithm, the B-mode and Doppler powers signals for a pixel are compared and the larger one is used to set the pixel grey level. This avoids blooming since a pixel will not display a power Doppler signal if the B-mode signal for that pixel is large. This comparison algorithm also reduces the nuisance value of any residual clutter since, where added tissue clutter is responsible for a power Doppler signal level exceeding that of the a B-mode signal, the affected pixel will merge relatively inconspicuously with those showing strong B-mode tissue signals.

In common with other techniques that use short (wide bandwidth) pulses (see Sect. 4.4.7.1), the centre frequency and bandwidth of the noise-limiting band-pass filter in the receiving system are progressively reduced to constantly match the changes in the echo spectra from deeper targets.

Adequate rejection of tissue clutter is difficult when using only a few interrogations of each line, since there only as many samples of the Doppler signal as there are interrogations. In conventional CFI, this is overcome to some extent by using a type of filter known as infinite impulse response (IIR) that effectively increases the number of samples by using output data from the filter well as input data. At the beginning of each sequence of samples there is no output to use, of course, so artificial "initialising" samples, based on extrapolation of the first few samples, are generated to precede each set of genuine samples. As the set of samples passes through the filter, these initialising signals are replaced by genuine output signals. There is, however, a transient artefact at the beginning of each sample sequence due to the imperfect nature of the initialising data. The technique works reasonably well with signals from blood, but there is a problem when using microbubble-based agents since the microbubble signal only exists for the first few pulses, after which too many of the microbubbles are destroyed. This filter transient therefore degrades tissue clutter rejection during the important early part of the interrogation when strong microbubble echoes are being generated.

An ingenious solution to the problem (SHIKI and MINE 2002b) is to store the whole set of Doppler data from all the lines in an image frame before processing them. During the clutter removal stage of processing, the samples for each pixel are read out in the reverse order, i.e. last sample first. The filter transient therefore degrades the last part of the signal rather than the first. The samples obtained when many microbubbles were still available to generate strong echoes are processed last, by which time the filter transient is over. Thus, transient-free efficient clutter removal is applied to the strong part of the Doppler signal. The time-reversal in this process means that positive Doppler frequencies are converted to negative ones, and vice versa, but this can be corrected by reversing the colour coding.

4.5.2
Pulse Subtraction

Alternative / associate names: Agent Detection Imaging (ADI), Rate Subtraction Imaging (RSI)

This technique involves the transmission of two identical high amplitude pulses, and the temporary storage of the two resulting echo sequences before the second is subtracted from the first. The two echo sequences from tissue are identical and so are cancelled on subtraction. Unlike pulse inversion techniques, this cancellation applies to the second harmonic as well as the fundamental components of tissue echoes. (Pulse inversion was introduced (Sect. 4.4.1) as a low MI techniques, but it can also be used with high MI pulses to suppress tissue echoes.) Microbubbles produce strong echoes from the first pulse but many are destroyed or substantially damaged in the process, so the echoes produced by the second pulse will be different. Subtraction of these two highly complex echo signals produces another complex signal, which is used to indicate the microbubbles distribution. Even if the transmissions have sufficient amplitude to completely destroy all the microbubbles in the beam on the first pulse, so that there are virtually no microbubble echoes from the second, subtraction will still produce a large difference signal.

The user can choose to display an image made up of either the subtracted echoes (microbubble signal only), the echoes from the second transmission (tissue only) or a combination of the two, with the contrast image presented as a coloured overlay on the tissue B-mode image.

4.5.3
1.5 Harmonic Imaging (1.5 HI)

Alternative / associated names: 1.5 Rate Subtraction Imaging (1.5 RSI), Power Contrast Imaging (PCI).

When a transmitted pulse has sufficient amplitude (e.g. more than 100 kPa or so) to rupture many or all of the microbubbles in the beam, the echoes produced have a broad spectrum (Fig. 4.22). The echoes from tissue, however, have a spectrum that is largely confined to two peaks, one centred on the fundamental frequency (f) and the other on the second harmonic frequency ($2f$). This method selects signals in the frequency band between these two peaks in order to take advantage of the larger ratio

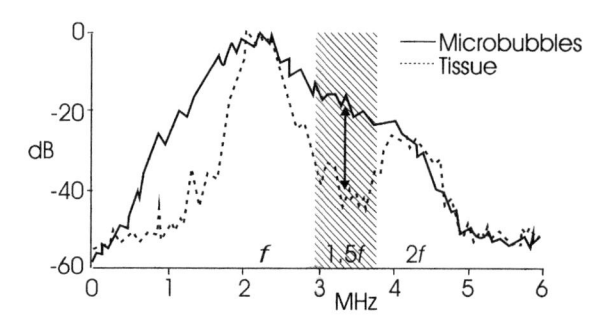

Fig. 4.22. Examples of echo spectra from microbubbles and tissue, normalised to the same peak value (adapted from KAWAGISHI 2004). The relative magnitude of the UCA signal is much greater in the hatched frequency band centred on 1.5 f, where f is the fundamental frequency of the transmitted pulse.

of microbubble signal to tissue signal there. This band has been labelled "1.5 f" (KAWAGISHI 2003). The technique can be used as part of either high-MI B-mode or Power Doppler Imaging procedures (KRISHNAN et al. 2001).

The larger ratio of microbubble signal to tissue signal in this band permits either improved tissue suppression for a given level of microbubble signal or, if a higher transmitted amplitude is used, increased sensitivity to microbubble echoes for the same level of background tissue signal. Experimental results show an improvement in sensitivity of 20 dB or more relative to second harmonic methods. Factors contributing to this improvement are that the 1.5 f frequency band is closer to the centre of the transducer frequency response, where transducer efficiency is greatest, and to the maximum of the broad microbubble spectrum, which is generally centred on the fundamental frequency. Uniformity with depth is also improved, as is penetration, because the lower frequency of this band means there is less attenuation in tissue.

The transmission circuitry must be able to produce a pulse with a very well controlled spectrum. Clearly, transmitted frequency components in the 1.5 f band would reduce contrast, but transmitted frequency components around 0.75 f would generate tissue harmonics in this band, irrespective of the presence of microbubbles, further reducing contrast. Generation of a suitable pulse, such as one with a Gaussian waveform, requires that each element be driven by a voltage waveform having a precisely controlled shape and amplitude. Careful filtering techniques are also needed to eliminate signals from the fundamental and second harmonic frequency bands whilst preserving those in the 1.5 f band.

1.5 H filtering may be used in combination with other methods for suppressing clutter from tissue. KAWAGISHI (2004) describes its use in combination with the pulse subtraction technique discussed in the previous section, where it suppresses any tissue signals that remain uncancelled due to tissue motion. Frequency bands below the fundamental and above the second harmonic frequency may also be allowed to contribute to the signal, in order to improve sensitivity.

4.6
Techniques for Imaging Perfusion and Flow in Very Small Vessels

Alternatice / associated names: Flash Contrast Imaging, Microvascular imaging, Micro View

Slow perfusion, such as in the vasculature of breast lesions, can be observed by monitoring the tracks of single microbubbles or microbubble clusters along very narrow vessels. A low-MI technique is necessary to avoid destroying the microbubbles, but there must also be excellent rejection of clutter, not only from moving tissue but also from movement of the probe, as this can be difficult to hold still over the observation period.

The pulse inversion technique is commonly used, as it allows the fundamental clutter signals from tissue to be rejected. Further discrimination is achieved by comparing consecutive frames with each other, pixel for pixel. If the content of a pixel has not changed from one frame to the next, it is rejected, leaving, ideally, only echoes from moving microbubbles. It can be difficult to identify a narrow vessel as such because of the sparse or irregular distribution of echo signals along its length. In order to help the eye to recognise the line of the vessel, the signals can be made to persist on the screen, either for a few seconds or to remain without appreciable fading, building up a complete cross-sectional view of the vascular structure. Different colours can be used to indicate the times at which echoes first appear – facilitating, for example, the differentiation of larger arteries from the capillary bed.

Where microbubbles continues to arrive over a long period, bursts of large amplitude pulses can be used to clear all the microbubbles from the imaged slice so that re-perfusion can be observed. It is also possible for the speed of individual microbubbles to be estimated from the distance moved between frames.

4.7
Techniques in Development

4.7.1
Subharmonic Imaging

When microbubbles are insonated at one frequency, some return echoes with a frequency component at half the insonation frequency, as well as at the fundamental frequency and the second, third and higher integer harmonics mentioned previously. The strength of this "subharmonic" signal is greatest, for a given transmitted pulse amplitude, if the natural resonance frequency of the microbubble is half that of the transmitted pulse. It is also greater for transmitted pulses containing a larger number of cycles. Two causes have been identified for the subharmonic signal (Krishna et al. 1999). One is the non-linear response of a microbubble to an incident pulse. The other is ringing (continuing oscillations) at the natural frequency of the bubble after the forced oscillation due to the incident pulse has stopped. Both will be particularly strong for those microbubbles in the injected bolus whose size makes them naturally resonant at half the incident frequency. Both effects are greater for more flexible microbubbles.

The strength of the subharmonic component in the scatter spectrum of microbubbles is greater than that of the second harmonic (Frinking et al. 2000). This, combined with the fact that non-linear propagation of ultrasound in tissue does not generate a subharmonic component, suggests that subharmonic detection might offer an imaging method with greater contrast between microbubble and tissue echoes.

The lower frequency of the subharmonic means attenuation is less, which would be an advantage when imaging deep-lying blood vessels. Against these advantages must be set the fact that pulses containing more cycles generate stronger subharmonic signals and such long pulses would not give good axial resolution. Lateral resolution would also be poorer due to the lower frequency of the signal.

Shi et al. (1999) have already succeeded in producing subharmonic images of a dog kidney using Optison (Amersham Health Inc., Princeton, NJ) and transmission pulses with eight cycles and a centre frequency of 6.6 MHz. The use of such a high transmitted frequency helps to limit the impairment of spatial resolution, but penetration is limited.

4.7.2
Release Burst Imaging

In the high-MI microbubble disruption techniques described previously, the pulse characteristics required for good spatial resolution are at variance to those required for efficient microbubble destruction and high sensitivity. An entirely different approach (Frinking et al. 2000) is to interrogate each scan line with a large amplitude "release burst" pulse to rupture the microbubbles, preceded and followed by other, lower amplitude, imaging pulses to detect the transient microbubble fragments and free gas bubbles thus released. This approach allows the properties of the release burst and the imaging pulses to be optimised separately for their distinct tasks. Thus, the imaging pulses can be short and of higher frequency to give good spatial resolution, and of moderate amplitude to minimise unwanted microbubble destruction. The release burst pulse, on the on the other hand, can contain more cycles, have a lower frequency and a larger amplitude, to increase microbubble destruction and hence increase sensitivity.

In applications where there is little tissue movement, one imaging pulse before and one imaging pulse after the release burst is sufficient. The echoes from the released gas bubbles can then be discriminated by simply subtracting the "before" from the "after" echo sequence. Where there is significant tissue movement, in the heart for example, a similar subtraction is performed, but several imaging pulses are transmitted before and after the release burst. The processing of the echoes from several pulses is effectively that of low-MI power Doppler imaging, so a Doppler clutter filter can be used to overcome the imperfect cancellation of tissue echoes caused by tissue motion (Kirkhorn et al. 2001). In either case, since the echoes from tissue before and after the release burst are cancelled by subtraction, it is possible to use the strong fundamental component of the echoes. This gives higher sensitivity than harmonic methods and means tissue harmonic signals do not degrade contrast.

Where flash artefacts due to moving tissue, or signals from intact microbubbles, cannot be entirely eliminated, they can, at least, be distinguished from genuine microbubble signals. To achieve this, separate images can be displayed side by side, one using release bursts and one where the release bursts are disabled. Without the release bursts, the process is equivalent to low-MI broadband power Doppler imaging. Of course, the release burst image may only be generated on an intermittent basis since it involves microbubble destruction, whereas the image without release bursts is real-time.

Acknowledgements

In particular, I would like to thank J. Powers (Philips) for his generously given time and expert advice. I am also grateful for the valuable help given by a number of other experts. These include M. Averkiou (Philips), P. Phillips, T. Jedrzejewicz and E. Bibby (Siemens), J. Schlegel, J. van de Kant and M. Beijer (Toshiba), D. Cosgrove and M. Blomley (Hammersmith Hospital, London), Jerome Borsboom (Erasmus MC, Rotterdam), and N. McDicken, V. Sboros and C. Moran (Edinburgh University).

References

Apfel RE, Holland KH (1991) Gauging the likelihood of cavitation from short pulse low duty cycle diagnostic ultrasound. Ultrasound Med Biol 17:179-185

Averkiou M, Powers J, Skyba D et al (2003) Ultrasound contrast imaging research. Ultrasound Quart 19:27-37

Becher H, Burns PN (2000) Handbook of contrast echocardiography. Springer, Berlin Heidelberg New York

Blomley MJK, Albrecht T, Wilson SR et al (1999) Improved detection of metastatic liver lesions using pulse inversion harmonic imaging with Levovist: a multi-center study. Radiology 213:1685

Borsboom J M G, Ting Chin C, de Jong N (2003) Nonlinear coded excitation method for ultrasound contrast imaging. Ultrasound Med Biol 29:285-292

Borsboom J, Ting Chin C, de Jong N (2004) Experimental evaluation of a non-linear coded excitation method for contrast imaging. Ultrasonics 42:671-675

Brock-Fisher GA, Poland MD, Rafter P (1996) Means for increasing sensitivity in non-linear ultrasound imaging systems. US patent no 5,577,505

Frinking PJ, Bouakaz A, Kirkhorn J et al (2000) Ultrasound contrast imaging: current and new potential methods. Ultrasound Med Biol 26:965-975

Holland KH, Apfel RE (1989) An improved theory for the prediction of micro-cavitation thresholds. IE Trans Ultrason Fairylike Freq Contr UFFI 36:139

Hope Simpson D, Powers J E, Schauf M, Villet C (2004) Ultrasonic diagnostic microvascular imaging. US patent no 6, 676, 606

Hunt TJ, Rafter PG, Brock-Fisher GA (2003) System and method for non-linear detection of ultrasonic contrast agents at a fundamental frequency. US patent no 6,652,463

Kawagishi T (2003) Technical description of 1.5-harmonic imaging, an effective technique for contrast-enhanced ultrasound diagnosis. Medical review 2003.3 Cardiology special issue, cardiac imaging and networking, toshiba medical systems

Kawagishi T (2004) Ultrasound diagnosis apparatus for imaging with a contrast agent. US patent no 6, 726, 630

Kirkhorn J, Frinking PJ, de Jong N, Torp H (2001) Three-stage approach to ultrasound contrast detection. IEEE Trans Ultrason Ferroelectr Freq Contr 48:1013-1022

Krishna PD, Shankar PM, Newhouse VL (1999) Subharmonic generation from ultrasonic contrast agents. Phys Med Biol 44:681-694

Krishnan S, Gardner EA, Holley G L et al (2001) Medical diagnostic ultrasound method and system for contrast specific frequency imaging. US patent no 6, 213, 951

Krishnan S, Phillips PJ, Holley GL et al (2003) Medical ultrasonic imaging pulse transmission method. US patent no 6,602,195

Kuntz-Hehner St, Tiemann K, Schlosser Th, Omran H, Luederitz B, Becher H (2002). Assessment of Myocardial Perfusion by Contrast Echocardiography Ready for Clinical Practice? J Clin Basic Cardiol 5: 145 148.

Meves SH, Wilkening W, Thies T et al (2002) Comparison between echo contrast agent-specific imaging modes and perfusion-weighted magnetic resonance imaging for the assessment of brain perfusion. Stroke 33:2433

Phillips PJ (2001) Contrast pulse sequencing (CPS): imaging nonlinear microbubbles. IEEE Ultrason Symp Proc, pp 1739-1741

Phillips PJ, Guracar IM, Ismayil M (2003) Dual process ultrasound contrast agent imaging. US patent no 6, 632, 177

Porter TR, Xie F (1995) Transient myocardial contrast after initial exposure to diagnostic ultrasound pressures with minute doses of intravenously injected microbubbles - demonstration and potential mechanisms. Circulation 92:2391-2395

Powers J, Porter TR, Wilson S et al (2000) Ultrasound contrast imaging research. Medica Mundi 44:26-36. Philips Medical Systems

Sato T (2003) Technological description of advanced dynamic flow in the aplio diagnostic ultrasound system. eMedical Review, Toshiba Corporation.

Sato T (2004) Apparatus and method for ultrasonic diagnostic imaging using a contrast medium. US patent no 6,814,703

Sato T, Oyanagi M, Mine Y (2003) Ultrasound diagnostic apparatus. US patent no 6,508,766

Shi WT, Forsberg F, Hall AL et al (1999) Subharmonic imaging with microbubble contrast agents: initial results. Ultrason Imaging 21:79-94

Shiki E, Mine Y (2002a) High resolution flow imaging for ultrasound diagnosis. US patent no 6,419,632

Shiki E, Mine Y (2002b) Ultrasound imaging using flash echo imaging technique. US patent no 6,450,961

Thomas LJ, Maslak SH, Phillips P, Holley GL (2002) Medical diagnostic ultrasound system using contrast pulse sequence imaging. US patent no 6,494,841

Whittingham TA (1997) New and future developments in ultrasonic imaging. Br J Radiol 70:S119-S132

Wilkening W, Krueger M, Emert H (2000) Phase-coded pulse sequence for non-linear imaging. Proceedings of the IEEE ultrasonics symposium ID-2

5 Contrast-Specific Imaging Techniques: Methodological Point of View

Emilio Quaia and Alessandro Palumbo

CONTENTS

5.1　Introduction　71
5.2　Modes of Injection of Microbubble-Based Contrast Agents　71
5.3　Modes of Scanning　72
5.3.1　High Acoustic Power Insonation　73
5.3.2　Low Acoustic Power Insonation　73
　　　References　75

5.1
Introduction

Microbubble-based ultrasound (US) contrast agents consist of bubbles of gases, covered by a shell of different composition, with a diameter of approximately 2–6 μm that enhance the US signal (Albrecht et al. 2000) and persist exclusively in the blood stream. The nature of microbubble interaction with the insonating US beam depends on the scanning parameters, principally the acoustic power of insonation and the US frequency.

The basic underlying principle of all microbubble-based contrast agents is the high difference in the acoustic impedance between the gas in the microbubble and the surrounding blood in vivo, which makes the microbubble highly reflective as a simple backscatterer in the range of insonation power below 100 KPa. Increasing the acoustic insonation power, the microbubbles show an increasingly non-linear response and the reflected US signal contains harmonic and sub-harmonic frequencies that are multiples and fractions of the insonating frequency (de Jong et al. 1994a,b; Burns et al. 1996; Kirkhorn et al. 2001). These non-linear signals are produced since less energy is required to expand the microbubble than to compress it. At yet higher insonation acoustic power, microbubbles are destroyed by the acoustic field, producing a strong signal, similar to a burst, with wideband harmonic frequencies.

E. Quaia, MD, Assistant Professor of Radiology;
A. Palumbo, MD
Department of Radiology, Cattinara Hospital, University of Trieste, Strada di Fiume 447, Trieste, 34149, Italy

Firstly, microbubbles have to be injected and this can be performed in two different ways, bolus or injection, according to the type of study the sonographer needs to perform. Secondly, microbubbles have to be correctly insonated and this can be performed by a low or high transmit power of insonation, according to the type of injected microbubble-based agent. Conventional grey-scale and colour Doppler US suffer as a result of limited sensitivity to harmonics signal and of colour signal saturation and blooming artefacts, respectively. Dedicated US contrast specific techniques were introduced to overcome these limitations and to selectively register the signal produced by microbubbles insonation. US contrast specific techniques are not of immediate application but a series of setting procedures have to be applied before and after microbubble injection. This chapter will describe the principal technical parameters which have to be correctly set to optimise microbubble insonation and harmonics registration.

5.2
Modes of Injection of Microbubble-Based Contrast Agents

Microbubble-based contrast agents may be injected intravenously as a bolus (2–4 ml/s) or as a slow infusion (0.2–1 ml/s). Intravenous bolus injection mode is usually performed manually and produces a transient increase in the blood backscattering. The echo-signal video-intensity exhibits a linear relation with the injected microbubble dose and the time-intensity curve (Fig. 5.1a) shows a first rapidly ascending tract followed by a progressive decay (Correas et al. 2000). The principal advantage is that the bolus injection mode is very easy to perform and is usually employed for all applications of microbubble-based agents, except for parenchymal or tumoral perfusion quantitation. The principal drawback of the bolus injection mode is artefact production, especially with colour or power Doppler US, which are markedly evident at the peak of the time-intensity curve and which are reduced if dedicated US contrast-specific techniques are employed.

Intravenous slow infusion of microbubble-based contrast agents is usually performed by dedicated automatic injectors. The time-intensity curve (Fig. 5.1b) shows a progressive increase in echo-signal video-intensity, followed by a stationary plateau phase from 1 to 2 min from the beginning of microbubble injection and which lasts the duration of microbubble injection, expressing the equilibrium kinetic between microbubble injection and washout (CORREAS et al. 2000). The time of achievement of the stationary phase is determined by the half-life of microbubbles in the blood (about four-fold the half-life of microbubbles). The principal advantage is that the slow infusion mode may be applied in the quantitative analysis of parenchymal or tumoral perfusion since it guarantees the achievement of a stationary state in microbubble concentration. The principal drawback is that it is not easy to perform and that dedicated automatic injection equipment needs to be used.

5.3
Modes of Scanning

Exposure to the US wave determines that microbubbles contract and expand their diameter several-fold at their resonant frequency. At low acoustic power microbubbles produce an US signal with the same frequency as the sound that excited them. By increasing the acoustic power microbubble expansion and contraction are non-linear and generate sub- and higher harmonics of the applied frequency (COSGROVE 2001; DAYTON et al. 1999). At further higher acoustic power of insonation the expansion/contraction eventually disrupts the microbubble shell resulting in the emission of a wideband frequencies signal.

Dedicated contrast specific US techniques may be employed by destructive or non-destructive mode according to the acoustic power. The acoustic power is variably related to the employed mechanical index

$$(MI) = \frac{P-}{\sqrt{f}},$$

with the peak negative acoustic pressure [P−] expressed in MPa (Pascal; 1 Pa = 1 Newton/m^2), and the frequency [f] in MHz. Actually, the MI value, which is displayed on all approved US scanners, ranging from 0.06 to 1.3, was introduced for protection purposes, expressing the potential for mechanical effects during a diagnostic US examination. It can be considered a practical index to express the intensity of the acoustic field. Actually, the MI is an unreliable predictor of microbubbles destruction, since at the same MI value different values of acoustic powers of insonation were measured in different US equipment (MERRITT et al. 2000). Of course, the higher the MI value, the higher the probability to produce microbubble destruction. In general, when the MI of the insonating beam is greater than 0.3 the microbubbles are increasingly destroyed, even though the threshold for microbubble destruction is

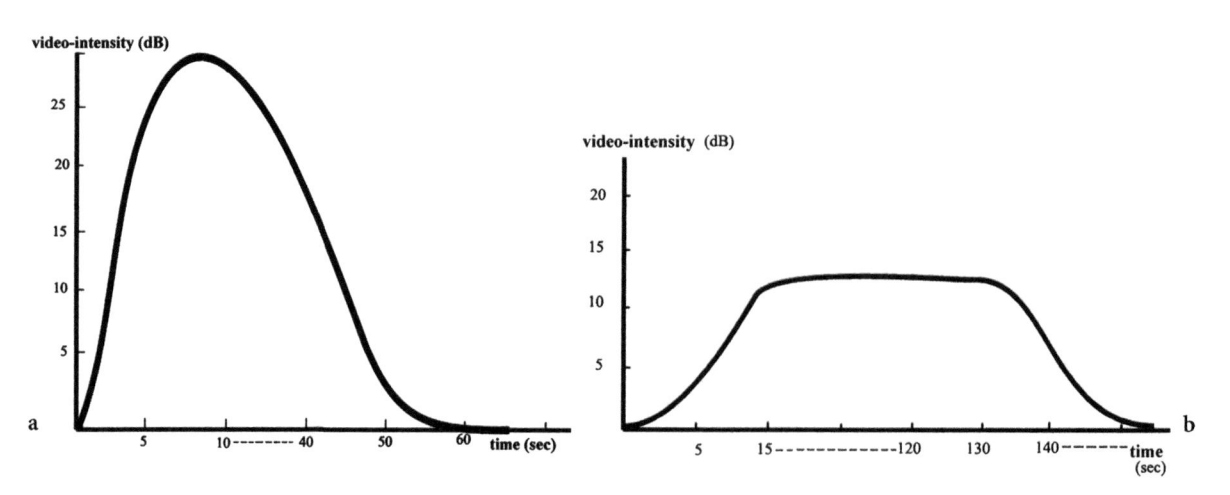

Fig. 5.1a,b. Bolus (a) versus infusion injection (b) profile of a microbubble-based contrast agent. After bolus injection (a), the microbubble concentration in the blood presents a rapid increase and a rapid decay. After slow continuous infusion (b), the microbubble blood concentration presents a progressive increase, a stationary state, which lasts according to the duration of microbubble injection, and a progressive decay when the microbubble infusion is stopped

variable and depends on many factors, such as the size and nature of the microbubble and the attenuation determined by the overlying tissues (KLIBANOV et al. 1998).

5.3.1
High Acoustic Power Insonation

The first mode, widely employed, made use of high-transmit acoustic power (Wo = peak negative pressure; 0.–2.5 MPa). Microbubble destruction produces the emission of a wideband frequency that includes both sub- and higher harmonics. Since MI value is limited, because of attenuation or safety regulations, the pulse length (K ~ 1/f) is the only parameter which can be further modified to increase the disruption efficiency (FRINKING et al. 1998; FRINKING 1999).

Microbubble destruction is a very fast process, taking place during a single or a few US pulses, during which a strong and highly non-linear signal is returned from microbubbles. This process is also called stimulated acoustic emission or transient scattering and may be considered as a sort of microbubble signature since it can be expressed exclusively by microbubbles. When colour Doppler is employed, microbubble destruction is displayed as a mosaic of randomly distributed pseudo-Doppler shifts that are independent of flow (BLOMLEY et al. 1998).

High acoustic power mode has to be employed with air-filled microbubbles, such as Levovist (SH U508A, Schering, Berlin, Germany) or Sonavist (SH U563A, Schering AG, Berlin, Germany), which present low harmonic behaviour (BLOMLEY et al. 1998, 1999; QUAIA et al. 2002). For this reason, the only way to produce harmonics is to destroy these types of microbubbles. High acoustic power mode is less suitable for new generation perfluorocarbon or sulphur hexafluoride-filled microbubbles which present an effective harmonic response even if insonated at low acoustic power. Anyway, some of the new generation microbubble-based agents, such as Sonazoid (NC100100, Amersham Health, Oslo, Norway), a perfluorocarbon-filled contrast agent, may be effectively insonated even at high acoustic power (FORSBERG et al. 2002).

High acoustic power mode may be employed continuously or intermittently (QUAIA et al. 2003). In continuous scanning, the frame rate has to be registered at the lowest level, with a lower time resolution, to minimise microbubble destruction, while the echo-signal persistence has to be switched off to visualise fresh undestroyed microbubbles in each new frame. Continuous insonation is usually applied to detect focal liver lesions in the liver or in the spleen since it allows the complete evaluation of the parenchyma. The focal zone has to be positioned at 10–12 cm from the abdominal surface to produce homogeneous contrast enhancement during insonation throughout the liver parenchyma.

In intermittent high acoustic power insonation different trains of between four and six high acoustic power US pulses are sent during the different parenchymal phases (arterial, portal and late phases in the liver or spleen; early and late corticomedullary phase in the kidney). The intermittent insonation is usually applied to characterise focal tumour in the liver, spleen or kidney, since it allows the tumour insonation during the different parenchymal phases.

The two principal advantages of high acoustic power mode over low acoustic power mode are the intense signals produced by microbubble insonation and the possibility to visualise the deep areas of the insonated parenchyma without signal attenuation from the superficial levels. Conversely, high acoustic power mode has four principal drawbacks. First, the destructive nature of this mode means that real-time scanning may be performed one single time and the largest amount of microbubbles are destroyed after the first sweep. For this reason, there is no possibility to assess the parenchymas with different acoustic windows at the same time. Second, liver scan has to be rapid and uniform to produce homogeneous microbubble rupture on liver parenchyma. In fact, the scanning irregularities, determined by a less than uniform free-hand sweep, or patient movements, during the emission of the two out phases US pulses, may produce artefacts (COSGROVE 2001; FORSBERG et al. 1994) simulating focal liver lesions. Third, at high acoustic power insonation the suppression of stationary tissue background is imperfect due to the harmonic signals produced by native tissues which present non-linear behaviour as microbubbles at high acoustic power, with a consequent production of significant tissue background on which bubble signal is superimposed.

5.3.2
Low Acoustic Power Insonation

The introduction of perfluorocarbon and sulphur hexafluoride-filled microbubbles, with effective harmonic properties, has made it possible to perform continuous low acoustic power insonation (Wo – peak negative pressure 100–600 KPa; MI below 0.2)

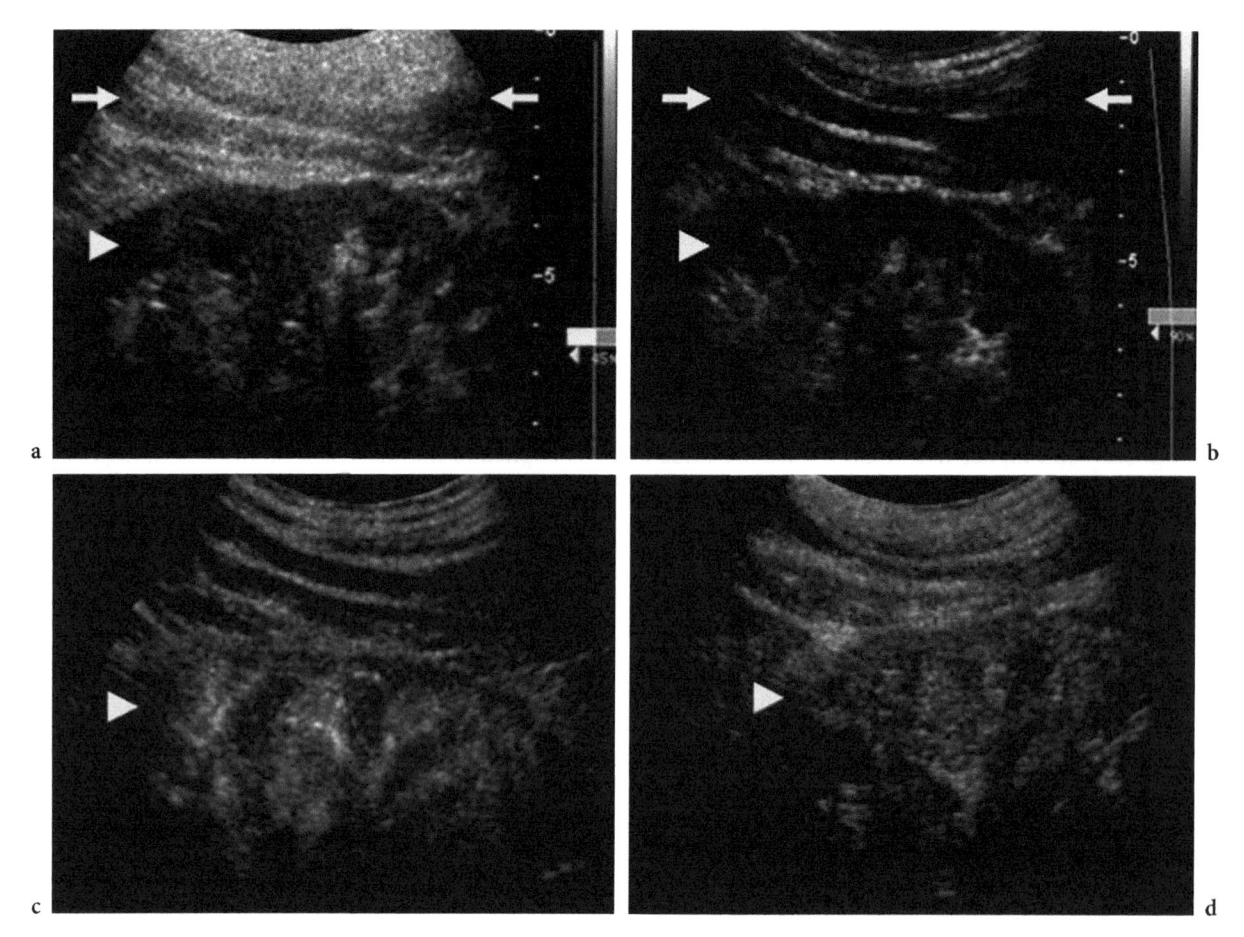

Fig. 5.2a-d. Kidney insonation (*arrowhead*). **a** Before microbubble injection, excessive signal gain is evident in the superficial planes (*arrows*). **b** Correct signal gain before microbubble injection. The signal gain is correctly set in the superficial planes (*arrows*) and appears uniform throughout the scanned parenchyma. The same signal gain is maintained after microbubble injection (**c,d**) providing the effective visualisation of contrast enhancement in renal parenchyma

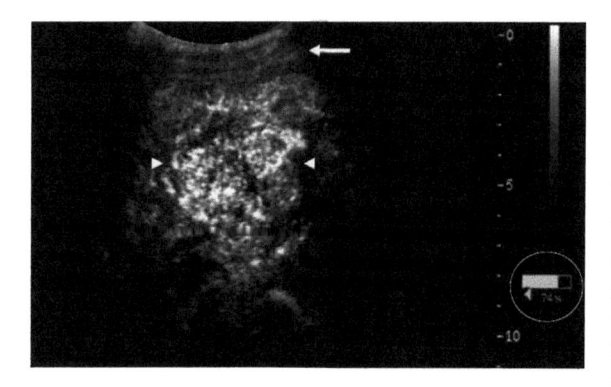

Fig. 5.3. The correct focal zone position (*circle*) at low acoustic power insonation. The focal zone has to be positioned below the focal liver lesion (*arrowheads*) to be characterised. The signal gain in the superficial planes (*arrow*) is correctly registered

which is the most employed scanning mode nowadays after microbubble administration (ALBRECHT et al. 2003; CORREAS et al. 2003; NICOLAU et al. 2003; HOHMANN et al. 2004; QUAIA et al. 2004).

Before microbubble-based agent injection, the background signal from stationary tissues has to be uniformly set at the lowest level, from the superficial (Figs. 5.2 and 5.3) to the deeper scanning levels (Fig. 5.4). The focal zone has to be positioned (Fig. 5.3) below the parenchymal region to be assessed, the echo-signal persistence should be turned off to reduce artefacts, while the frame rate should be registered at the lowest level to minimise microbubble destruction (which does occur, even though at a much lower level than with high acoustic power insonation).

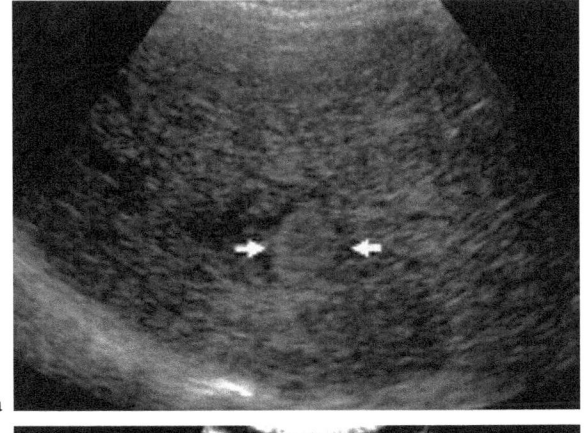

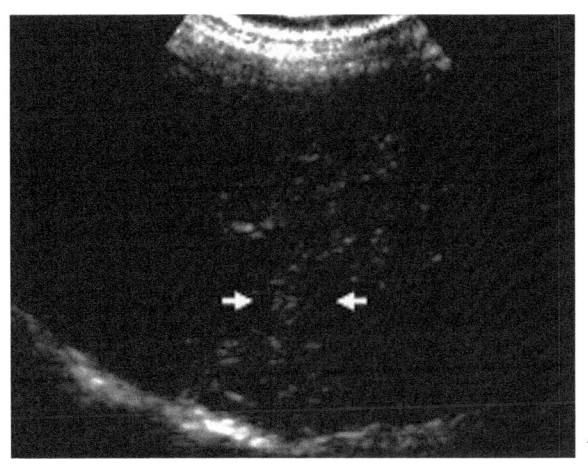

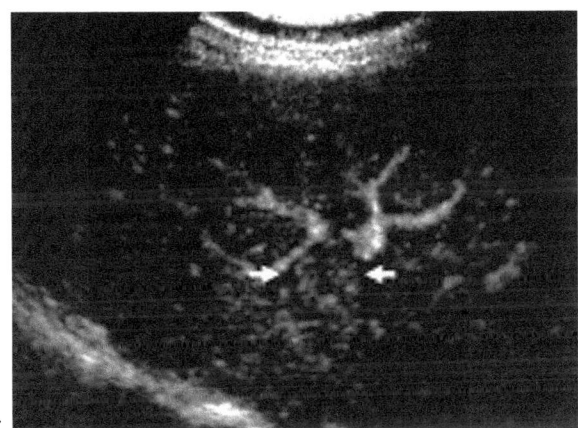

Fig. 5.4a–c. The correct signal gain before microbubble injection in the liver by using low acoustic power insonation. a A focal liver lesions (*arrows*) is identified in the liver at baseline conventional greyscale US. b Before microbubble injection, the acoustic power and the echo-signal gain have to be registered at the lowest level to suppress the background signal from stationary tissues and to make the signal intensity in the different scanning phases uniform. c After microbubble injection, diffuse increase in the echo-signal intensity, due to parenchymal contrast enhancement, is visualised

The two principal advantages of low over high power mode is, firstly, to minimise microbubble rupture allowing the continuous real-time evaluation of contrast enhancement and, secondly, to allow the effective suppression of the stationary tissue background and the selective registration of harmonic signals produced by microbubbles with improved contrast-to-noise-ratio. The only limitation of low power mode is the lower reliability in assessing the deep parenchymal regions, since harmonics present a lower intensity than with high power mode. However, this limitation has been almost completely resolved in state of the art US equipment and by multi-pulse contrast specific techniques which present an increased sensitivity to microbubble harmonic signals.

References

Albrecht T, Hoffmann CW, Schettler S et al (2000) B-mode enhancement at phase-inversion US with air-based microbubble contrast agent: initial experience in humans. Radiology 216:273-278

Albrecht T, Oldenburg A, Hohmann J et al (2003) Imaging of liver metastases with contrast-specific low-MI real time ultrasound and SonoVue. Eur Radiol 13 [Suppl 3]:N79-N86

Blomley M, Albrecht T, Cosgrove D et al (1998) Stimulated acoustic emission in liver parenchyma with Levovist (letter). Lancet 351:568-569

Blomley MJ, Albrecht TA, Cosgrove DO et al (1999) Improved detection of liver metastases with stimulated acoustic emission in late phase of enhancement with the US contrast agent SH U 508: early experience. Radiology 210:409-416

Burns P, Powers JE, Simpson DH et al (1996) Harmonic imaging principles and preliminary results. Clin Radiol 51 [Suppl]:50-55

Correas JM, Burns PN, Lai X, Qi X (2000) Infusion versus bolus of an ultrasound contrast agent: in vivo dose-response measurements of BR1. Invest Radiol 35:72-79

Correas JM, Claudon M, Tranquart F, Hélenon O (2003) Contrast-enhanced ultrasonography: renal applications. J Radiol 84:2041-2054

Cosgrove DO (2001) Ultrasound contrast agents. In: Meire H, Cosgrove DO, Dewbury K, Farrant P (eds) Clinical ultrasound – a comprehensive text. Abdominal and general ultrasound. Churchill Livingstone, London, pp 67-79

Dayton PA, Morgan KE, Klibanov L et al (1999) Optical and acoustical observations of the effects of ultrasound on contrast agents. IEEE Trans Ultrason Ferroelect Freq Contr 46:220-232

De Jong N, Cornet R, Lance CT (1994a) Higher harmonics of

vibrating gas-filled microspheres. I. Simulations. Ultrasonics 32:447-453

De Jong N, Cornet R, Lance CT (1994b) Higher harmonics of vibrating gas-filled microspheres. II. Measurements. Ultrasonics 32:455-459

Forsberg F, Liu JB, Burns P et al (1994) Artefacts in ultrasonic contrast agent studies. J Ultrasound Med 13:357-365

Forsberg F, Piccoli CW, Liu JB et al (2002) Hepatic tumor detection: MR imaging and conventional US versus pulse-inversion harmonic US of NC100100 during its reticuloendothelial system-specific phase. Radiology 222:824-829

Frinking PJA (1999) Ultrasound contrast agents: acoustic characterization and diagnostic imaging. Optima Grafische Communicatie, Rotterdam

Frinking PJA, Céspedes EI, de Jong N (1998) Multi-pulse ultrasound contrast imaging based on a decorrelation detection strategy. Proc IEEE Ultrason Symp 2:1787-1790

Hohmann J, Skrok J, Puls R, Albrecth T (2004) Characterization of focal liver lesions with contrast-enhanced low MI real time ultrasound and SonoVue. Fortschr Rontgenstr 176:1-9

Kirkhorn J, Frinking PJA, de Jong N, Torp H (2001) Three-stage approach to ultrasound contrast detection. IEEE Trans Ultrason Ferroelect Freq Contr 48:1013-1021

Klibanov AL, Ferrara KW, Hughes MS et al (1998) Direct video-microscopic observation of the dynamic effects of medical ultrasound on ultrasound contrast microspheres. Invest Radiol 33:863-870

Merritt CR, Forsberg F, Shi WT et al (2000) The mechanical index: an inappropriate and misleading indicator for destruction of ultrasound microbubble contrast agents. Radiology 217:395

Nicolau C, Catalá V, Brú C (2003) Characterization of focal liver lesions with contrast-enhanced ultrasound. Eur Radiol 13 [Suppl 3]:N70-N78

Quaia E, Blomley MJK, Patel S et al (2002) Initial observations on the effect of irradiation on the liver-specific uptake of Levovist. Eur J Radiol 41:192-199

Quaia E, Bertolotto M, Calderan L et al (2003) US characterization of focal hepatic lesions with intermittent high acoustic power mode and contrast material. Acad Radiol 10:739-750

Quaia E, Calliada F, Bertolotto M et al (2004) Characterization of focal liver lesions by contrast-specific US modes and a sulfur hexafluoride-filled microbubble contrast agent: diagnostic performance and confidence. Radiology 232:420-430

6 Biological Effects of Microbubble-Based Ultrasound Contrast Agents

Diane Dalecki

CONTENTS

6.1 Introduction 77
6.2 Acoustic Mechanisms for Bioeffects 77
6.3 Hemolysis 78
6.4 Effects on Blood Vessels 79
6.5 Cardiac Effects 81
6.6 Lithotripsy 82
6.7 Summary 83
References 84

6.1 Introduction

Ultrasound (US) is used widely in medicine and has a long history of safety and efficacy in diagnostic imaging. Microbubble-based contrast agents are providing new opportunities to enhance the capabilities of diagnostic US imaging. US contrast agents consist of stabilized, gas-filled microbubbles. These microbubbles circulate through the vasculature and provide effective backscatter to enhance diagnostic images. Innovative imaging modalities that rely on the characteristics of the interaction of the sound field with the microbubbles have been developed specifically for use with US contrast agents. Ongoing development of novel diagnostic imaging techniques employing contrast agents, combined with efforts to design new types of contrast agents, may widen the role of contrast agents in diagnostic US imaging. As an example, research on the development of targeted contrast agents aims to provide site-specific localization of the contrast agent and may expand the application of diagnostic US to areas of molecular imaging (e.g., Klibanov 1999).

D. Dalecki, PhD
Assistant Professor, Department of Biomedical Engineering and the Rochester Center for Biomedical Ultrasound, University of Rochester, 309 Hopeman Building, PO Box 270168, Rochester, NY 14627, USA

The combination of US and microbubble contrast agents also has the potential to provide unique avenues for a variety of new, noninvasive therapies. Although still in research and development, US contrast agents show promise for applications of US for drug delivery (e.g., Unger et al. 2001a), tumor therapy (e.g., Simon et al. 1993), thrombolysis (e.g., Birnbaum et al. 1998; Culp et al. 2001), and gene therapy (e.g., Unger et al. 2001b; Greenleaf et al. 1998).

US exposures used for diagnostic imaging are designed to minimize the interaction of the sound field with the tissue. In comparison, therapeutic applications often depend upon the interaction of the sound with the biological system to produce the desired effect. The presence of microbubble-based agents can influence the interaction of US with biological tissues through various acoustic mechanisms. For either diagnostic or therapeutic applications, increased knowledge of the interaction of US and contrast agents in tissues is important in order to avoid potential adverse bioeffects or to produce desired therapeutic endpoints. A complete understanding of the interaction of US and contrast agents with biological tissues in vivo is still needed for microbubble-based agents to achieve their full potential use in biomedical US.

6.2 Acoustic Mechanisms for Bioeffects

US can produce a wide variety of biological effects in vitro and in vivo through thermal and nonthermal mechanisms (for review see NCRP 2002 and AIUM 2000). Nonthermal interactions of US and tissue include mechanisms such as acoustic cavitation, radiation force, and acoustic streaming. The presence of microbubble contrast agents can potentially influence many of these acoustic mechanisms. Acoustic cavitation is widely studied and various bioeffects in vitro and in vivo can be attributed to activity associated with acoustic cavitation.

In general, acoustic cavitation describes the interaction of an acoustic field with an existing gas cavity. When exposed to a sound field, a bubble in a liquid will oscillate around an equilibrium radius. Although a comprehensive discussion of acoustic cavitation is beyond the scope of this chapter, various theoretical models can be used to describe the response of a gas bubble to a sound field (e.g., see YOUNG 1989; LEIGHTON 1994). The maximum response of a bubble occurs when it is exposed at its resonance frequency. For frequencies relevant to diagnostic imaging, resonance-sized bubbles are on the order of a few micrometers in radius. Noninertial cavitation describes repetitive oscillations of a bubble where the maximum expansion typically does not exceed twice the equilibrium radius. These acoustically driven bubble oscillations can result in localized heat production, microstreaming of fluid near the bubble, and localized shear stresses. Under appropriate exposure conditions, a bubble may expand to a maximum radius greater than twice its initial radius and then collapse to a fraction of its initial radius. This process is termed inertial cavitation. The response of the inertial cavity is highly nonlinear and depends upon parameters including acoustic frequency, pressure amplitude, and initial bubble radius. Various physical phenomena can be associated with inertial cavitation. Inertial collapse of a gas bubble can result in the production of localized high temperatures and pressures, as well as the generation of acoustic shock waves and free radicals. Bubbles near boundaries can collapse asymmetrically, resulting in the formation of high-speed, liquid microjets. These phenomena associated with inertial cavitation are typically localized spatially near the collapsing microbubble and are limited temporally to the duration of the collapse.

Tissues that contain gas naturally are susceptible to bioeffects from exposure to US. For example, exposure of the gas-filled intestines can result in the production of petechiae through mechanisms associated with acoustic cavitation (DALECKI et al. 1995, 1996). The introduction of microbubble contrast agents into the vasculature can provide nuclei for the generation of acoustic cavitation under appropriate exposure conditions. Tissues that are typically free of damage from US exposure can become susceptible to localized biological effects when microbubble-based agents are present. The response of stabilized microbubble contrast agents to US exposure differs in some ways from the classical models of the response of a free bubble in an infinite fluid medium. In addition, our understanding of the response to US of microbubble-based agents confined in the microvasculature in tissues is limited. Current investigations indicate that the presence of microbubbles in the blood can increase the likelihood of occurrence of some US bioeffects, such as hemolysis, capillary rupture, effects on cardiac rhythm, and localized delivery of drugs or genetic material. Not all reported bioeffects of US and microbubble-based agents have been performed under diagnostically relevant exposure conditions with clinical contrast agent doses.

The sections that follow review current research on the interaction of US with tissues containing microbubble-based agents. Since microbubbles are injected intravascularly, the summaries below focus mainly on the effects of US and contrast agents on red blood cells, blood vessels, and the heart in vivo. Most investigations in vivo have been performed with small laboratory animals. There have been no reports of any adverse clinical consequences of the use of US and microbubbles. It is important to note that the bioeffects of US and microbubbles are localized (typically occurring on microscale) and any medical significance of these effects has not been identified. In general, the extent of bioeffects produced by the combination of US and microbubble-based agents can be reduced by using lower pressure amplitudes, higher acoustic frequencies, and lower contrast agent doses.

6.3
Hemolysis

Many investigations have demonstrated that US exposure can produce hemolysis in vitro when US contrast agents are present in the blood (for a review see NCRP 2002). Hemolysis in vivo with Albunex in the blood was reported to occur in murine hearts exposed to pulsed US at 1.15 MHz (10-µs pulse duration, 100-Hz pulse repetition frequency, 5 min exposure duration) (DALECKI et al. 1997a). At evenly spaced times during the exposure, four boluses of Albunex were injected into the tail vein for a total volume of ~0.1 ml of Albunex. This contrast agent dose exceeds that used clinically. Under these conditions, the threshold at 1.15 MHz for hemolysis occurred at an amplitude of 3.0 MPa positive pressure and 1.9 MPa negative pressure. This threshold is near the upper limits of diagnostic imaging devices. The percent hemolysis for mice exposed at the highest amplitude in the absence of contrast agent was comparable to that of sham-exposed animals, indicating that the presence of microbubble nuclei in normal blood in vivo is rare. When contrast agent was present, the threshold for hemolysis increased with increasing frequency such that no measurable hemolysis was produced for exposure at 2.4 MHz for diagnostically relevant exposure amplitudes. This dependence of the threshold for hemolysis on frequency is consistent with the lack of observed hemolysis in rabbits in vivo exposed to the fields of a 5-MHz diagnostic imaging device when the contrast agent Optison (Amerham Health Inc., Princeton, NJ) was present in the vasculature (KILLAM et al. 1998). In summary, the relatively high threshold for hemolysis at 1.15 MHz combined with the strong dependence of the effect on frequency suggests a low likelihood of significant US-induced hemolysis in vivo for clinical diagnostic procedures.

6.4
Effects on Blood Vessels

Microbubble-based contrast agents are designed to be of an appropriate size such that they easily circulate through the capillary beds and also provide effective backscatter to enhance diagnostic imaging techniques. As discussed above, acoustic cavitation describes the oscillation of an existing gas cavity about its equilibrium radius in response to exposure to an US field. Physical phenomena associated with acoustic cavitation (e.g., microstreaming, localized fluid jets, shock wave generation, etc.) can potentially produce effects on biological tissues. Since contrast agents are in close proximity to blood vessels, it is important to understand the effects of the interaction of contrast agents and microvessels in vivo. Although the number of studies to date is limited, several investigations demonstrate that localized capillary rupture can be produced in laboratory animals exposed to diagnostic US when microbubbles are present in the blood. This section summarizes results from several studies that have investigated the effects of US and microbubble-based agents on the microvasculature of tissues such as the intestine, muscle, kidney, lung, and brain.

The intestine contains gas naturally and is susceptible to damage from exposure to US even without contrast agents (DALECKI et al. 1995). However, the presence of a microbubble-based agent in the blood has been shown to significantly increase the extent of vascular damage in laboratory animals (MILLER and GIES 1998, 2000). In mice exposed to pulsed US at 1.09 MHz, the production of intestinal petechiae and hemorrhage was significantly greater in animals injected with contrast agent (10 ml/kg dose of Albunex) than in control animals (MILLER and GIES 1998). The enhancement of the bioeffect was significant in that there was a 30-fold increase in the number of petechiae in mice injected with Albunex and exposed to US (10-µs pulse duration, 1-ms PRP, 100-s exposure) compared to controls (MILLER and GIES 1998). Larger doses of Albunex resulted in greater numbers of US-induced petechiae. In mice injected with Albunex, the threshold for petechiae was 0.8 MPa and the threshold for hemorrhage was 2.4 MPa for exposure at 1.09 MHz (10-µs pulse duration, 0.01 duty factor) (MILLER and GIES 1998). A second study that investigated the dependence of threshold on frequency determined that for pulsed exposures (10-µs pulse duration, 1-kHz pulse repetition frequency, 100-s exposure duration), the threshold for production of intestinal petechiae when Albunex was injected into the vasculature was 0.42, 0.85, and 2.3 MPa for exposure at 0.4, 1.09, and 2.4 MHz, respectively (MILLER and GIES 2000). When four different contrast agents that contained either air or perfluorocarbon microbubbles (Albunex, Optison, PESDA and Levovist) were investigated, it was found that the contrast agents that contained perfluorocarbon gases produced more intestinal petechiae than did contrast agents containing air-filled microbubbles (MILLER and GIES 2000).

Diagnostic imaging devices can also produce capillary damage in muscle when contrast agent is present in the vasculature (SKYBA et al. 1998; MILLER and QUDDUS 2000). One study (SKYBA et al. 1998) used intravital microscopy to directly observe the effects of US on the microvasculature of exteriorized spinotrapezius muscle in rats when the contrast agent Optison was present in the blood. Using a diagnostic phased-array system operated in harmonic imaging mode (2.3-MHz transmit), destruction of microbubbles and capillary rupture were observed in rats exposed to US with outputs ranging from mechanical index (MI) values of 0.4 to 1.0. The number of capillary rupture sites increased monotonically with increasing MI. A second study (MILLER and QUDDUS 2000) also reported production of petechial hemorrhage in murine abdominal muscle exposed to fields generated by a diagnostic imaging device (2.5-MHz transmit) when Optison was present in the vasculature. In general, the number of abdominal and intestinal petechiae increased with increasing pressure amplitude and with increasing dose of Optison (0.05–5 ml/kg) (MILLER and QUDDUS 2000). Abdominal petechiae were also observed from exposure to only a single scan, suggesting that damage produced by cavitation in vivo occurs quickly. For exposure at 2.5 MHz, MILLER and QUDDUS (2000) determined a threshold for the generation of abdominal petechiae of 0.64 MPa (i.e., MI of 0.4). This threshold is consistent with results reported by SKYBA et al. (1998).

The combination of microbubble-based contrast agents and diagnostic US has also been reported to produce microvessel damage to renal tissue in vivo (WIBLE et al. 2002). In this study, rat kidneys were exposed using a clinical imaging device with either a continuous mode (30 Hz) or intermittent (1 Hz) technique. Frequencies of 1.8, 4, and 6 MHz were investigated for MI values ranging from 0.4 to 1.6. Petechiae and areas of hemorrhage were observed in rat kidneys exposed to US when contrast was present. Extravasation of red blood cells in the glomerular space and proximal convoluted tubules was observed under histological examination. For exposures at 1.8 MHz, statistically significant damage was observed, with intermittent imaging for MI values greater than 0.8 (measured negative pressure of 1.26 MPa). Intermittent imaging produced significantly more damage than continuous imaging, and lower frequencies were more effective in producing vascular damage than higher frequencies. Although several types of contrast agents (all containing perfluorocarbon gas but different stabilizing shells) were investigated, all agents produced similar damage, indicating that the shell material had little effect on the production of this bioeffect.

Many reports have demonstrated lung hemorrhage in laboratory animals exposed to diagnostically relevant US (see AIUM 2000; NCRP 2002). Although the sensitivity of the lung is related to the presence of gas (HARTMAN et al. 1990), the role of cavitation as a mechanism for US-induced lung hemorrhage is unclear (CARSTENSEN et al. 2000). RAEMAN et al. (1997) investigated the influence of contrast agents on murine lungs exposed to 1.2-MHz pulsed US. Exposures were performed at an amplitude well above the threshold for US-induced lung hemorrhage. The extent of lung hemorrhage in exposed mice injected with Albunex (0.1 ml) was compared to that in mice injected with saline. The size of the lesion area on the surface of the lung was not statistically different for mice injected with Albunex compared to mice injected with saline (RAEMAN et al. 1997). These results are consistent with the concept that inertial cavitation in the vasculature is not the mechanism for US-induced lung hemorrhage (CARSTENSEN et al. 2000). Although current output levels of diagnostic imaging devices are within the threshold for US-induced lung hemorrhage in laboratory animals, the presence of contrast agents in the vasculature does not appear to increase the sensitivity of the lung to US-induced damage.

SCHLACHETZKI et al. (2002) investigated the effects of contrast agents (Levovist or Optison) on the blood-brain barrier in humans exposed to a clinical diagnostic imaging device. In this study, transcranial exposures were performed for 3 min at maximum output (MI ~1.9 and pressure amplitude ~2.7 MPa) using a clinical phased array (2–3.5 MHz). Opening of the blood-brain barrier was assessed using gadolinium-enhanced MR imaging. No T1-weighted signal enhancement due to extravasation of MR imaging contrast agent was observed for any subjects exposed to US for either microbubble-based contrast agent. In this study, diagnostic transcranial imaging of the brain when US contrast agents were present in the blood did not result in observable opening of the blood-brain barrier. However, transient opening of the blood-brain barrier with contrast agents has been demonstrated in laboratory animals exposed to US with pulse durations significantly greater than those used by diagnostic imaging devices (HYNYNEN et al. 2001). In this study, brains of rabbits were exposed to 1.6 MHz US following a bolus injection of Optison (0.05 ml/kg). The total US exposure was 20 s. Burst durations of 10 or 100 ms were employed with a pulse repetition frequency of 1 Hz and pressure amplitudes from 0 to 5 MPa. Opening of the blood-brain barrier was evaluated using T1-weighted MR images. Presence of Optison in the vasculature significantly increased the opening of the blood-brain barrier, and signal intensity of the T1-weighted images increased with increasing acoustic exposure amplitude. Histology indicated extravasation of red cells and damage to the brain in 70% of animals exposed at 5 MPa and 25% of animals exposed at 2–3 MPa. This study (HYNYNEN et al. 2001) indicates that US can transiently and reversibly open the blood-brain barrier and demonstrates the feasibility of the use of US for local, noninvasive delivery of drugs or genetic material to the brain.

Indeed, production of localized capillary damage by US and contrast agents may provide opportunities for various potential therapeutic applications of US. Since the production of capillary permeability or rupture is highly localized, the combination of US and microbubble-based agents provides a potential means for noninvasive therapies. Targeted contrast agents may produce site-specific localization of contrast. Active research is ongoing in applications of US and contrast agents for drug delivery, tumor therapy, thrombolysis, and gene therapy. In addition, capillary rupture resulting from the interaction of US and contrast agents has been demonstrated to increase the number of arterioles, arteriole diameter, and nutrient blood flow in skeletal muscle (SONG et al. 2002).

In summary, studies with laboratory animals indicate that diagnostic US in combination with microbubble contrast agents can produce microvessel damage in various tissues, such as the intestine, kidney, muscle, and heart. Exposures and contrast agent doses used in these studies are within those used for diagnostic imaging. The observed capillary damage is localized and the clinical significance of such microvessel damage is not clear. Capillary rupture is reduced or eliminated with the use of lower acoustic pressures and frequencies (i.e. low MI), and lower doses of contrast agent. In some instances, US-induced increases in vascular permeability may be desirable for therapeutic effects. The studies detailed above that have characterized the acoustic parameters necessary to produce capillary bioeffects will likely be useful in the design of US techniques for site-specific drug or gene delivery.

6.5
Cardiac Effects

Under appropriate exposure conditions, US either with or without contrast agents can produce premature cardiac contractions (Fig. 6.1). This section begins with a review of the effects of US on the heart without the use of microbubbles. This is followed by a summary of recent reports that have begun to investigate the effects of the interaction of US and contrast agents in cardiac tissues.

Early studies with lithotripter fields demonstrated that acoustic pulses directed to the heart can produce premature cardiac contractions (DALECKI et al. 1991; DELIUS et al. 1994). When the lithotripter pulse is delivered during the most sensitive phase of the cardiac cycle (i.e., TP segment, diastole), the threshold for producing a premature contraction is on the order of 5 MPa (DALECKI et al. 1991; DELIUS et al. 1994). A series of repetitive acoustic pulses delivered to the heart can capture and pace the heart in laboratory animals (DALECKI et al. 1991). Although the threshold for premature contractions is below clinical lithotripsy pressure amplitudes, in clinical practice the delivery of the acoustic pulses is synchronized with the ECG to avoid effects on cardiac rhythm.

Premature cardiac contractions can also result from exposure to pulsed US. A single burst of high-intensity US delivered to the heart in vivo during diastole (TP segment) can produce a premature contraction in laboratory animals (DALECKI et al. 1993a,b, 1997b; MACROBBIE et al. 1997). A pulse of US delivered during systole (QRS complex) can produce a reduction in developed aortic pressure (DALECKI et al. 1993a) and this effect appears related to radiation force (DALECKI et al. 1997b). In the murine heart, the threshold for US-induced premature contractions is ~2 MPa for exposure at 1.2 MHz with a single 5-ms burst of US (MACROBBIE et al. 1997). This threshold increases with decreasing pulse duration and increasing frequency. Thus, with the short duration pulses used in diagnostic US, there is no evidence for production of these effects from exposure to diagnostic imaging devices. However, recent studies detailed below indicate that the presence of microbubble-based agents in the vasculature significantly reduces the threshold for US-induced effects on the heart such that premature contractions can be produced with exposure to diagnostic US.

In one study (VAN DER WOUW et al. 2000), premature ventricular contractions were reported to occur in humans injected with an experimental contrast agent (AIP 101, Andaris Ltd) and exposed to diagnostic US. A diagnostic imaging device operated in triggered harmonic imaging mode with a fundamental frequency of 1.66 MHz was used for exposures. In subjects who received contrast, a significant increase in the production of premature ventricular contractions was observed for end-systolic triggering with an MI=1.5 but not with an MI=1.1. No premature ventricular contractions were reported in subjects injected with contrast and exposed with

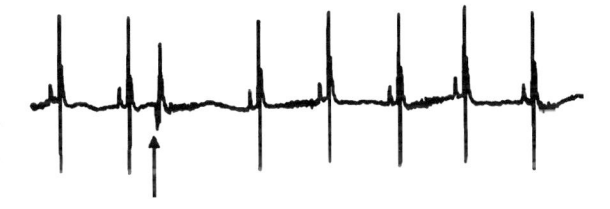

Fig. 6.1. Mouse ECG illustrating a US-induced premature contraction when microbubble contrast agents are present in the blood. The arrow denotes the delivery to the heart of a US pulse (10 µs, 1.2 MHz) at pressure amplitude above threshold.

end-diastolic triggering (MI=1.5) or in subjects exposed without contrast agents. The production of premature ventricular contractions increased with increasing pressure amplitude and contrast agent dose. These results are consistent with observations of a lack of production of premature contractions in myocardial contrast echocardiography performed with an MI of less than 1.0 (RAISINGHANI et al. 2003). Myocardial damage in humans has not been reported to result from the interaction of US and contrast agents (BORGES et al. 2002).

Although isolated premature contractions have been reported to occur in humans from exposure to diagnostic US with contrast agents, further characterization of this effect and greater insight into the mechanisms for cardiac bioeffects will likely arise from investigations with laboratory animals. LI et al. (2003, 2004) investigated effects of US and contrast agents on cardiac rhythm and vascular permeability in rats in vivo. In these studies, US exposures were performed with a commercial diagnostic imaging device operated with a transmit frequency of 1.7 MHz. Contrast agent was injected prior to US exposure. Numbers of premature ventricular contractions were counted prior to and during US exposure. Evans blue dye was also injected into the rats to serve as an indicator of microvessel permeability. Effects on the microvasculature were quantified by measuring area of Evans blue dye coloration and by counting the number of petechiae on the surface of the heart. No premature ventricular contractions, petechiae, or microvessel leakages were detected in rats exposed to US without contrast agent. In comparison, when contrast agent was present in the vasculature, clear effects on cardiac rhythm and microvessel damage were observed. The occurrence of premature ventricular contractions and effects on microvasculature increased with increasing pressure amplitude (LI et al. 2003, 2004). This is consistent with a report of cardiac arrhythmia and myocardial damage in rats injected with contrast and exposed to US at acoustic pressures that exceeded those used for clinical diagnosis (ZACHARY et al. 2002). The pressure threshold for the production of US-induced premature contractions in rats with Optison was ~1.0 MPa and the threshold for production of petechiae was ~0.5 MPa (LI et al. 2003, 2004). Production of premature ventricular contractions and capillary rupture increased with increasing contrast agent dose over the range of 25–500 µl/kg (LI et al. 2003). End-systolic triggering was more effective in producing cardiac effects than end-diastolic imaging (LI et al. 2003). A study comparing Definity, Imagent, and Optison demonstrated that premature ventricular contractions can result from the interaction of US and all three agents for exposures using a clinical imaging device operated at 1.7 MHz with peak rarefactional pressure amplitude of 1.9 MPa (LI et al. 2004).

6.6
Lithotripsy

Lithotripsy is an application of US that has dramatically altered the clinical treatment of kidney stone disease. In lithotripsy procedures, high-amplitude acoustic pulses are focused noninvasively on a kidney stone to produce stone fragmentation through both cavitation and mechanical mechanisms. The acoustic characteristics of a typical clinical lithotripter pulse are significantly different than exposure parameters used for diagnostic US. High-amplitude, clinical lithotripter fields can produce focal tissue damage (e.g., DELIUS et al. 1988, 1990). However, when microbubble-based agents are present, even relatively low-amplitude lithotripter fields can produce significant damage to the microvasculature of many organs and tissues. Investigations using laboratory animals have demonstrated that the presence of US contrast agents dramatically increases tissue damage produced by lithotripter fields (e.g., DALECKI et al. 1997c; MILLER and GIES 1999). In one investigation (DALECKI et al. 1997c), mice injected with Albunex (~0.1 ml) were exposed to 200 lithotripter pulses, each with a peak positive pressure amplitude of 2 MPa. For comparison, a group of mice were exposed to the same lithotripter fields but were not injected with contrast agent. Mice that were exposed to the lithotripter field alone exhibited damage to the lung and intestine only. This damage was minimal and consistent with investigations that have demonstrated the sensitivity of gas-containing tissues, such as the lung and intestine, to US exposure. In contrast, the mice injected with Albunex during the exposure had extensive vascular damage to the fat, muscle, mesentery, stomach, intestine, kidney, bladder, and seminal vesicles. The total length of damage along the intestine was two orders of magnitude greater when Albunex was present compared to mice without contrast. The sensitivity of tissues to lithotripter exposures can persist for hours after an initial injection of contrast agent (DALECKI et al. 1997d). These results indicate that contrast agents can serve as cavitation nuclei in vivo and produce damage to many tissues exposed to lithotripter fields at pressure amplitudes that are at least an order of magnitude less than those used in clinical lithotripsy.

MILLER and GIES (1999) also reported increased intestinal damage from lithotripter exposure when US contrast agents were present in the vasculature of mice. In this study, each lithotripter pulse had a peak positive pressure of 24.4 MPa and a negative pressure of 5.2 MPa. When microbubble-based agents were present, petechiae were also observed in tissues such as skin, muscle, fat, mesentery, and bladder. The total number of intestinal petechiae increased with increasing dose of Albunex. This study also observed that the presence of contrast agent reduced the 24-h survival rate of mice exposed to the lithotripter field.

The dramatic increase in damage to many tissues exposed to lithotripter fields when contrast agents are present in the blood provides evidence that the damage results from cavitation in vivo. A report that damage produced from negative pressure pulses is greater than that produced by positive pressure pulses provides further evidence that vascular damage from exposure to lithotripter fields when contrast agent is present is a result of cavitation (DALECKI et al. 2000). The enhanced sensitivity of many tissues to damage from lithotripter fields when contrast agents are present contraindicates the use of contrast agents with clinical lithotripsy procedures. However, the ability of the combination of contrast agents and lithotripter fields to produce localized microvessel rupture and permeabilization may provide unique avenues for cancer treatment and site-specific delivery of drugs or genetic material (e.g., MILLER and SONG 2002).

6.7
Summary

This chapter has reviewed investigations to date on the biological effects of US exposure of various tissues containing microbubble contrast agents. Figure 6.2 provides a summary of thresholds for bioeffects produced by US and contrast agents in laboratory animals in vivo. The solid line in the figure corresponds to the current US output limit for diagnostic imaging devices of an MI equal to 1.9. Although, US-induced hemolysis can be produced in laboratory animals in vivo with contrast agents in the blood, the relatively high threshold and frequency dependence of the effect indicate a minimal likelihood of any significant US-induced hemolysis for current diagnostic output levels. Under appropriate conditions, exposing the heart to US with end-systolic triggering can result in isolated premature ventricular contrac-

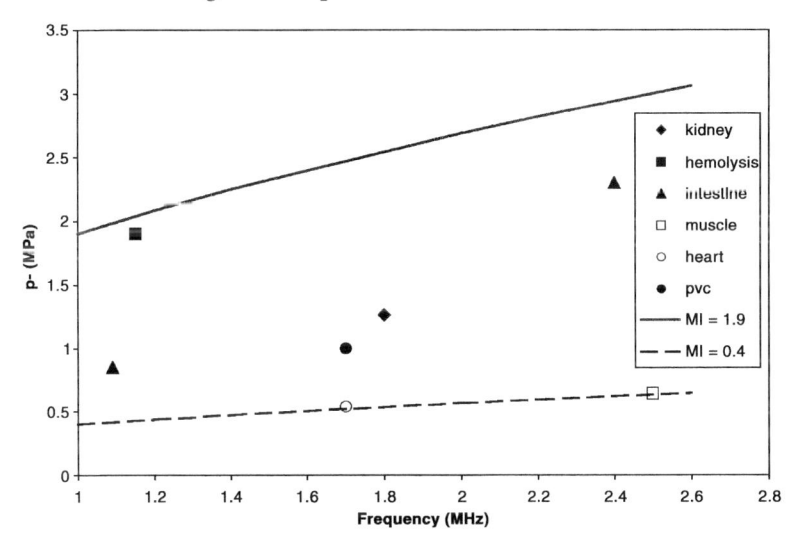

Fig. 6.2. Summary of reported thresholds for bioeffects in laboratory animals in vivo produced by US and contrast agents. Thresholds are reported in terms of negative acoustic pressure (MPa) versus exposure frequency (MHz). Data are for the following bioeffects from the indicated studies. solid diamond, kidney petechiae (WIBLE et al. 2002); solid square, hemolysis (DALECKI et al. 1997a); solid triangle, intestinal petechiae (MILLER and GIES 2000); open square, abdominal petechiae (MILLER and QUDDUS 2000); open circle, capillary rupture in myocardium (LI et al. 2003, 2004); solid circle, premature ventricular contractions (pvc) (LI et al. 2003, 2004). The equivalent mechanical index (MI) is calculated as the negative acoustic pressure divided by the square root of frequency. The dashed line corresponds to MI=0.4 and the solid line to the current output limit of MI=1.9 for diagnostic imaging devices.

tions when contrast agents are present. US-induced, localized petechiae can occur in tissues, such as intestine, kidney, myocardium, and skeletal muscle, in laboratory animals infused with contrast agents. The lowest threshold reported for capillary rupture in mice occurred at an equivalent MI of 0.4. The clinical significance of localized capillary rupture is not yet clear and there is no evidence that this effect occurs in humans. However, enhanced permeability of the microvasculature produced by the combination of US and contrast agents may provide opportunities for localized drug and gene delivery. In general, effects of US and contrast agents are reduced or eliminated through the use of lower pressure amplitudes, higher frequencies, and lower doses of contrast agent. Further research is required to clarify the biological effects of US and microbubble-based agents.

Microbubble-based contrast agents are enhancing the use of diagnostic US imaging techniques and are providing new possibilities for the use of US in therapy. Under appropriate exposure conditions, the combination of US and microbubble-based agents can affect cells and tissues. Expanding our knowledge of the mechanisms for the biological effects of US and microbubble-based agents will provide vital information for advancing the use of US contrast agents in medicine.

Acknowledgements

This work was supported in part by a grant from the National Institutes of Health.

References

AIUM (American Institute of Ultrasound in Medicine) (2000) Mechanical bioeffects from diagnostic ultrasound: AIUM consensus statements. J Ultrasound Med 19:120-142

Birnbaum Y, Luo H, Nagai T et al (1998) Noninvasive in vivo clot dissolution without a thrombolytic drug: recanalization of thrombosed iliofemoral arteries with transcutaneous ultrasound combined with intravenous infusion of microbubbles. Circulation 97:130-134

Borges AC, Walde T, Reibis RK et al (2002) Does contrast echocardiography with Optison induce myocardial necrosis in humans? J Am Soc Echocardiogr 15:1080-1086

Carstensen EL, Gracewski S, Dalecki D (2000) The search for cavitation in vivo. Ultrasound Med Biol 26:1377-1385

Culp WC, Porter TR, Xie F et al (2001) Microbubble potentiated ultrasound as a method of declotting thrombosed dialysis grafts: experimental study in dogs. Cardiov Intervent Radiol 24:407-412

Dalecki D, Keller BB, Carstensen EL et al (1991) Thresholds for premature ventricular contractions in frog hearts exposed to lithotripter fields. Ultrasound Med Biol 17:341-346

Dalecki D, Keller BB, Raeman CH, Carstensen EL (1993a) Effects of pulsed ultrasound on the frog heart. I. Thresholds for changes in cardiac rhythm and aortic pressure. Ultrasound Med Biol 19:385-390

Dalecki D, Raeman CH, Carstensen EL (1993b) Effects of pulsed ultrasound on the frog heart. II. An investigation of heating as a potential mechanism. Ultrasound Med Biol 19:391-398

Dalecki D, Raeman CH, Child SZ, Carstensen EL (1995) Intestinal hemorrhage from exposure to pulsed ultrasound. Ultrasound Med Biol 21:1067-1072

Dalecki D, Raeman CH, Child SZ, Carstensen EL (1996) A test for cavitation as a mechanism for intestinal hemorrhage in mice exposed to a piezoelectric lithotripter. Ultrasound Med Biol 22:493-496

Dalecki D, Raeman CH, Child SZ et al (1997a) Hemolysis in vivo from exposure to pulsed ultrasound. Ultrasound Med Biol 23: 307-313

Dalecki D, Raeman CH, Child SZ, Carstensen EL (1997b) Effects of pulsed ultrasound on the frog heart. III. The radiation force mechanism. Ultrasound Med Biol 23:275-285

Dalecki D, Raeman CH, Child SZ et al (1997c) The influence of contrast agents on hemorrhage produced by lithotripter fields. Ultrasound Med Biol 23:1435-1439

Dalecki D, Raeman CH, Child SZ et al (1997d) Remnants of Albunex nucleate acoustic cavitation. Ultrasound Med Biol 23:1405-1412

Dalecki D, Child SZ, Raeman CH et al (2000) Bioeffects of positive and negative acoustic pressures in mice infused with microbubbles. Ultrasound Med Biol 26:1327-1332

Delius M, Enders F, Xuan ZR et al (1988) Biological effects of shock waves: kidney damage by shock waves in dogs – dose dependence. Ultrasound Med Biol 14:117-122

Delius M, Jordan M, Liebich HG, Brendel W (1990) Biological effects of shock waves: effect of shock waves on the liver and gallbladder wall of dogs - administration rate dependence. Ultrasound Med Biol 16:459-466

Delius M, Hoffman G, Steinbeck G, Conzen P (1994) Biological effects of shock waves: induction of arrhythmia in piglet hearts. Ultrasound Med Biol 20:279-285

Greenleaf WF, Golander ME, Sarkar G et al (1998) Artificial cavitation nuclei significantly enhance acoustically induced cell transfection. Ultrasound Med Biol 24:587-595

Hartman C, Child SZ, Mayer R et al (1990) Lung damage from exposure to the fields of an electrohydraulic lithotripter. Ultrasound Med Biol 16:675-679

Hynynen K, McDannold N, Vykhodtseva N, Jolesz FA (2001) Noninvasive MR imaging-guided focal opening of the blood-brain barrier in rabbits. Radiology 220:640-646

Killam AL, Greener Y, McFerran BA et al (1998) Lack of bioeffects of ultrasound energy after intravenous administration of FS069 (Optison) in the anesthetized rabbit. J Ultrasound Med 17:349-356

Klibanov AL (1999) Targeted delivery of gas-filled microsphere, contrast agents for ultrasound imaging. Adv Drug Deliv Rev 37:139-157

Leighton TG (1994) The acoustic bubble. Academic, London

Li P, Cao L-Q, Dou C-Y et al (2003) Impact of myocardial contrast echocardiography on vascular permeability: an in vivo dose response study of delivery mode, pressure amplitude and contrast dose. Ultrasound Med Biol 29:1341-1349

Li P, Armstrong WF, Miller D (2004) Impact of myocardial contrast echocardiography on vascular permeability:

comparison of three different contrast agents. Ultrasound Med Biol 30:83-91

MacRobbie AG, Raeman CH, Child SZ, Dalecki D (1997) Thresholds for premature contractions in murine hearts exposed to pulsed ultrasound. Ultrasound Med Biol 23:761-765

Miller DL, Gies RA (1998) Gas-body-based contrast agent enhances vascular bioeffects of 1.09 MHz ultrasound on mouse intestine. Ultrasound Med Biol 24:1201-1208

Miller DL, Gies RA (1999) Consequences of lithotripter shockwave interaction with gas body contrast agent in mouse intestine. J Urol 162:606-609

Miller DL, Gies RA (2000) The influence of ultrasound frequency and gas-body composition on the contrast agent-mediated enhancement of vascular bioeffect in mouse intestine. Ultrasound Med Biol 26:307-313

Miller DL, Quddus J (2000) Diagnostic ultrasound activation of contrast agent gas bodies induces capillary rupture in mice. Proc Natl Acad Sci USA 97:10179-10184

Miller DL, Song J (2002) Lithotripter shock waves with cavitation nucleation agents produce tumor growth reduction and gene transfection in vivo. Ultrasound Med Biol 28:1343-1348

National Council on Radiation Protection and Measurements (NCRP) (2002) Exposure Criteria for Medical Diagnostic Ultrasound. II. Criteria based on all known mechanisms. NCRP, Besthesda, MD

Raeman CH, Child SZ, Meltzer RS, Carstensen EL (1997) Albunex® does not increase the sensitivity of the lung to pulsed ultrasound. Echocardiography 14:553-557

Raisinghani A, Wei KS, Crouse L et al (2003) Myocardial contrast echocardiography (MCE) with triggered ultrasound does not cause premature ventricular complexes: evidence from PB127 MCE studies. J Am Soc Echocardiogr 16:1037-1042

Schlachetzki F, Holscher T, Koch HJ, Draganski B, May A, Schuierer G, Bogdahn U (2002) Observation on the integrity of the blood-brain barrier after microbubble destruction by diagnostic transcranial color-coded sonography. J Ultrasound Med 21:419-429

Simon RH, Ho SY, Lange SC et al (1993) Applications of lipid-coated microbubble contrast to tumor therapy. Ultrasound Med Biol 19:123-125

Skyba DM, Price RJ, Linka AZ et al (1998) Direct in vivo visualization of intravascular destruction of microbubbles by ultrasound and its local effects on tissues. Circulation 98:290-293

Song J, Qi M, Kaul S, Price RJ (2002) Stimulation of arteriogenesis in skeletal muscle by microbubble destruction with ultrasound. Circulation 106:1550-1555

Unger EC, Hersh E, Vannan M et al (2001a) Local drug delivery through microbubbles. Prog Cardio Dis 44:45-54

Unger EC, Hersh E, Vannan M, McCreery T (2001b) Gene delivery using ultrasound contrast agents. Echocardiography 18:355-361

Van der Wouw PA, Brauns AC, Bailey SE et al (2000) Premature ventricular contractions during triggered imaging with ultrasound contrast. J Am Soc Echocardio 13:288-294

Wible JH, Galen KP, Wojdyla JK et al (2002) Microbubbles induce renal hemorrhage when exposed to diagnostic ultrasound in anesthetized rats. Ultrasound Med Biol 28:1535-1546

Young F (1989) Cavitation. McGraw-Hill, New York

Zachary JF, Hartleben S, Frizzell LA, O'Brien WD (2002) Arrhythmias in rat hearts exposed to pulsed ultrasound after intravenous injection of a contrast agent. J Ultrasound Med 21:1347-1356

Vascular Applications

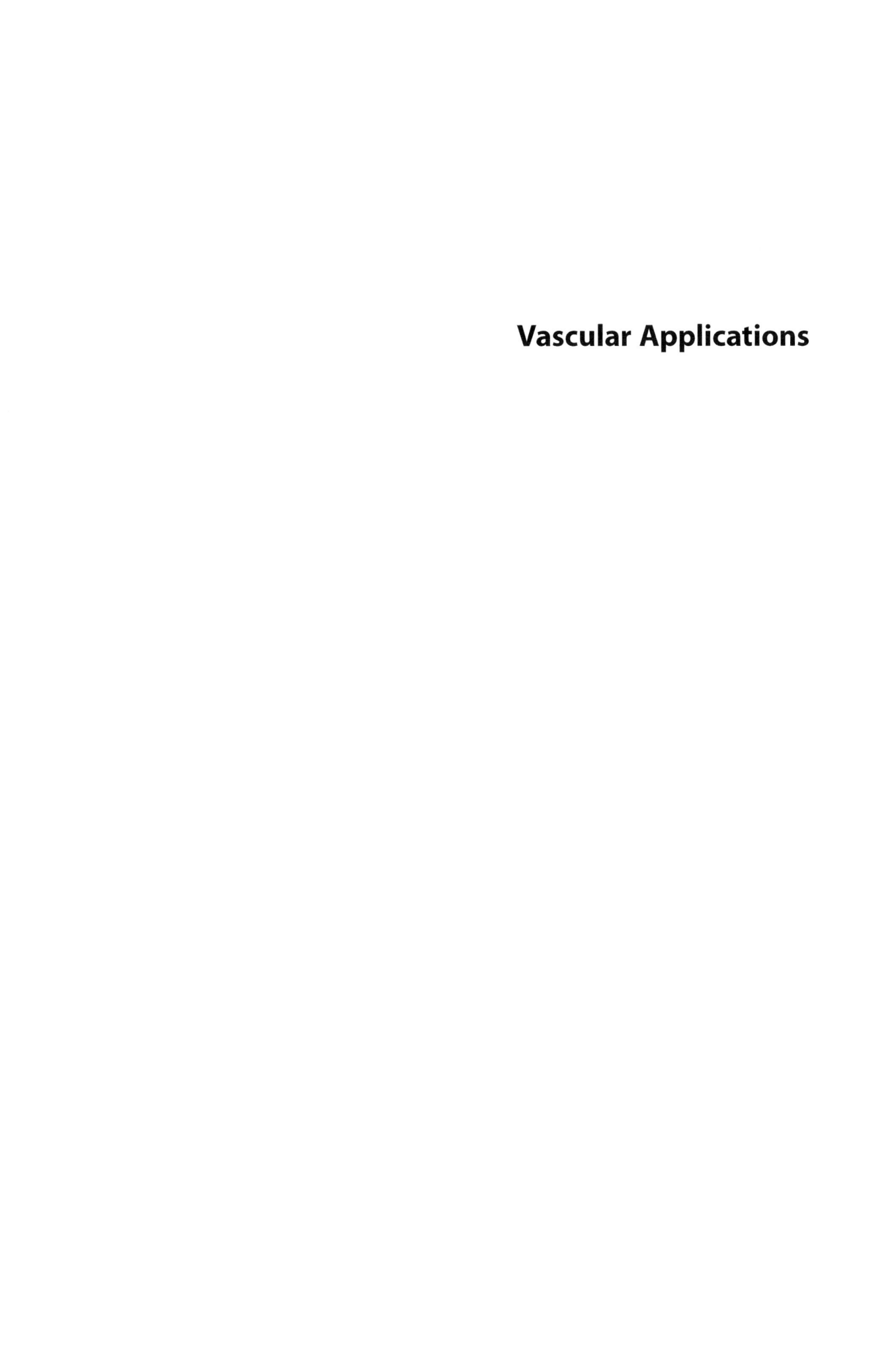

7 Cerebral Vessels

Giuseppe Caruso, Giuseppe Salvaggio, Fortunato Sorrentino, Giuseppe Brancatelli, Antonio Nicosia, Giuseppe Bellissima, and Roberto Lagalla

CONTENTS

7.1 Introduction 89
7.2 Principles and Technique 89
7.3 Velocity Measurement 90
7.4 Brain Perfusion 91
7.4.1 Injection Techniques 91
7.4.2 Data Acquisition and Processing Technique 92
7.5 Stroke 93
7.5.1 Arterial Occlusion 93
7.5.2 Arterial Stenosis 94
7.6 Arteriovenous Malformations 94
7.7 Aneurysms 96
References 98

7.1 Introduction

Transcranial color Doppler ultrasound (US), introduced by Aaslid et al. (1982), provides a noninvasive real-time method to assess intracranial hemodynamics. Microbubble-based contrast agents were first applied in the evaluation of the central nervous system in 1993 (Becker et al. 1993; Bogdahn et al. 1993). Transcranial color Doppler US depicts intracranial vessels and parenchymal structures with high spatial resolution (Seidel et al. 1995; Zipper and Stolz 2002; Baumgartner et al. 1997a), and it is a reliable technique for noninvasive assessment of cerebral arteries (Seidel et al. 1995; Baumgartner et al. 1996). The study of the cerebral structures is often possible through the temporal bone, where the skull thickness is very thin. In approximately 16–20% of patients an insufficient temporal bone window is found (Seidel et al. 1995; Baumgartner et al. 1997b), while about 20-30% of patients in the age range at risk for stroke present a small and thick

G. Caruso, MD, Associate Professor of Radiology;
G. Salvaggio, MD; F. Sorrentino, MD;
G. Brancatelli, MD; A. Nicosia, MD; G. Bellissima, MD;
R. Lagalla, MD, Professor of Radiology;
Department of Radiology, University of Palermo, Via del Vespro 127, 90127 Palermo, Italy

transtemporal acoustic window (Baumgartner et al. 1997a; Gahn et al. 2000). Microbubbles provide a backscatter surface that increases the US reflection coefficient to 0.99, whereas soft biological tissues present a reflection coefficient of about 0.03 (Zipper and Stolz 2002); this results in better visualization of cerebral vessels.

The principal indication for microbubble-based contrast agents in transcranial color Doppler US is poor visibility of cerebral vessels at baseline scan, especially when flow is absent or slow (Seidel and Meyer 2002). In these cases, microbubble based contrast agents markedly improve vessel identification in 90% of cases (Zipper and Stolz 2002) and may identify very slow blood flow velocities and low flow volume (small vessels, vessel pseudo-occlusion, microcirculation) (Seidel et al. 2002) and some pathological conditions, such as cerebral artery occlusion, stenosis, or collateral pathways (Postert et al. 1999a; Droste et al. 2000). Moreover, the use of microbubbles, which present blood pool features, allows the study of perfusion, as with other imaging techniques.

7.2 Principles and Technique

Phased-array probes with a low-frequency emission (2–2.5 MHz) and high-intensity emission up to 200 mW/cm^2 are employed to transmit US through the temporal bone. The temporal window lies between the zygomatic arch and the inferior temporal edge. Three different locations of the temporal acoustic windows are identified: (a) anterior, located posterior to the frontal process of the zygomatic bone; (b) posterior, located just anterior to the ear; (c) middle, located between the anterior and posterior temporal windows.

The temporal axial mesencephalic or orbitomeatal plane is identified by landmarks such as the butterfly-shaped hypoechoic mesencephalon surrounded by the echogenic basal cistern, the highly echogenic sphenoid bone, and the lateral fissure. By an upward movement of the transducer at 10° from the mesencephalic axial plane, the diencephalic plane is visualized (Fig. 7.1). These are the two planes used for vascular study, and minimal movements of the transducer are necessary to optimize the visualization of the intracranial vessels. After microbubble-based agents injection one can see the middle cerebral artery (M1 segment), the anterior cerebral artery (A1 segment) (Fig. 7.2), and the posterior cerebral artery (P1 and P2 segments).

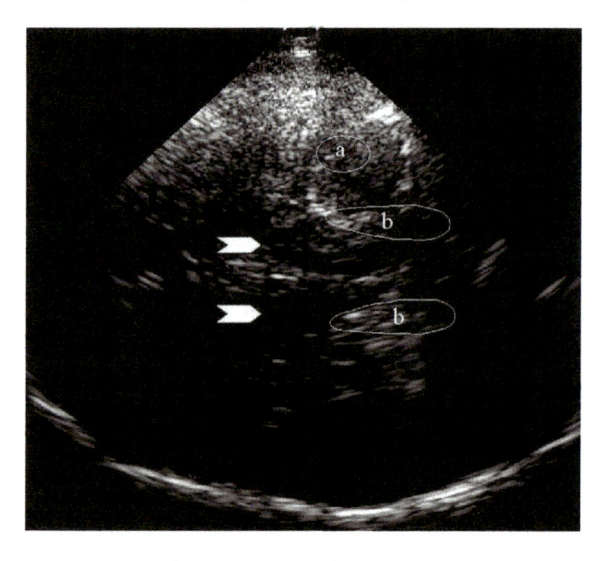

Fig. 7.1. Diencephalic plane. B-mode imaging shows the frontal horns of the lateral ventricles (*arrowheads*). The white matter (*a*) and the thalamic zone (*b*) are also identified.

Cerebral vein imaging is restricted by anatomic factors such as the depth, the low blood flow velocities, the unfavorable insonation angles, and the low-frequency probes. Nevertheless, microbubble-based contrast agent injection leads to an improvement in cerebral vein visualization. In fact, STOLTZ et al. (1999) confirmed the improved visibility of the deep middle cerebral vein, the basal vein, the vein of Galen, and part of the superior sagittal sinus. The transforaminal plane is used to study V3 and V4 vertebral artery segments. The basilar artery origin is demonstrated in 84% of cases, while the distal segment is seen in less than 50% of cases, even after administration of microbubble-based agents.

7.3
Velocity Measurement

Color Doppler US allows the combination of gray-scale imaging and depiction of vascular structures. It permits the correct positioning of the spectral Doppler sample volume and the calculation of blood flow velocities, providing information on turbulent flow, increased flow, systolic and diastolic velocities, and flow direction.

Initial studies in vitro and in animal models have shown a variable increase in the peak systolic velocity (FORSBERG et al. 1994; ABILDGAARD et al. 1996; PETRIK et al. 1997). KHAN et al. (2000), after bolus administration of a microbubble-based contrast

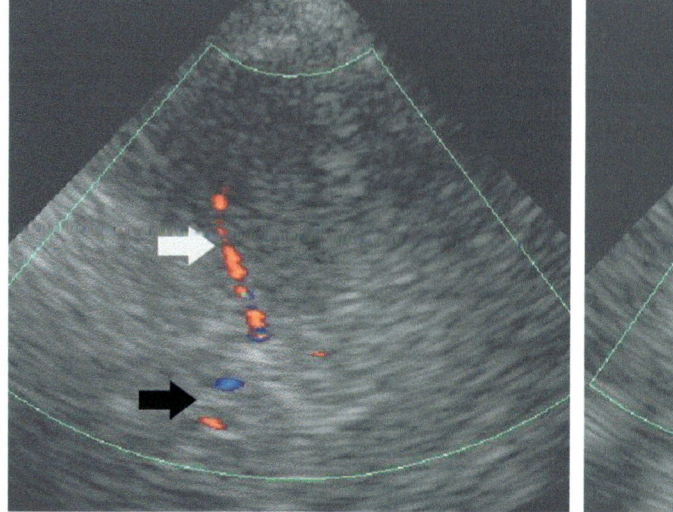

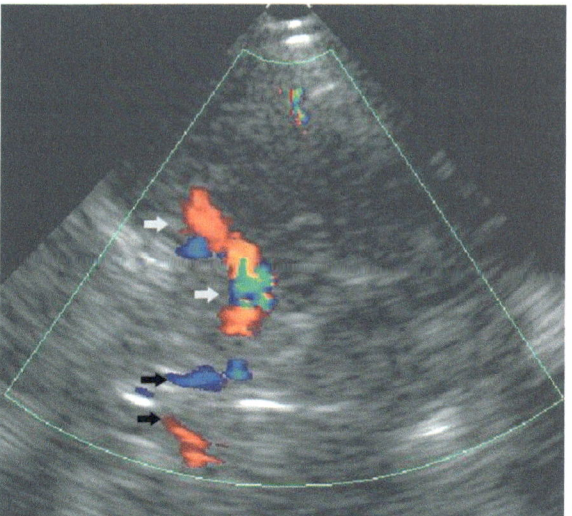

Fig. 7.2. a Transcranial color Doppler in a healthy subject. An ineffective temporal bone window precludes the correct visualization of circle of Willis. White arrow, middle cerebral artery; black arrow, anterior cerebral artery. b Injection of a microbubble-based agent allows better visualization of the middle cerebral artery (*white arrows*) and both anterior cerebral arteries (*black arrows*).

agent, found increasing peak systolic velocities in the middle cerebral artery compared with baseline velocities. For this reason, peak systolic velocities, which were normal before the administration of contrast material, could exceed a velocity threshold, falsely suggesting abnormality. The reduction of Doppler gain can easily compensate for this artifact (PETRICK et al. 1997), even though it is necessary to standardize gain reduction after microbubble-based contrast agent administration. ALBRECHT et al. (1998) investigated the effects of continuous infusion of microbubble-based contrast agents, and the infusion technique was found to result in a low increase in peak systolic velocity that did not significantly interfere with the use of current peak systolic velocity thresholds.

In conclusion, when a bolus technique is used, the effect of increasing velocity needs to be taken into account if peak systolic velocity thresholds, developed for disease detection at baseline scan, are employed after microbubble injection. This technical artifact needs to be considered when velocity criteria are employed in the classification of stenoses.

7.4
Brain Perfusion

Transcranial color Doppler US is able to identify large vessels, but it cannot visualize small vessels or vessels involved in parenchymal perfusion owing to the reduced dimensions. The ability of US to measure capillary blood flow and tissue perfusion by means of microbubble-based contrast agents was improved by the development of low-frequency scanners and dedicated contrast-specific modes.

Studies by POSTERT et al. (1999b), FEDERLEIN et al. (2000), and SEIDEL et al. (2000b) have demonstrated the ability of second harmonic imaging (BURNS 1996) to evaluate human brain perfusion after microbubble injection, and destructive imaging techniques are considered the most sensitive tool. High pulse repetition frequency and wall filters are applied in loss of correlation imaging or stimulated acoustic emission (SCHLACHETKI et al. 2001), harmonic B-mode imaging (POSTERT et al. 1999a; SEIDEL et al. 2003), pulse inversion harmonic imaging (EYDING et al. 2003a), contrast burst imaging, and time variance imaging (POSTERT et al. 2000; EYDING et al. 2003b).

Contrast burst imaging and time variance imaging are derived from power Doppler, in which pulses are broadband with high acoustic power. The changes in microbubble shape and size are reflected in the amplitude and spectral energy distribution of echoes, so that short sequences of six to ten pulses per line can reveal the presence of microbubbles. The changes are then detected as broadband noise in the Doppler spectrum in contrast burst imaging or as characteristic features of microbubbles using dedicated algorithms in time variance imaging (WILKENING et al. 1998).

7.4.1
Injection Techniques

Two main injection techniques are employed when using microbubbles for perfusion measurements: bolus administration and continuous administration.

a) Bolus administration. In bolus administration, the contrast material is injected over a few seconds, modifying imaging and the time-intensity curve. This technique was developed for perfusion measurement for ultrafast CT (AXEL 1980; GOBBEL et al. 1991) and was adapted for US imaging. The mean duration of diagnostically adequate enhancement is dose dependent and ranges from 73 to 368 s (TOTARO et al. 2002). Color Doppler US is compromised by blooming artifacts: the vessels appear large or merge if near each other, requiring down-regulation of the gain settings. B-mode imaging shows an increase in intensity in the circle of Willis and, after some seconds, in the parenchymal tissue. In the bolus approach, the time-intensity curve reaches maximum intensity, and a typical mono-exponential washout is delineated: a rapid increase in contrast enhancement is followed by a short peak of strong enhancement with a subsequent slow exponential fall-off, explained by the normal degradation of the microbubbles, within a few minutes (OTIS et al. 1995; SCHMINKE et al. 2001). This kinetics approach allows the calculation of values like peak intensity, time to peak intensity, and peak width. With this approach it is often necessary to perform several injections of contrast material in order to achieve an adequate duration of diagnostic enhancement.

b) Continuous administration by slow infusion. Microbubbles are administered intravenously, using a specially configured infusion pump, at a constant rate. Microbubbles are destroyed by high acoustic power and, subsequently, nondestructive imaging is used to observe the slow refilling of the microcircle. Constant administration should therefore lead to a steady-state concentration in the blood pool at a level lasting over 10 min and therefore useful for diagnosis. Microbubbles are destroyed in the insonation plane, while new microbubbles progressively fill the insonated parenchymal volume, depending on the time interval between two destructive pulses. Assuming that the microbubble concentration in the tissue is related to the intensity of scattered US, the intensity is related to the velocity of the contrast agent in the microcirculation. SEIDEL et al. (2001) and SEIDEL and MEYER (2002) demonstrated in their studies that assessment of cerebral microcirculation is possible by analyzing the refill kinetics after microbubble destruction.

A sufficiently extended period of enhancement is often required, and continuous intravenous infusion is a suitable solution (ALBRECHT et al. 1998; HOLSHER et al. 2001; TOTARO et al. 2002). Continuous infusion of contrast could further optimize three-dimensional (3D) reconstruction of power Doppler frames which provides spatial orientation of the intracranial vessels, thereby improving the detection of stenoses, intracranial aneurysms, and angiomas (DELCKER and TEGELER 1998; SCHMINKE et al. 2000).

7.4.2
Data Acquisition and Processing Technique

Perfusion study is based on a dynamic data acquisition after bolus injection. At the end of the examination, a region of interest (ROI) is selected. ROIs are most commonly placed over the basal nuclei (i.e., lentiform nucleus), thalamus, white matter, cortical structures, and principal arteries. Time-intensity curves are calculated by proprietary dedicated software. POSTERT et al. (1998) and FEDERLEIN et al. (2000) described three characteristic phases in time-intensity curves: (1) a baseline period before contrast agent administration, (2) a sudden acoustic intensity peak increase, and (3) a slow decrease in acoustic intensity (Fig. 7.3). The curves obtained are influenced by microbubble destruction and by the use of high concentrations of microbubbles (EYDING et al. 2002). Several time-intensity curve parameters were studied: peak intensity, time to peak intensity, peak width, area under the curve, and peak intensity/time to peak intensity ratio (positive gradient).

The main disadvantage of all US techniques is that physical properties, such as the nonlinear relationship between microbubble concentration and optic intensities (WIENCEK et al. 1993) and the depth-dependent attenuation of the received harmonic signals, makes absolute quantification of peak intensities impossible (EYDING et al. 2003a; HARRER and KLOTZSCH 2002). In all studies the peak intensity showed wide variation and depth-dependent differences, with higher intensities in the region closer to the probe. EYDING et al. (2003a) showed no significant differences between gray and white matter regions for time to peak intensity.

Even though time to peak intensity is influenced by various factors such as heart rate, heart ejection fraction, and position of the venous cannula, its potential to demonstrate hemodynamic impairment of cerebral perfusion in acute stroke conditions has been shown in perfusion-MR imaging (NEUMANN-HAEFELIN et al. 1999). MEVES et al. (2002), in a comparison between US and perfusion-MR examinations, demonstrated that time to peak intensity and peak width provide reliable parameters in US perfusion examinations because they are not depth-dependent parameters. Finally, area under curve and positive gradient showed a large intra- and inter-individual variation which could have been the result of different insonation conditions.

As previously demonstrated (POSTERT et al. 2000; SEIDEL et al. 2000a), these parameters can be evaluated only qualitatively, because of specific physical

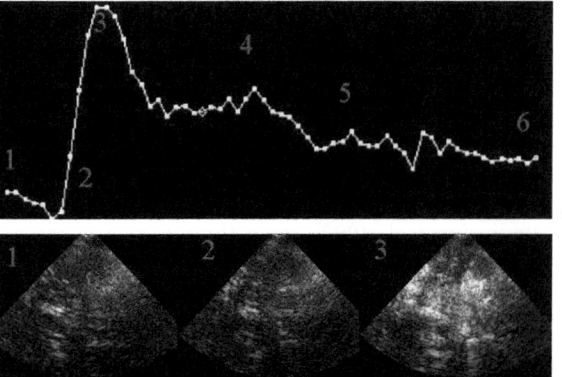

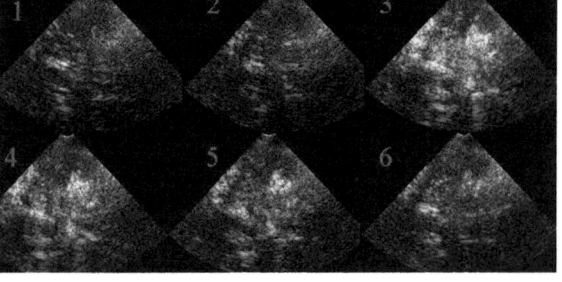

Fig. 7.3. a Time-intensity curve measured in a healthy subject, with the different phases of contrast enhancement after microbubble injection. b Corresponding gray-scale appearance of the brain. *1* baseline, *2, 3* 30-40 s after microbubble injection with increase in acoustic intensity, *4-6* progressive decrease in acoustic intensity.

properties such as depth-dependent attenuation of the US signals, heterogeneous temporal bone window, and nonlinear relation between echo contrast concentration and video intensity (Bos et al. 1995).

7.5
Stroke

Cerebrovascular disease is the third most frequent cause of death after cardiovascular disease and cancer. It is possible to classify three kinds of major vascular attacks: (1) ischemic stroke, (2) hemorrhagic stroke, and (3) subarachnoid hemorrhage.

Ischemic stroke can be occlusive or nonocclusive. Occlusive causes can be divided into embolic cardiovascular, vascular atherothrombotic, and nonatherothrombotic, such as arteritis. Nonocclusive, or hemodynamic, stroke is caused by a critical reduction in the cerebral perfusion pressure that can be worsened by stenotic arteries (Bonavita et al. 1996). Arterial lesions preferentially involve carotid arteries in white people, and intracranial large arteries in patients of Asian, African, or Hispanic ancestry (Wong et al. 2000). Early identification of the occlusive artery allows a reduction in mortality and morbidity, and aggressive treatment such as fibrinolysis has been developed and has proved effective in improving outcome (Gahn et al. 2001).

MR imaging may show both vascular occlusion and the mismatch between necrosis and ischemic zone (Gahn and von Kummer 2001). If MR imaging is not available within 24 h, evaluation is based on CT, which provides information exclusively about parenchymal ischemic damage (von Kummer and Weber 1997).

Transcranial contrast-enhanced color Doppler US can fill the diagnostic vascular gap owing to the potential improvement in identification of the circle of Willis collateral pathways (Gahn and von Kummer 2001). Koga et al. (2002) showed that unenhanced transcranial color Doppler US is able to visualize normal basilar artery flow through the transforaminal window in only 76.4% of the patients, and that use of a contrast agent can improve its detection to 98.2% (Fig. 7.4a,b).

7.5.1
Arterial Occlusion

Diagnostic criteria of middle cerebral artery occlusion are: (1) missing or discontinued color-coded signal of the middle cerebral artery and lack of pulsed-wave Doppler signal; (2) detection of the anterior cerebral artery, the posterior cerebral artery, or both vessels of the affected side; (3) visualization of the middle cerebral artery on the contralateral side (Postert et al. 1999a). In cases of suspected middle cerebral artery occlusion, if the vessels of the circle of Willis can be accounted for except for the middle cerebral artery, the findings are essentially pathognomonic of middle cerebral artery occlusion (Gahn et al. 2000).

Finally, contrast-enhanced transcranial color Doppler US shows a sensitivity and specificity of about 100% and 83%, respectively, in the detec-

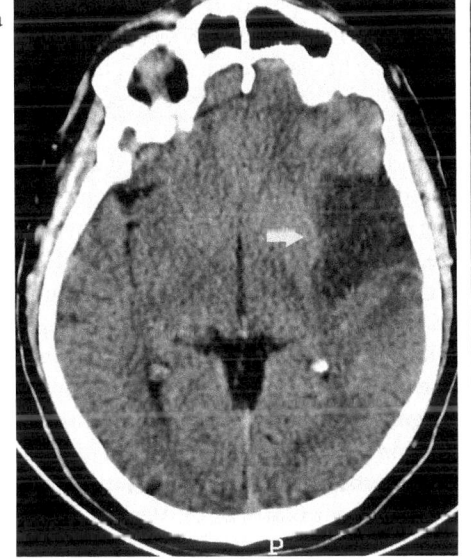

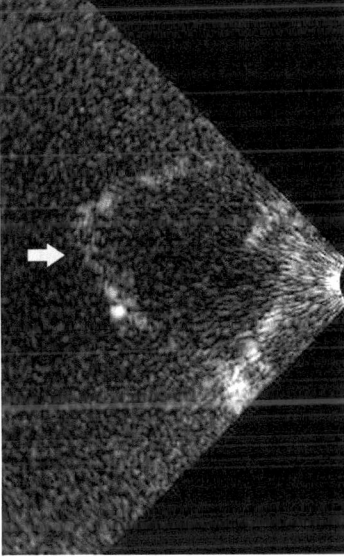

Fig. 7.4. a A 47-year-old patient. CT scan of the brain shows a large hypodense area involving the temporal lobe. b Trans-cranial contrast-enhanced US shows a hypovascular region (*arrow*) surrounded by hyperechoic parenchyma corresponding to reperfused cerebral areas.

tion of middle cerebral artery occlusion, compared with conventional angiography (SEIDEL and MEYER 2002). POSTERT et al. (1999a), in a series of 90 patients, investigated the diagnostic potential of contrast-enhanced transcranial color Doppler US in patients with ischemia in the field of the middle cerebral artery, and correlated these findings with clinical, angiographic, and CT results. In territorial middle cerebral artery infarctions, the size of the ischemic lesions was correlated with a decrease in flow velocities or middle cerebral artery occlusion on the initial contrast-enhanced transcranial color Doppler examination. In particular, large infarctions (exceeding two-thirds of the middle cerebral artery territory) and medium-sized infarctions (encompassing one- to two-thirds of the middle cerebral artery territory) were associated with a middle cerebral artery occlusion or decreased flow velocities. In those patients with a small infarction (less than one-third of the middle cerebral artery territory), lacunae, or no CT lesions, no middle cerebral artery occlusions were found, and normal flow velocities were observed in 75% of individuals.

In patients with extracranial artery occlusion, contrast-enhanced transcranial color Doppler was found to have a sensitivity and specificity of 92% and 94%, respectively, for the detection of the intracranial collateral pathways (DROSTE et al. 2000).

7.5.2
Arterial Stenosis

Diagnostic criteria for arterial stenosis are: (1) identification of localized aliasing phenomena, (2) poststenotic flow turbulence with decreased flow velocities, and (3) local modification of flow characteristics (BAUMGARTNER et al. 1999). Modification of flow characteristics has been analyzed by several authors. KLOTZSCH et al. (2002) classified stenoses according to whether luminal narrowing was less or more than 50%. The cut-off value of minimal peak velocities for stenoses of less than 50% and more than 50% were, respectively: anterior cerebral artery, 120 and 155 cm/s; middle cerebral artery, 155 and 220 cm/s; posterior cerebral artery, 100 and 145 cm/s; basilar artery, 100 and 140 cm/s.

ZUNKER et al. (2002) considered the following to be US criteria for intracranial stenoses: a segmental flow acceleration of 50% from baseline, a side difference of >30 cm/s (V_{mean}) between corresponding intracranial arteries, and absolute V_{mean} values of >80 cm/s for the middle cerebral artery and internal carotid artery, >75 cm/s for the anterior cerebral artery, >60 cm/s for the posterior cerebral artery, and >65 cm/s for the basilar artery.

We must take into account that modifications of peak systolic velocities, as compared with baseline, are possible after contrast agent administration, as found by KHAN et al. (2000). BAUMGARTNER et al. (1997a) found that the peak systolic velocity cut-off values used for contrast-enhanced transcranial color Doppler diagnosis of stenosis are 23% higher than those used for nonenhanced investigations.

Identification of intracranial pathways via the anterior or posterior communicating artery showed a sensitivity of 89% and a specificity of 79% for contrast-enhanced transcranial color Doppler as compared with angiography (GAHN et al. 2001) in patients with extracranial stenoses.

7.6
Arteriovenous Malformations

Vascular malformations of the brain have been classified by RUSSEL and RUBINSTEIN (1989) into four major pathologic types: arteriovenous malformations, cavernous angioma, capillary telangiectasia, and venous angioma. Arteriovenous malformations represent the most common clinically symptomatic cerebrovascular malformation (PERRET and NISHIOKA 1966). Arteriovenous malformations are congenital anomalies of blood vessel development that result from direct communication between arterial and venous channels without an intervening capillary network (KAPLAN et al. 1961). The incidence in the general population is approximately 0.14%. According to YASARGIL (1987), arteriovenous malformations may be classified as small, medium-sized, or large when the diameter is, respectively, <2 cm, 2–4 cm, and >4 cm.

SPETZLER and MARTIN (1986) proposed a simple scheme for grading intracranial arteriovenous malformations in order to improve surgical planning, based on the size of the nidus, the location of the nidus, and the venous drainage pattern. The nidus size is scored as small (<3 cm), medium (3–6 cm), or large (>6 cm). The location of the nidus is determined to be within either eloquent regions (sensorimotor, visual, or language cortex, internal capsule, thalamus, hypothalamus, brainstem, cerebellar peduncles, and deep cerebellar nuclei: all with a score of 1) or noneloquent areas (score of 0). Venous drainage is classified as either superficial (score of 0), if

Cerebral Vessels

drainage is entirely into the cortical venous system, or deep (score of 1), if any or all drainage enters the deep system. Based on these parameters, intracranial arteriovenous malformations can be graded from I to V (more surgically difficult lesions).

The most common initial symptom is related to acute intracranial hemorrhage, although larger arteriovenous malformations are more likely to present with seizures (Waltimo 1973). Intracranial hemorrhage is most often intraparenchymal and occurs during the second or third decade (Brown et al. 1988; Ondra et al. 1990). According to Heros and Korosue (1990), data suggest a rate of hemorrhage in the range of 2–4% per year. The long-term prognosis of untreated arteriovenous malformations is unfavorable (Vinuela 1992). Therefore surgery, radiosurgery, embolization, or a combination thereof is used to reduce morbidity and mortality (Steiner et al. 1993).

Transcranial color Doppler US allows the direct or indirect visualization of intracranial arteriovenous malformations by identifying the location and the dominant feeding vessel (Baumgartner et al. 1996; Uggowitzer et al. 1999). In direct visualization, transcranial color Doppler US shows the nidus of arteriovenous malformations as a mixed color area with a mosaic-like appearance in color mode because of the convolution of vessels with different flow directions (Zipper and Stolz 2002) (Fig. 7.5a). Moreover, transcranial color Doppler US can demonstrate the principal feeding artery and the main draining vein with pulsatile, low-resistance flow within it (Krejza et al. 2000) (Fig. 7.5b).

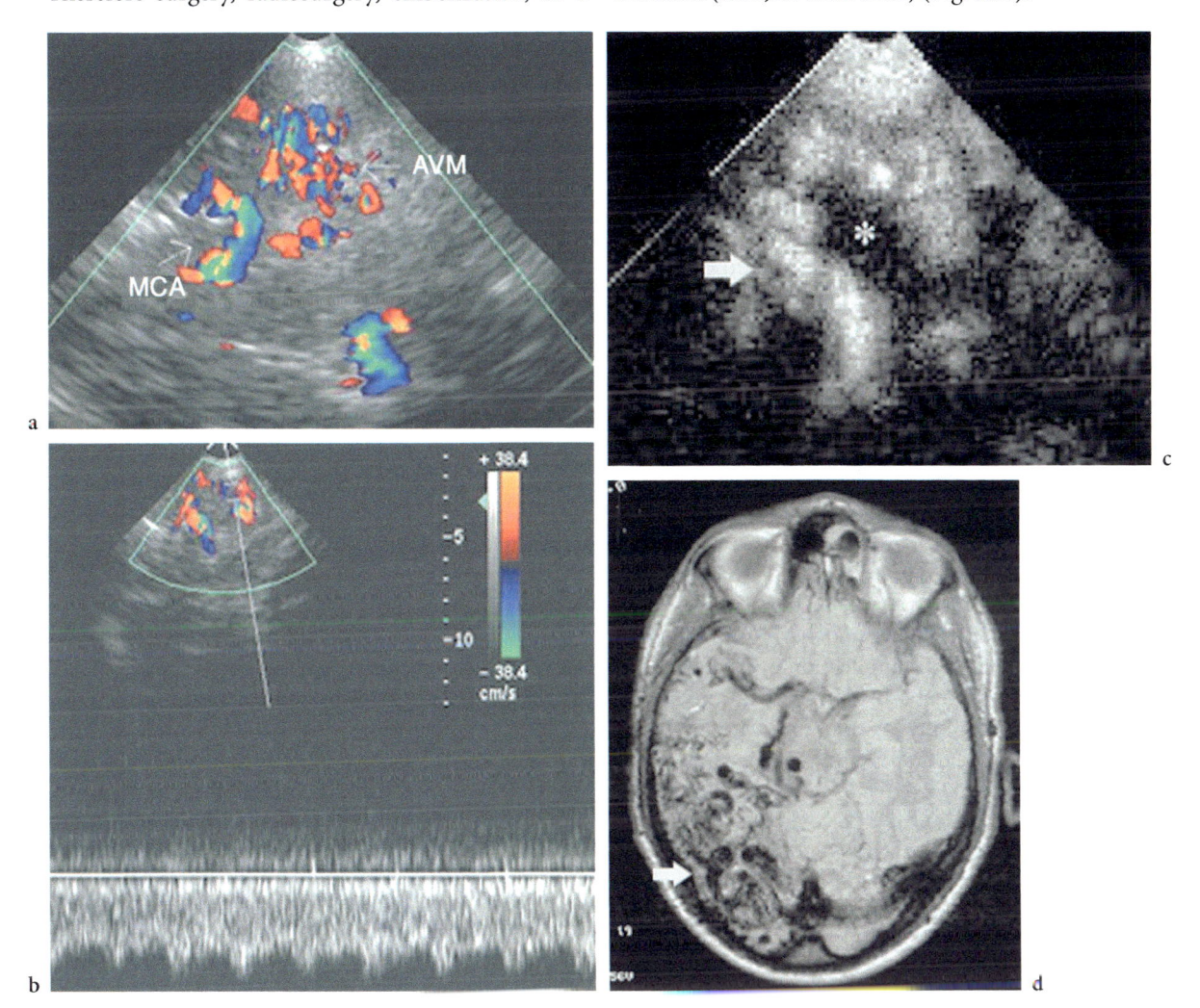

Fig. 7.5. a Control of large embolized arteriovenous malformation (*AVM*) involving parietal region of the brain. Transcranial color Doppler shows the vessel loops in the AVM nidus as a mixed color area with a "mosaic-like appearance." *MCA* middle cerebral artery. b Pulsed Doppler of a feeding artery makes it possible to identify high flow velocities and decreased pulsatility and resistance indices. c Contrast agent administration permits differentiation between the embolized (*) and the vascular zone (*arrow*). d Corresponding MR image. The arteriovenous malformation (*arrow*) is clearly visualized.

Several studies (e.g., Mast et al. 1995; Zipper and Stolz 2002) have shown an inverse correlation between arteriovenous malformation size and peak mean systolic velocity in the feeding arteries. Even when a lesion cannot be visualized with transcranial color Doppler, it might be assessed in terms of hemodynamic differences. The indirect diagnostic criteria are: increased peak systolic and end-diastolic flow velocities, a low pulsatility in the feeding arteries, and increased flow velocities in the draining veins. Hemodynamic parameters such as peak systolic velocities and resistive index of the feeding arteries must be compared with the values assessed in the corresponding contralateral segment. However, Mast et al. (1995) reported that unenhanced transcranial color Doppler has limited sensitivity in the detection of small lesions. In fact, the size of an arteriovenous malformation is the main factor determining the volume of shunting, the flow velocity in the feeders, and thus the frequency of sonographic detection using hemodynamic criteria. Using these criteria, most arteriovenous malformations with a diameter of >2 cm, as well as about two-thirds of those with a diameter of <2 cm can be detected with transcranial color Doppler (Baumgartner et al. 1996). The authors of the latter study identified 79% of arteriovenous malformations due to detection of feeding arteries, visualizing all large and medium-sized arteriovenous malformations. By comparison, Klotzsch et al. (1995) revealed 71% of arteriovenous malformations and their main feeders with transcranial color Doppler. Unfortunately in 20–30% of patients undergoing transcranial color Doppler, insufficient acoustic properties are responsible for inconclusive examinations (Uggowitzer et al. 1999).

An insufficient signal-to-noise ratio is the principal indication for the application of microbubble-based contrast agents in intracranial investigations with sonography (Seidel and Meyer 2002). Uggowitzer et al. (1999) found contrast-enhanced transcranial color Doppler to have a sensitivity of 92% in the detection of arteriovenous malformations. Uggowitzer et al. (1999) correctly identified the location and the dominant arterial feeder of the lesions but slightly underestimated the size of malformations. In particular, they observed that use of a microbubble-based contrast agent resulted in a diagnostic improvement in the detection of small arteriovenous malformations (<2.5 cm) and lesions located in areas difficult to insonate. Peak systolic velocities values are significantly higher and resistive index values are lower in the lesion's feeding arteries than in the corresponding contralateral vessel. However, markedly overlapping values, as well as the possible occurrence of bilateral arteriovenous malformations, make the use of side-to-side differences in peak systolic velocity and resistive index unadvisable as a diagnostic tool.

Nevertheless, sensitivity in the detection of arteriovenous malformations is strictly dependent on their location, and in the case of arteriovenous malformations located in the posterior fossa, the differentiation of feeding arteries is unreliable because of the close proximity of the vessels (Klotzsch et al. 2002). Scanning of supratentorial blood vessels is considerably limited by the extent and site of the temporal bone window, which limits the area of insonation (Seidel and Meyer 2002).

Some authors, such as Klotzsch et al. (2002), have suggested the use of transcranial color Doppler as a screening method for arteriovenous malformations in patients with cryptogenic intracranial hemorrhage or frequent monomorphic migraine attacks, even though a negative transcranial color Doppler examination does not exclude arteriovenous malformations. Krejza et al. (2000) suggested the use of transcranial color Doppler in screening patients with intracerebral hematoma to detect possible underlying arteriovenous malformations and thereby improve surgical planning.

In conclusion, there is no agreement as to the most appropriate method for screening the general population for cerebral arteriovenous malformations. Transcranial color Doppler would be useful as a noninvasive monitoring system for follow-up examinations during stepwise treatment of arteriovenous malformations (Petty et al. 1990; Diehl et al. 1994).

Contrast-enhanced transcranial color Doppler US seems to be a promising technique for the diagnosis, assessment, localization, and follow-up of arteriovenous malformations (Fig. 7.5c,d). However, unfavorable lesion location and an insufficient acoustic window currently limit the role of this method, and further investigation is needed.

7.7
Aneurysms

Rinkel et al. (1998) in a systematic review, reported that the prevalence of unruptured intracranial aneurysms varies between 3.6% and 6%. Their incidence increases in patients over 30, and they are more common in women. According to the INTERNATIONAL STUDY OF UNRUPTURED INTRACRANIAL ANEURYSM INVESTIGATORS (1998), the rupture rate of small aneurysms is only 0.05% per year in patients with no prior clinical history of subarachnoid hemorrhage, and 0.5% per year for large aneurysms (>1 cm diameter) and for all aneurysms with previous subarachnoid hemorrhage. WARDLAW and WHITE (2000) classified cerebral aneurysms as follows: (1) symptomatic aneurysms, i.e., those causing subarachnoid hemorrhage following rupture or symptoms due to a space-occupying effect; (2) asymptomatic aneurysms, i.e., additional aneurysms found in patients with a symptomatic aneurysm which are not responsible for the clinical presentation, or aneurysms found in patients investigated because they are at risk; and (3) incidental aneurysms, i.e., those found unexpectedly in patients undergoing investigation for other suspected pathology. Aneurysm location varies in the studies reported. TURNER et al. (2003) found aneurysms in the posterior circulation in 58% of patients, while BONILHA et al. (2001) and FORGET et al. (2001) reported 73% of aneurysms to occur in the anterior circulation. In recent years, there has been increasing interest in the possibility of detection and treatment of intracranial aneurysms prior to rupture.

The gold standard for identification of an intracranial aneurysm is digital subtraction angiography, as reported by MAYBERG et al. (1994). However, digital subtraction angiography is invasive, costly and carries the risk of complications. For these reasons, it is unsuitable as a screening test. In recent years there has been increasing interest in the use of noninvasive imaging methods, such as magnetic resonance imaging, computer tomography, and transcranial color Doppler US, for the diagnosis of intracranial aneurysms (WARDLAW and WHITE 2000).

Typically, transcranial color Doppler US depicts aneurysms as round or oval structures originating from arterial segments with zones of opposite flow direction within the structure (coffee-bean shape) (ZIPPER and STOLZ 2002). After microbubble administration, the aneurysm becomes visible as an area of increased echogenicity (GAILLOUD et al. 2002) (Fig 7.6). WARDLAW and WHITE (2000), using color Doppler and power Doppler US, found an overall sensitivity of 80% and a specificity of 87.5% for aneurysm detection, and sensitivity increased to 91% in patients who had an adequate bone temporal window. The use of microbubble-based agents and 3D US may improve accuracy in aneurysm detection. KLOTZSCH et al. (1999) reported a sensitivity of 87% and a specificity of 100% in a series of 30 patients with aneurysms ranging in diameter from 3 to 16 mm.

The reported sensitivities and specificities must be interpreted with caution, however; in fact, publication bias could be present: studies showing a greater accuracy are more likely to be submitted and published than those showing a poorer accuracy. Contrast-enhanced transcranial color Doppler US offers a noninvasive method for monitoring progressive intra-aneurysmal thrombosis following coil embolization and for follow-up of patients with untreatable fusiform aneurysms. Using combined

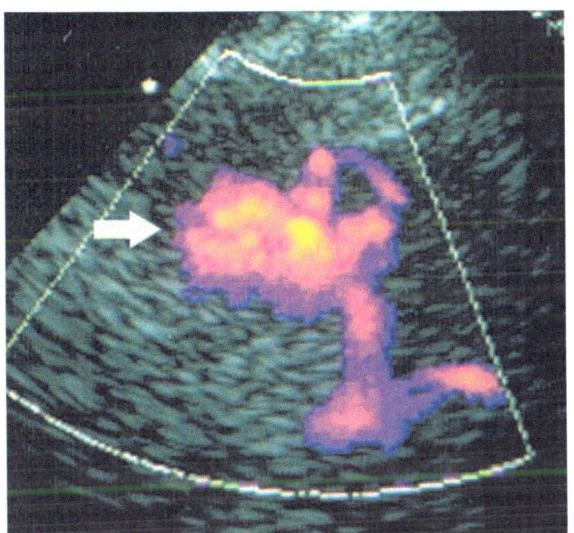

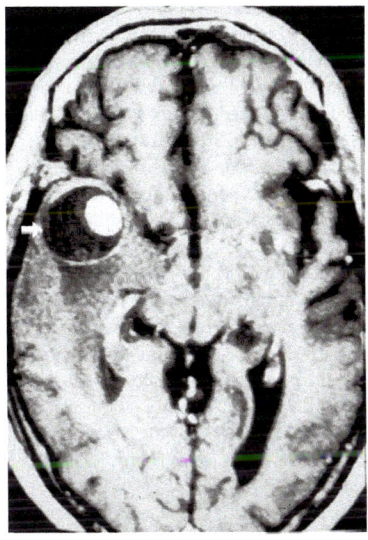

Fig. 7.6. a Transverse plane. Contrast-enhanced transcranial color Doppler reveals a large aneurysm (*arrow*) of the middle cerebral artery. **b** Corresponding MR image. The cerebral aneurysm (*arrow*) is clearly visualized.

contrast-enhanced and non-contrast-enhanced transcranial color Doppler, TURNER et al. (2003) studied 46 patients with intracranial aneurysms treated with coils. They identified aneurysms with complete occlusion with a sensitivity of 95% and a specificity of 84%; aneurysms with minimal residual flow with a sensitivity of 40% and a specificity of 97%; aneurysms with moderate residual flow with a sensitivity of 100% and a specificity of 95%; and extensive residual flow with a sensitivity of 96% and a specificity of 100%.

Contrast-enhanced transcranial color Doppler US is a promising modality for the evaluation of intracranial aneurysms, for screening the general population or first-degree relatives of subarachnoid hemorrhage patients, for surveillance of coiled aneurysms, or as an imaging technique for follow-up examinations.

References

Aaslid R, Markwalder TM, Nornes H (1982) Non invasive transcranial Doppler ultrasound recording of flow velocity in basal cerebral arteries. J Neurosurg 57:769-774

Abildgaard A, Egge TS, Klow NE, Jakobsen JA (1996) Use of sonicated albumin (Infoson) to enhance arterial spectral and color Doppler imaging. Cardiovasc Intervent Radiol 19:265-271

Albrecht T, Urbank A, Mahler M et al (1998) Prolongation and optimization of Doppler enhancement with microbubble US contrast agent by using continuous infusion: preliminary experience. Radiology 207:339-347

Axel L (1980) Cerebral blood flow determination by rapid-sequence computed tomography: theoretical analysis. Radiology 137:679-686

Baumgartner RW, Mattle HP, Schroth G (1996) Transcranial colour-coded duplex sonography of cerebral arteriovenous malformations. Neuroradiology 38:734-737

Baumgartner RW, Arnold M, Gönner F et al (1997a) Contrast-enhanced transcranial color-coded duplex sonography in ischemic cerebrovascular disease. Stroke 28:2473-2478

Baumgartner RW, Baumgartner I, Mattle HP, Schroth G (1997b) Transcranial color-coded duplex sonography in the evaluation of collateral flow through the circle of Willis. AJNR Am J Neuroradiol 18:127-133

Baumgartner RW, Mattle HP, Schroth G (1999) Assessment of >/=50% and <50% intracranial stenoses by transcranial color-coded duplex sonography. Stroke 30:87-92

Becker G, Lindner A, Bogdahn U (1993) Imaging of the vertebrobasilar system by transcranial color-coded real-time sonography. J Ultrasound Med 12:395-401

Bogdahn U, Becker G, Schlief R et al (1993) Contrast-enhanced transcranial color-coded real-time sonography. Results of a phase-two study. Stroke 24:676-684

Bonavita V, Di Costanzo A, Tedeschi G (1996) Cerebrovascular disease. In: Bonavita V, di Iorio G (eds) Clinical neurology: diagnosis and therapy. Edizioni Medico Scientifiche, Torino, pp 595-650

Bonilha L, Marques EL, Carelli EF et al (2001) Risk factors and outcome in 100 patients with aneurysmal subarachnoid hemorrhage. Arq Neuropsiquiatr 59:676-680

Bos LJ, Piek JJ, Spaan JAE (1995) Background subtraction from time-intensity curves in videodensitometry: a pitfall in flow assessment using contrast echocardiography. Ultrasound Med Biol 21:1211-1218

Burns PN, Powers JE, Simpson DH et al. (1996) Harmonic imaging: principles and preliminary results. Clin Radiol 51(Suppl):50-55

Brown RD Jr, Wiebers DO, Forbes G et al (1988) The natural history of unruptured intracranial arteriovenous malformations. J Neurosurg 68:352-357

Delcker A, Tegeler C (1998) Entwicklung und Einsatz der 3D Sonographie in der Neurologie. Akt Neurol 25:56-62

Diehl RR, Henkes H, Nahser HC et al (1994) Blood flow velocity and vasomotor reactivity in patients with arteriovenous malformations. A transcranial Doppler study. Stroke 25:1574-1580

Droste DW, Jürgens R, Weber S et al (2000) Benefit of echocontrast-enhanced transcranial color-coded duplex ultrasound in the assessment of intracranial collateral pathways. Stroke 31:920-923

Eyding J, Wilkening W, Postert T (2002) Brain perfusion and ultrasonic imaging techniques. Eur J Ultrasound 16:91-104

Eyding J, Krogias C, Wilkening W et al (2003a) Parameters of cerebral perfusion in phase-inversion harmonic imaging (PIHI) ultrasound examinations. Ultrasound Med Biol 29:1379-1385

Eyding J, Wilkening W, Reckhardt M et al (2003b) Contrast burst depletion imaging (CODIM): a new imaging procedure and analysis method for semiquantitative ultrasonic perfusion imaging. Stroke 34:77-83

Federlein J, Postert T, Meves S et al (2000) Ultrasonic evaluation of pathological brain perfusion in acute stroke using second harmonic imaging. J Neurol Neurosurg Psychiatry 69:616-622

Forget TR Jr, Benitez R, Veznedaroglu E et al (2001) A review of size and location of ruptured intracranial aneurysm. Neurosurgery 49:1322-1326

Forsberg F, Liu JB, Burns PN et al (1994) Artifacts in ultrasonic contrast agent studies. J Ultrasound Med 13:357-365

Gahn G, von Kummer R (2001) Ultrasound in acute stroke: a review. Neuroradiology 43:702-711

Gahn G, Gerber J, Hallmeyer S et al (2000) Contrast enhanced transcranial color-coded duplex sonography in stroke patients with limited bone windows. AJNR Am J Neuroradiol 21:509-514

Gahn G, Hahn G, Hallmeyer-Elgner S et al (2001) Echo-enhanced transcranial colour coded duplex sonography to study collateral blood flow in patients with symptomatic obstructions of the internal carotid artery and limited acoustic bone windows. Cerebrovasc Dis 11:107-112

Gailloud P, Khan HG, Albayram S et al (2002) Pooling of echographic contrast agent during transcranial Doppler sonography: a sign in favor of slow-flowing giant saccular aneurysms. Neuroradiology 44:21-24

Gobbel GT, Cann CE, Iwamoto HS, Fike JR (1991) Measurement of regional cerebral blood flow in the dog using ultrafast computed tomography. Experimental validation. Stroke 22:772-779

Harrer JU, Klotzsch C (2002) Second harmonic imaging of the human brain: the practicability of coronal insonation

planes and alternative perfusion parameters. Stroke 33:1530-1535
Heros RC, Korosue K (1990) Arteriovenous malformations of the brain. Curr Opin Neurol Neurosurg 3:63-67
Holscher T, Schlachetzki F, Bauer A et al (2001) Echo-enhanced transcranial color-coded US: clinical usefulness of intravenous infusion versus bolus injection of SH U 508A. Radiology 219:823-827
International Study of Unruptured Intracranial Aneurysm Investigators (1998) Unrupted intracranial aneurysms -- risk of rupture and risks of surgical intervention. N Engl J Med 339:1725-1733
Kaplan HA, Aronson SM, Browderes EJ (1961) Vascular malformations of the brain. An anatomical study. J Neurosurg 18:630-635
Khan HG, Gailloud P, Bude RO et al (2000) The effect of contrast material on transcranial Doppler evaluation of normal middle cerebral artery peak systolic velocity. AJNR Am J Neuroradiol 21:386-390
Klotzsch C, Henkes H, Nahser HC et al (1995) Transcranial color-coded duplex sonography in cerebral arteriovenous malformations. Stroke 26:2298-2301
Klotzsch C, Bozzato A, Lammers G et al (1999) Three-dimensional transcranial colour-coded sonography of cerebral aneurysms. Stroke 30:2285-2290
Klotzsch C, Bozzato A, Lammers G et al (2002) Contrast-enhanced three-dimensional transcranial color-coded sonography of intracranial stenosis. Am J Neuroradiol AJNR 23:208-212
Koga M, Kimura K, Minematsu K, Yamaguchi T (2002) Relationship between findings of conventional and contrast-enhanced transcranial color-coded real-time sonography and angiography in patients with basilar artery occlusion. AJNR Am J Neuroradiol 23:568-571
Krejza J, Mariak Z, Bert RJ (2000) Transcranial colour Doppler sonography in emergency management of intracerebral haemorrhage caused by an arteriovenous malformation: case report. Neuroradiology 42:900-904
Mast H, Mohr JP, Thompson JL et al (1995) Transcranial Doppler ultrasonography in cerebral arteriovenous malformations. Diagnostic sensitivity and association of flow velocity with spontaneous hemorrhage and focal neurological deficit. Stroke 26:1024-1027
Mayberg MR, Batjer HH, Dacey R et al (1994) Guidelines for the management of aneurysmal subarachnoid hemorrhage. A statement for healthcare professionals from a special writing group of the Stroke Council, American Heart Association. Stroke 25:2315-2328
Meves SH, Wilkening W, Thies T et al (Ruhr Center of Competence for Medical Engeneering) (2002) Comparison between echo contrast agent-specific imaging modes and perfusion-weighted magnetic resonance imaging for the assessment of brain perfusion. *Stroke* 33:2433-2437
Neumann-Haefelin T, Wittsack HJ, Wenserski F et al (1999) Diffusion- and perfusion-weighted MRI. The DWI/PWI mismatch in acute stroke. Stroke 30:1591-1597
Ondra SL, Troupp H, George ED, Schwab K (1990) The natural history of symptomatic arteriovenous malformations of the brain: a 24-year follow-up assessment. J Neurosurg 73:387-391
Otis S, Rush M, Boyajian R (1995) Contrast-enhanced transcranial imaging. Results of an American phase-two study. Stroke 26:203-209
Perret G, Nishioka H (1966) Report on cooperative study of intracranial aneurysms and subarachnoid hemorrhage. Section VI. Arteriovenous malformations. An analysis of 545 cases for cranio-cerebral arteriovenous malformations and fistulae reported to the cooperative study. J Neurosurg 25:467-490
Petty GW, Massaro AR, Tatemichi TK et al (1990) Transcranial Doppler ultrasonographic changes after treatment for arteriovenous malformations. Stroke 21:260-266
Petrik J, Zomack M, Schlief R (1997) An investigation of the relationship between ultrasound echo enhancement and Doppler frequency shift using a pulsatile arterial flow phantom. Invest Radiol 32:225-235
Postert T, Muhs A, Meves S et al (1998) Transient response harmonic imaging: an ultrasound technique related to brain perfusion. Stroke 29:1901-1907
Postert T, Braun B, Meves S et al (1999a) Contrast-enhanced transcranial color-coded sonography in acute hemispheric brain infarction. Stroke 30:1819-1826
Postert T, Federlein J, Weber S et al (1999b) Second harmonic imaging in acute middle cerebral artery infarction. Preliminary results. Stroke 30:1702-1706
Postert T, Hoppe P, Federlein J et al (2000) Contrast agent specific imaging modes for the ultrasonic assessment of parenchymal cerebral echo contrast enhancement. J Cereb Blood Flow Metab 20:1709-1716
Rinkel GJ, Djibuti M, Algra A, van Gijn J (1998) Prevalence and risk of rupture of intracranial aneurysm: a systematic review. Stroke 29:251-256
Russell DS, Rubinstein LJ (1989) Pathology of tumors of the nervous system, 5th edn. Williams and Wilkins, Baltimore
Schlachetzki F, Hoelscher T, Dorenbeck U et al (2001) Sonographic parenchymal and brain perfusion imaging: preliminary results in four patients following decompressive surgery for malignant middle cerebral artery infarct. Ultrasound Med Biol 27:21-31
Schminke U, Motsch L, von Smekal U et al (2000) Three-dimensional transcranial color-coded sonography for the examination of the arteries of the circle of Willis. J Neuroimaging 10:173-176
Schminke U, Motsch L, Bleiss A et al (2001) Continuous administration of contrast medium for transcranial colour-coded sonography. Neuroradiology 43:24-28
Seidel G, Meyer K (2002) Impact of ultrasound contrast agents in cerebrovascular diagnostics. Eur J Ultrasound 16:81-90
Seidel G, Kaps M, Gerriets T (1995) Potential and limitations of transcranial color-coded sonography in stroke patients. Stroke 26:2061-2066
Seidel G, Algermissen C, Christoph A et al (2000a) Harmonic imaging of the human brain. Visualization of brain perfusion with ultrasound. Stroke 31:151-154
Seidel G, Algermissen C, Christoph A et al (2000b) Visualization of brain perfusion with harmonic gray scale and power doppler technology: an animal pilot study. Stroke 31:1728-1734
Seidel G, Claassen L, Meyer K, Vidal-Langwasser M (2001) Evaluation of blood flow in the cerebral microcirculation: analysis of the refill kinetics during ultrasound contrast agent infusion. Ultrasound Med Biol 27:1059-1064
Seidel G, Meyer K, Metzler V et al (2002) Human cerebral perfusion analysis with ultrasound contrast agent constant

infusion: a pilot study on healthy volunteers. Ultrasound Med Biol 28:183-189
Seidel G, Albers T, Meyer K, Wiesmann M (2003) Perfusion harmonic imaging in acute middle cerebral artery infarction. Ultrasound Med Biol 29:1245-1251
Spetzler RF, Martin NA (1986) A proposed grading system for arteriovenous malformations. J Neurosurg 65:476-483
Steiner L, Lindquist C, Cail W et al (1993) Microsurgery and radiosurgery in brain arteriovenous malformations. J Neurosurg 79:647-652
Stolz E, Kaps M, Kern A et al (1999) Transcranial colour-coded duplex sonography of intracranial veins and sinuses in adults. Reference data from 130 volunteers. Stroke 30:1070-1075
Totaro R, Baldassarre M, Sacco S et al (2002) Prolongation of TCD-enhanced Doppler signal by continuous infusion of Levovist. Ultrasound Med Biol 28:1555-1559
Turner CL, Higgins JN, Kirkpatrick PJ (2003) Assessment of transcranial colour-coded duplex sonography for the surveillance of intracranial aneurysms treated with Guglielmi detachable coils. Neurosurgery 53:866-872
Uggowitzer MM, Kugler C, Riccabona M et al (1999) Cerebral arteriovenous malformation: diagnostic value of echo-enhanced transcranial Doppler sonography compared with angiography. AJNR Am J Neuroradiol 20:101-106
Vinuela F (1992) Functional evaluation and embolization of intracranial arteriovenous malformations. In: Vinuela F, van Halback V, Dion JE (eds) Interventional neuroradiology. Raven, New York, pp 77-86
Von Kummer R, Weber J (1997) Brain and vascular imaging in acute ischemic stroke: the potential of computed tomography. Neurology 49:S52-S55
Waltimo O (1973) The relationship of size, density and localization of intracranial arteriovenous malformations to the type of the initial symptom. J Neurol Sci 19:13-19
Wardlaw JM, White PM (2000) The detection and management of unruptured intracranial aneurysm. Brain 123:205-221
Wiencek JG, Feinstein SB, Walker R, Aronson S (1993) Pitfalls in quantitative contrast echocardiography: the steps to quantitation of perfusion. J Am Soc Echocardiogr 6:395-416
Wilkening W, Lazenby JC, Ermert H (1998) A new method for detecting echoes from microbubble contrast agent based on time-variance. Proc IEEE Ultrasonics Symp 1823-1826
Wong KS, Li H, Chan YL et al (2000) Use of transcranial Doppler ultrasound to predict outcome in patient with intracranial large-artery occlusive disease. Stroke 31:2641-2647
Yasargil MG (1987) Pathological consideration. In : Yasargil MG (ed) Microneurosurgery, vol IIIA. AVM of the brain, history, embryology, pathological considerations, hemodinamics, diagnostic studies, microsurgical anatomy. Thieme, Stuttgart, pp 49-211
Zipper SG, Stolz E (2002) Clinical application of transcranial colour-coded duplex sonography -- a review. Eur J Neurol 9:1-8
Zunker P, Wilms H, Brossmann J et al (2002) Echo contrast-enhanced transcranial ultrasound: frequency of use, diagnostic benefit and validity of results compared with MRA. Stroke 33:2600-2603

8 Carotid Arteries

Emilio Quaia, Fabio Pozzi Mucelli, and Antonio Calgaro

CONTENTS

8.1 Introduction *101*
8.2 Carotid and Vertebrobasilar Color Doppler US *102*
8.3 Contrast-Enhanced US of the Carotid Arteries *102*
8.4 Advantages of Contrast-Enhanced US Compared to Baseline Color Doppler US *103*
8.4.1 Quantification of Internal Carotid Artery Stenosis *103*
8.4.2 Assessment of the Distal Internal Carotid Artery *104*
8.4.3 Characterization of Atherosclerotic Plaques and Detection of Carotid Plaque Ulceration *104*
8.5 Limitations of Contrast-Enhanced US in the Assessment of Carotid Arteries *108*
References *110*

8.1 Introduction

According to clinical trials in symptomatic (North American Symptomatic Carotid Endarterectomy Trial Collaborators 1991) or asymptomatic patients (Executive Committee for the Asymptomatic Carotid Atherosclerosis Study 1995), the prevalence of significant (>50%) stenosis of the carotid bifurcation in symptomatic patients is 18–20%, while that in asymptomatic patients referred for carotid imaging is 14%. The prevalence of internal carotid artery disease (Grant et al. 2003) in the asymptomatic group, therefore, approaches that found in symptomatic patients. Both the above-mentioned studies proved the benefit of carotid endarterectomy in patients with severe symptomatic carotid artery stenosis. Recent publications have demonstrated that subgroups of patients with a 50%–69% stenosis may also expect a small benefit from carotid endarterectomy (European Carotid Surgery Trialists' Collaborative Group 1991).

Color Doppler ultrasound (US) has dramatically increased the accuracy and feasibility of US carotid examination and is now the screening examination of choice in the detection of extracranial carotid artery stenosis (Grant et al. 2003). Considerable gains have been made in the quality of US examinations of the carotid arteries, such as improved gray-scale resolution due to use of speckle-reducing modes, tissue harmonic and compound imaging, and Doppler methods with improved sensitivity to slow flows. Nevertheless, color Doppler US is nondiagnostic in a small but significant number of cases. The more frequent causes of nondiagnostic color Doppler US are borderline stenosis or preocclusive internal carotid artery stenosis.

Intra-arterial digital subtraction angiography (DSA) is considered the reference procedure in the assessment of carotid stenosis, and DSA has become the standard of reference for selecting patients for carotid surgery (Nederkorn et al. 2003). However, DSA has several drawbacks, e.g., patient discomfort, its invasive nature, and the risk of complications. According to previous reports there is a 4% risk of transient ischemic attack or minor stroke, a 1% risk of major stroke, and even a small (<1%) risk of death (Hankey et al. 1990; Davies and Humphrey 1993). Therefore, noninvasive or minimally invasive techniques such as three-dimensional (3D) time-of-flight (TOF) magnetic resonance (MR) angiography and contrast-enhanced MR angiography (Back et al. 2000; Nederkorn et al. 2003) are increasingly being used as supplements to duplex US in the diagnosis of carotid artery stenosis. Recently, contrast-enhanced US, performed after the injection of a microbubble-based agent, has been proposed for the assessment of carotid artery stenosis (Kono et al. 2004).

E. Quaia, MD
Assistant Professor of Radiology, Department of Radiology, Cattinara Hospital, University of Trieste, Strada di Fiume 447, 34149 Trieste, Italy
F. Pozzi Mucelli, MD; A. Calgaro, MD
Department of Radiology, Cattinara Hospital, University of Trieste, Strada di Fiume 447, 34149 Trieste, Italy

8.2
Carotid and Vertebrobasilar Color Doppler US

The NASCET (1991) and ECST trials (1991) showed the strong benefit of endarterectomy in appropriate symptomatic patients with 70-90% internal carotid artery stenoses. In the NASCET method, the smallest internal carotid artery lumen diameter is compared to the distal internal carotid artery diameter, while in ECST the smallest internal carotid artery lumen diameter is compared with the estimated lumen diameter of the normal carotid bulb.

Numerous imaging and Doppler parameters are currently used at various laboratories for the evaluation of internal carotid artery stenosis, including peak systolic velocity (PSV), end-diastolic velocity (EDV), the ratio of PSV of the internal and the common carotid artery, EDV in the common carotid artery, and the ratio of EDV in the internal and the common carotid artery. The PSV measured in the internal carotid artery stenosis and the presence of plaque on gray-scale and/or color Doppler US are the parameters that should be used when diagnosing and grading stenosis (GRANT et al. 2003). The other parameters may be employed when the PSV may not be representative of the extent of disease owing to technical or clinical factors such as the presence of tandem lesions, contralateral high-grade stenosis, discrepancy between visual assessment of plaque and the PSV in the internal carotid artery, elevated velocity in the common carotid artery, hyperdynamic cardiac state, or low cardiac output (GRANT et al. 2003).

Analysis of the spectral Doppler waveforms has been successful in the detection of stenosis even though this is an indirect method of evaluating the degree of narrowing. Color and power Doppler US provide angiographic-like images of the carotid arteries that help delineate the lumen but are limited by low temporal or spatial resolution, angle dependence, and susceptibility to artifacts (KONO et al. 2004). Although Doppler imaging is reasonable in a number of situations, the represented flow and the vessel wall do not overlap in conditions in which flow is turbulent or disturbed by plaque or clot or when vascular tortuosity is present. Furthermore, regions of slow or small-volume flow, as occur in very tight stenoses and long narrow channels, may be invisible at Doppler imaging.

8.3
Contrast-Enhanced US of the Carotid Arteries

Microbubble-based contrast agents may be imaged by dedicated gray-scale contrast-specific modes such as phase inversion or multipulse techniques. The phase-inversion harmonic technique was found to be superior to the second harmonic technique for vascular imaging because of its higher spatial resolution, more effective tissue suppression, and higher sensitivity to flow (STEINBACH 1999).

Gray-scale filling of vessels with a microbubble-based agent was shown to be more reliable and more accurate than filling of vessels with color Doppler signal both in vitro and in an animal model (SIRLIN et al. 2001), and in humans (MATTREY and KONO 1999). The normal carotid bulb and the internal and external carotid arteries (Fig. 8.1) are clearly depicted by contrast-enhanced US, with accurate delineation of the external and internal borders of the carotid wall (Fig. 8.2).

High-frequency (5–10 MHz) linear-array transducers have to be employed to assess carotid arteries,

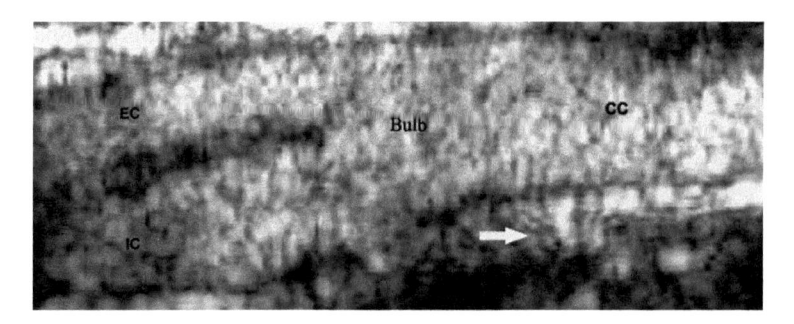

Fig. 8.1. Contrast-enhanced US angiography of the normal carotid bulb. Contrast-tuned imaging (Esaote, Genoa, Italy) with a high-frequency (3–10 MHz) linear transducer and low acoustic power insonation after the injection of sulfur hexafluoride-filled microbubbles. The common carotid (*CC*), internal carotid (*IC*), and external carotid (*EC*) arteries are clearly depicted by enhancing the acoustic backscattering from blood. A moderately high acoustic power (mechanical index = 0.3) is employed to increase the signal produced by microbubbles, in part from microbubble resonance and in part from microbubble destruction. However, the increased insonation power results in incomplete suppression of the background signal from stationary tissues (*arrow*).

Carotid Arteries

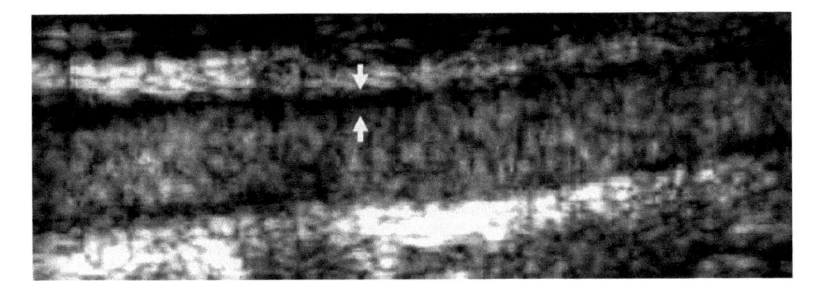

Fig. 8.2. Contrast-enhanced US angiography of the normal common carotid artery. Contrast-tuned imaging (Esaote, Genoa, Italy) with a high-frequency (3–10 MHz) linear transducer and low acoustic power insonation after the injection of sulfur hexafluoride-filled microbubbles. The vessel wall of the common carotid artery, at both the intimal and the adventitial side, is accurately delineated by the enhanced acoustic backscattering from blood owing to the microbubbles.

including after the injection of microbubble-based agents (Fig. 8.1). Nowadays, high-frequency linear-array transducers display lower sensitivity to microbubble resonance than do low-frequency curved-array transducers. This is because the resonance frequency is related to the diameter of the microbubbles, and most microbubbles present a resonance frequency of around 3–3.7 MHz, which is closer to the center frequency transmitted by low-frequency transducers than to that transmitted by high-frequency transducers. Consequently, the insonation produced by a high-frequency transducer results in the resonance of fewer microbubbles with a smaller diameter, and in the production of a lower signal. For these reasons, in contrast-enhanced US of carotid arteries it is reasonable to slightly increase the acoustic power of insonation (e.g., mechanical index of 0.3–0.4) in order to increase the signal, produced partly from microbubble destruction and partly from microbubble resonance. Nevertheless, this results in an incomplete suppression of the background signal from the stationary tissues (Fig. 8.1), which produce signal if the acoustic power insonation presents a mechanical index exceeding 0.15–0.2.

8.4
Advantages of Contrast-Enhanced US Compared to Baseline Color Doppler US

8.4.1
Quantification of Internal Carotid Artery Stenosis

Correct quantification of the percentage reduction in the carotid lumen by a plaque may be obtained by contrast-enhanced US (Figs. 8.3, 8.4). Correct quantification of internal carotid artery stenosis may be

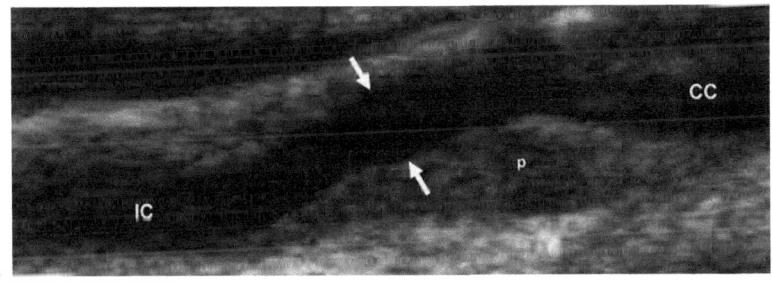

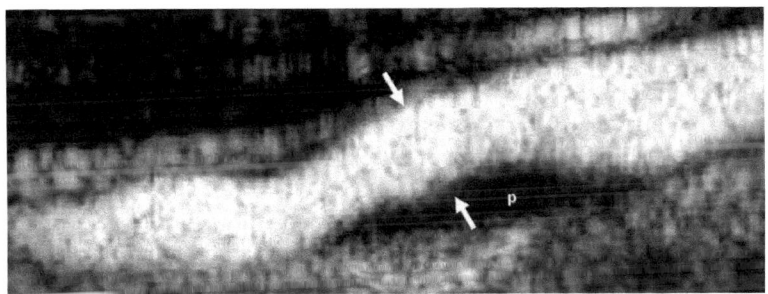

Fig. 8.3a,b. Contrast-enhanced US angiography of a fibrous plaque (*p*) in the carotid bulb. Baseline US (**a**) and contrast-enhanced US (**b**) after the injection of sulfur hexafluoride-filled microbubbles. Longitudinal plane. The residual lumen (*arrows*) of the vessel is clearly depicted by the enhanced acoustic backscattering from blood owing to the microbubbles. *CC* common carotid artery, *IC* internal carotid artery.

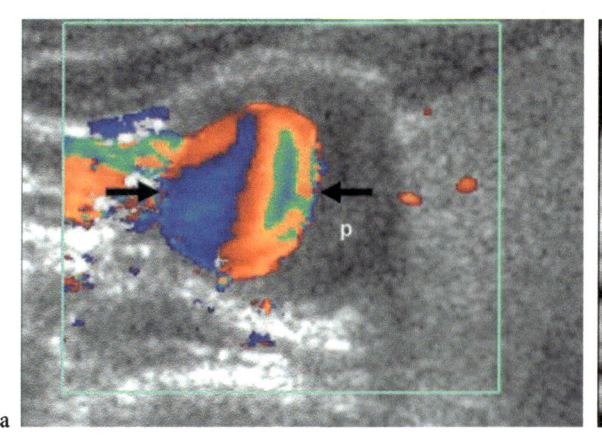

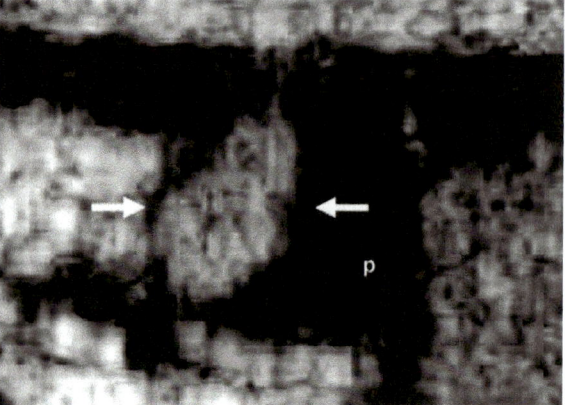

Fig. 8.4a,b. Contrast-enhanced US angiography of a fibrous plaque (*p*) in the carotid bulb. Baseline color Doppler US (a) and contrast-enhanced US (b) after the injection of sulfur hexafluoride-filled microbubbles. Axial plane. The residual lumen (*arrows*) of the vessel is clearly delineated by both color Doppler US and contrast enhanced US.

achieved by means of contrast-enhanced US after microbubble injection. According to the NASCET method (1991), the smallest internal carotid artery lumen diameter at the stenosis level is compared to the distal internal carotid artery diameter (Figs. 8.5, 8.6). Significant agreement has been shown between contrast-enhanced US and intra-arterial digital subtraction angiography in the quantification of internal carotid artery stenosis (Kono et al. 2004).

The ability to visualize the entire internal carotid artery lumen allows the accurate depiction of stenoses, with percentage stenosis values that are highly correlated with those obtained using conventional DSA (Kono et al. 2004). Furthermore, because US images also show the outer wall, the full thickness of the plaque is displayed (Fig. 8.4), which allows accurate monitoring of disease regression or progression (Sirlin et al. 2001).

The ability to depict the outer and inner margins in the transverse plane allows the measurement of percentage area reduction at the point of maximal narrowing. Percentage area narrowing values are more reliable than the percentage diameter stenosis because they are measured at the point of interest rather than at the distal vessel, where findings may or may not be normal (Kono et al. 2004). Furthermore, because stenoses can be eccentric, one would expect them to be more accurately measured on two-dimensional projections, as has been demonstrated by ex vivo measurements of resected carotid plaque at MR imaging (Kono et al. 2004).

The principal application of contrast-enhanced US in carotid artery disease is in differentiating tight stenoses from complete occlusion (Fig. 8.7). In particular, regions of slow flow or small-volume flow, such as channels in recanalized clots or very tight preocclusive stenoses, may not be identified by Doppler but are clearly depicted by contrast-enhanced US due to its higher spatial and time resolution (Sirlin et al. 1997). The correct differentiation of a preocclusive internal carotid artery stenosis from internal carotid artery occlusion is of fundamental importance for the decision on whether to adopt a surgical or a conservative approach.

8.4.2
Assessment of the Distal Internal Carotid Artery

Contrast-enhanced US also allows more effective assessment of the distal part of the internal carotid artery in comparison with color Doppler US. In particular, the part of the internal carotid artery immediately outside the cranium may be effectively assessed by contrast-enhanced US (Fig. 8.5c,d). Although contrast-enhanced US is not impaired by artifacts, such as the blooming that occurs in color Doppler US, acoustic shadowing or signal attenuation may be identified if a large dose of microbubbles has been employed (Kono et al. 2004).

8.4.3
Characterization of Atherosclerotic Plaques and Detection of Carotid Plaque Ulceration

Color Doppler US does not allow correct assessment of the surface of thrombotic atherosclerotic plaques owing to the limited spatial resolution, the presence

Carotid Arteries

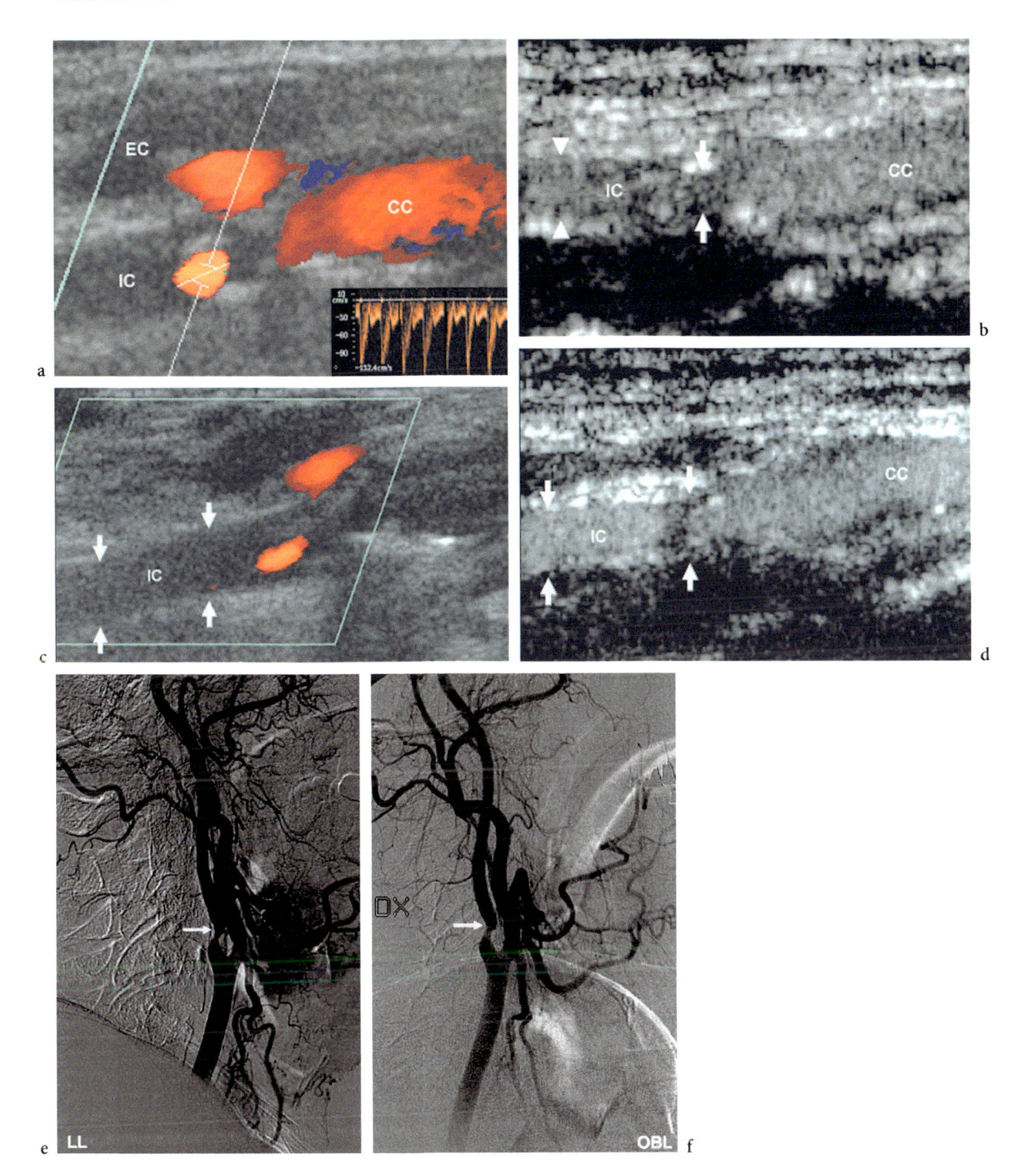

Fig. 8.5a–f. Improvement in the assessment of internal carotid artery stenosis and of the distal arterial segment by contrast-enhanced US in comparison with baseline color Doppler US. a Baseline power Doppler US does not allow accurate assessment of the right internal carotid (*IC*) artery stenosis (*arrows*) for the presence of a fibrocalcific plaque in the carotid bulb. b Contrast-enhanced US after the injection of sulfur hexafluoride-filled microbubbles allows assessment of the residual lumen of the internal carotid artery. Quantitation of internal carotid artery stenosis is performed by comparing the smallest diameter (*arrows*) of the arterial stenotic segment to the diameter of the distal internal carotid artery (*arrowheads*) according to the NASCET method (about 60% stenosis). c Baseline color Doppler US does not allow evaluation of the right internal carotid artery segment (*arrows*) distal to the fibrocalcific plaque in the bulb. d Contrast-enhanced US clearly depicts the distal internal carotid artery, revealing normal patency. e, f Right lateral (e) and oblique (f) intra-arterial digital subtraction angiography confirms the stenosis (about 60%) (*arrow*). *CC* common carotid artery, *EC* external carotid artery.

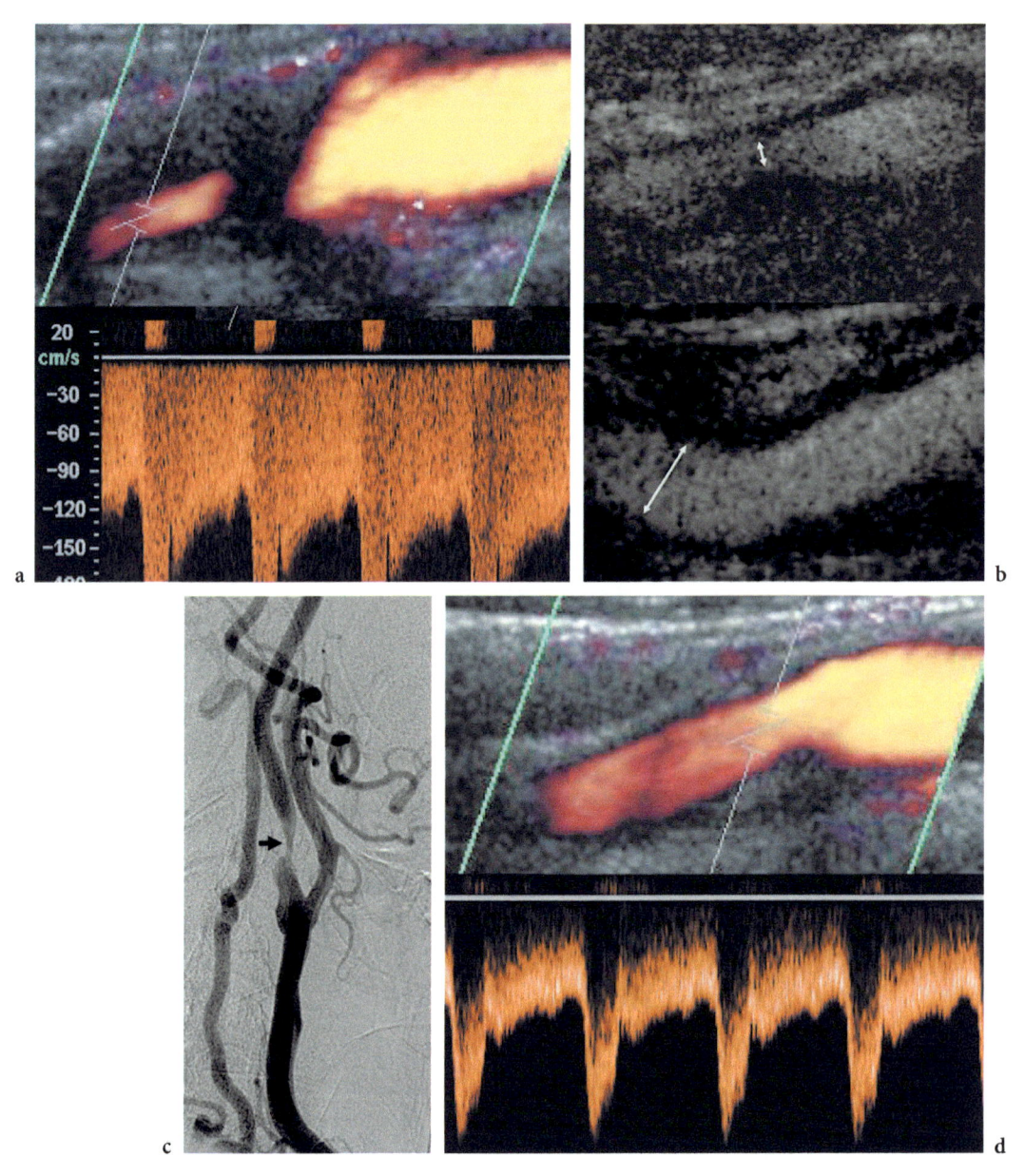

Fig. 8.6a–f. Further examples of improvement in the assessment of internal carotid artery stenosis and of the distal arterial segment by contrast-enhanced US in comparison with baseline color Doppler US. **a** Baseline power Doppler US does not allow assessment of the right internal carotid artery stenosis for the presence of a fibrocalcific plaque in the carotid bulb. Doppler interrogation (Doppler volume) is possible exclusively downstream of the calcific plaque, revealing high peak systolic velocity with spectral trace broadening. **b** Contrast-enhanced US after the injection of sulfur hexafluoride-filled microbubbles allows assessment of the residual lumen (*arrows*) of the internal carotid artery. By comparing the internal carotid artery lumen diameter at the stenosis (above) to the downstream internal carotid artery diameter (below), according to the NASCET method, the right internal carotid artery stenosis is quantified as 90%. **c** Lateral view of the right internal carotid artery on intra-arterial digital subtraction angiography. The high-grade stenosis (90%) of right internal carotid artery (*arrow*) is confirmed. **d** Baseline color Doppler US identifies a moderate stenosis caused by a fibrotic plaque in the left internal carotid artery (Doppler volume).

Carotid Arteries

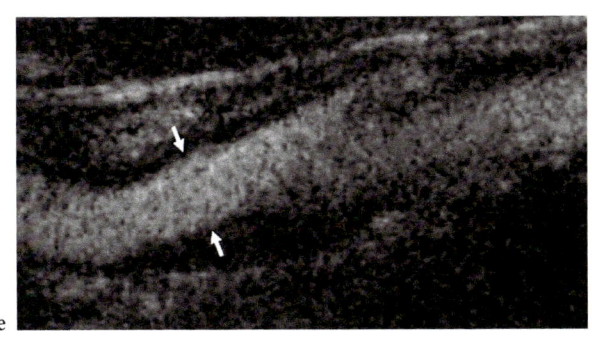

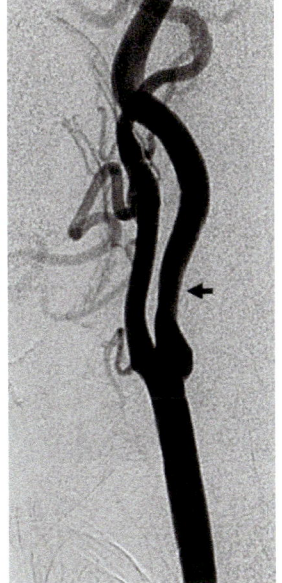

continued Fig. 8.6. e Contrast-enhanced US allows a clear depiction of the residual lumen of the left internal carotid artery. The stenosis is quantified as 40%. **f** Lateral view of the left internal carotid artery on intra-arterial digital subtraction angiography. The low-grade stenosis of the left internal carotid artery (*arrow*) is confirmed.

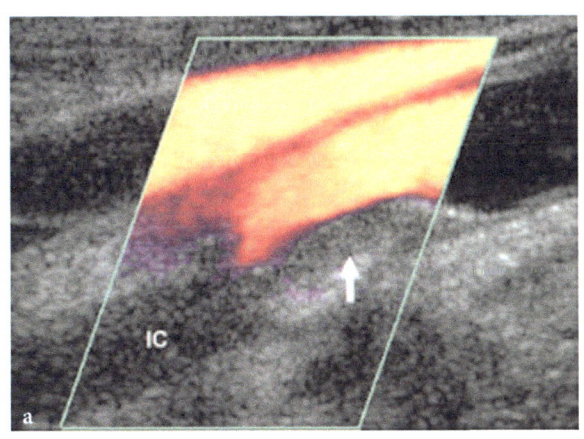

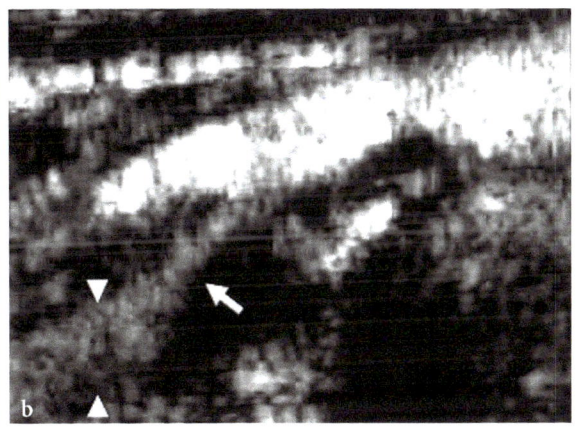

Fig. 8.7a–d. Improvement in the assessment of preocclusive internal carotid artery stenosis by contrast-enhanced US in comparison with baseline color Doppler US. **a** Baseline power Doppler US reveals a fibrous plaque (*arrow*) in the right carotid bulb without revealing the residual lumen of the internal carotid (*IC*) artery. **b** Contrast-enhanced US after the injection of sulfur hexafluoride-filled microbubbles allows correct visualization of the residual lumen of the internal carotid artery (*arrow*), revealing a reduction in the lumen diameter of about 90–95%. The quantitation is performed by comparing the smallest diameter (*arrow*) of the stenotic segment to the diameter (*arrowheads*) of the distal internal carotid artery according to the NASCET method. **c, d** Right anteroposterior (c) and laterolateral (d) intra-arterial digital subtraction angiography confirms preocclusive internal carotid artery stenosis (about 95%) (*arrow*).

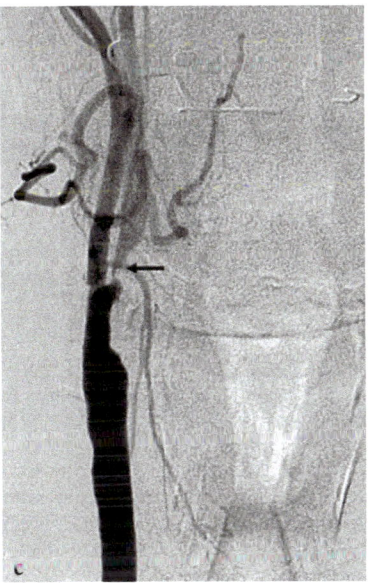

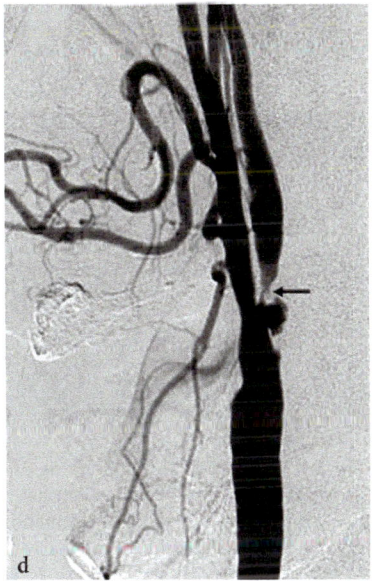

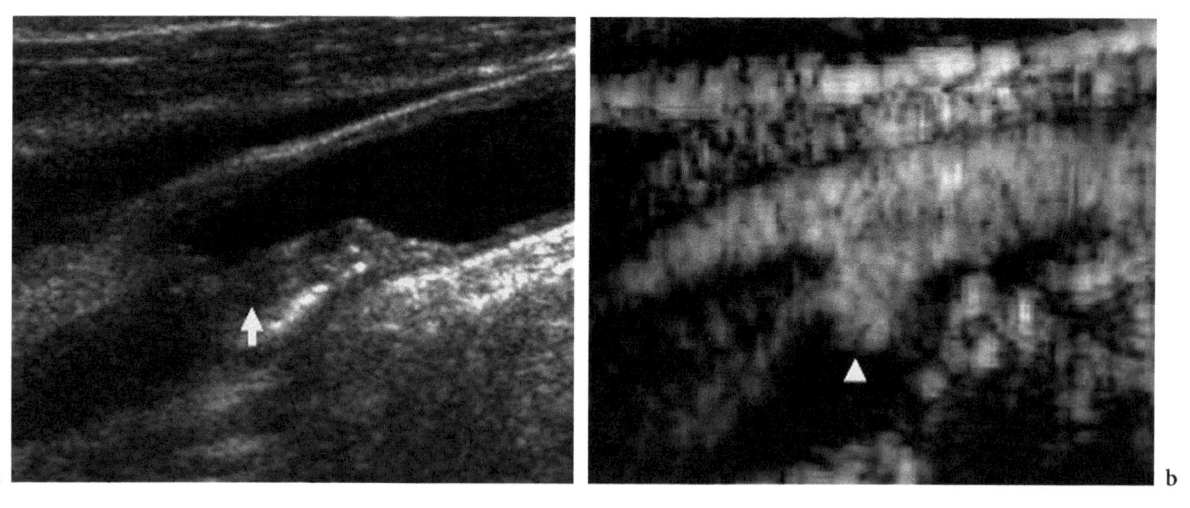

Fig. 8.8. a Baseline US reveals a fibrotic plaque in the right carotid bulb (*arrow*). **b** Contrast-enhanced US after injection of sulfur hexafluoride-filled microbubbles reveals ulceration (*arrowhead*) in the plaque in the carotid bulb.

of artifacts and superimposition of color pixels at the plaque borders. Nowadays, contrast-specific modes offer high spatial resolution and permit the elimination of artifacts. For these reasons, the border of a complicated plaque, such as an ulcerative or hemorrhagic plaque (Fig. 8.8), may be effectively identified and characterized after microbubble injection.

Contrast-enhanced US can clearly depict plaque ulcerations and recanalization not detected on Doppler US images because of the effect of turbulence, flow disturbance, or slow flow (Kono et al. 2004). Moreover, contrast-enhanced US has further advantages over color Doppler US, such as independence from the angle of incidence and absence of the technical parameters necessary for optimal filling of vessels on color Doppler US (Kono et al. 2004).

8.5
Limitations of Contrast-Enhanced US in the Assessment of Carotid Arteries

Contrast-enhanced US of the carotid arteries does have various limitations. First, like color Doppler US, contrast-enhanced US is of limited value in the presence of grossly calcific plaque, the only possible solution being to examine the vessels before and after the acoustic shadowing caused by the plaque. This limitation is obvious, given that US transmission is almost completely arrested behind a calcific interface, and severe calcifications hinder full visualization of the residual carotid lumen even in comparison with color Doppler US (Figs. 8.9, 8.10).

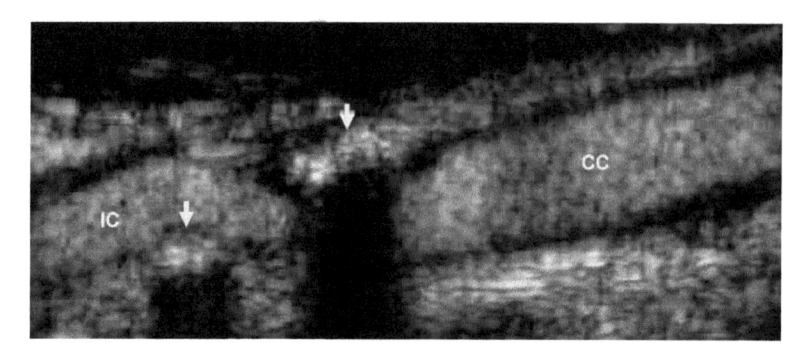

Fig. 8.9. Example of the limitations of contrast-enhanced US angiography in the presence of extensively calcified plaques (*arrows*) of the carotid bulb. Contrast-tuned imaging (Esaote, Genoa, Italy) with a high-frequency (3–10 MHz) linear transducer and low acoustic power insonation after injection of sulfur hexafluoride-filled microbubbles. At the level of carotid blub, the lumen of the vessel cannot be assessed owing to the posterior acoustic shadowing caused by the calcific component of the plaque. *CC* common carotid artery, *IC* internal carotid artery.

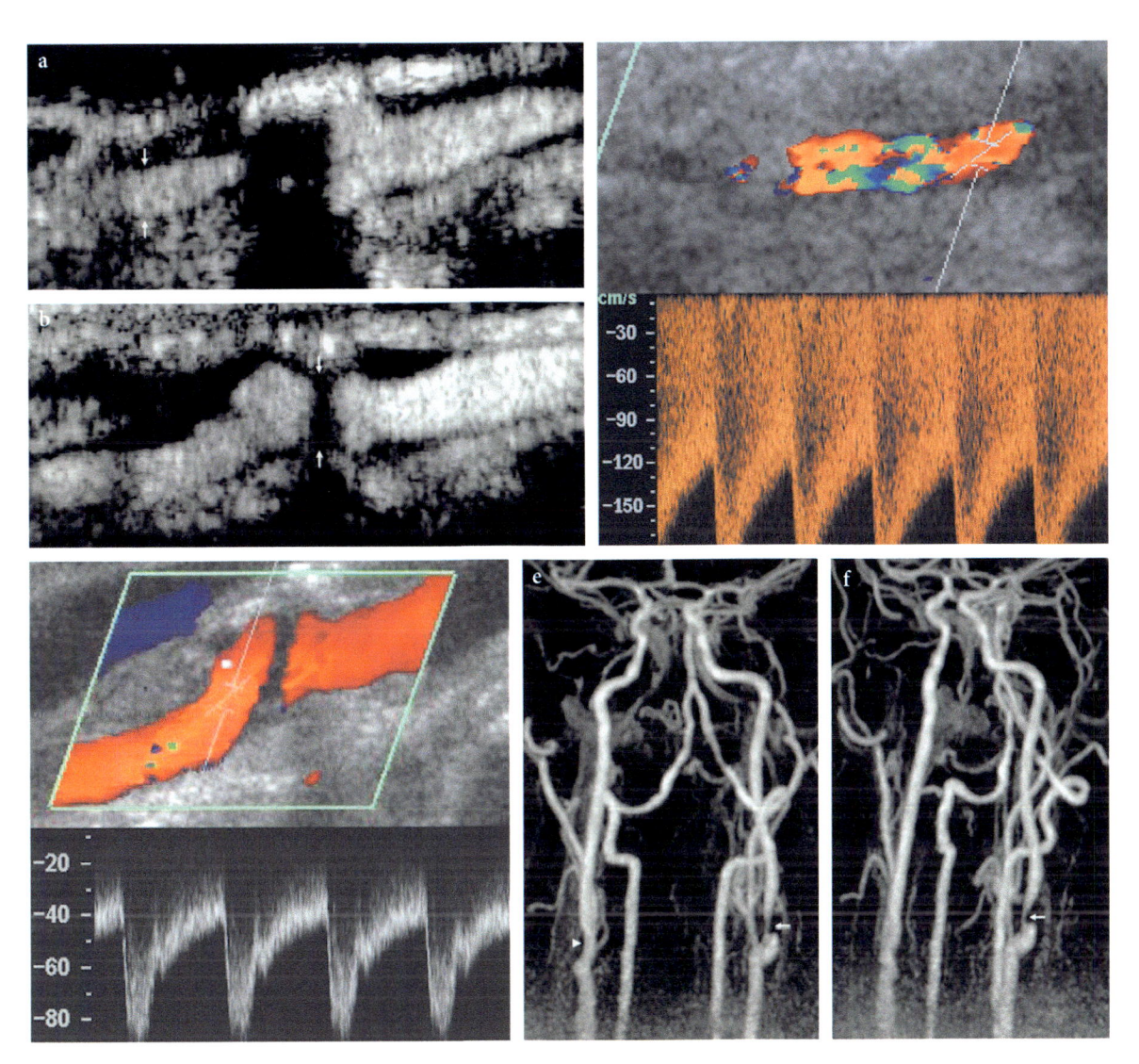

Fig. 8.10a–f. Further example of the limitations of contrast-enhanced US angiography in the presence of extensively calcified plaques of the carotid bulb. a, b Contrast-enhanced US angiography after the injection of sulfur hexafluoride-filled microbubbles. The tight stenosis of the left internal carotid artery (a) cannot be assessed owing to the posterior acoustic shadowing caused by the calcified component of the plaque, while the distal tract of the internal carotid artery (*arrows*) is clearly depicted. The presence of a calcified plaque in the right carotid bulb (b) resulted in posterior acoustic shadowing. c Color Doppler US of the left internal carotid artery with Doppler interrogation of the arterial segment immediately distal to the calcified plaque. The spectral broadening with an increase in the peak systolic velocity reveals a tight stenosis (about 90%). d Color Doppler US of the right internal carotid artery with Doppler interrogation. The regular Doppler trace allows exclusion of a significant stenosis. e, f Contrast-enhanced MR angiography confirms a tight stenosis of the left internal carotid artery (*arrow*) and a nonstenosing plaque (*arrowhead*) in the right bulb.

Second, contrast-enhanced US cannot assess velocimetric parameters related to the grade of stenosis but only geometric parameters related to carotid lumen reduction. Velocimetric parameters still have to be evaluated by Doppler interrogation of the vessels.

Third, dedicated contrast-specific modes have to be employed after the injection of microbubble-based agents. The use of contrast-enhanced color Doppler US is still not acceptable because of the presence of many artifacts, such as color blooming and spike artifacts in the Doppler trace (Fig. 8.11).

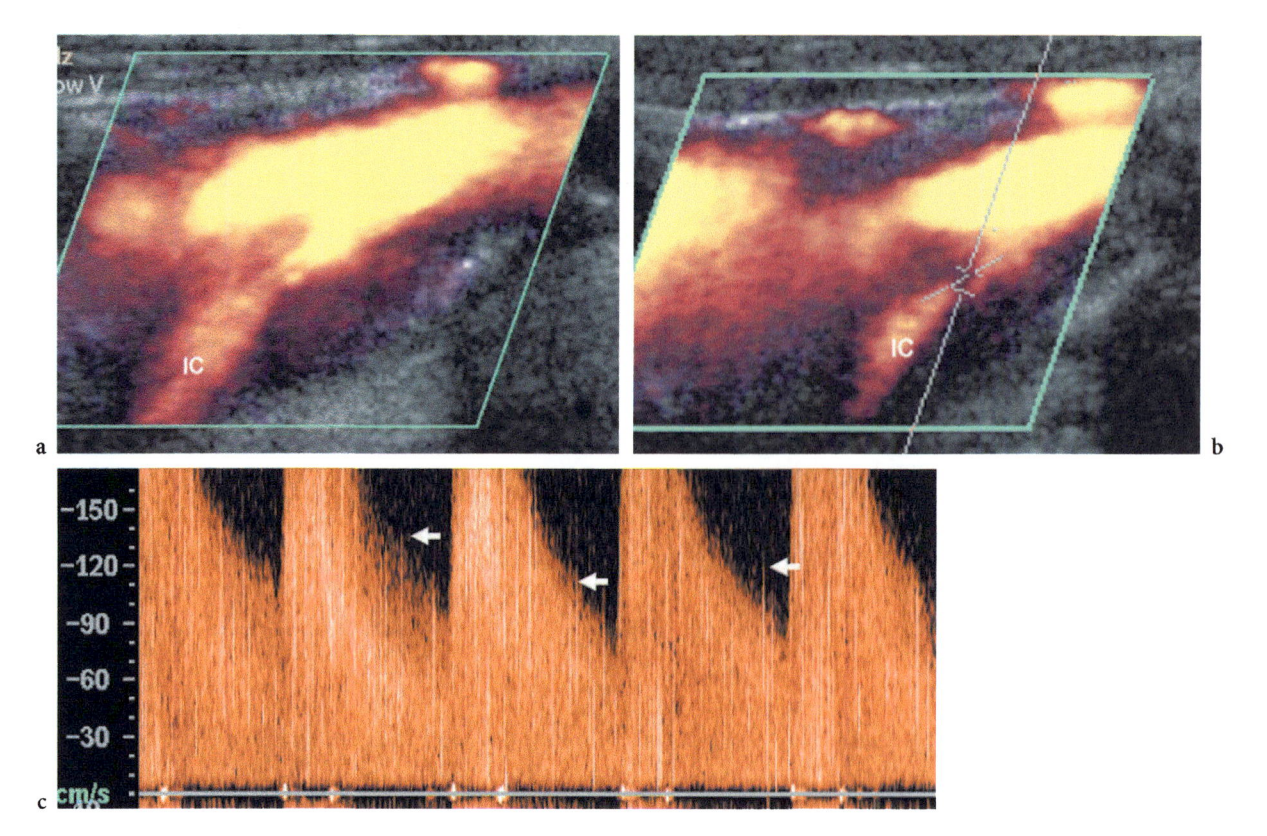

Fig. 8.11a–c. Power Doppler US with Doppler interrogation of the internal carotid artery after microbubble injection reveals spectral broadening with a markedly increased peak systolic velocity at the internal carotid artery. Extensive blooming artifacts, with color signal outside the vessel wall, are visible. Moreover, spike artifacts (*arrows*) from macrobubble aggregates or microbubble collapse are identifiable in the spectral trace (c).

References

Back MR, Wilson JS, Rushing G et al (2000) Magnetic resonance angiography is an accurate imaging adjunct to duplex ultrasound scan in patient selection for carotid endarterectomy. J Vasc Surg 32:429-438

Davies KN, Humphrey PR (1993) Complications of cerebral angiography in patients with symptomatic carotid territory ischaemia screened by carotid ultrasound. J Neurol Neurosurg Psychiatry 56:967-972

European Carotid Surgery Trialists' Collaborative Group (1991) MRC European Carotid Surgery Trial: interim results for symptomatic patients with severe (70–99%) or with mild (0–29%) carotid stenosis. Lancet 337:1235-1243

Executive Committee for the Asymptomatic Carotid Atherosclerosis Study (1995) Endarterectomy for asymptomatic carotid artery stenosis. JAMA 273:1421-1428

Grant EG, Benson CB, Moneta GL et al (2003) Carotid artery stenosis: gray-scale and Doppler US diagnosis - Society of Radiologists in Ultrasound Consensus Conference. Radiology 229:340-346

Hankey GJ, Warlow CP, Sellar RJ (1990) Cerebral angiographic risk in mild cerebrovascular disease. Stroke 21:209-222

Kono Y, Pinnell SP, Sirlin CB et al (2004) Carotid arteries: contrast-enhanced US angiography - preliminary clinical experience. Radiology 230:561-568

Mattrey RF, Kono Y (1999) Contrast-specific imaging and potential vascular applications. Eur Radiol 9 [Suppl 3]:S353-S358

Nederkoorn PJ, Elgersma OEH, van der Graaf Y et al (2003) Carotid artery stenosis: accuracy of contrast-enhanced MR angiography for diagnosis. Radiology 228:677-682

North American Symptomatic Carotid Endarterectomy Trial collaborators (1991) Beneficial effect of carotid endarterectomy in symptomatic patients with high-grade carotid stenosis. N Engl J Med 325:445-453

Sirlin CB, Steinbach GC, Girard MS et al (1997) Improved visualization of the arterial luminal surface in replicas of diseased human carotids using ultrasound contrast media. J Ultrasound Med 16:S62

Sirlin CB, Lee YZ, Girard MS et al (2001) Contrast-enhanced B-mode US angiography in the assessment of experimental in vivo and in vitro atherosclerotic disease. Acad Radiol 8:162-172

Steinbach GC (1999) Contrast-specific instrumentation and its potential applications. In: Thomsen HS, Muller R, Mattrey RF (eds) Trends in contrast media. Medical radiology: diagnostic imaging and radiation oncology series. Springer, Berlin Heidelberg New York, pp 321-332

9 Detection of Endoleak After Endovascular Abdominal Aortic Aneurysm Repair

Emilio Quaia

CONTENTS

9.1 Introduction 111
9.2 Contrast-Enhanced US 112
References 114

9.1 Introduction

Endovascular abdominal aortic aneurysm repair is considered an accepted alternative to standard open surgery. Endoleaks are defined as areas of persistent blood flow outside the lumen of the endograft after endovascular aortic aneurysm repair, either within the aneurysm sac or within connected vascular segments bypassed by the graft (White et al. 1997). Persistent leaks are associated with outflow vessels that contribute to the patency of leaks (Görich et al. 2000). The evidence of blood flow in the aneurysm sac (perigraft leak or endoleak) is a meaningful predictor of clinical outcome after successful endovascular aneurysm repair (Rozenblit et al. 2003). Persistent perigraft flow within an abdominal aortic aneurysm remains the most common complication of endovascular graft placement and is considered a failure of the procedure since it is associated with aneurysm enlargement and even rupture (van Marrewijk et al. 2002; Corriere et al. 2004). The incidence of endoleaks ranges from 5% to 65% (Greenberg 2003; Corriere et al. 2004; Dalainas et al. 2004; Engellau et al. 2004; Napoli et al. 2004). Following endovascular abdominal aortic aneurysm repair, lifelong surveillance by imaging is required to identify leaks since patients with endoleak may require additional endovascular interventions or conversion to open repair (Corriere et al. 2004). No criteria currently exist for cessation or reduction in frequency of screening imaging studies (Corriere et al. 2004).

E. Quaia, MD
Assistant Professor of Radiology, Department of Radiology, Cattinara Hospital, University of Trieste, Strada di Fiume 447, 34149 Trieste, Italy

Endoleaks are classified into four types: type I, failure to obtain a complete seal at a proximal or distal graft attachment site; type II, retrograde reconstitution of the excluded aneurysmal portion of the aorta from collateral arterial branches, such as lumbar and mesenteric artery branches (White et al. 1997); type III, graft disruption (White et al. 1997); and type IV, graft porosity (White et al. 1998). Types III and IV are rarer than types I and II. Type I and type III endoleaks are associated with an increased risk of rupture of the aneurysm (Buth et al. 2003) and should be corrected, preferably by endovascular means. If endovascular repair is not possible, then open conversion should be considered. Type IV endoleak is also correlated with an increased need for secondary interventions. These types of endoleak need to be treated without delay, and when no other possibilities are present, an open conversion to eliminate the risk of rupture should be considered. Small reconstitution type II endoleaks do not pose an indication for urgent treatment since many of them will occlude spontaneously (Greenfield et al. 2002). However, they may not be harmless, because there is a frequent association with enlargement of aneurysm and reinterventions. Intervention is primarily indicated if expansion of the aneurysm is documented (Buth et al. 2003).

Those cases of aneurysm enlargement in which no cause is identified by imaging modalities have been classified as endotension or type V endoleak (White et al. 1999; White 2001; Lin et al. 2003). They are caused by pressure transmission through the thrombus at the attachment site or by very low flow endoleak. The treatment of type V endoleak is controversial.

Although color Doppler ultrasound (US) may detect substantial perigraft leaks (Greenfield et al. 2002; Raman et al. 2003), contrast-enhanced computed tomography (CT) is considered the reference imaging procedure for detecting the origin of the perigraft leak, the outflow vessels, and the complications related to endoluminal treatment of aortic aneurysms (Golzarian et al. 1998, 2002;

Thurnher and Cejna 2002). Recently, contrast-enhanced MR imaging has also been proposed for the follow-up of endovascular abdominal aneurysm repair (Cejna et al. 2002; Ayuso et al. 2004; Ersoy et al. 2004).

Examinations performed to screen patients for endoleaks after stent graft placement commonly include contrast-enhanced CT angiography (Rozenblit et al. 2003). CT angiography is an operator-independent, reproducible examination and is not limited by the presence of bowel gas, which is often a problem for duplex US in the early postoperative period. Delayed scan at 2–3 min after injection of iodinated contrast agent improves endoleak detection (Rozenblit et al. 2003). Recognized limitations of serial CT angiographic examinations include repeated radiation exposure, the need to use intravenous contrast material with potential risk of allergy and nephrotoxicity, the relatively high cost (D'Auddiffret et al. 2001), and the impossibility of depicting the velocity or direction of the blood flow causing the endoleak.

Contrast-enhanced US has displayed good capabilities in revealing the perigraft endoleak after endovascular repair of aortic aneurysm (McWilliams et al. 1999, 2002; Aiani et al. 2004; Napoli et al. 2004), allowing identification of the blood flow direction and providing information regarding the origin and mechanisms of the endoleak.

9.2
Contrast-Enhanced US

From 20 to 25 s after microbubble-based agent injection, the entire aorta has to be scanned in both the longitudinal and the transverse plane, from the diaphragm to below the iliac limb attachment sites (Napoli et al. 2004). The limits of the endoluminal graft are well identified after microbubble-based agent injection (Fig. 9.1).

The presence of endoleak is identified through the evidence of active staining of the aortic lumen outside the graft after microbubble injection. This may be identified at the proximal or the distal graft attachment site (Fig. 9.2) or outside the lateral tract of the aortic graft, through collateral arterial branches or graft disruption or porosity (Fig. 9.3). As for contrast-enhanced CT (Rozenblit et al. 2003), delayed scans at 2–4 min after microbubble injection may improve endoleak detection (Fig. 9.3).

The main advantages of contrast-enhanced US over CT are the absence of radiation exposure and the avoidance of iodinated contrast agent injection in patients who frequently present with a reduced renal function. These are important advantages for an imaging procedure which has to be employed in lifelong follow-up, and the latter precludes the risk of allergy and nephrotoxicity associated with iodinated contrast agents. Moreover, contrast-enhanced US is noninvasive and fast and has a higher temporal resolution (time required to produce an image) and a higher sensitivity to the contrast material than CT. Contrast-enhanced US also offers the possibility of detecting dynamically the origin of endoleak if low transmit power insonation is employed. The only limitation is that contrast-enhanced US can be performed for the analysis of only one defined area of the aneurysm with continuous imaging. If the site of endoleak is not known at the time of scanning, a second bolus of microbubble-based agent may be required to image the aneurysm at a different level (Napoli et al. 2004).

Because of its advantages, contrast-enhanced US is becoming a very important diagnostic tool in the evaluation of patients with suspected endoleak at contrast-enhanced CT.

Detection of Endoleak After Endovascular Abdominal Aortic Aneurysm Repair 113

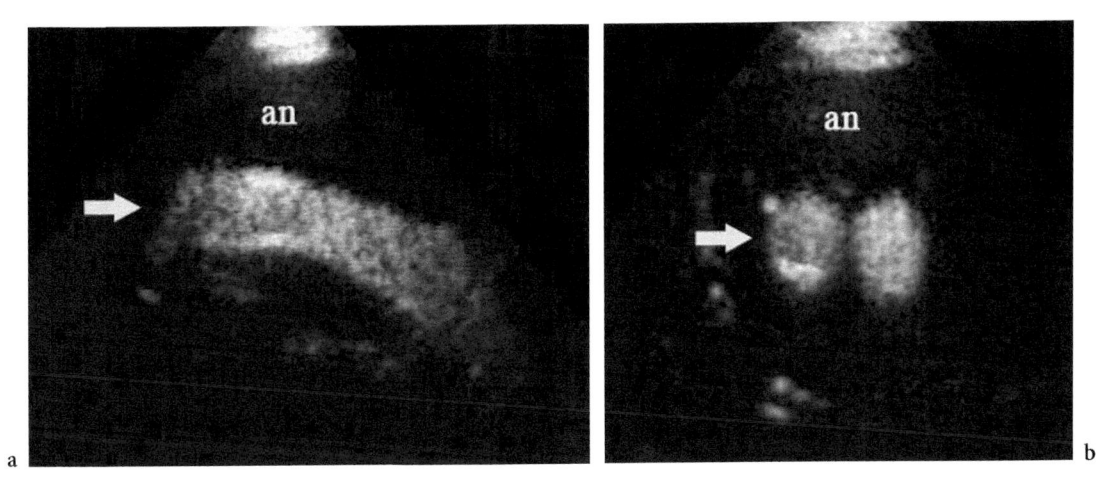

Fig. 9.1a,b. Normal endoluminal staining of the aortic graft (*arrow*) after microbubble-based agent injection at low acoustic power insonation. In the longitudinal plane (**a**) the graft is represented in its aortic branch (*arrow*), while the transverse scan (**b**) represents both branches (*arrow*) of the graft positioned in the common iliac arteries. *an* aneurysm.

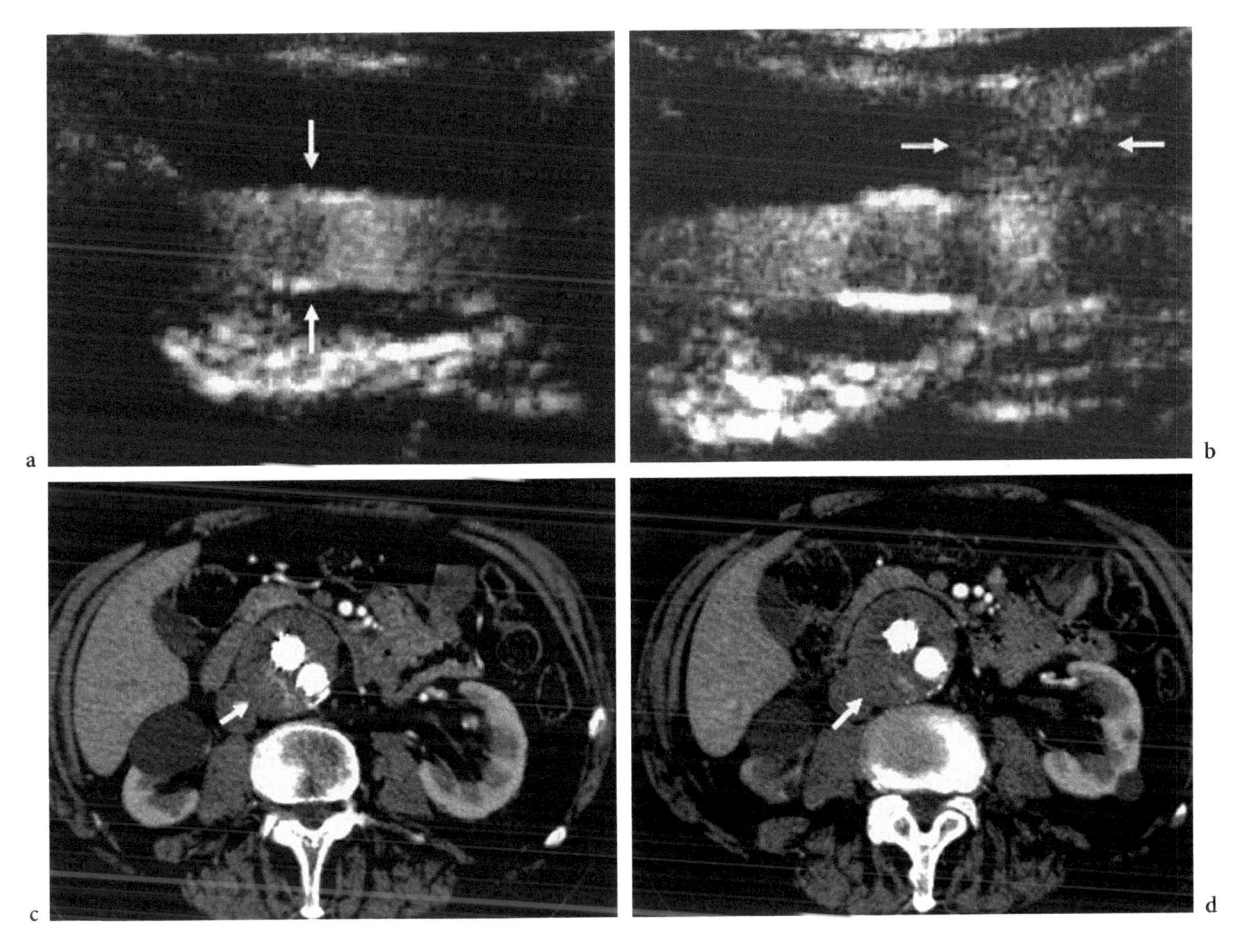

Fig. 9.2a–d. Evidence of endoleak through the distal graft attachment site of the endoluminal graft. Type I endoleak. **a, b** Contrast-enhanced US after the injection of sulfur hexafluoride filled microbubbles. The graft (*arrows*) shows complete filling after microbubble injection (**a**), and there is an endoleak at the level of the distal portion of the graft corresponding to the common iliac arteries. **c, d** Contrast-enhanced CT confirms the US findings. Endoleak is identified in the distal portion of the aortic aneurysm at the level of the common iliac arteries.

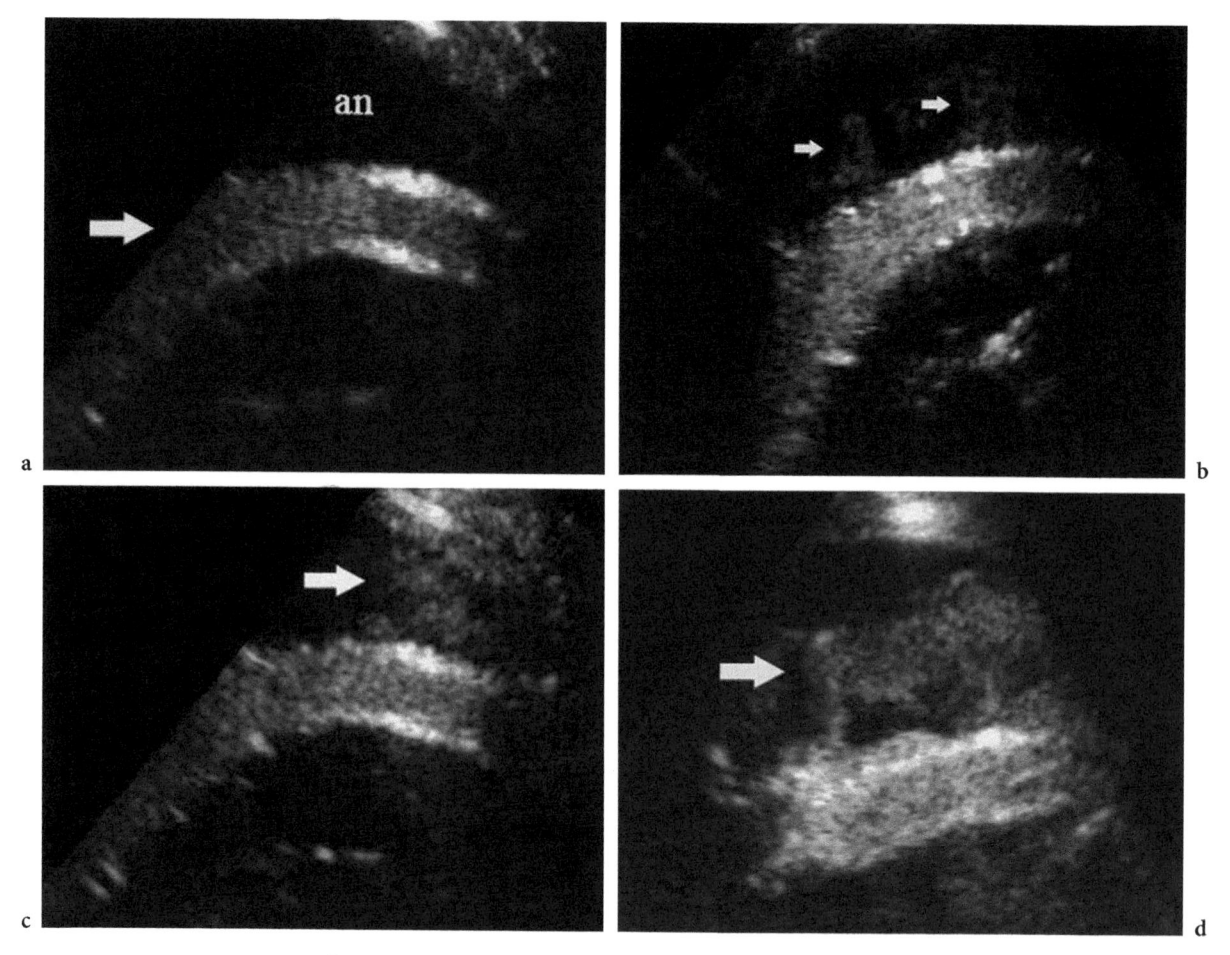

Fig. 9.3a–d. Type I endoleak: evidence of endoleak due to graft porosity. **a** Filling of the graft after microbubble injection (*arrow*). **b** Evidence of endoleak via graft porosity 40 s after microbubble injection. **c, d** Endoleak becomes more evident on delayed scan performed 2 min after microbubble injection.

References

Aiani L, del Favero C, Sopransi M et al (2004) Follow-up of aortic percutaneous endoprostheses with contrast-enhanced ultrasound (CEUS) performed at low mechanical index (MI) and with a II generation contrast agent (abstract). RSNA 2004

Ayuso JR, de Caralt TM, Pages M, et al (2004) MRA is useful as a follow-up technique after endovascular repair of aortic aneurysms with nitinol endoprostheses. J Magn Reson Imaging 20:803-810

Buth J, Harris PL, van Marrewijk C, Fransen G (2003) The significance and management of different types of endoleaks. Semin Vasc Surg 16:95-102

Cejna M, Loewe C, Schoder M et al (2002) MR angiography vs CT angiography in the follow-up of nitinol stent grafts in endoluminal treated aortic aneurysms. Eur Radiol 12:2443-2450

Corriere MA, Feurer ID, Becker SY et al (2004) Endoleak following endovascular abdominal aortic aneurysm repair: implications for duration of screening. Ann Surg 239:800-807

Dalainas I, Nano G, Casana R, Tealdi Dg D (2004) Mid-term results after endovascular repair of abdominal aortic aneurysms: a four-year experience. Eur J Vasc Endovasc Surg 27:319-323

D'Audiffret A, Desgranges P, Kobeiter DH et al (2001) Follow-up evaluation of endoluminally treated abdominal aortic aneurysms with duplex ultrasonography: validation with computed tomography. J Vasc Surg 33:42-50

Engellau L, Albrechtsson U, Norgren L, Larsson EM (2004) Long-term results after endovascular repair of abdominal aortic aneurysms with the Stentor and Vanguard stent-graft. Acta Radiol 45:275-283

Ersoy H, Jacobs P, Kent CK, Prince MR (2004) Blood pool MR angiography of aortic stent-graft endoleak. AJR Am J Roentgenol 182:1181-1186

Golzarian J, Dussaussois L, Abada HT et al (1998) Helical CT of aorta after endoluminal stent-graft repair: value of biphasic acquisition. AJR Am J Roentgenol 171:329-331

Golzarian J, Murgo S, Dussaussois L et al (2002) Evaluation of abdominal aortic aneurysm after endoluminal treatment. AJR Am J Roentgenol 178:623-628

Görich J, Rilinger N, Kramer S et al (2000) Angiography of leaks after endovascular repair of infrarenal aortic aneurysms. AJR Am J Roentgenol 174:811-814

Greenfield AL, Halpern EJ, Bonn J (2002) Application of duplex US for characterization of endoleaks in abdominal aortic stent-grafts: report of five cases. Radiology 225:845-851

Greenberg R; Zenith Investigators (2003) The Zenith AAA endovascular graft for abdominal aortic aneurysms: clinical update. Semin Vasc Surg 16:151-157

Lin PH, Bush RL, Katzman JB et al (2003) Delayed aortic aneurysm enlargement due to endotension after endovascular abdominal aortic aneurysm repair. J Vasc Surg 38:840-842

McWilliams RG, Martin J, White D et al (1999) Use of contrast-enhanced ultrasound in follow-up after endovascular aortic aneurysm repair. J Vasc Interv Radiol 10:1107-1114

McWilliams RG, Martin J, White D et al (2002) Detection of endoleak with enhanced ultrasound imaging: comparison with biphasic computed tomography. J Endovasc Ther 9:170-179

Napoli V, Bargellini I, Sardella SG et al (2004) Abdominal aortic aneurysm: contrast-enhanced US for missed endoleaks after endoluminal repair. Radiology 233:217-225

Raman KG, Missig Carroll N, Richardson T et al (2003) Color-flow duplex ultrasound scan versus computed tomographic scan in the surveillance of endovascular aneurysm repair. J Vasc Surg 38:645-651

Rozenblit AM, Patlas M, Rosenbaum AT et al (2003) Detection of endoleaks after endovascular repair of abdominal aortic aneurysm: value of unenhanced and delayed helical CT acquisitions. Radiology 227:426-433

Thurnher S, Cejna M (2002) Imaging of aortic stent graft and endoleaks. Radiol Clin North Am 40:799-833

Van Marrewijk C, Buth J, Harris PL et al (2002) Significance of endoleaks after endovascular repair of abdominal aortic aneurysms: the EUROSTAR experience. J Vasc Surg 35:461-473

White GH (2001) What are the causes of endotension? J Endovasc Ther 8:454-456

White GH, Yu W, May J et al (1997) Endoleak as a complication of endoluminal grafting of abdominal aortic aneurysms: classification, incidence, diagnosis, and management. J Endovasc Surg 4:152-168

White GH, May J, Waugh RC et al (1998) Type III and type IV endoleak: toward a complete definition of blood flow in the sac after endoluminal AAA repair. J Endovasc Surg 5:305-309

White GH, May J, Petrasek P et al (1999) Endotension: an explanation for continued AAA growth after successful endoluminal repair. J Endovasc Surg 6:308-315

10 Renal Arteries

Emilio Quaia

CONTENTS

10.1 Introduction 117
10.2 Baseline Color and Power Doppler US 117
10.3 Contrast-Enhanced US 118
References 121

10.1
Introduction

Renal arterial stenosis, normally associated with widespread atherosclerosis, may manifest in different clinical situations and is the most frequent cause of secondary hypertension. It may be a causal factor in renovascular hypertension and renal insufficiency, and it accounts for up to 15% of cases of chronic renal failure. The documented prevalence of renal arterial stenosis varies from 0.5% to over 20% and depends on many factors, including the age of the patient and the degree of investigation (BERGLUND et al. 1976). Nevertheless, the prevalence of detected renal arterial stenosis is likely to increase with the age of the population and the widespread use of noninvasive screening tests (HAVEY et al. 1985).

Renal artery stenosis is potentially curable with percutaneous transluminal angioplasty, endovascular stent placement, or surgical revascularization. For this reason, many noninvasive imaging methods have been applied to screen renal artery stenosis. Although to date the definitive diagnosis of renal arterial stenosis has been made by means of intra-arterial digital subtraction angiography, color Doppler ultrasound (US), helical computed tomographic (CT) angiography, captopril renography, and magnetic resonance (MR) angiography have all been assessed in the diagnosis of renal arterial stenosis. While these techniques have been reported to have a sensitivity and specificity exceeding 90% in selected cases, they all have limitations (DAVIDSON and WILCOX 1992) and none of them fulfill the ideal criteria of being noninvasive and cheap and having a high sensitivity and high negative predictive value (CORREAS et al. 1999).

10.2
Baseline Color and Power Doppler US

The pathology of the renal artery (main or accessory) includes stenosis and obstruction. The detection of renal artery stenosis usually arises from a clinical or laboratory context in which the presence of renovascular hypertension is strongly suspected. Baseline color Doppler US is often employed as the first-line procedure to detect renal artery stenosis (CORREAS et al. 2003) in patients at risk for renovascular hypertension. Doppler US is cheap, easy to perform, widely available, and noninvasive (CORREAS et al. 1999). The diagnostic performance of color Doppler US in renal artery stenosis relies principally on perfect knowledge of the diagnostic criteria and the limitations of the imaging procedure (HELENON et al. 1998) and is operator dependent (CORREAS et al. 1999). A screening strategy based on Doppler US appears to be cost-effective; it decreases the number of diagnostic angiographic procedures and increases the number of patients with renovascular hypertension who can benefit from an appropriate renovascularization procedure (CORREAS et al. 1999). Morphological findings at color Doppler US of renal artery stenosis include focal narrowing, thickening, and calcification of the arterial wall, indicating an atherosclerotic lesion, and a typical beady appearance in cases of fibromuscular dysplasia (CORREAS et al. 1999). Color Doppler US was found to be effective in the identification of renal artery aneurysm, arteriovenous fistula,

E. QUAIA, MD
Assistant Professor of Radiology, Department of Radiology, Cattinara Hospital, University of Trieste, Strada di Fiume 447, 34149 Trieste, Italy

and distal occlusive disease (HELENON et al. 1995). Power Doppler US has a reduced angle dependence compared to color Doppler and is usually employed in technically challenging cases (HELENON et al. 1998). Moreover, power Doppler allows better morphologic appreciation of atherosclerotic changes in the renal artery wall, resulting in an improved diagnostic performance especially in hemodynamically nonsignificant plaques and in the differentiation between subocclusive renal artery stenosis and occlusion (HELENON et al. 1998).

There are two methods to identify renal artery stenosis. The first method corresponds to Doppler interrogation of the renal artery/arteries to detect direct signs of stenosis, while the second is Doppler assessment of the arterial waveform in intrarenal vessels for the identification of abnormalities suggestive of a more proximal stenosis involving the main renal artery. It is appropriate to employ both methods of evaluation to detect renal artery stenosis.

Velocimetric analysis of the Doppler trace derived from renal arteries is of primary importance to identify renal artery stenosis. Direct Doppler criteria have been proposed for the detection of renal arterial stenosis, including an increased peak systolic velocity (>150–180 cm/s) and end-diastolic velocity at the level of the stenosis (CORREAS et al. 1999; GRANT and MELANY 2001), post-stenotic flow disturbance resulting in spectral broadening and reversed flow (CORREAS et al. 1999), increased ratio (≥3.5) of peak systolic velocity in the renal artery and aorta (renal-aortic ratio), and presence of turbulence within the renal artery (DESBERG et al. 1990; HELENON et al. 1995). Although this technique is easy to perform, its accuracy is questionable because the lack of an early systolic peak has a low sensitivity for moderate stenoses, and the waveform is dependent on the maintenance of vessel compliance, which limits its effectiveness in elderly patients and patients with atherosclerosis (BUDE et al. 1994; BUDE and RUBIN 1995).

Downstream hemodynamic repercussions of renal artery stenosis in the distal intrarenal arterial bed may be identified by Doppler US and may provide an indirect diagnosis of renal artery stenosis. Numerous parameters are still being debated (CORREAS et al. 1999) except in cases of critical stenosis (>80%). In fact, even though examination of intraparenchymal arteries is technically easier than evaluation of the main renal artery, Doppler US findings in interlobar and arcuate renal cortical arteries are less reliable than those at the stenotic site. This is because downstream repercussions are absent in 20% of cases of tight stenosis (>80%) of the main renal artery when there is a well-developed collateral blood supply. When a hemodynamically significant renal artery stenosis is present, the Doppler trace measured at the poststenotic or intrarenal part of the renal artery reveals a "tardus et parvus" profile (STAVROS et al. 1992; BUDE et al. 1994), consisting in an increased time to reach the peak of the trace (acceleration time >70 ms) with loss of early systolic peak and a decreased acceleration index (<300 cm/s2). Poststenotic pulsus tardus is caused by the compliance of the poststenotic vessel wall in conjunction with the stenosis, which produces the tardus effect by damping the high-frequency components of the arterial waveform. This information allows the identification of those conditions which may produce false-positive or false-negative results when the tardus phenomenon is used to predict hemodynamically significant upstream stenosis (BUDE et al. 1994). This happens in the loss of vascular compliance in severe diffuse atherosclerosis, which may prevent the tardus and parvus phenomenon decreasing the sensitivity of color Doppler US (GRANT and MELANY 2001). Among the other findings which may be observed in the intraparenchymal arteries in the presence of renal artery stenosis is a reduction in the resistive indices in interlobar and arcuate renal cortical arteries, with an increased side difference of more than 10% (CORREAS et al. 1999).

Color Doppler US shows a sensitivity of 84–89% and a specificity of 97–99% for the detection of renal artery stenosis or occlusion (HELENON et al. 1995; GRANT and MELANY 2001). Nevertheless, the technical failure rate in evaluating renal artery is high due to obesity, overlying bowel gas, respiratory motion, deep renal artery location, tortuosity and number of renal arteries, and the presence of nephropathy (CORREAS et al. 1999). Obesity and overlying bowel gas are probably the most important causes of unsuccessful examinations, accounting for 30–40% of the failures (BERLAND et al. 1990; DESBERG et al. 1990).

10.3
Contrast-Enhanced US

New diagnostic opportunities have been created by the increased sensitivity of the latest US equipment and by microbubble-based contrast agents, which improve the visualization of renal arteries. The principal drawback of the use of contrast-enhanced

Doppler US to evaluate renal arteries is the frequent presence of artifacts, with spectral Doppler dispersion, pseudo-acceleration of the peak systolic flow, and blooming (CORREAS et al. 2003). Slow intravenous infusion (e.g., 1 ml/min) of the microbubbles can be used to produce a flatter profile of the time–concentration curve and thereby reduce artifacts at Doppler analysis.

The main renal artery is often difficult to detect on baseline color Doppler US owing to its perpendicular position in relation to the sound and its depth. The injection of microbubble-based contrast agents improves the overall quality of the procedure by increasing the visibility of the main renal artery (Figs. 10.1, 10.2) or the accessory renal arteries and the signal to noise ratio in the spectral Doppler analysis (CORREAS et al. 1999, 2003). Since accessory renal arteries occur in up to 25% of patients and may contain stenoses that result in renovascular hypertension (GRANT and MELANY 2001), the visibility of these vessels is very important for complete diagnostic work-up. Microbubble-based agents allow more accurate placement of the pulsed Doppler sample volume in the lumen of the main renal artery (Fig. 10.3) and provide reliable angle-adjusted velocity measurements (CORREAS et al. 1999).

Contrast-enhanced Doppler US significantly improves the overall quality of the examination and reduces the examination time in complex anatomical situations (Fig. 10.4) (CORREAS et al. 2003), e.g., in patients who are obese or in the presence of interposing bowel gas. It also reduces the frequency of technical failures, particularly in the juxtaostial and middle segments of the main renal artery.

The results of a European multicenter study (CLAUDON et al. 2000) showed that the number of examinations with successful results increased following contrast-enhanced Doppler US examination, including in patients with obesity (Fig. 10.4) or renal dysfunction, and that diagnostic agreement between Doppler US and intravenous digital subtraction angiography in the diagnosis or exclusion of renal arterial stenosis improved after the injection of microbubble-based agents. Similarly, in another study the overall diagnostic performance and reliability of color Doppler US in the diagnosis of renal artery stenosis were found to improve after microbubble-based agent injection (Fig. 10.5) (GRANT and MELANY 2001).

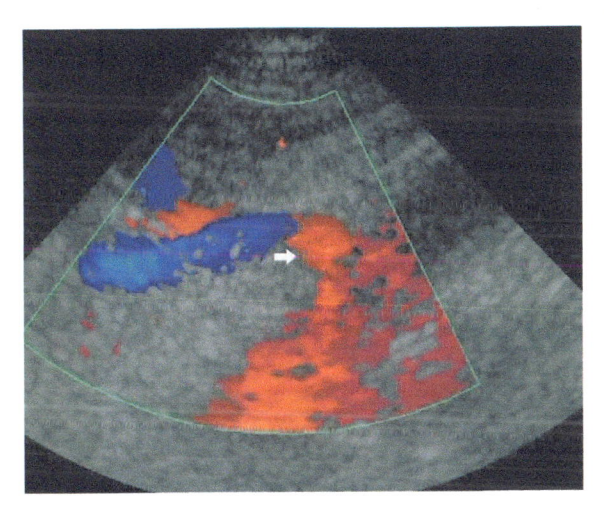

Fig. 10.1. Optimal visibility of the left renal artery on color Doppler US after the injection of microbubble-based agents both at the ostium (*arrow*) and in the middle portion (*blue*).

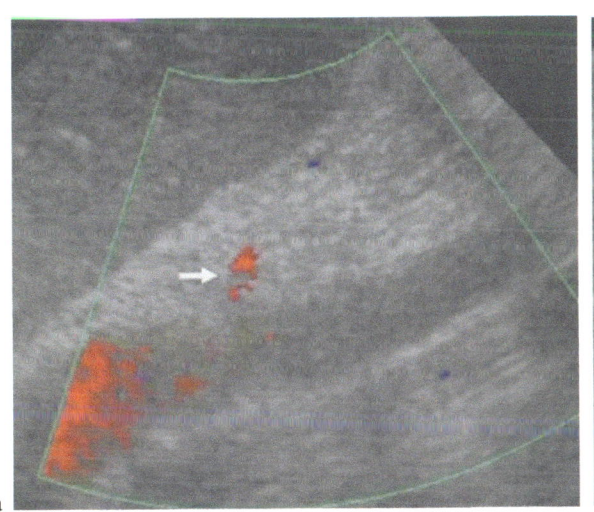

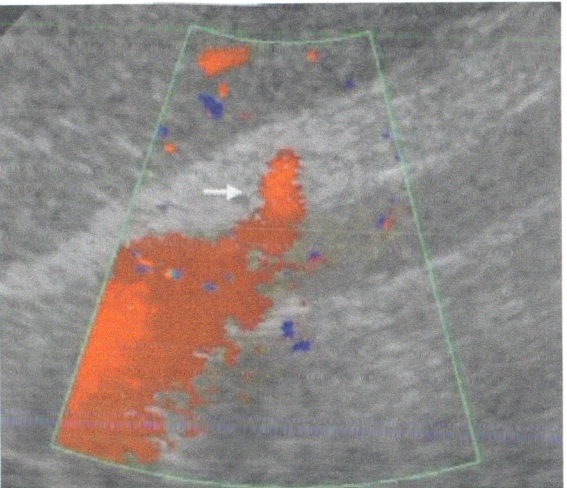

Fig. 10.2a,b. Poor visibility of the right renal artery in a 75-year-old male patient. a Baseline color Doppler US does not allow satisfactory visualization of the right renal artery (*arrow*). b The artery is visualized after injection of the microbubble-based agent.

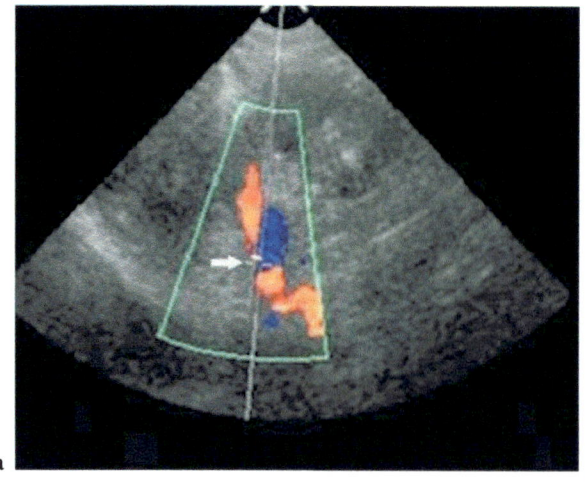

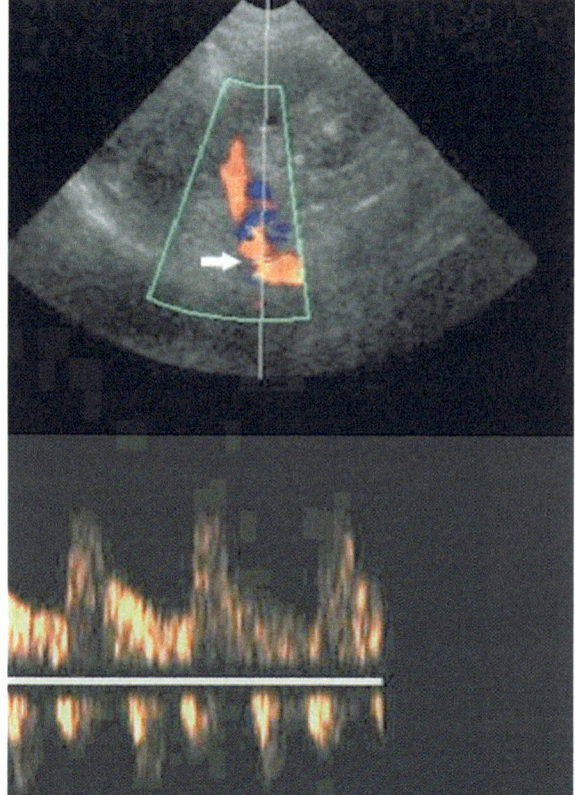

Fig. 10.3. a Microbubble-based agent injection allows correct placement of the pulsed Doppler sample window (*arrow*) at the lumen of the main renal artery. b Doppler trace is obtained with a correct angle correction (*arrow*).

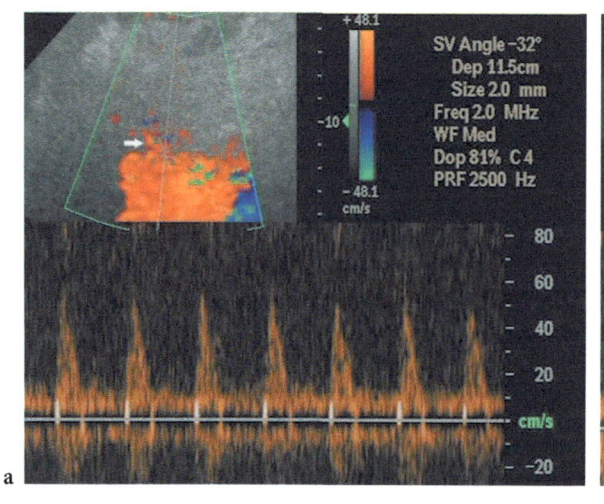

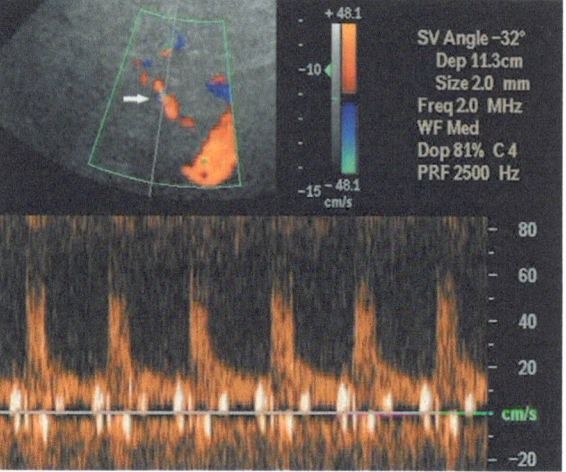

Fig. 10.4. a The right renal artery (*arrow*) is incompletely visualized on baseline color Doppler US in an obese patient. b Microbubble-based agent injection allows complete visualization of the main renal artery and correct placement of the Doppler sample window (*arrow*).

Moreover, contrast-enhanced Doppler improves the characterization of the lesions responsible for renal artery stenosis, in particular in the diagnosis of arterial fibrodysplasia (Correas et al. 2003).

The injection of microbubble-based agents also increases confidence in the diagnosis of renal obstruction (Correas et al. 2003) when no color Doppler signal is identified around the renal ostium or in the intrarenal vessels. Microbubble-based agents may also improve the differentiation of partial from complete occlusion of the main renal artery (Correas et al. 1998).

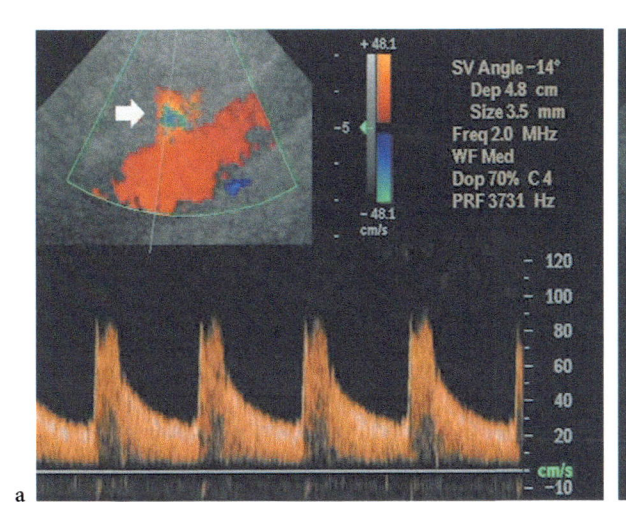

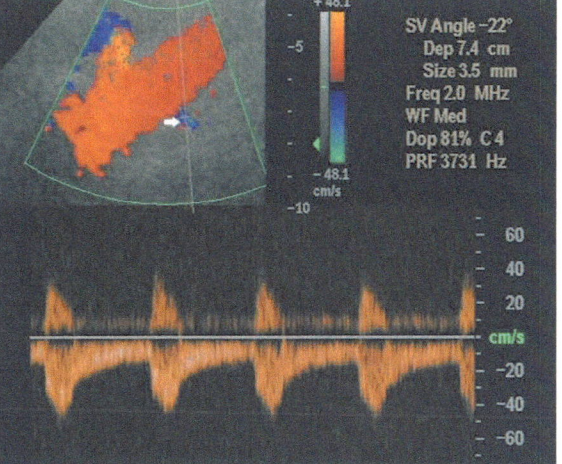

Fig. 10.5a,b. Improved visibility of renal artery stenosis. Baseline color Doppler US scan did not allow satisfactory visualization of the stenotic right renal artery. **a** After injection of the microbubble-based agent, aliasing artifact (*arrow*) is observed at the proximal segment of the right renal artery, with a slight increase in the peak systolic velocity (compared to the other side) and spectral broadening of the Doppler trace. A 60% renal artery stenosis was shown at digital angiography. **b** The left renal artery (*arrow*) is visualized by employing the same acoustic window as was employed to visualize the right renal artery.

References

Berglund G, Andersson O, Wilhelmsen L (1976) Prevalence of primary and secondary hypertension: studies in a random population sample. Br Med J 2:554-556

Berland LL, Koslin DB, Routh WD et al (1990) Renal artery stenosis: prospective evaluation of diagnosis with color duplex US compared with angiography. Radiology 174:421-423

Bude RO, Rubin JM (1995) Detection of renal artery stenosis with Doppler sonography: it is more complicated than originally thought (editorial). Radiology 196:612-613

Bude RO, Rubin JM, Platt JF et al (1994) Pulsus tardus: its cause and potential limitations in detection of arterial stenosis. Radiology 190:779-784

Claudon M, Plouin PF, Baxter GM, et al (2000) Renal arteries in patients at risk of renal arterial stenosis: multicenter evaluation of the echo-enhancer SH U 508A at color and spectral Doppler US. Radiology 214:739-746

Correas JM, Menassa L, Helenon O et al (1998) Diagnostic improvement of renal ultrasonography in humans after IV injections of Perflenapent emulsion. Acad Radiol 5: S185-S188

Correas JM, Helenon O, Moreau JF (1999) Contrast enhanced ultrasonography of native and transplant kidney diseases. Eur Radiol 9 [Suppl 3]:394-400

Correas JM, Claudon M, Tranquart F, Hélenon O (2003) Contrast-enhanced ultrasonography: renal applications. J Radiol 84:2041-2054

Davidson RA, Wilcox CS (1992) Newer tests for the diagnosis of renovascular disease. JAMA 268:3353-3358

Desberg AL, Paushter DM, Lammert GK et al (1990) Renal artery stenosis: evaluation with color Doppler flow imaging. Radiology 177:749-753

Grant EG, Melany ML (2001) Ultrasound contrast agents in the evaluation of the renal arteries. In: Goldberg BB, Raichlen JS, Forsberg F (eds) Ultrasound contrast agents. Basic principles and clinical applications, 2nd edn. Dunitz, London, pp 289-295

Havey RJ, Krumlowsky F, deGreco F, Martin HG (1985) Screening for renovascular hypertension. JAMA 254:388-393

Helenon O, Rody EL, Correas JM et al (1995) Color Doppler US of renovascular disease in native kidneys. Radiographics 15:833-854

Helenon O, Correas JM, Chabriais J et al (1998) Renal vascular Doppler imaging: clinical benefits of power mode. Radiographics 18:1441-1454

Stavros AT, Parker SH, Yakes WF et al (1992) Segmental stenosis of the renal artery: pattern recognition of tardus and parvus abnormalities with duplex sonography. Radiology 184:487-492

Abdominal Applications: Liver and Spleen

11 Characterization of Focal Liver Lesions

Emilio Quaia, Mirko D'Onofrio, Tommaso Vincenzo Bartolotta,
Alessandro Palumbo, Massimo Midiri, Fabrizio Calliada, Sandro Rossi,
and Roberto Pozzi Mucelli

CONTENTS

11.1 Introduction 125
11.2 Scanning Technique for Focal Hepatic Lesions 126
11.2.1 Preliminary Baseline Scan 126
11.2.2 Scanning Modes After Microbubble Injection 127
11.2.3 Dynamic Phases After Microbubble Injection 129
11.2.4 Contrast Enhancement Patterns 132
11.3 Benign Focal Liver Lesions 133
11.3.1 Hemangioma 133
11.3.2 Focal Nodular Hyperplasia 137
11.3.3 Hepatocellular Adenoma 140
11.3.4 Macroregenerative and Dysplastic Nodules 143
11.3.5 Focal Fatty Sparing and Focal Fatty Changes 147
11.3.6 Other Benign Focal Liver Lesions 148
11.4 Malignant Focal Liver Lesions 151
11.4.1 Hepatocellular Carcinoma 151
11.4.2 Metastases 154
11.4.3 Intrahepatic Cholangiocellular Carcinoma 158
11.4.4 Other Malignant Focal Liver Lesions 158
11.5 Clinical Results 159
11.6 When Should Microbubble-Based Agents Be Employed? 160
References 161

E. Quaia, MD, Assistant Professor of Radiology;
A. Palumbo, MD
Department of Radiology, Cattinara Hospital, University of Trieste, Strada di Fiume 447, 34149 Trieste, Italy
R. Pozzi Mucelli, MD, Professor of Radiology;
M. D'Onofrio, MD, Assistant Professor of Radiology
Department of Radiology, Hospital GB Rossi, University of Verona, Piazza L.A. Scuro 10, 37134 Verona, Italy
T. V. Bartolotta, MD, Assistant Professor of Radiology;
M. Midiri, MD, Professor of Radiology,
Department of Radiology, University of Palermo, Via del Vespro 129, 90127 Palermo, Italy
F. Calliada, MD, Professor of Radiology
Department of Radiology, San Matteo Hospital, University of Pavia, Piazzale Golgi 1, 27100 Pavia, Italy
S. Rossi, MD
Operative Unit for Interventional US, San Matteo Hospital, University of Pavia, Piazzale Golgi 1, 27100 Pavia, Italy

11.1 Introduction

Focal liver lesions may be identified incidentally, e.g., during an abdominal ultrasound (US) scan performed for clinical reasons unrelated to the liver lesion or during staging or follow-up procedures for a primary neoplasm or liver cirrhosis. Focal liver lesions may be characterized by baseline gray-scale US and color Doppler US when a typical pattern is identified, as in the case of homogeneously hyperechoic hemangiomas (Vilgrain et al. 2000) or focal nodular hyperplasia with a spoke-wheel shaped central vascular pattern on color Doppler US (Wang et al. 1997). Even though color Doppler US may improve diagnostic confidence in the characterization of focal liver lesions (Taylor et al. 1987; Hosten et al. 1999a; Tanaka et al. 1990; Nino-Murcia et al. 1992; Numata et al. 1993; Reinhold et al. 1995; Lee et al. 1996; Gonzalez-Anon et al. 1999), it does have important limitations since benign and malignant lesions may show a similar appearance on both gray-scale and color Doppler US.

It has been shown that the visibility of peripheral and intratumoral vessels may be improved on color and power Doppler US after the injection of microbubble-based contrast agents (Hosten et al. 1999b; Kim et al. 1999; Lee et al. 2002; Leen et al. 2002). Nevertheless, color signal saturation, motion and blooming artifacts, insensitivity to the flow of capillary vessels and limited sensitivity to the signal produced by microbubble-based agents represent important limitations of color Doppler US.

Microbubble-based contrast agents (Gramiak and Shah 1968) and dedicated US contrast-specific modes were introduced to overcome the limitations of baseline gray-scale and color Doppler US. Air-, perfluorocarbon- or sulfur hexafluoride-filled microbubbles may be employed to characterize focal liver lesions, though the technique of scanning differs according to the employed agent.

Levovist (SH U 508A, Schering, Berlin, Germany) is an air-filled microbubble contrast agent covered by a shell of galactose and palmitic acid. Since Levovist presents a low acoustic nonlinear response and low production of harmonic frequencies when insonated at a low acoustic transmit power, insonation with high acoustic power is necessary to produce microbubble destruction with emission of a wideband frequency signal detectable by dedicated contrast-specific techniques. Destructive imaging requires intermittent scanning and a limited number of sweeps to minimize bubble rupture and, consequently, does not allow prolonged evaluation of liver contrast enhancement. In comparison with baseline US, the injection of Levovist has been shown to allow the identification of tumoral vessels, to differentiate benign and malignant focal liver lesions according to the enhancement pattern (BERTOLOTTO et al. 2000; BURNS et al. 2000; KIM TK et al. 2000; WILSON et al. 2000; BLOMLEY et al. 2001; NUMATA et al. 2001; DILL-MACKY et al. 2002; VON HERBAY et al. 2002; KIM EA et al. 2003; MIGALEDDU et al. 2004; WEN et al. 2004), and to improve the characterization of focal liver lesions in terms of both overall accuracy and diagnostic confidence (TANAKA et al. 2001; ISOZAKI et al. 2003; VON HERBAY et al. 2002; BRYANT et al. 2004). The late liver-specific phase of Levovist (BLOMLEY et al. 1998, 1999; QUAIA et al. 2002b), beginning from 3 to 5 min after injection, has been demonstrated to be the most important dynamic phase for the characterization of focal liver lesions (BLOMLEY et al. 2001; BRYANT et al. 2004). During the late phase, benign liver lesions present similar microbubble uptake to the adjacent liver, while malignant liver lesions present lower microbubble uptake (BERTOLOTTO et al. 2000; BURNS et al. 2000; BLOMLEY et al. 2001; BRYANT et al. 2004).

New generation perfluorocarbon- or sulfur hexafluoride-filled microbubbles covered by a phospholipid shell, such as SonoVue (BR1, Bracco, Milan, Italy), Definity (MRX 115, Bristol-Myers Squibb, North Billerica, MA, NY, USA), and Sonazoid (NC100100, Nycomed Amersham, Oslo, Norway), present a nonlinear response with production of harmonic and subharmonic frequencies (SCHNEIDER et al. 1995; MOREL et al. 2000; CORREAS et al. 2000, 2001; COSGROVE et al. 2002) at low acoustic power insonation, allowing the employment of nondestructive imaging and the real-time evaluation of contrast enhancement in focal liver lesions (ALBRECHT et al. 2003; BRANNIGAN et al. 2004; NICOLAU et al. 2003a; HOHMANN et al. 2003; QUAIA et al. 2004). Preliminary experimental and clinical investigations proved the safety and efficacy of SonoVue in vascular and parenchymal diagnostic applications (QUAIA et al. 2003, 2004).

Besides commercial microbubble-based contrast agents, direct intra-arterial CO_2 injection into the proper hepatic artery after selective hepatic arteriography and superior mesenteric arteriography has been proposed for the assessment of vascularity in hepatic tumors and particularly in hepatocellular carcinoma (CHEN et al. 2002; KUDO et al. 1992).

11.2 Scanning Technique for Focal Hepatic Lesions

11.2.1 Preliminary Baseline Scan

Before microbubble injection, sonologists must perform a complete and accurate assessment of the liver parenchyma and of each identified focal liver lesion. The baseline scan includes the assessment of lesion appearance on gray-scale and color Doppler US, with the employment of tissue harmonic imaging and compound imaging (CLAUDON et al. 2002) and of state-of-the-art US equipment provided by wideband frequency transducers. Although tissue harmonic imaging was originally developed for microbubble-based contrast agents (BURNS et al. 1996; WARD et al. 1997), it also allows a clear enhancement of the image quality in native tissues. This is achieved by improvement of contrast resolution, particularly in patients who are difficult to image with conventional techniques, by reduction of the artifacts that degrade conventional sonograms, and by improvement in the differentiation between solid and liquid components. Compound imaging may combine multiple coronal images obtained from different spatial orientations, i.e., spatial compound imaging (JESPERSEN et al. 1998), or may involve the acquisition of images of the same object at different frequencies, combining them into a single image, i.e., frequency compound imaging (GATENBY et al. 1989). The result is the generation of a single image with better delineated margins and curved surfaces, fewer image artifacts, speckles (echoes from subresonation scatterers), and noise, and improved image contrast.

Baseline color Doppler US is performed by using slow-flow settings (pulse repetition frequency 800–1,500 Hz, wall filter of 50 Hz, high levels of color versus echo priority, and color persistence). Color gain is varied dynamically during the examination to enhance color signals and avoid excessive noise, with the size of the color box being adjusted

Characterization of Focal Liver Lesions

to include the entire lesion in the field of view of the color image. Spectral analysis of central and peripheral vessels is performed by pulsed Doppler to reveal continuous venous or pulsatile arterial flows.

11.2.2
Scanning Modes After Microbubble Injection

Two different insonation modes, destructive and nondestructive, may be employed after microbubble injection according to the acoustic power output, which is related to the employed mechanical index (MI) value. The MI value is a practical index to express the intensity of the acoustic field, even though it is an unreliable predictor of microbubble destruction, since the same MI value corresponds to different powers of the transmitted US beam in different US systems (MERRITT et al. 2000). The destructive mode has to be performed using the highest available MI to achieve extensive bubble rupture and production of a wideband frequency signal.

a) Destructive high acoustic power intermittent mode. This technique employs high acoustic power insonation to achieve microbubble destruction with emission of a transitory broadband frequency signal. It is suitable for agents with a late liver-specific postvascular phase, such as Levovist (BLOMLEY et al. 1998, 2001; QUAIA et al. 2002b) and Sonavist (SH U563 A, Schering AG, Berlin, Germany), because it allows effective assessment and characterization of focal liver lesions during the late phase: malignant liver lesions typically do not retain microbubbles while benign lesions present persistent microbubble uptake (BLOMLEY et al. 1998; BRYANT et al. 2004). To minimize microbubble rupture, destructive imaging requires intermittent scanning and a limited number of sweeps. Moreover, the high acoustic power of insonation produces a marked mixture of tissue harmonics and microbubble harmonics (COSGROVE et al. 2002), with production of a significant tissue background on which the bubble signal is superimposed.

Intermittent scanning may be manually or ECG triggered or it may be turned on simply by defreez-

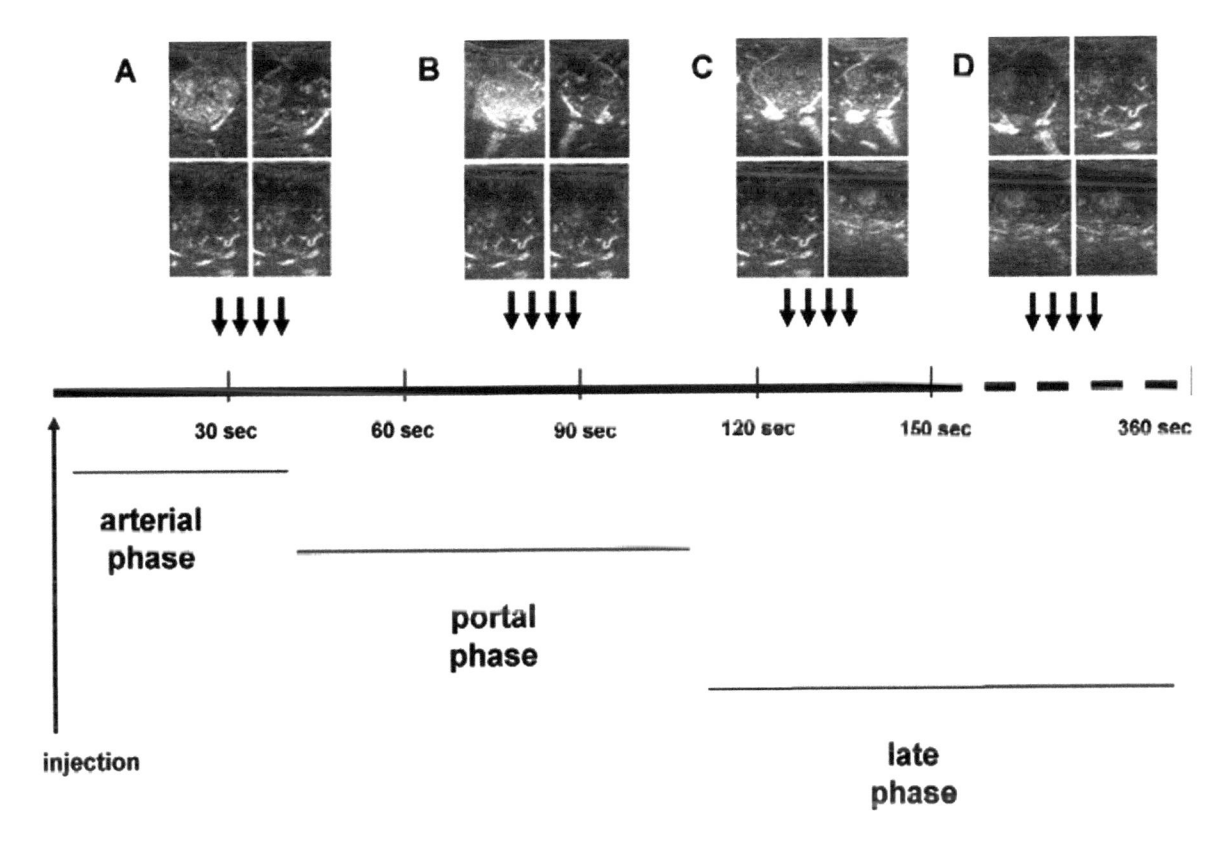

Fig. 11.1. Scheme of intermittent high acoustic power insonation for the characterization of focal liver lesions. Different trains of four high acoustic power US pulses are sent during the arterial, portal, and late phases. During the arterial phase, which is brief, a single train is transmitted. During the portal and late phases, which are longer than the arterial phase, two trains for each phase may be transmitted.

ing imaging for 1–2 s. Different trains with four to six high acoustic power US pulses may be employed (Fig. 11.1). The gray-scale gain is set immediately below the noise threshold, with one focal zone positioned just below the lesion. The delay time between the first and second destructive pulses of each train, corresponding to 110–140 ms (0.110–0.140 s = 1/frame rate = 1/7–1/9), is long enough to allow bubble refilling in large tumor vessels with fast flow but too brief to allow refilling in tumoral capillary and microvessels with slow flows. Since bubbles are rapidly destroyed from the first to the second frame, altering image contrast from a fractional blood volume-weighted image (first frame, Fig. 11.2) to a fractional blood flow-weighted image (second and subsequent frames, Fig. 11.2), the first frame represents both large and small tumor vessels and shows the pattern of contrast enhancement, while the second frame selectively represents large arterial/venous vessels with fast flow and permits assessment of tumor vessel appearance and distribution. The following two frames obtained from each train do not add any significant findings; they appear very similar to the second frame and are characterized only by a progressive reduction in bubble content due to bubble rupture.

b) Nondestructive low acoustic power continuous mode. This mode of insonation was allowed by the introduction of a new generation of perfluorocarbon- or sulfur hexafluoride-filled microbubbles and of multipulse scanning modes showing increased sensitivity to the nonlinear harmonic responses of the microbubbles and more effective suppression of tissue signals. A frequency corresponding to the microbubble resonance frequency is transmitted, and

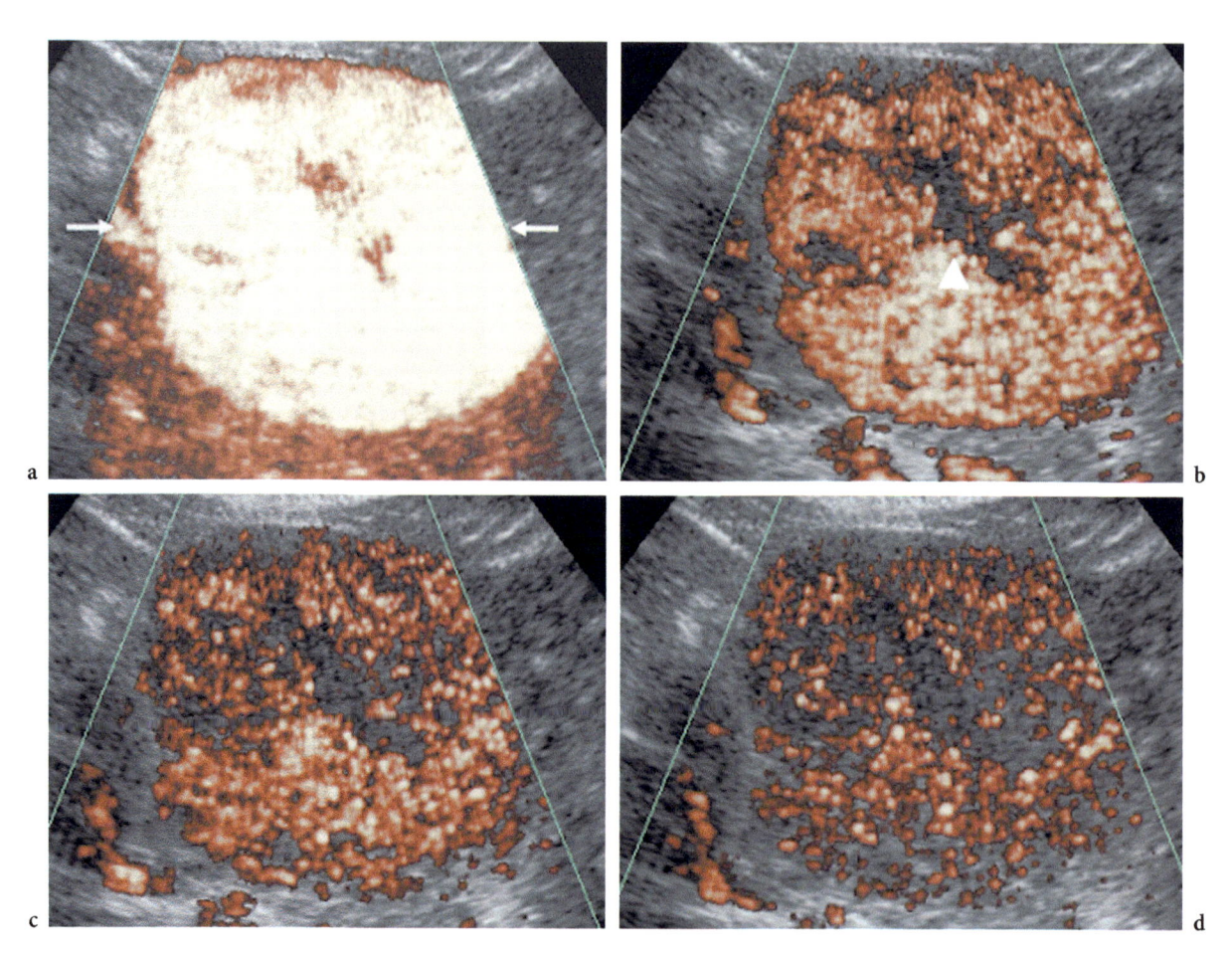

Fig. 11.2a–d. Stimulated acoustic emission after air-filled microbubble injection at high acoustic power insonation. Agent Detection Imaging (Philips-ATL, WA, USA). Four frames were obtained from high transmit power insonation. Diffuse contrast enhancement (*arrows*) is evident in the late phase (**a**) in the first frame of the train. In the subsequent frames of the train (**b–d**), contrast enhancement decreases progressively due to microbubble destruction, with evidence of a central scar spared by contrast enhancement.

harmonic frequencies are generated from nonlinear behavior of microbubbles (COSGROVE et al. 2002). Harmonic frequencies that present a value double that of the fundamental frequency may be detected by using dedicated contrast-specific imaging modes.

The nondestructive mode has several advantages over the destructive mode. First, it allows the effective suppression of tissue background signal since the stationary native tissue does not produce harmonic signals when insonated at low acoustic power. Second, the nondestructive mode allows assessment of contrast enhancement in real time, avoiding scan delay; it even offers better temporal resolution than contrast-enhanced CT and MR imaging. Third, this technique permits the acoustic window to be changed after microbubble injection. Possible disadvantages of nondestructive as compared with destructive imaging are a lower signal-to-noise ratio and the narrower dynamic range caused by the lower acoustic power of insonation.

Insonation should encompass all the arterial phase and must be extended to the first part (20 s) of the portal phase (Fig. 11.3). During the following seconds of the portal phase and during the late phase, the sonologist should perform brief insonations of 5–10 s and then resume the contrast-specific mode for 20–30 s to allow lesion replenishment by microbubbles (Fig. 11.3). These brief insonations should number at least two for the portal phase and three for the late phase. During the late phase each lesion should be scanned up to microbubble disappearance from the microcircle (6–8 min).

11.2.3
Dynamic Phases After Microbubble Injection

Different dynamic phases of contrast enhancement may be identified in the liver parenchyma after the injection of microbubble-based contrast agents, as for computed tomography (CT) or magnetic resonance (MR) imaging after the injection of iodinated or paramagnetic agents (VAN LEEUWEN et al. 1996).

The arterial (vascular) phase is very brief. It begins at about 10–20 s after microbubble injection (Figs. 11.4a, 5a–d) and lasts up to 25–35 s from the

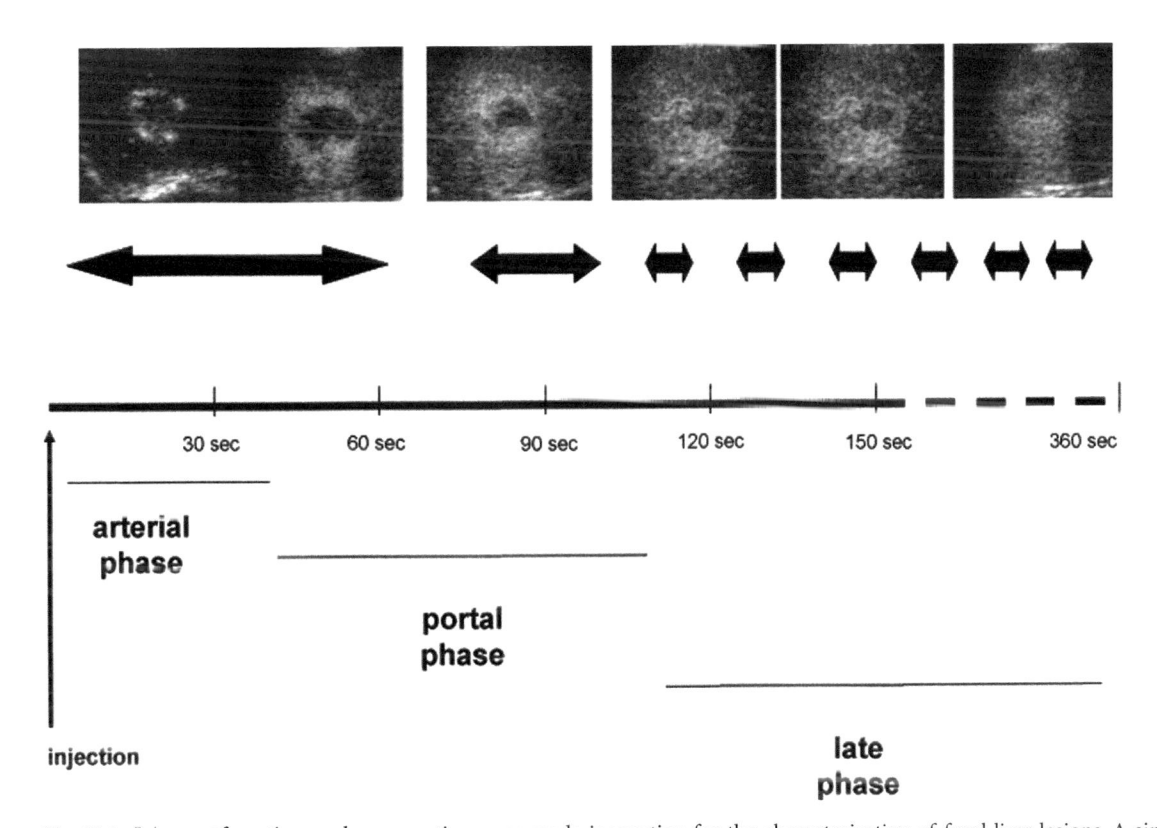

Fig. 11.3. Scheme of continuous low acoustic power mode insonation for the characterization of focal liver lesions. A single continuous scan has to be performed during the arterial phase, while several brief scans may be employed during the portal and late phases. For the latter purpose, insonations of 5–10 s are performed, with subsequent resumption of the contrast-specific mode for 20–30 s

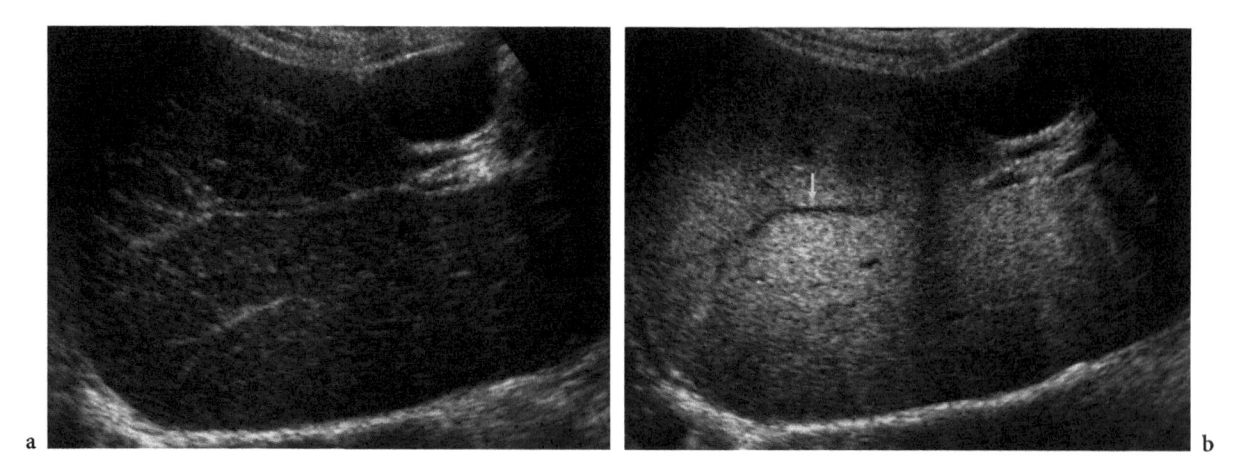

Fig. 11.4a,b. Transverse scan. Appearance of the liver during the arterial (**a**) and late (**b**) phases after Levovist (air-filled microbubble agent) injection at high acoustic power insonation. Intense contrast enhancement is demonstrated during the late liver-specific phase (**b**) 5 min after microbubble injection) owing to microbubble destruction. During the late liver-specific phase, microbubbles are pooling in liver sinusoids without evidence of microbubbles in the portal vessels (*arrow*), which appear as voids in the diffusely enhancing liver parenchyma.

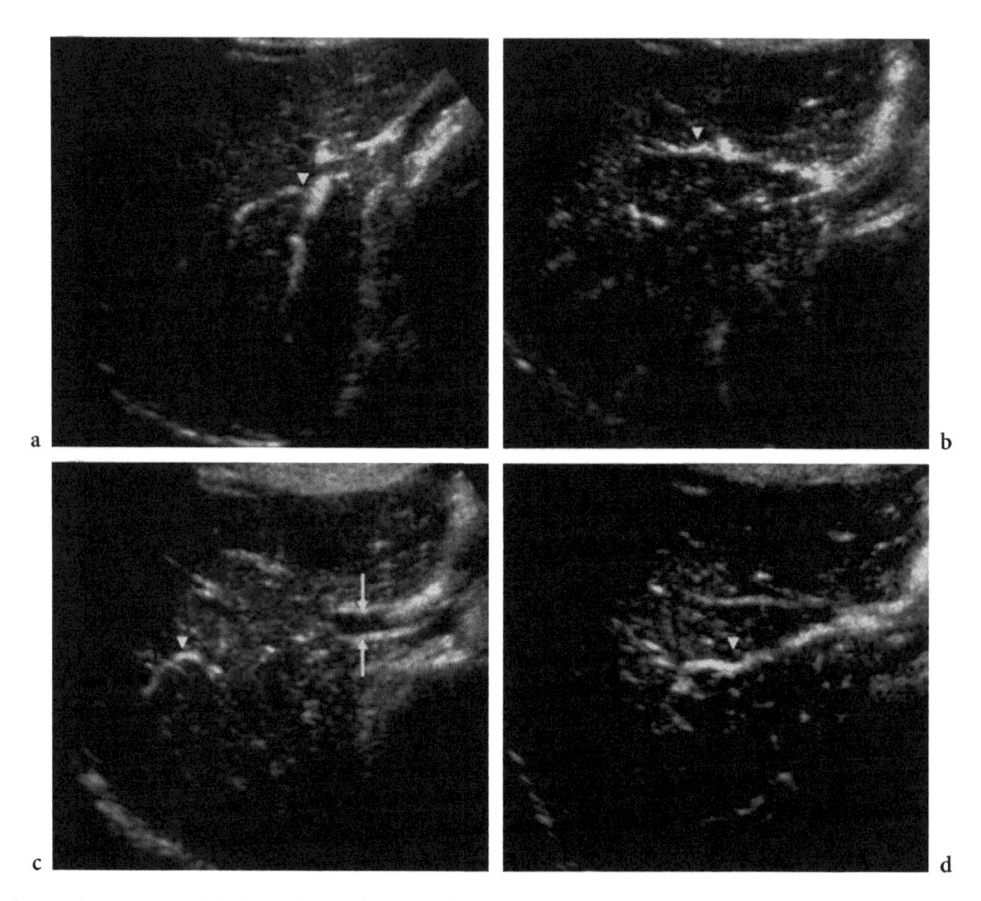

Fig. 11.5a–l. Longitudinal scan. Appearance of the liver during the arterial (**a–d**), portal (**e–h**), and late (**i–n**) phases after SonoVue (sulfur hexafluoride-filled microbubble agent) injection at low acoustic power insonation. During the arterial phase (**a–d**), 15 s after microbubble injection, microbubbles fill the hepatic arterial vessels (*arrowheads*), sparing the portal vein (*arrows*) and portal intrahepatic vessels. During the portal phase (**e–h**), 45 s after microbubble injection, microbubbles fill the portal vessels (*arrows*), progressively filling the liver sinusoids. In the late phase (**i–l**), 120 s after microbubble injection, microbubbles fill the liver sinusoids, giving rise to diffuse contrast enhancement in the liver parenchyma.

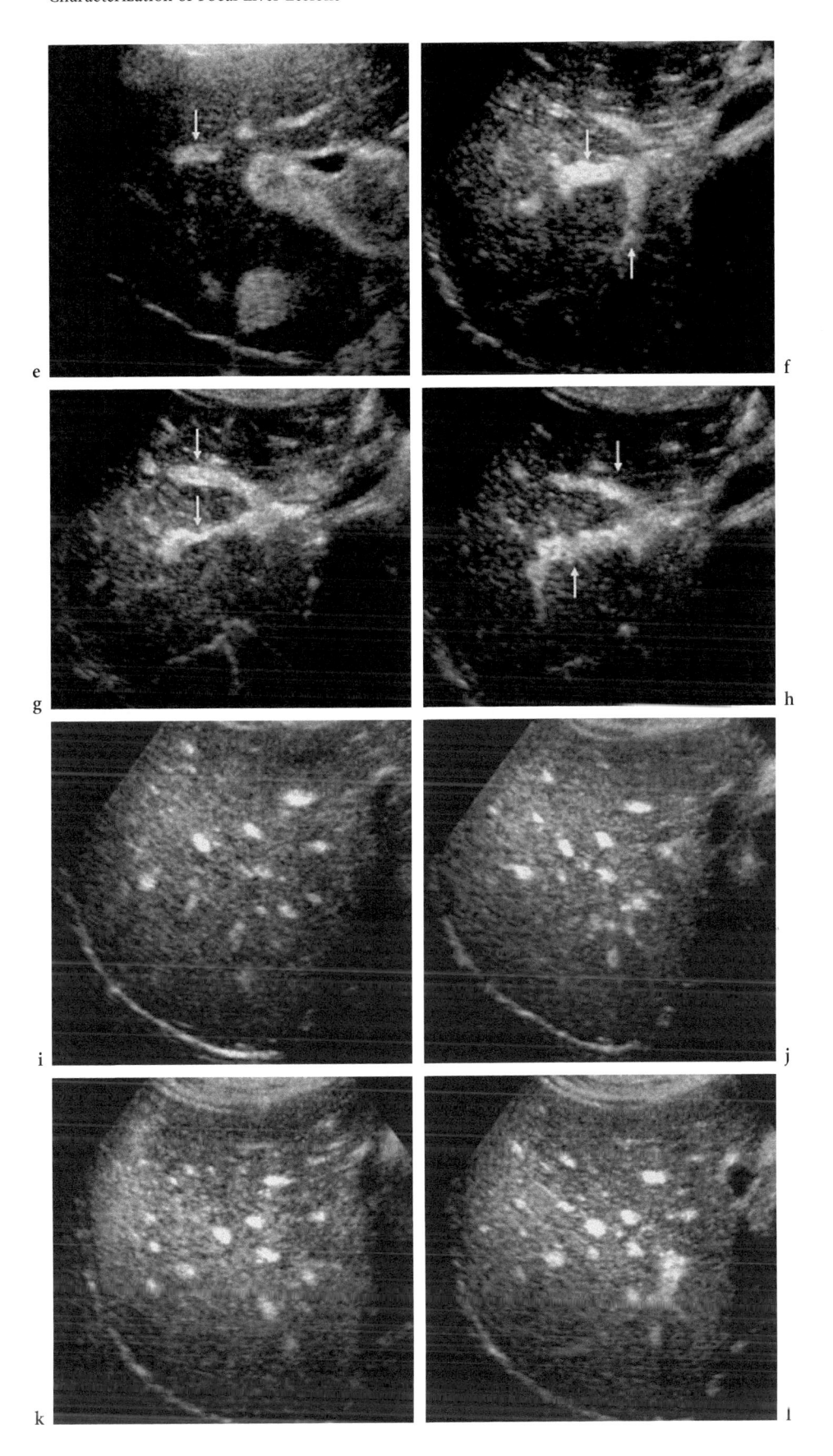

Characterization of Focal Liver Lesions

131

time of injection according to the circulation time (ALBRECHT et al. 2003; LEE et al. 2003). The arterial phase is necessary to evaluate lesion perfusion: diffuse and intense contrast enhancement is observed in hypervascular focal liver lesions whereas hypovascular focal liver lesions are characterized by absent or dotted contrast enhancement.

The portal and late phases (Figs. 11.4b, 11.5e-n) are much longer. The portal phase begins at 30-35 s and lasts up to 100-110 s from the beginning of microbubble injection. In liver cirrhosis, altered hepatic blood flow dynamics are frequently found, resulting in increased arterial flow and decreased portal vein flow to the liver (QUIROGA et al. 2001). Therefore, patients with advanced cirrhosis often have inadequate, and sometimes transient, hepatic parenchymal enhancement during the portal phase (CHEN et al. 1999). It is likely that in CT and MR imaging the portal phase has limited usefulness for the characterization of hepatic neoplasms.

The late (delayed or parenchymal) phase begins after the portal phase and lasts about 5-8 min, up to the time of disappearance of the microbubbles from the peripheral circulation. The late phase of microbubble agents is different from the equilibrium phase of non-liver-specific CT and MR contrast agents, since microbubble-based contrast agents do not present an interstitial (equilibrium or postvascular) phase and are pure intravascular agents. For this reason, microbubbles circulate in liver sinusoids during the late phase and different agents display different persistence in sinusoids.

After blood pool clearance, air-filled agents, such as Levovist or Sonavist, and perfluorocarbon-filled agents, such as Sonazoid (NC100100, Amersham Health, Oslo, Norway), have also been demonstrated to show hepatosplenic-specific parenchymal affinity in the late phase, during which the microbubbles are stationary in liver and spleen, in part pooled in sinusoids and in part phagocytosed by the reticuloendothelial system (HAUFF et al. 1997; BLOMLEY et al. 1998; QUAIA et al. 2002a; KINDBERG et al. 2003). This phase is comparable to the late phase of liver-specific MR agents such as gadobenate dimeglumine (Gd-BOPTA; Multihance; Bracco Imaging, Milan, Italy).

The late phase, with or without liver specificity, has been shown to be the most important for the characterization of focal liver lesions since benign lesions typically present persistent microbubble uptake with a hyper- or isovascular appearance relative to the adjacent liver while malignant lesions typically display microbubble washout with a hypovascular appearance (BLOMLEY et al. 2001; ALBRECHT et al. 2003; NICOLAU et al. 2003a,b; BRYANT et al. 2004; QUAIA et al. 2004). For these reasons, the late phase is the most important in the characterization of focal liver lesions, as with liver-specific MR agents (GRAZIOLI et al. 2001a,b).

11.2.4
Contrast Enhancement Patterns

The echogenicity of focal liver lesions on baseline gray-scale US and the tumoral vascularity and staining after microbubble-based contrast agent injection have to be compared with the adjacent liver. Lesions with a homogeneous or slightly heterogeneous echo intensity distribution are defined as hyper-, iso-, or hypoechoic (or hyper-, iso-, or hypovascular), depending on whether they display a prevalently higher, similar, or lower echogenicity relative to the adjacent liver parenchyma. In all other cases, lesions are defined as heterogeneous.

According to the lesion appearance during the arterial phase, contrast enhancement patterns (Fig. 11.6) are classified as: (a) absent (no difference before and after microbubble injection), (b) dotted (tiny separate spots of enhancement distributed throughout the lesion), (c) rim-like (continuous ring of peripheral contrast enhancement), (d) nodular (discontinuous or continuous peripheral enhancement with nodular appearance), (e) central (enhancement of the central portion of the lesion, defined as spoke-wheel shaped if the central vessel appears to branch toward the periphery of the lesion), or diffuse (enhancement of the whole lesion) with either (f) a homogeneous or (g) a heterogeneous appearance.

It has been proposed (TANAKA et al. 2001), the diffuse heterogeneous enhancement in hepatocellular carcinomas should be defined as mosaic-like if only some parts of the tumor show enhancement during the arterial phase and reticular if net-like enhancement appears throughout the tumor during the portal and late phases.

According to the lesion appearance during the late phase, contrast enhancement patterns (Fig. 11.7) are classified as: (h) hypoechoic (compared to the echogenicity of adjacent liver parenchyma), (i) residual (central hypoechoic area in a lesion with a persistent hyper- or isoechoic appearance), (l) hyperechoic (compared to the echogenicity of adjacent liver parenchyma), or (m) heterogeneous (prevalently hypoechoic or hyperechoic).

Characterization of Focal Liver Lesions

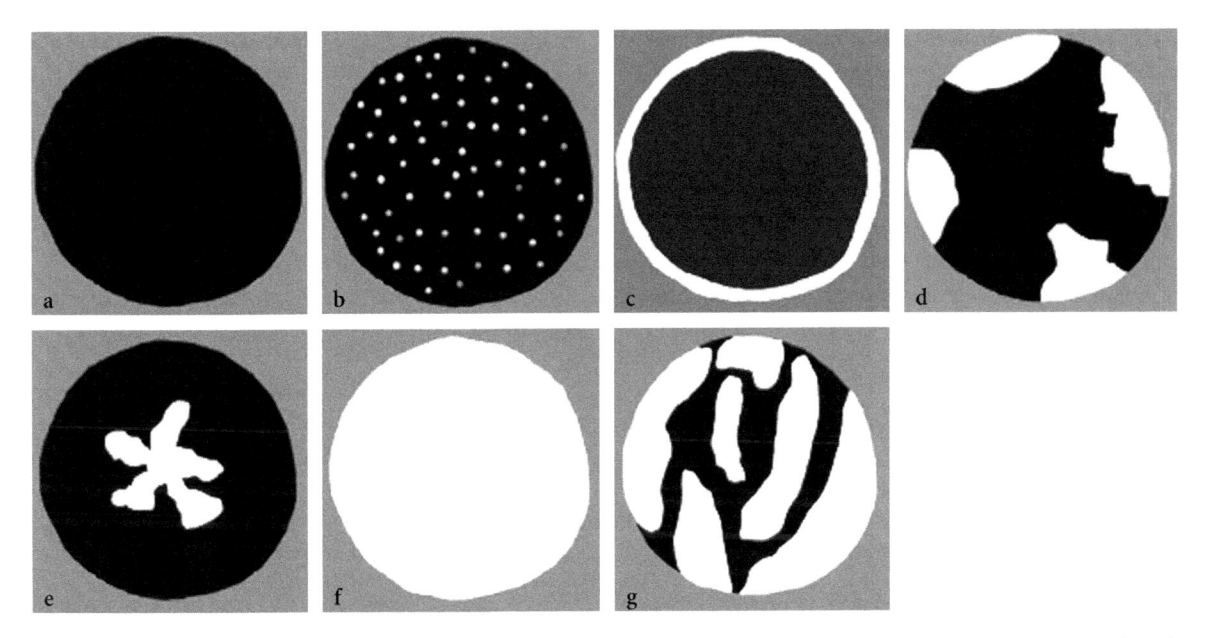

Fig. 11.6a–g. The different patterns of contrast enhancement in focal liver lesions during the arterial phase: **a** absent, **b** dotted, **c** peripheral rim-like, **d** peripheral nodular, **e** central with a spoke-wheel shape, **f** diffuse homogeneous, **g** diffuse heterogeneous.

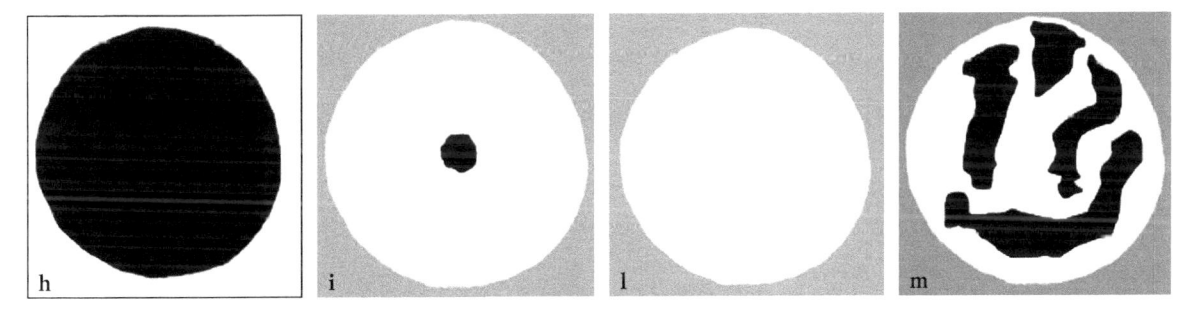

Fig. 11.7h–m. The different patterns of contrast enhancement in focal liver lesions during the late phase: **h** hypoechoic (or hypovascular), **i** residual central hypoechoic area in a lesion with a persistent iso- to hyperechoic (or iso- to hypervascular) appearance, **l** hyperechoic (hypervascular), **m** heterogeneous.

11.3
Benign Focal Liver Lesions

11.3.1
Hemangioma

Epidemiology and histopathologic features. Hemangiomas are the most common benign tumors of the liver (Ros 1990), with an incidence in the general population ranging from 0.4% to 20% (Edmondson 1958; Karhunen 1986). Although hemangiomas occur more frequently in women, they are not particularly prevalent at any age. Hemangiomas show an association with focal nodular hyperplasia, and the two lesions may coexist in the same liver (Vilgrain et al. 2003).

Multimodality imaging - US and color Doppler US. Liver hemangiomas may display a typical appearance on baseline gray-scale US consisting in a hyperechoic and homogeneous or centrally heterogeneous pattern, with or without posterior acoustic enhancement and well-defined regular margins (Vilgrain et al. 2000). Besides their typical appearance, liver hemangiomas may also present atypical and therefore indeterminate patterns on baseline US, appearing either homogeneous or heterogeneous, hypoechoic or isoechoic, and with or without a thin peripheral echoic border (Vilgrain et al. 2000; Quaia et al 2002a). Even though typical liver hemangiomas do not need further confirmatory studies, both benign (focal fatty change, hepatocellular adenoma, focal nodular hyperplasia, lipoma) and malignant (hepato cellular carcinoma and metastasis) focal liver lesions may present a similar appearance to hemangiomas on baseline gray-scale US. Like baseline gray-scale US, color Doppler US shows only moderate accuracy in the characterization of liver hemangiomas and may also be limited by motion artifacts and low sensitivity to slow flows. Absence of flow or a small number of intratumoral color spots may be observed in smaller hemangiomas, while intratumoral vessels, mostly with a venous flow, are seen in larger hemangiomas (QUAIA et al. 2002a).

Multimodality imaging – CT and MR imaging. The imaging procedures most frequently employed to characterize liver hemangiomas are CT and MR imaging, performed after contrast agent administration during different dynamic phases (arterial, portal, equilibrium, and late phases). The typical contrast enhancement pattern of hemangiomas consists in peripheral nodular enhancement with progressive centripetal fill-in (NINO-MURCIA et al. 2000). Nevertheless, a variety of less frequent or less typical contrast enhancement patterns may be observed, such as diffuse contrast enhancement in hypervascular hemangiomas or absence of contrast enhancement in fibrotic hemangiomas, which are frequently detected in cirrhotic patients (BRANCATELLI et al. 2001a).

Contrast-enhanced US. Various contrast enhancement patterns may be observed in liver hemangiomas after the administration of microbubble-based contrast agents.

Most liver hemangiomas display peripheral nodular enhancement (Fig. 11.8) during the arterial

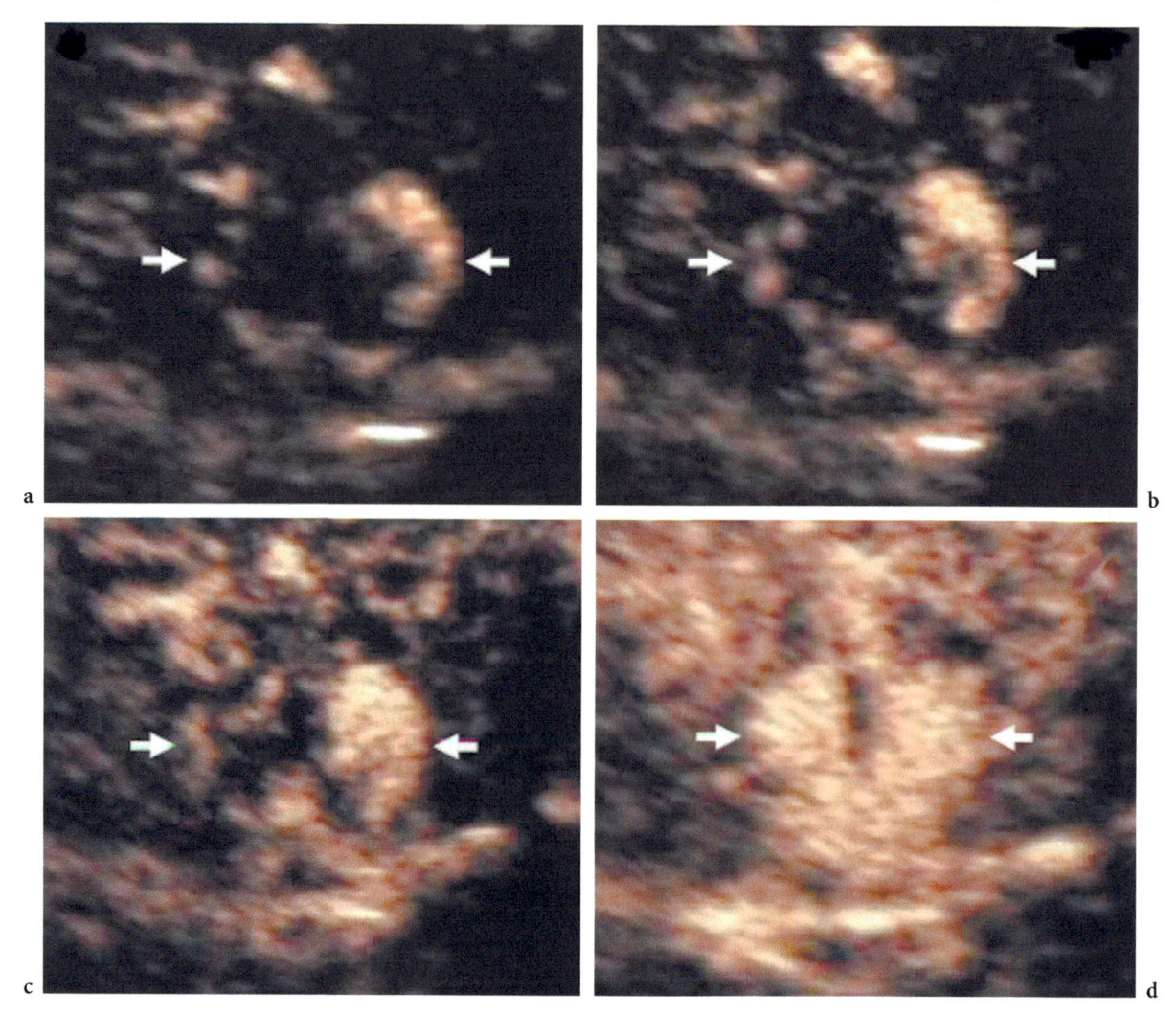

Fig. 11.8a–d. Hemangioma: typical peripheral nodular contrast enhancement pattern with progressive fill-in. Contrast-specific mode: Cadence Contrast Pulse Sequence (Siemens-Acuson, CA, USA) with low acoustic power insonation. Peripheral nodular enhancement is demonstrated during the arterial phase (**a**), with progressive centripetal fill-in during the portal (**b, c**) and late (**d**) phases.

phase, with progressive centripetal fill-in from 50 to 280 s after injection. During the late phase, the centripetal fill-in appears complete in 40–50% of cases (LEE et al. 2002; NICOLAU et al. 2003a), and partial in the remainder (owing to the presence of intratumoral areas of fibrosis or thrombosis).

Hyperechoic liver hemangiomas may also show progressive fill-in without evidence of centripetal progression (Fig. 11.9) and with an iso- or hyperechoic appearance relative to the adjacent liver in the late phase. In these hemangiomas the progressive fill-in involves both the periphery and the center of the lesion at the same time during the arterial and late phases.

Hypervascular liver hemangiomas usually display rapid fill-in with diffuse contrast enhancement (Figs. 11.10, 11.11) during the arterial phase (QUAIA et al. 2002a, 2004). Rapidly filling hemangiomas usually measure less than or equal to 3 cm, and correspond to roughly 16% of all hemangiomas

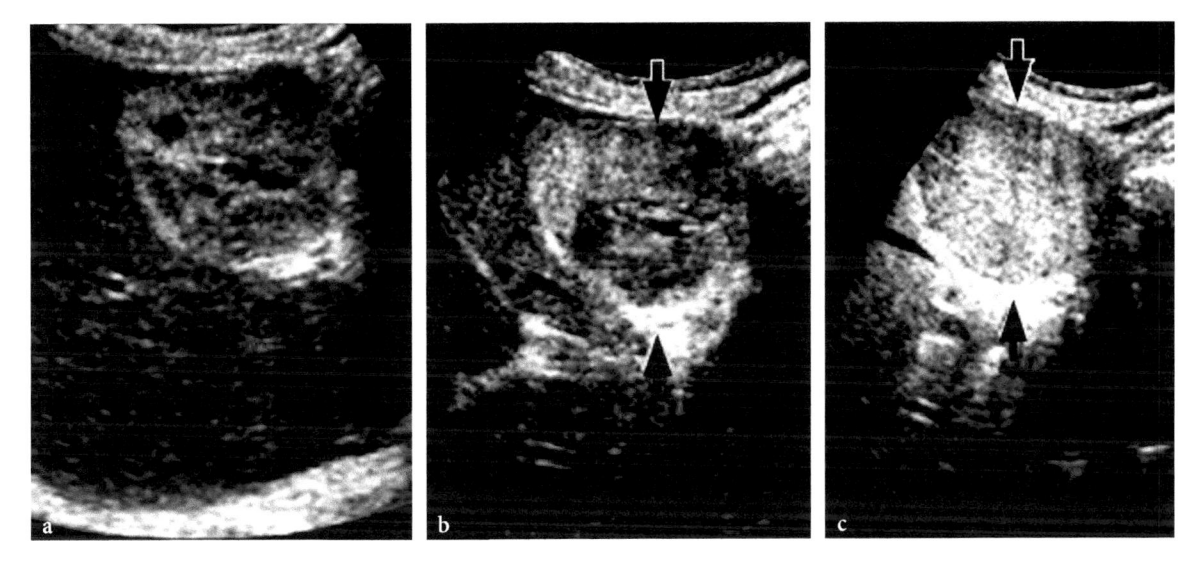

Fig. 11.9a–c. Hemangioma: progressive fill-in without nodular enhancement during the arterial phase. Longitudinal plane. a Baseline US. The hemangioma (*arrows*) appears hyperechoic and slightly heterogeneous. b, c Contrast-enhanced US. Contrast-specific mode: Pulse Inversion Mode (Philips-ATL, WA, USA) with high acoustic power insonation. Progressive centripetal fill-in without evidence of peripheral enhancement is demonstrated during the arterial (b) and late (c) phases.

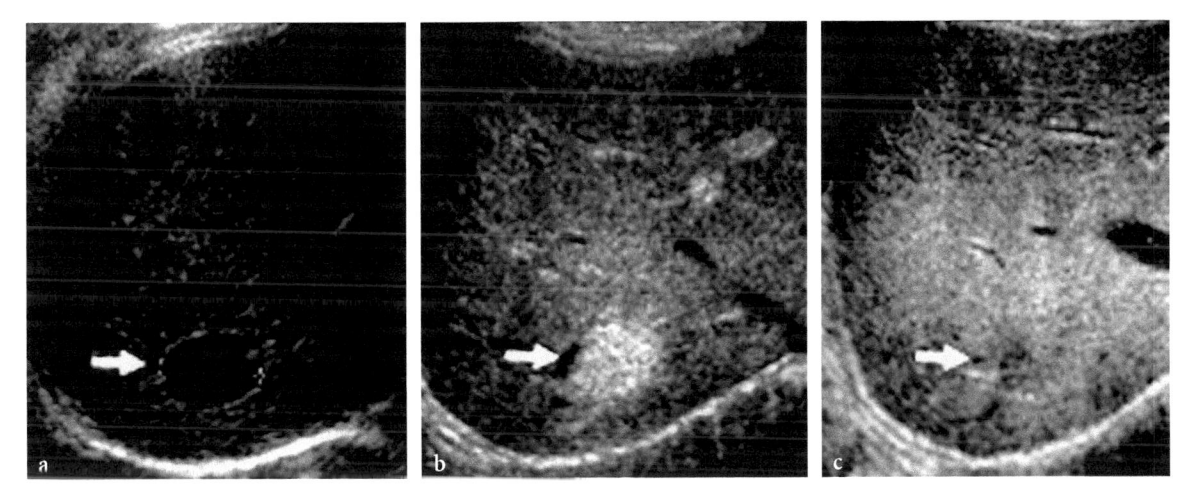

Fig. 11.10a–c. Hypervascular hemangioma: diffuse contrast enhancement. a Baseline US. A hypoechoic lesion (*arrow*) is demonstrated in a bright liver. b, c Contrast-enhanced US. Contrast-specific mode: Pulse Inversion Mode (Philips-ATL, WA, USA) with low acoustic power insonation. Diffuse homogeneous contrast enhancement demonstrated in the arterial phase (b) persists during the late phase (c), with a hyperechoic appearance in comparison to the adjacent liver parenchyma. Hemangioma was proved by US-guided biopsy.

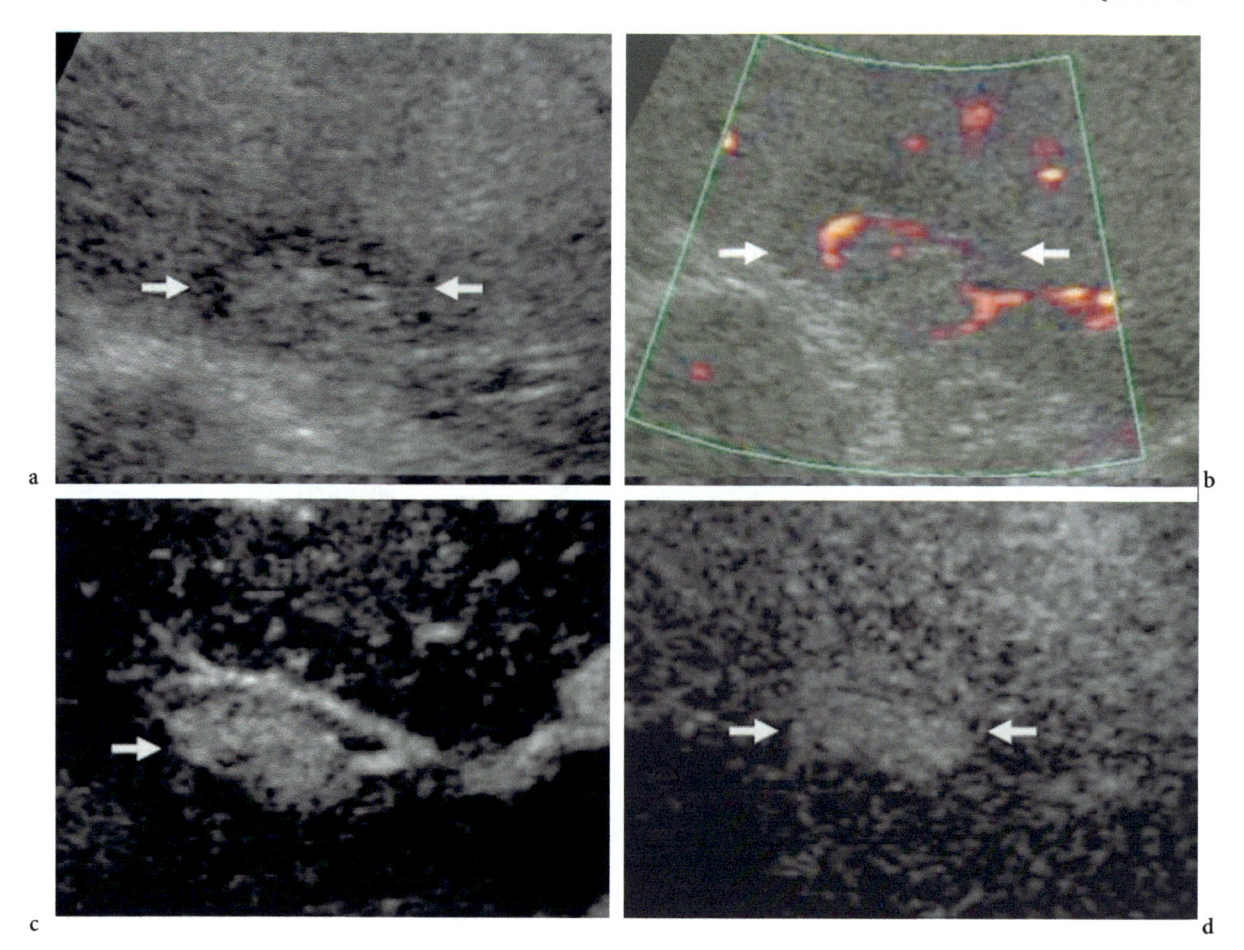

Fig. 11.11a–d. Hypervascular hemangioma: diffuse contrast enhancement. a Baseline US. A heterogeneous lesion (*arrows*) is demonstrated in a bright liver with some intratumoral vessels on baseline power Doppler US (b). c, d Contrast-enhanced US. Contrast-specific mode: Pulse Inversion Mode (Philips-ATL, WA, USA) with low acoustic power insonation. Diffuse homogeneous contrast enhancement is demonstrated during the arterial phase (c) and persists during the late phase (d), with an isoechoic appearance in comparison to the adjacent liver parenchyma. Hemangioma was proved by US-guided biopsy.

(VILGRAIN et al. 2000); such hemangiomas are most commonly identified in cirrhotic patients (BRANCATELLI et al. 2001a). This enhancement pattern is similar to that observed on contrast-enhanced CT after the injection of iodinated contrast agents (BRANCATELLI et al. 2001a).

Persistent dotted contrast enhancement (Fig. 11.12) with an isovascular appearance relative to the adjacent liver may be observed in liver hemangiomas. This pattern is particularly frequent in liver hemangiomas with a hyperechoic appearance on baseline US (QUAIA et al. 2002a) and is due to the difficulty in appreciating the vascularity and contrast enhancement in hyperechoic lesions (KODA et al. 2004). This pattern is quite frequent in hyperechoic liver hemangiomas after air-filled microbubble injection and intermittent high acoustic power insonation (QUAIA et al. 2002a). It is more rarely observed after perfluorocarbon- or sulfur hexafluoride-filled microbubble injection at low acoustic power insonation, since this mode allows more effective suppression of the echo intensity of stationary tissues, thereby increasing the sensitivity to microbubble signals.

After microbubble injection, liver hemangiomas may also present a persistent hypoechoic appearance due to absence of contrast enhancement (Fig. 11.13), with or without rim-like peripheral enhancement. This enhancement pattern is frequently observed in thrombosed, fibrosclerotic, or hyalinized atypical liver hemangiomas, as proven using contrast-enhanced CT (BRANCATELLI et al. 2001a). In atypical liver hemangiomas, peripheral nodular enhancement with centripetal fill-in is often observed (Fig. 11.14).

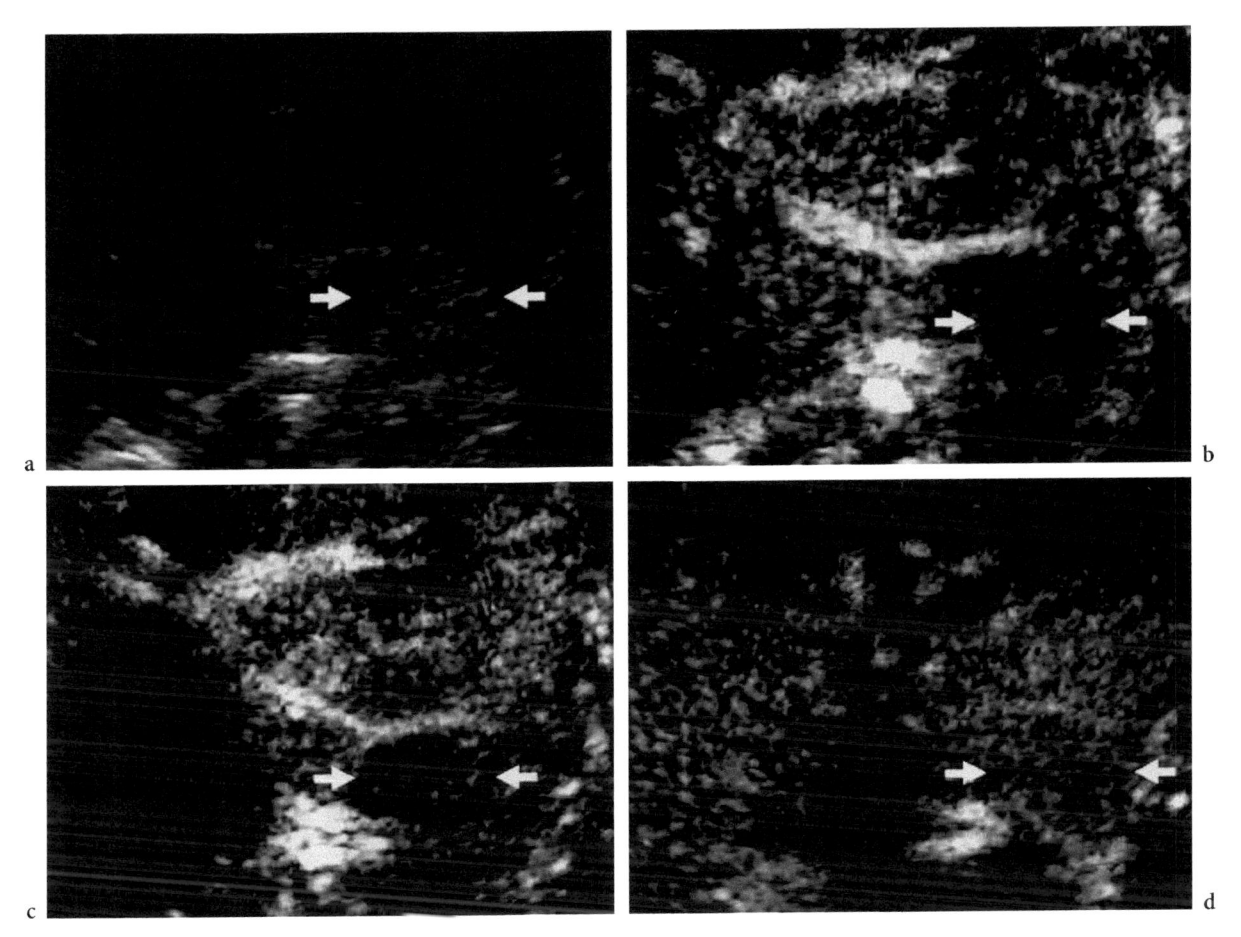

Fig. 11.12a-d. Hemangioma: dotted contrast enhancement. a Baseline US. A hyperechoic homogeneous lesion (*arrows*) is demonstrated. b-d Contrast-enhanced US. Contrast-specific mode: Contrast Tuned Imaging (Esaote, Genoa, Italy) with low acoustic power insonation. Dotted contrast enhancement is demonstrated in the arterial (**b**) and portal (**c**) phases, while there is an isoechoic appearance relative to the surrounding liver in the late phase (**d**).

11.3.2
Focal Nodular Hyperplasia

Epidemiology and histopathologic features. Focal nodular hyperplasia is the second most common benign tumor of the liver after liver hemangiomas, with an incidence of 1-3% (KARHUNEN 1986). Focal nodular hyperplasia is usually discovered as an asymptomatic incidental mass in young women who are undergoing imaging examinations for unrelated reasons and is multiple in 20% of cases. Focal nodular hyperplasia is up to eight times more common in women than in men, typically presents in the third to fifth decade, and measures less than 5 cm in size. The association of focal nodular hyperplasia with contraceptives is not definitely proven, even though pregnancy and oral contraceptive use can induce lesion growth. Focal nodular hyperplasia is probably caused by a hyperplastic response to a localized vascular abnormality (WANLESS et al. 1985). Although focal nodular hyperplasia deserves conservative management, it may simulate the imaging characteristics of some malignant liver masses; therefore, correct preoperative diagnosis is essential. Focal nodular hyperplasia presents intratumoral hemorrhage or necrosis in up to 6% of cases (SANDLER et al. 1980).

Histologically, focal nodular hyperplasia is composed of normal hepatic structures (hepatocytes, Kupffer cells, and bile ducts) which are abnormally arranged, and it is usually not capsulated. A distinct central scar and radiating fibrous septa are detected in the majority of cases (70-80%) upon analysis of the gross specimen. A fibromyxoid or fibrotic com-

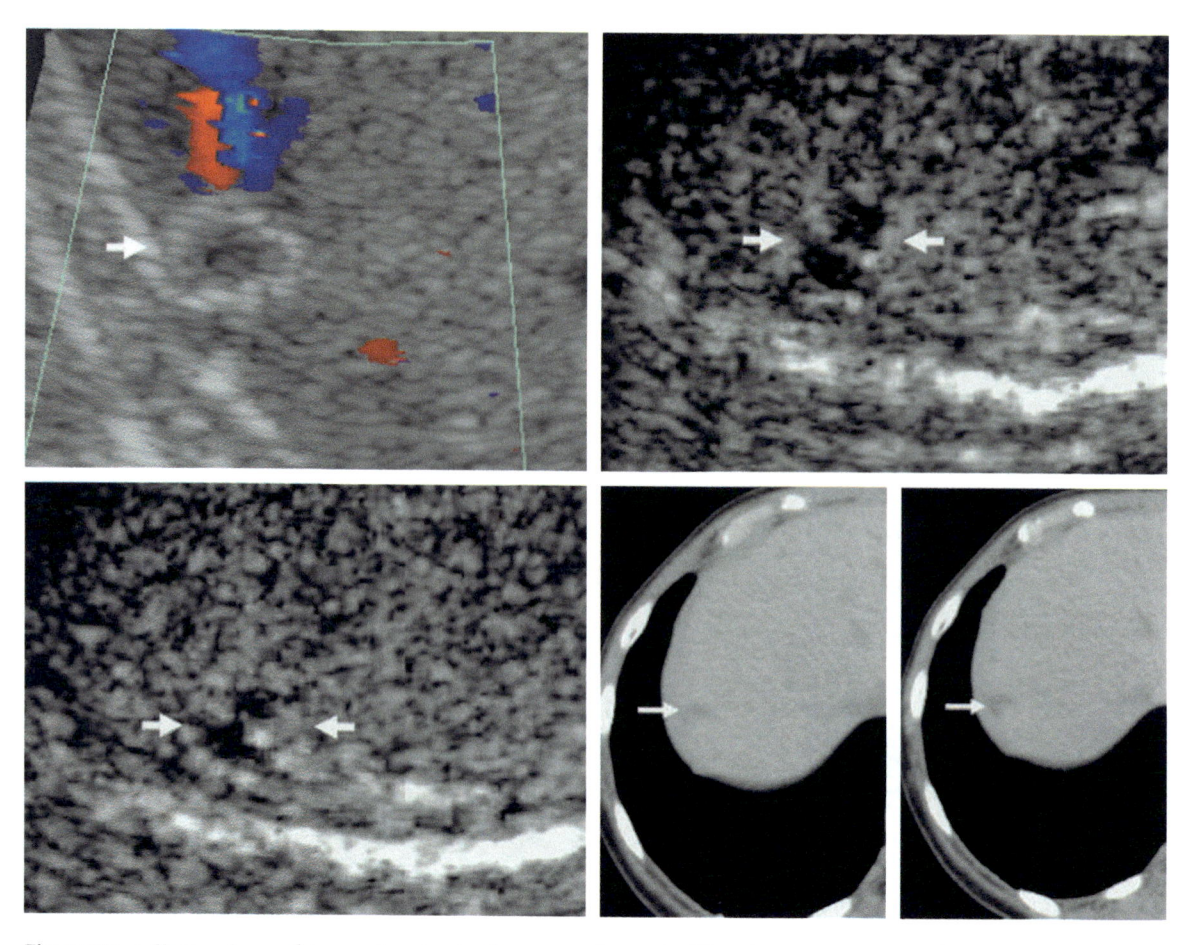

Fig. 11.13a-e. Hemangioma: absence of contrast enhancement in atypical liver hemangioma. a Baseline color Doppler US. A hypoechoic lesion with a peripheral hyperechoic rim and without evidence of peripheral or intralesional vessels is identified. b, c Contrast-enhanced US. Contrast-specific mode: Contrast Tuned Imaging (Esaote, Genoa, Italy) with low acoustic power insonation. There is no contrast enhancement during either the arterial (b) or the late (c) phase, and the lesion has a hypoechoic appearance relative to the surrounding liver. d, e Contrast-enhanced CT. Again, there is no evidence of contrast enhancement after iodinated contrast agent injection, the lesion having a hypodense appearance during both the arterial (d) and the late (e) phase. Hemangioma was proved by US-guided biopsy.

ponent may be present, depending on the degree of the liquid component, and there may be gross calcifications. In other cases, fibrous bands may be seen organizing the parenchymal architecture into lobules (BRANCATELLI et al. 2001b). Usually intratumoral calcifications, fat, and areas of necrosis are not identified.

Multimodality imaging – US and color Doppler US. Focal nodular hyperplasia usually appears homogeneously isoechoic or only slightly hyper- or hypoechoic compared to the adjacent liver. The characteristic spoke-wheel shaped pattern, with the central vessel radiating from the center to the periphery, can be identified at baseline color Doppler US. This pattern (WANG et al. 1997) is considered highly specific for focal nodular hyperplasia; however, its sensitivity is low since it is found in only 50% of cases, most frequently in larger lesions (BRANCATELLI et al. 2001b).

Multimodality imaging - CT. Focal nodular hyperplasia presents ill-defined smooth borders and a slightly hypodense or isodense appearance on nonenhanced CT, sometimes with evidence of the hypodense central scar. The lesion is frequently subcapsular and may present a mass effect with displacement of the adjacent blood vessels. Exophytic growth or distortion of the hepatic contour may be observed in about one-third of the lesions. After the injection of an iodinated contrast agent, the intratumoral feeding arteries, peripheral draining veins, and a peripheral pseudocapsule may be observed. During the arterial phase, focal nodular hyperplasia

Characterization of Focal Liver Lesions

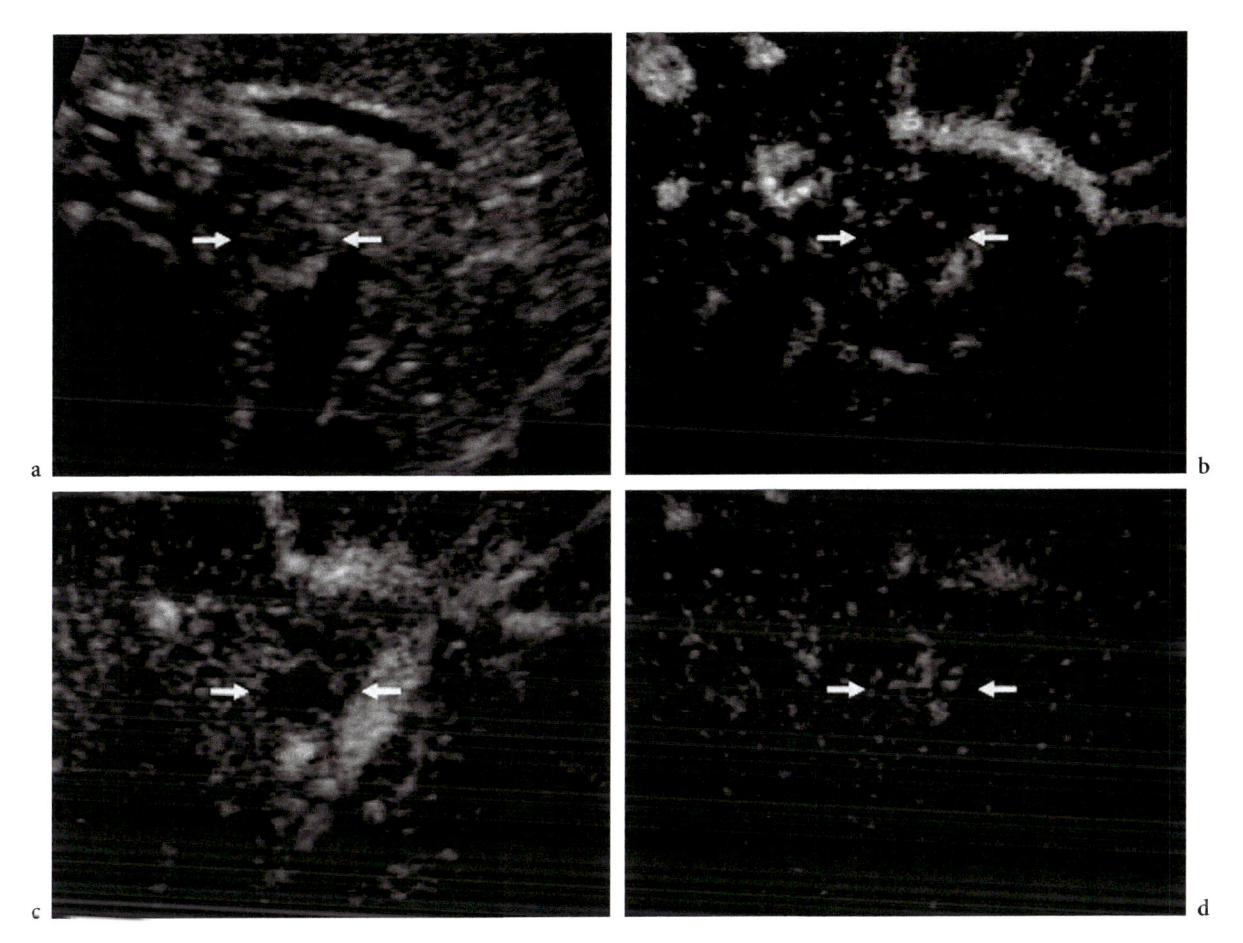

Fig. 11.14a–d. Hemangioma: peripheral nodular enhancement with centripetal fill-in in atypical liver hemangioma. **a** Baseline US. Atypical liver hemangioma with peripheral hyperechoic rim (*arrows*). **b–d** Contrast-enhanced US. Contrast-specific mode: Pulse Inversion Mode (Philips-ATL, WA, USA) with low acoustic power insonation. Peripheral nodular enhancement is demonstrated during the arterial phase (**b**), with progressive centripetal fill-in during the portal (**c**) and late (**d**) phases.

typically appears hyperattenuating relative to the adjacent liver, with a central hypoattenuating scar; the appearance is usually iso- or hyperattenuating during the portal and late phase scans. In the late phase, during the interstitial phase of iodinated contrast agent in the fibromyxoid tissue, the central scar more frequently appears hyper- or isoattenuating (BRANCATELLI et al. 2001b) in comparison with the rest of the lesion.

Multimodality imaging - MR. Focal nodular hyperplasia presents an isointense or slightly hyper- or hypointense appearance on nonenhanced T2-weighted sequences, while the central scar may appear hyper- or hypointense according to the liquid content of the fibromyxoid component. After the injection of a paramagnetic gadolinium-based contrast agent, the lesion appears hyperintense during the arterial phase due to diffuse contrast enhancement. A progressive reduction in contrast enhancement, leading to isointensity, is identified in the portal venous and late phases.

Administration of the liver-specific agent gadobenate dimeglumine (Gd-BOPTA) is essential to properly differentiate focal nodular hyperplasia from hepatocellular adenoma and malignant focal hepatic lesions (GRAZIOLI et al. 2001b). Gd-BOPTA is a paramagnetic gadolinium-based contrast agent with a vascular–interstitial distribution in the initial minutes after injection and late biliary excretion of 2–4% of the administered dose after uptake by functioning hepatocytes (KIRCHIN et al. 1998; SPINAZZI et al. 1999). At least 1 h after Gd-BOPTA administration, focal nodular hyperplasia appears generally hyperintense (the central scar is hypointense) compared with adjacent liver, while other lesions appear isointense or slightly hypointense (GRAZIOLI et al. 2001b). This hyperintensity is due to the prolonged and excessive hepatocellular accumulation of Gd-BOPTA in focal nodular hyperplasia, which lacks a well-formed bile canalicular system to allow normal excretion.

The administration of superparamagnetic iron oxide-based particulate agents, such as ferumoxides or ferucarbotran, which are taken up by the cells of the reticuloendothelial system, results in signal intensity loss on T2-weighted MR images (BLUEMKE et al. 2003; M.G. KIM et al. 2003) in focal nodular hyperplasia and other benign liver tumors containing reticuloendothelial cells. No such loss occurs in malignant liver tumors, with the exception of hepatocellular carcinomas with a reticuloendothelial intratumoral component.

Contrast-enhanced US. After the injection of air-filled microbubbles in the intermittent high acoustic power mode, focal nodular hyperplasia typically shows diffuse homogeneous contrast enhancement during the arterial phase. The intermittent insonation usually does not allow identification of the central spoke-wheel shaped contrast enhancement in the arterial phase. During the late phase, focal nodular hyperplasia typically shows persistent microbubble uptake similar to the adjacent liver (BLOMLEY et al. 2001). This is due to the liver-specific properties of some air-filled microbubbles such as Levovist or Sonavist, which probably pool in sinusoids or are phagocytosed by Kupffer cells, in a manner similar to that observed when using sulfur colloid for scintigraphy or liver-specific contrast agents for MR imaging (BLUEMKE et al. 2003; M.G. KIM et al. 2003). During the late phase, the central scar, being devoid of sinusoids and Kupffer cells, is often evident since it is spared by microbubble uptake (Fig. 11.15).

After the administration of new generation sulfur hexafluoride- or perfluorocarbon-filled microbubbles for low acoustic power imaging, focal nodular hyperplasia may display central spoke-wheel shaped contrast enhancement (Fig. 11.16) during the first 10–15 s post injection (ALBRECHT et al. 2003; NICOLAU et al. 2003a; QUAIA et al. 2003, 2004), often with evidence of peripheral tortuous draining vessels. During the following seconds there is persistent diffuse homogeneous contrast enhancement, with a hyper- or isoechoic appearance relative to the adjacent liver during the late phase (QUAIA et al. 2004). In cases of focal nodular hyperplasia smaller than 3 cm, the central spoke-wheel shaped contrast enhancement is more rarely observed, and diffuse contrast enhancement is immediately seen during the whole arterial phase. In the late phase the central scar may appear evident as a central hypoechoic region (Fig. 11.17) spared by microbubbles (ALBRECHT et al. 2003; NICOLAU et al. 2003a; QUAIA et al. 2003, 2004). This is because microbubble-based agents are purely intravascular agents and do not present any leakage into the interstitium during the late phase, a process that causes scar enhancement on contrast-enhanced CT and MR imaging.

11.3.3
Hepatocellular Adenoma

Epidemiology and histopathologic features. Hepatocellular adenoma is a rare benign hepatic neoplasm. Risk factors are use of estrogen- or androgen-containing steroid medications (the risk being related to the dose and duration) and the presence of type I glycogen storage disease (GRAZIOLI et al. 2001a). The clinical presentation is usually pain due to mass effect (40%) or intratumoral or intraperitoneal hemorrhage (40%); it is an asymptomatic incidental finding in the remaining 20% of cases. Hepatocellular adenomas usually measure 8–10 cm at presentation, may be multiple (more than 10), are frequently encapsulated, and may be difficult to differentiate from other benign or malignant hepatic tumors (ICHIKAWA et al. 2000). Adenomas present intratumoral hemorrhage or necrosis in up to 60% of cases (SANDLER et al. 1980).

Adenoma cells are larger than normal hepatocytes and contain large amounts of glycogen and lipid, which gives the characteristic yellow appearance of the cut surface. The propensity to hemorrhage reflects the histologic characteristics of adenomas, which consist of large plates of cells separated by dilated sinusoids that are perfused by arterial pressure since adenomas lack a portal venous supply and are fed solely by peripheral arterial feeding vessels. The extensive sinusoids and feeding arteries account for the hypervascular nature of hepatocellular adenoma, and the poor connective tissue support also predisposes to hemorrhage. Bile ductules are notably absent, as are Kupffer cells, a key histologic feature that helps distinguish hepatocellular adenoma from focal nodular hyperplasia. Malignant trans-

Characterization of Focal Liver Lesions

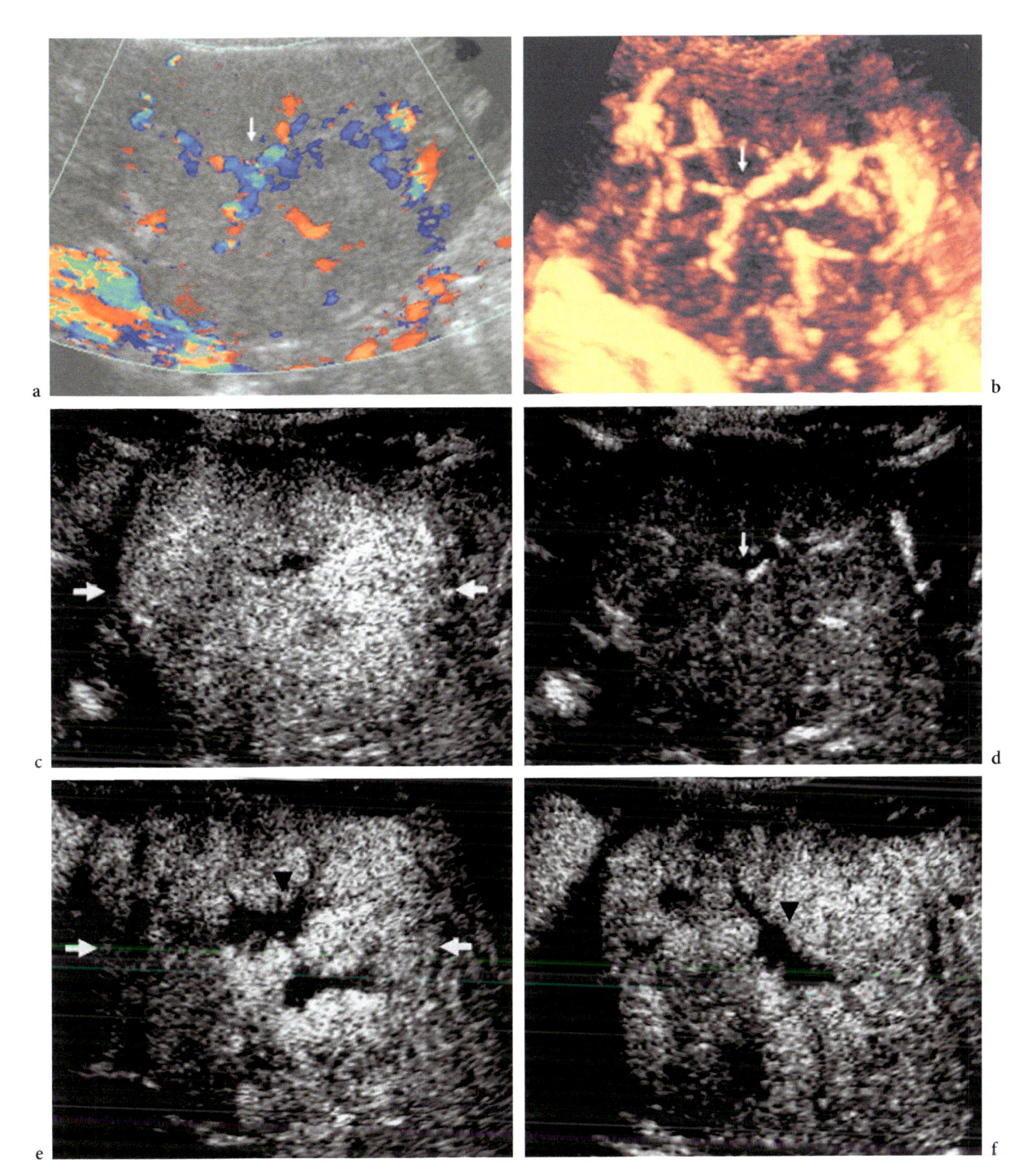

Fig. 11.15a–f. Focal nodular hyperplasia: spoke-wheel shaped contrast enhancement. **a, b** Baseline color (**a**) and power (**b**) Doppler. The central spoke-wheel shaped pattern (*arrow*) is identified, with a central vessel branching toward the periphery. **c–f** Contrast-enhanced US. Contrast-specific mode: Pulse Inversion Mode (Philips-ATL, WA, USA) after air-filled microbubble injection with high acoustic power insonation and production of four frames after each insonation. Diffuse homogeneous (*arrows*) contrast enhancement is evident during the arterial phase in the first frame of the train (**c**), while intratumoral vessels with a spoke-wheel shaped appearance (*arrow*) are identified in the second frame of the train (**d**). Diffuse contrast enhancement (*arrows*) persists in the late phase (**e, f**), sparing a central hypoechoic region (*black arrowhead*) that corresponds to the central scar.

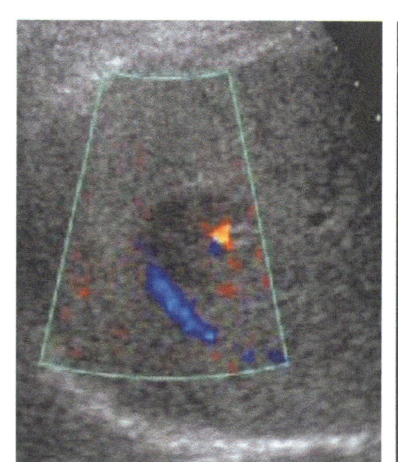

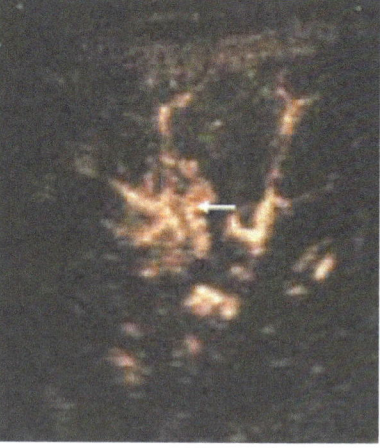

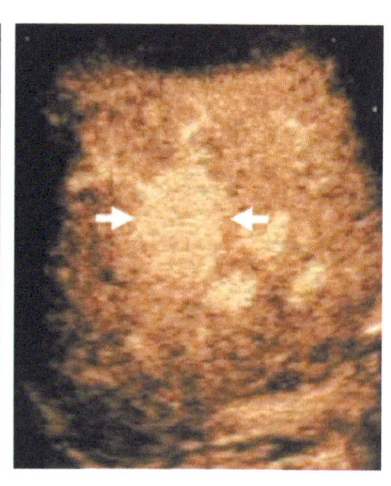

Fig. 11.16a–c. Focal nodular hyperplasia: central spoke-wheel shaped contrast enhancement pattern. Axial plane. **a** Baseline color Doppler US. Central vessels are identified in a hypoechoic focal liver lesion. **b, c** Contrast-enhanced US. Contrast-specific mode: Cadence Contrast Pulse Sequence (Siemens-Acuson, CA, USA). Central spoke-wheel shaped (*arrow*) contrast enhancement is evident 12 s after SonoVue injection (**b**). During the late phase (**c**), contrast enhancement remains diffuse, the lesion appearing isoechoic (*arrows*) relative to the surrounding liver.

Fig. 11.17a–c. Focal nodular hyperplasia: diffuse contrast enhancement pattern. Axial plane. **a** Baseline US. A slightly hyperechoic lesion (*arrows*) is identified. **b, c** Contrast-enhanced US. Contrast-specific mode: Coherent Contrast Imaging (Siemens-Acuson, CA, USA). Diffuse (*arrows*) contrast enhancement is evident 20 s after SonoVue injection (**b**), with evidence of some peritumoral tortuous draining vessels. In the late phase (**c**), contrast enhancement remains diffuse and the lesion has a hyperechoic appearance with evidence of a central hypoechoic region, corresponding to the central scar (*arrow*).

formation into hepatocellular carcinoma has been described (BRANCATELLI et al. 2002a).

Multimodality imaging – US and color Doppler US. The sonographic appearance of hepatocellular adenoma is variable and nonspecific. Most commonly it appears as a well-defined hyperechoic mass that is heterogeneous in terms of size and presence of hemorrhage and necrosis. The high lipid content of hepatocytes may result in variable to uniform hyperechogenicity within the lesion. No vascular pattern is considered specific for hepatocellular adenomas on color Doppler US (GOLLI et al. 1994), though subcapsular peripheral arteries and intranodular veins have been described (BARTOLOZZI et al. 1997).

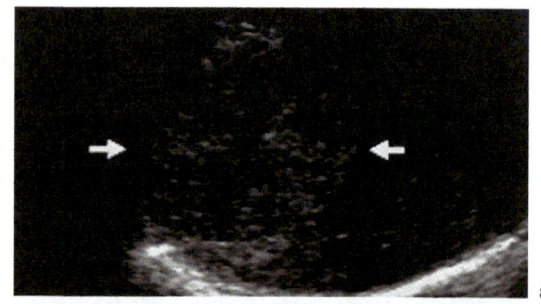

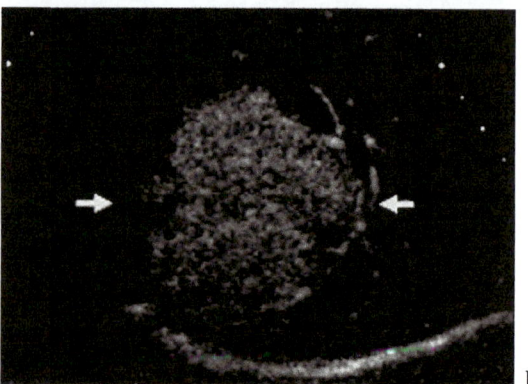

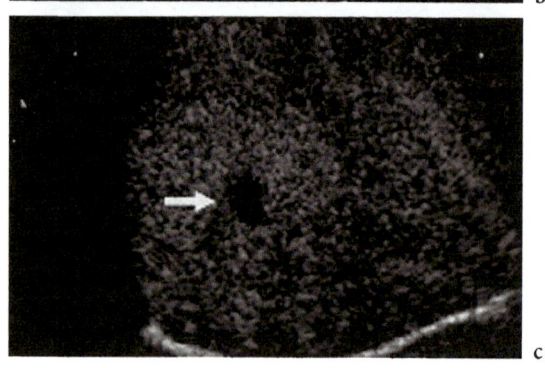

Multimodality imaging - CT. Histotype diagnosis of hepatocellular adenoma is often difficult with CT even though it may reveal some typical features (MATHIEU et al. 1986; WELCH et al. 1985; ICHIKAWA et al. 2000). The areas of fat may be identified on nonenhanced CT as low-attenuation intratumoral components, while areas of acute tumoral or subcapsular hemorrhage appear as heterogeneous hyperattenuating fluid. Necrosis and hemorrhage are identified in about one-fourth of hepatocellular adenomas (ICHIKAWA et al. 2000). Calcifications are rare and appear as large, coarse calcific opacities within areas of hemorrhage or necrosis.

The attenuation of the adenoma relative to the surrounding liver parenchyma varies depending on the composition of the tumor and that of the liver, as well as the phase of contrast enhancement after injection of iodinated contrast agent.

In patients with fatty liver, hepatocellular adenoma usually appears hyperattenuating during all phases of contrast enhancement. In normal liver, hepatocellular adenoma appears hyperattenuating during the arterial phase and isodense to the liver during the portal and late phases. It may have a homogeneous or heterogeneous appearance, the latter being particularly frequent when the lesion size exceeds 3 cm, and there is often evidence of a hyperattenuating tumoral capsule.

Multimodality imaging **MR.** Hepatocellular adenoma shows diffuse contrast enhancement during the arterial phase after paramagnetic contrast agent injection, often with a heterogeneous appearance due to the intratumoral hemorrhagic or necrotic component. A hypointense appearance compared to adjacent liver 1 h after administration of Gd-BOPTA is considered typical since this lesion is devoid of biliary structures (GRAZIOLI et al. 2001a).

Contrast-enhanced US. After microbubble injection, hepatocellular adenoma displays diffuse homogeneous or heterogeneous contrast enhancement. It may show either a persistent iso- or slightly hyperechoic appearance relative to the adjacent liver up until the late phase or a heterogeneous appearance. Whether hepatocellular adenomas display a homogeneous (Fig. 11.18) or heterogeneous (Fig. 11.19) appearance during each dynamic phase depends on the extent of the hemorrhagic and necrotic intratumoral component. Pericapsular feeding blood vessels are best visualized in the early arterial phase, while in the portal and late phases hepatocellular adenoma usually presents the same vascular behavior as the surrounding liver parenchyma (QUAIA et al. 2004).

11.3.4
Macroregenerative and Dysplastic Nodules

Epidemiology and histopathologic features. Liver cirrhosis is preceded by varying pathologic parenchymal changes, including steatosis, inflammation, and edema, before the irreversible stages of fibro-

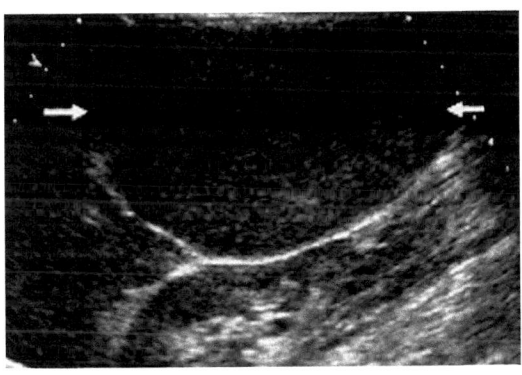

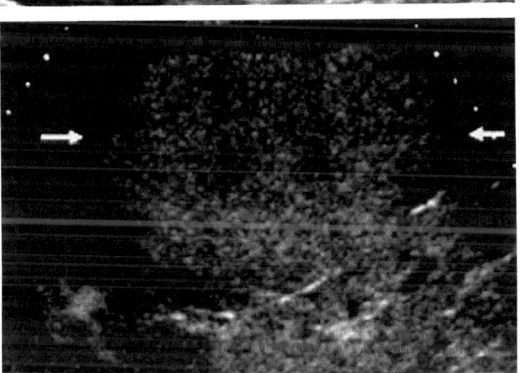

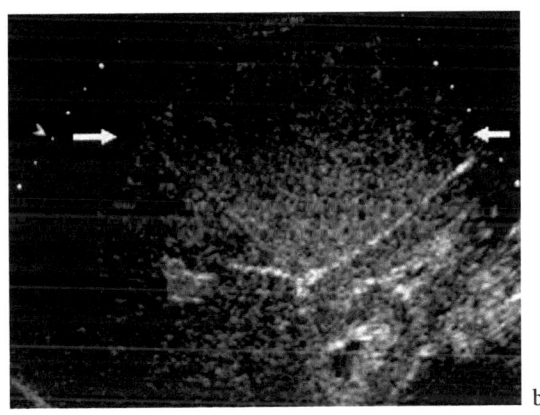

Fig. 11.18a–c. Hepatocellular adenoma: homogeneous appearance on contrast-enhanced US. Longitudinal plane. a Baseline US. A large hypoechoic lesion is identified in the left lobe of the liver (*arrows*). b, c Contrast-specific mode: Coherent Contrast Imaging (Siemens-Acuson, CA, USA). After the injection of sulfur hexafluoride-filled microbubbles, the lesion shows diffuse and homogeneous contrast enhancement during the arterial phase (b). Microbubble uptake persists during the late phase (c), and the lesion has a hyperechoic appearance relative to the adjacent liver.

144   E. Quaia et al.

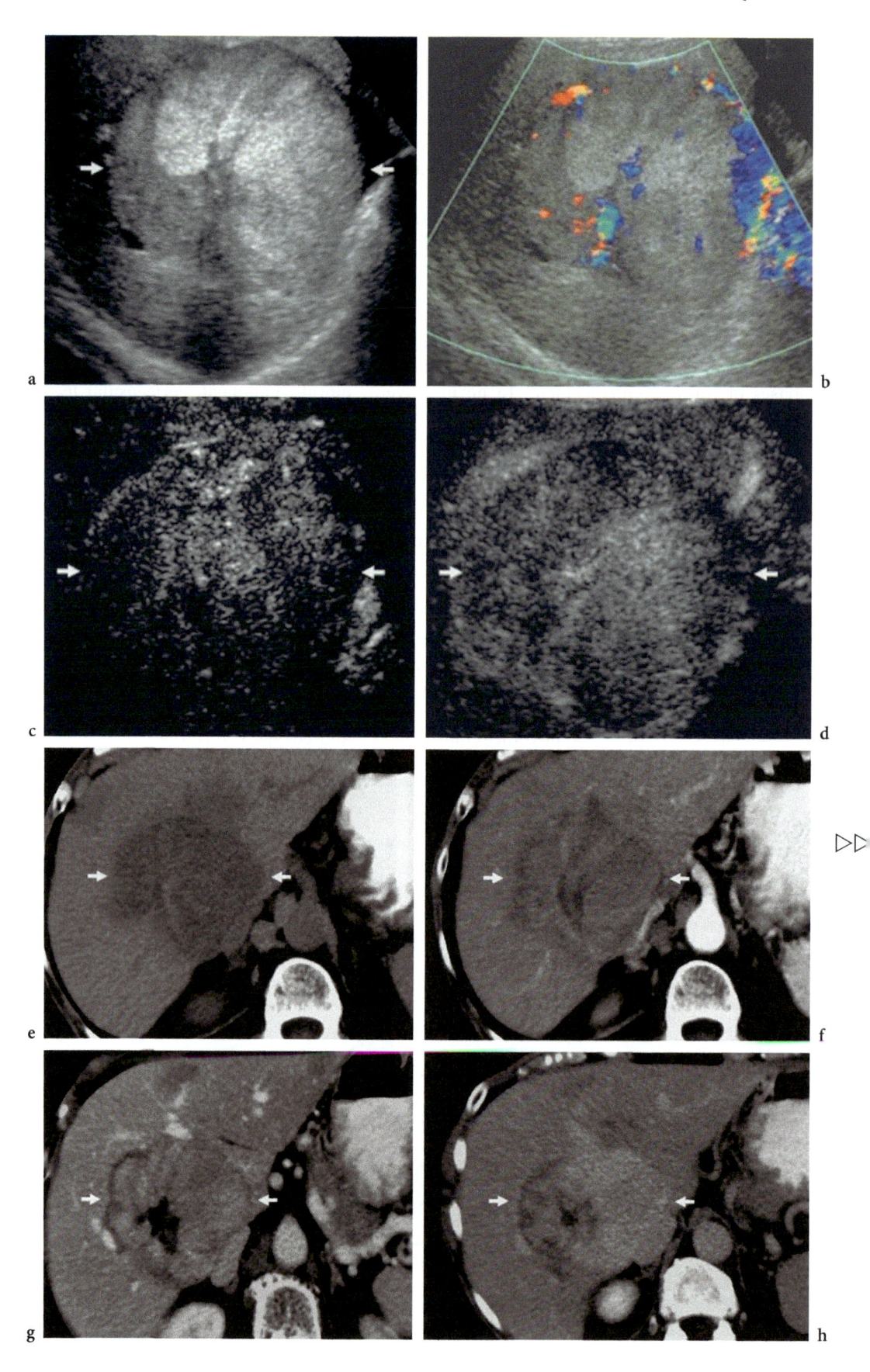

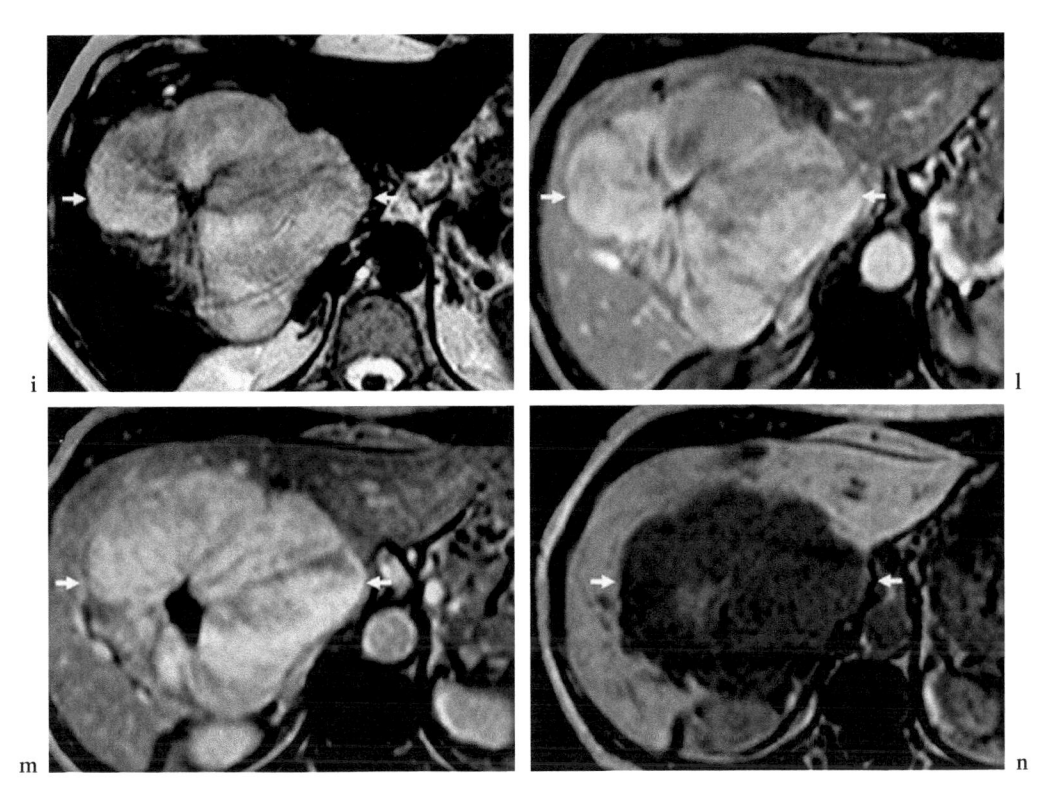

Fig. 11.19a-n. Hepatocellular adenoma: heterogeneous appearance on contrast-enhanced US. Axial plane. **a, b** Baseline US and color Doppler US. The lesion (*arrows*) has a heterogeneous appearance on baseline US (**a**) and peripheral and intratumoral vessels are demonstrated on color Doppler US (**b**). **c, d** Contrast-specific mode: Pulse Inversion Mode (Philips-ATL, WA, USA) after the injection of sulfur hexafluoride-filled microbubbles. Diffuse and heterogeneous contrast enhancement (*arrows*) appears 20 s after microbubble injection (**c**). The lesion (*arrows*) shows persistent microbubble uptake during the late phase (**d**), with a heterogeneous appearance. **e-h** Nonenhanced (**e**) and iodinated contrast-enhanced (**f-h**) CT scan. The hepatocellular adenoma (*arrows*) appears heterogeneous on the nonenhanced scan (**e**) and presents persistent and heterogeneous contrast enhancement during the arterial (**f**), portal (**g**), and late (**h**) phases. **i-n** Nonenhanced (**i**) and Gd-BOPTA-enhanced (**l-n**) MR scan. The hepatocellular adenoma (*arrows*) appears hyperintense on T2-weighted turbo spin echo nonenhanced scan (**i**) and presents diffuse and heterogeneous contrast enhancement during the arterial (**l**) and portal (**m**) phases. A diagnostic hypointense appearance is seen at 1 h post injection on the delayed scan (**n**).

sis and nodular regeneration occur (BARON and PETERSON 2001).

Nodular lesions within the liver parenchyma can be separated into three broad categories: regenerative, dysplastic, or neoplastic. Regenerative nodules represent a region of parenchyma enlarged in response to necrosis, altered circulation, or other stimuli and may be observed both in noncirrhotic liver pathologies and in cirrhosis. The correct term for nodules larger than 5 mm in diameter is macroregenerative nodules or large regenerative nodules. Nodules smaller than 5 mm are usually not identified by imaging, even though they may give rise to a heterogeneous appearance of liver parenchyma.

In the absence of surrounding fibrous stroma, such nodules are also known as nodular regenerative hyperplasia (BARON and PETERSON 2001). Nodular regenerative hyperplasia is frequently observed in many hepatic vascular disorders or systemic conditions such as Budd-Chiari syndrome (BRANCATELLI et al. 2002a), autoimmune disease, myeloproliferative disorders, and lymphoproliferative disorders.

When the macroregenerative nodule is surrounded by fibrous septa and constitutes the entire region banded by septa, it is also called a regenerative nodule on the basis of surrounding parenchymal attributes. When larger than 2 cm, macroregenerative nodules are usually dysplastic and contain cellular atypia without frank malignant changes (BARON and PETERSON 2001).

Dysplastic nodules in the liver are nodular hepatocellular proliferations lacking the definite histopathologic criteria for malignancy (KIM et al. 2002). They contain cellular atypia without frank malignant changes and are sometimes precursors to frank hepatocellular carcinoma. Low-grade (adenomatous hyperplasia) and high-grade (atypical adenomatous hyperplasia) dysplastic nodules may be identified, and a prevalently portal blood flow in macroregenerative nodules and arterial blood flow in dysplastic nodules has been reported (KIM et al. 2002). Although low-grade dysplastic nodules have a somewhat higher prevalence of portal blood supply than high-grade dysplastic nodules, the portal and arterial supplies are very variable (LIM et al. 2000; KIM et al. 2002).

Multimodality imaging. Macroregenerative nodules usually show a hypoechoic appearance on baseline US, and often they appear heterogeneous. On color Doppler US, macroregenerative nodules display peripheral arterial and venous vessels (QUAIA et al. 2002c).

Findings on CT during arterial portography and CT during hepatic arteriography correlated positively with histologic grading. An overlap in appearance with dysplastic nodules and hepatocellular carcinomas was observed (HAYASHI et al. 1999, 2002).

Macroregenerative nodules may appear hyperdense on nonenhanced CT. After the injection of iodinated contrast agent they usually display a hypodense appearance during the arterial phase, and progressively appear isodense relative to adjacent liver parenchyma during the late phase (BARON and PETERSON 2001). Typically, macroregenerative nodules show low signal intensity on T2-weighted MR images, variable signal intensity on T1-weighted images, and no enhancement on arterial phase dynamic gadolinium-enhanced images (HUSSAIN et al. 2002).

Dysplastic nodules appear hyperdense on nonenhanced CT and become isoattenuating during the portal phase on contrast-enhanced CT (BARON and PETERSON 2001). Dysplastic nodules may display diffuse contrast enhancement and may simulate hepatocellular carcinoma. MR imaging of large dysplastic nodules may show a distinct pattern of homogeneous high signal intensity on T1-weighted images and very low signal intensity on T2-weighted images due to the high iron content (BARON and PETERSON 2001).

Contrast-enhanced US. After microbubble injection, most macroregenerative nodules show absent or persistent dotted contrast enhancement, with a

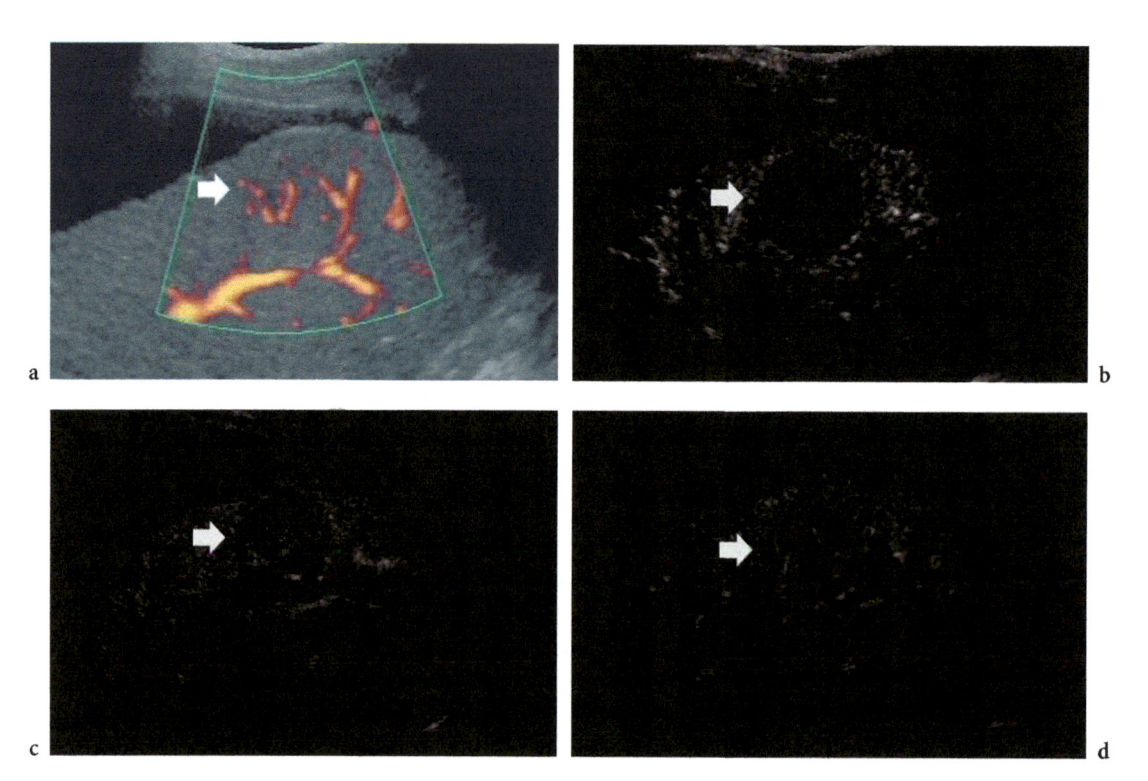

Fig. 11.20a-d. Macroregenerative nodule. **a** Baseline power Doppler US. An isoechoic lesion (*arrow*) with some intratumoral vessels is identified. **b-d** Contrast-enhanced US. Pulse Inversion Mode (Philips-ATL, WA, USA) with low acoustic power after injection of sulfur hexafluoride-filled microbubbles. There is absence of contrast enhancement in the arterial phase, the lesion having a hypovascular appearance (**b**). Progressively the lesion appears isoechoic relative to the adjacent liver during the portal (**c**) and late phases (**d**).

hypovascular or isovascular appearance during the arterial phase followed by an isovascular appearance during the late phase (Fig. 11.20) (Quaia et al. 2002b, 2004).

Dysplastic macroregenerative nodules may display diffuse (Quaia et al. 2004) contrast enhancement during the arterial phase. In relation to the adjacent liver, they appear iso- or hyperechoic in the arterial phase and isoechoic in the late phase (Fig. 11.21). A predominantly arterial blood flow is frequently present, this being the cause of the diffuse contrast enhancement (Kim et al. 2002). When diffuse contrast enhancement pattern is observed, consideration must be given to differentiation between dysplastic macroregenerative nodules and well-differentiated hepatocellular carcinomas, which may be difficult or even impossible, including at histologic assessment (Longchampt et al. 2000). Absence of contrast enhancement (Wen 2004) is related to a prevalently portal blood supply and arterial hypovascularity, as has been shown by other studies (Matsui et al. 1991). Development of hepatocellular carcinoma within high-grade dysplastic nodules of the liver may be identified by contrast-enhanced US (Nomura et al. 1993), on the basis of focal nodular intratumoral enhancement in the tumoral zone with malignant transformation ("nodule in nodule" pattern).

11.3.5
Focal Fatty Sparing and Focal Fatty Changes

Epidemiology and histopathologic features. Fatty infiltration of the liver is a well-characterized entity caused by accumulation of triglycerides within hepatocytes (Alpers and Isselbachers 1975). Fatty changes can be diffuse, even though heterogeneous distribution of fat is also frequently found. Nondiffuse fatty change of the liver, involving focal fatty deposition (Baker et al. 1985; Brawer et al. 1980; Halvorsen et al. 1982) and focal spared areas (Hirohashi et al. 2000; Kissin et al. 1986), appear as skip focal areas.

Multimodality imaging. On baseline US, focal fatty infiltration and focal fatty sparing are most commonly found adjacent to the gallbladder wall, the hepatic hilum, or the falciform ligament. Both focal

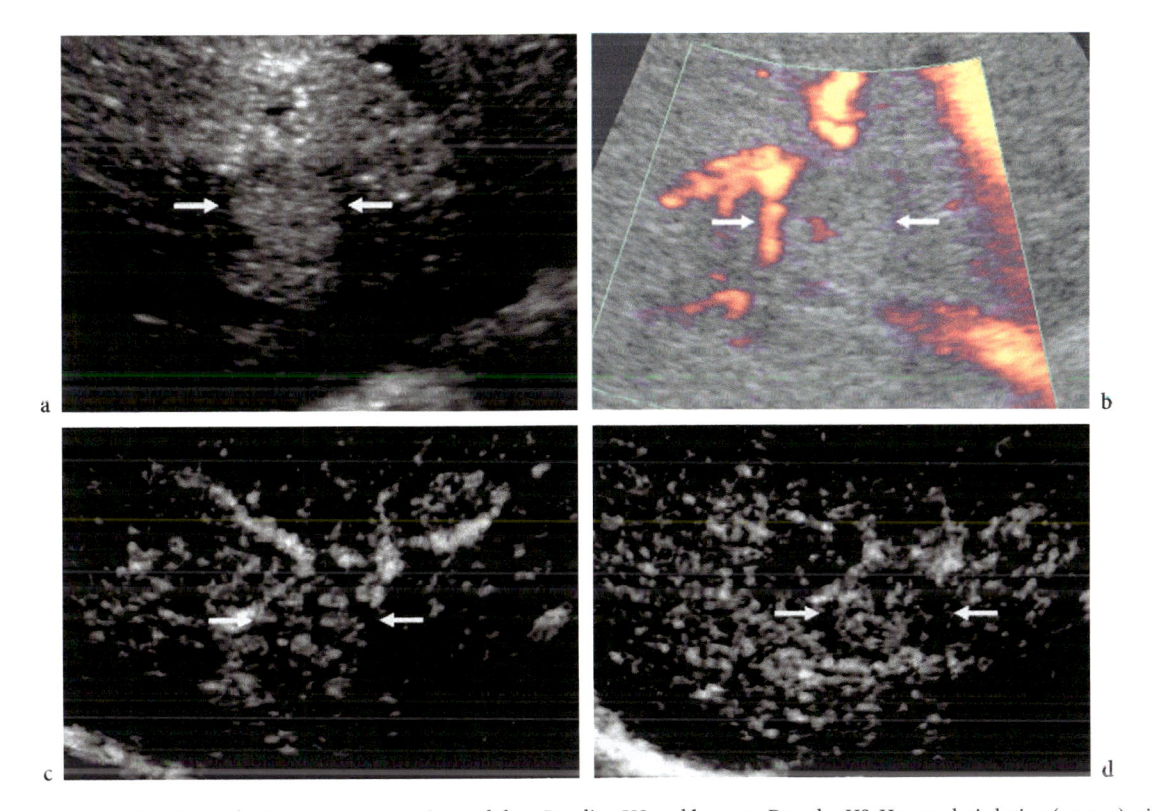

Fig. 11.21a–d. Dysplastic macroregenerative nodule. a Baseline US and b power Doppler US. Hyperechoic lesion (*arrows*) with one intratumoral vessel flow signal is identified. c, d Contrast-enhanced US. Contrast Tuned Imaging (Esaote, Genoa, Italy) with low acoustic power after the injection of sulfur hexafluoride-filled microbubbles. Diffuse contrast enhancement (*arrows*) is identified during the arterial phase (c), while the lesion has an isoechoic appearance relative to the adjacent liver in the late phase (d).

fatty infiltration and focal sparing may present a nodular or pseudonodular pattern which has to be differentiated from other focal liver lesions. Color Doppler US typically identifies normal vessels that run unaltered throughout the liver areas. On CT and MR imaging, both entities are easily differentiated from real tumors by the lack of a mass effect, undistorted vessels in the suspected area, and a similar grade of enhancement compared to the adjacent liver (HALVORSEN et al. 1982; KANE et al. 1993).

Contrast-enhanced US. After microbubble injection, focal fatty sparing and focal fatty changes display homogeneous contrast enhancement with the same echo intensity as the adjacent normal liver parenchyma in the arterial, portal, and late phases (Fig. 11.22) (NICOLAU et al. 2003a; QUAIA et al. 2004).

11.3.6
Other Benign Focal Liver Lesions

Hepatic abscess. Hepatic abscesses are usually pyogenic (88%), amoebic (10%), or fungal (2%); 50% are multiple. On baseline US, colliquative liver abscess present an anechoic appearance with multiple heterogeneous spots at different levels. After microbubble injection, liver abscesses may present a similar appearance to hepatic malignancies since they show a hypoechoic appearance during the late phase (ALBRECHT et al. 2003) that may or may not be preceded by rim-like peripheral enhancement during the arterial phase (Fig. 11.23). The principal difference between liver abscesses and hepatic malignancies relates to the lesion shape and margins, which are coalescent and sharp in abscesses and round and ill-defined in malignancies (KIM et al. 2004a). Another important difference is the complete absence of vessels and enhancement in the central liquid portion of abscesses: even hypovascular metastases display some spots of weak contrast enhancement in the center of the lesion, except in the case of completely necrotic lesions (ALBRECHT et al. 2003).

Solitary necrotic hepatic nodule. This is a rare benign focal liver lesion which is often an incidental finding on US and may mimic a metastases (DE LUCA et al. 2000; COLAGRANDE et al. 2003). Most reported cases of solitary necrotic nodule have been in males, and the majority of these lesions have occurred in the right hepatic lobe (KOEA et al. 2003). At histologic analysis the solitary necrotic nodule is characterized by central coagulative necrosis, often partly calcified and surrounded by a dense hyalinized fibrous capsule containing elastin fibers (KOEA et al. 2003). On US, the necrotic nodule usually appears hypoechoic or target-like with a hyperechoic center, while on contrast-enhanced CT and MR imaging no contrast enhancement is identified. After microbubble injection, the absence of contrast enhancement is evident (Fig. 11.24).

Other rare benign focal liver lesions may be identified and scanned after the injection of microbubble-based agents, e.g., inflammatory pseudotumor (chronic inflammatory cell infiltration and fibrosis), intrahepatic extramedullary hemato-

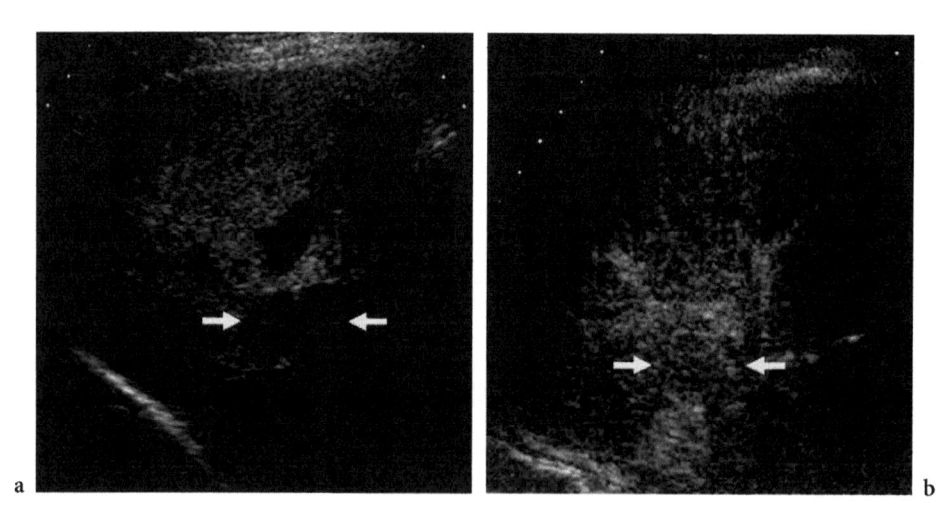

Fig. 11.22a,b. Region of focal fatty sparing. **a** Baseline US and **b** contrast-enhanced US during the late phase, 2 min after the injection of sulfur hexafluoride-filled microbubbles. The lesion (*arrows*) appears hypoechoic in a bright liver on baseline US but isoechoic during the late phase after microbubble injection.

Characterization of Focal Liver Lesions

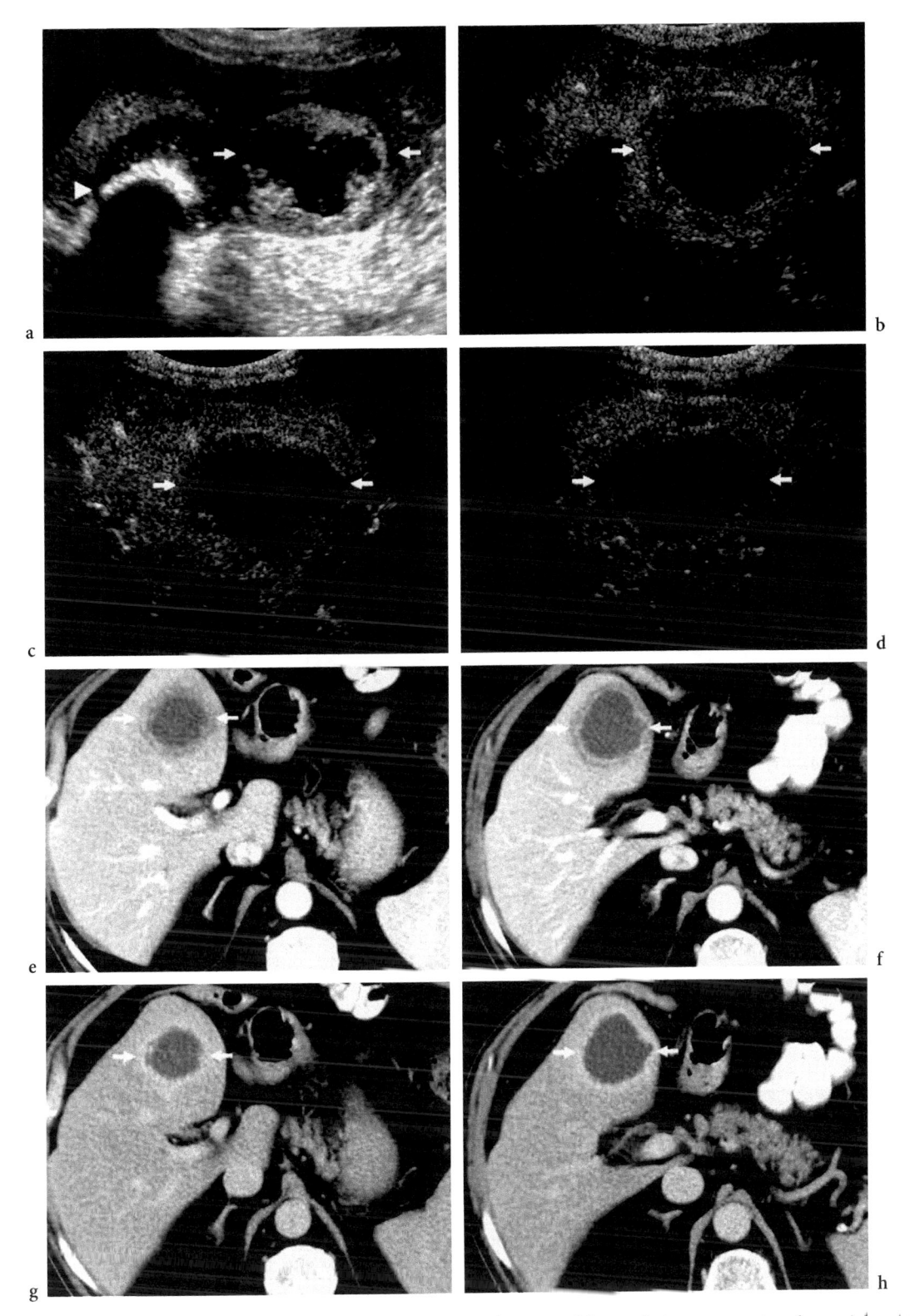

Fig. 11.23a–h. Liver abscess. a A heterogeneous lesion with a central hypoechoic component and a peripheral hyperechoic component adjacent to a calculous gallbladder is identified on baseline US. b–d After microbubble injection, the abscess demonstrates peripheral capsular enhancement sparing the central liquid portion. e–h On contrast-enhanced CT (iodinated contrast agent), the peripheral capsule displays progressively increasing contrast enhancement with a hyperdense appearance during the late phase, sparing the central liquid portion.

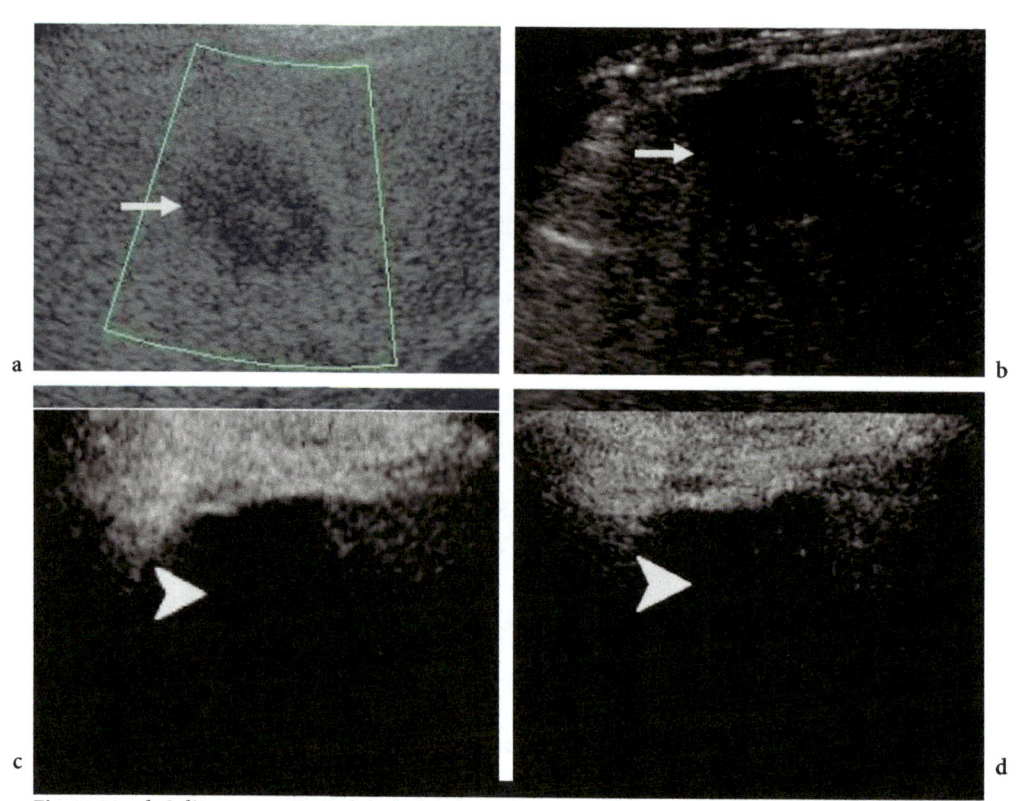

Fig. 11.24a–d. Solitary necrotic nodule. Axial plane. Contrast-enhanced US. Contrast-specific mode: Contrast Tuned Imaging (Esaote, Genoa, Italy) after the injection of sulfur hexafluoride-filled microbubbles. The lesion (*arrows*) appears hypoechoic on baseline US (**a**), with intratumoral vessels visible on color Doppler US (**b**). Contrast enhancement is absent in both the arterial (**c**) and the late phase (**d**). The lesion has a persistent hypoechoic appearance during the late phase (*arrowheads*).

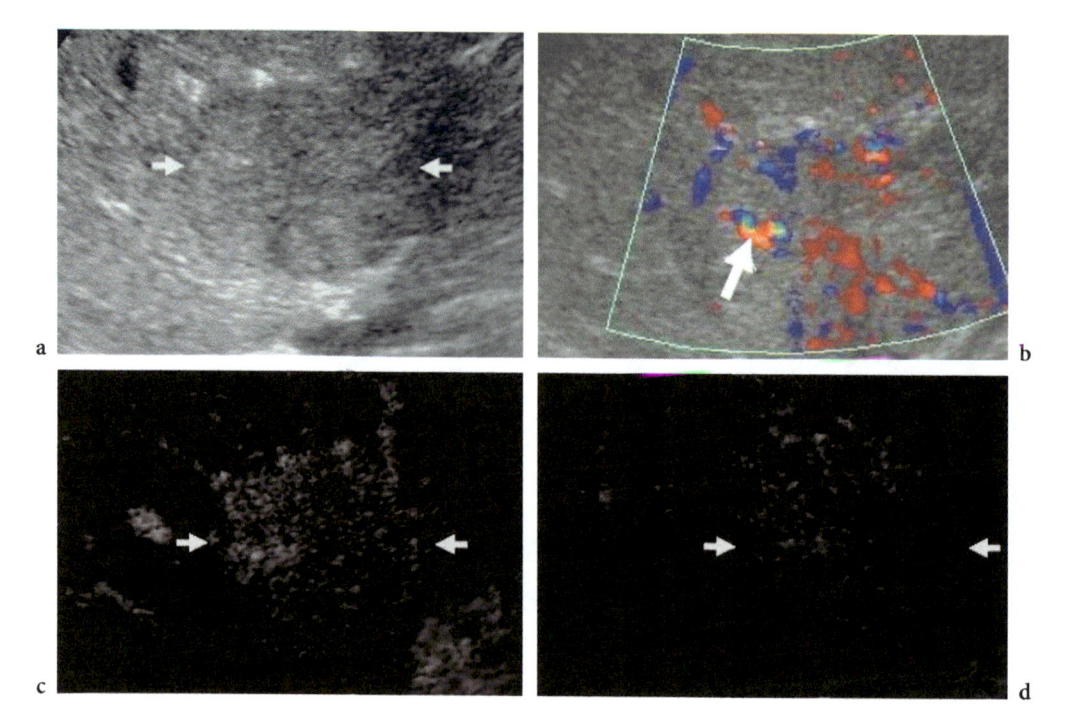

Fig. 11.25a–d. Intrahepatic extramedullary hematopoiesis. Axial plane. Contrast-enhanced US. Contrast-specific mode: Pulse Inversion Mode (Philips-ATL, WA, USA) after the injection of sulfur hexafluoride-filled microbubbles. The lesion (*arrows*) appears hypoechoic on baseline US (**a**), with intratumoral vessels (*arrow*) on color Doppler US (**b**). Diffuse contrast enhancement is identified during the arterial phase (**c**) and persists into the late phase (**d**), when the lesion continues to appear slightly hyperechoic relative to the surrounding liver.

poiesis (Fig. 11.25), and hepatic angiomyolipoma (Fig. 11.26). These lesions usually display a hypervascular pattern during the arterial phase, with persistent microbubble uptake in the late phase, as for the other benign focal liver lesions.

11.4
Malignant Focal Liver Lesions

11.4.1
Hepatocellular Carcinoma

Epidemiology and histopathologic features. Hepatocellular carcinoma is the most common primary liver malignancy and its incidence is increasing, particularly in Asia and Africa. The prevalence of hepatocellular carcinoma has been reported to be 14% among transplant recipients with cirrhosis in whom there was no suspicion of tumor before referral for transplantation (PETERSON et al. 2000). Accordingly, it is strongly associated with cirrhosis (80% of patients) and also with chronic viral hepatitis, the greatest increase in risk being observed among patients with hepatitis B or C (PETERSON et al. 2000; BARON and PETERSON 2001). Hepatocellular carcinoma shows a propensity for venous invasion, with involvement of the portal vein (in 30–60% of cases) or hepatic vein (in 15%) and inferior vena cava. HCC may occur in three forms: solitary, multiple, and diffuse infiltrative (LARCOS et al. 1998).

Multimodality imaging – US and color Doppler US. The appearance of hepatocellular carcinoma on baseline US is variable but there is a relationship with size. Hepatocellular carcinomas <3 cm (EBARA et al. 1986) predominantly appear hypoechoic, though small tumors may appear echogenic due to the presence of fatty changes or sinusoidal dilatation (YOSHIKAWA et al. 1988). A hypoechoic rim may be observed around small echogenic HCCs owing to the presence of a fibrous capsule; this assists in the differentiation from other focal liver lesions in the cirrhotic liver, such as hemangiomas. Large (>5 cm) hepatocellular carcinomas are predominantly hyperechoic and heterogeneous due to the presence of hemorrhage, fibrosis, and necrosis.

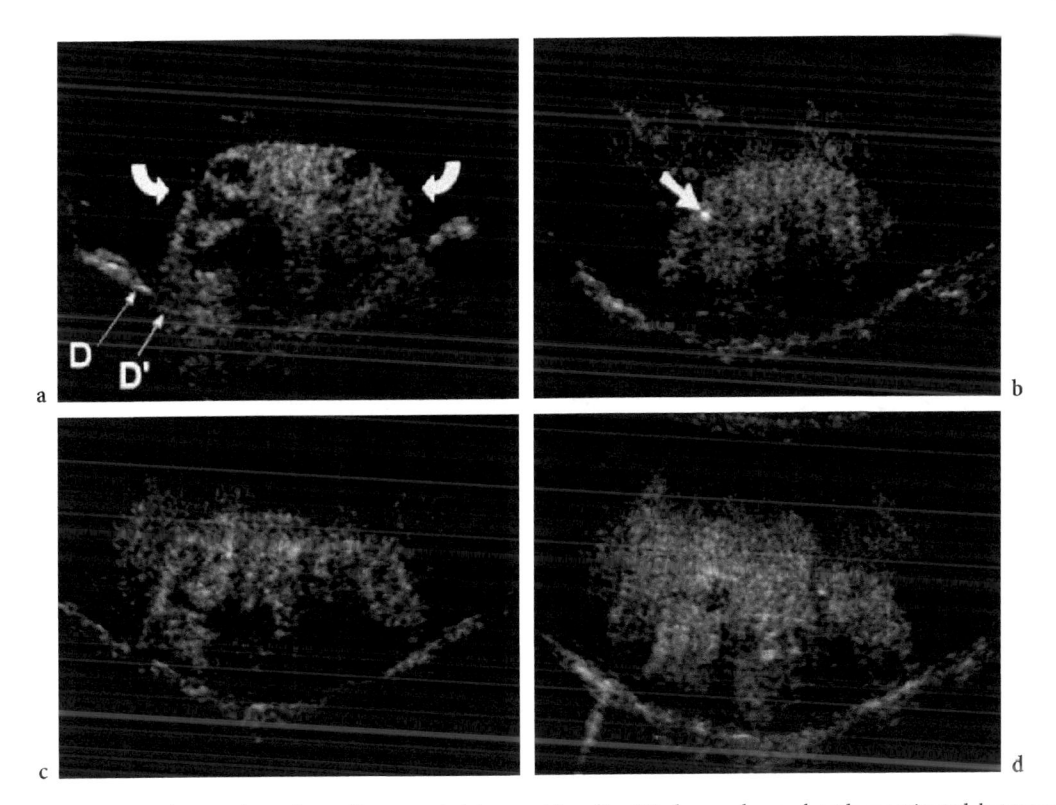

Fig. 11.26a–d. Hepatic angiomyolipoma. a Axial scan at baseline US shows a large, sharply marginated, heterogeneous and predominantly hyperechoic mass (*curved arrows*) with diffuse posterior acoustic enhancement. The segment of the diaphragm (*D'*) posterior to the hepatic mass appears displaced away from the rest of the diaphragm (*D*). This is due to an artifact caused by the lower US velocity in the fat of the angiomyolipoma compared with the adjacent liver parenchyma. b–d Contrast enhanced US, 25 s (b), 60 s (c), and 120 s (d) after the injection of air-filled microbubbles. Heterogeneous contrast enhancement is identified, with evidence of intralesional vessels (*arrow* in b).

It has been demonstrated that color Doppler US can accurately assess the vascularity of hepatocellular carcinomas (LENCIONI et al. 1996) for the purposes of differential diagnosis, choice of treatment, and assessment of therapeutic response. Color Doppler US with Doppler examination of tumor vessels shows high systolic and diastolic signals due to arteriovenous shunts and low-resistance vasculature. The basket pattern (TANAKA et al. 1992), consisting in peripheral arterial vessels branching toward the center of the lesion, is observed in about 75% of cases.

Multimodality imaging – CT and MR. Most hepatocellular carcinomas <3 cm are hypervascular and present diffuse contrast enhancement on CT and MR imaging, with contrast material washout in the portal venous phase (NINO-MURCIA et al. 2000; HUSSAIN et al. 2002). A minority of hepatocellular carcinomas <3 cm are hypovascular, with low or absent enhancement during the arterial phase (HAYASHI et al. 2002); such cases are best identified on portal venous phase or equilibrium phase imaging as hypodense lesions. Large (>5 cm) hepatocellular carcinomas are heterogeneous, with characteristic findings such as the mosaic pattern (different well-demarcated tumoral zone with different density) (STEVENS et al. 1996), a tumoral capsule, necrosis, and fatty metamorphosis (HUSSAIN et al. 2002). A tumoral capsule is in fact present in 60–82% of large hepatocellular carcinomas (HUSSAIN et al. 2002) and, typically, presents a hyperdense appearance during the late phase.

The signal intensity of hepatocellular carcinoma is variable on both T1-weighted and T2-weighted MR imaging sequences. Some hepatocellular carcinomas show a high signal intensity on T1-weighted images due to the presence of fat, copper, or glycoproteins (BARON and PETERSON 2001; HUSSAIN et al. 2002). After paramagnetic contrast agent injection, as on contrast-enhanced CT, enhancement is diffuse in smaller hepatocellular carcinomas and heterogeneous in larger cases. The evolution of a dysplastic nodule to hepatocellular carcinoma can be seen on MR imaging by virtue of the so-called nodule-in-a-nodule appearance (MITCHELL et al. 1991; HUSSAIN et al. 2002), with evidence of intratumoral contrast enhancement in the tumoral zone upon malignant transformation.

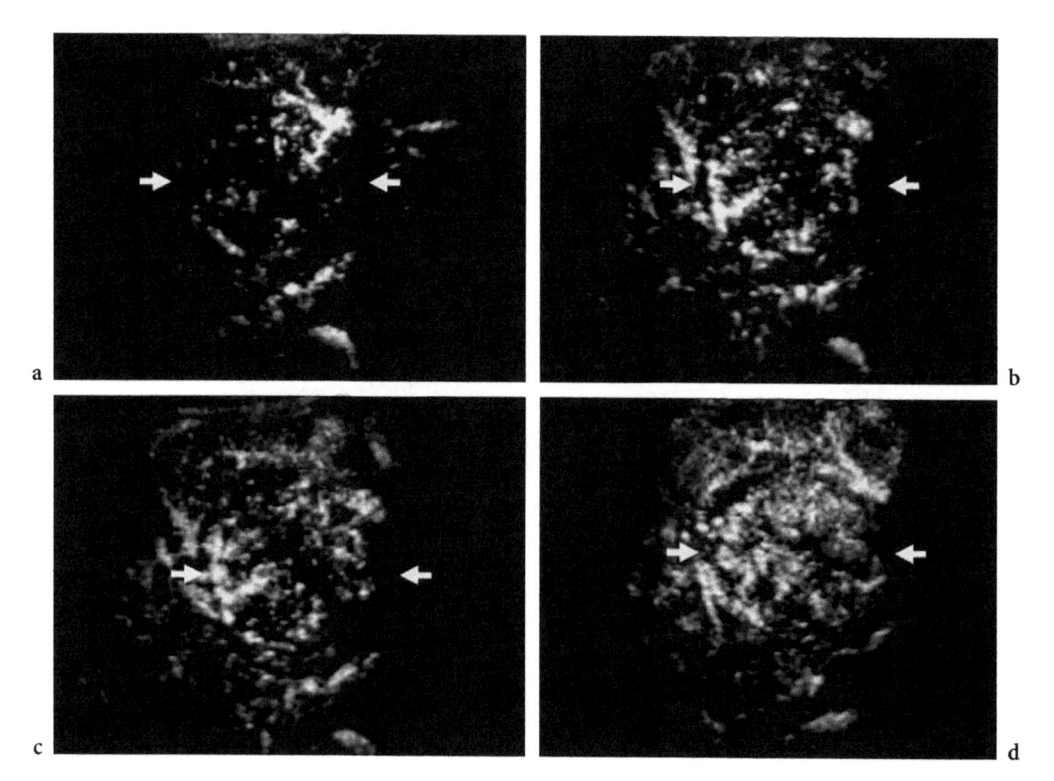

Fig. 11.27a–d. Hepatocellular carcinoma vascularity during the arterial phase after microbubble injection. Contrast-specific mode: Pulse Inversion Mode (ATL-Philips, WA, USA) with low acoustic power after the injection of sulfur hexafluoride-filled microbubbles. Within the hepatocellular carcinoma (*arrows*), peripheral and penetrating arterial vessels are observed during the first 15 (**a**) to 20 (**b**) s of the arterial phase. During the following seconds of the arterial phase (**c, d**), smaller intratumoral vessels also display contrast enhancement.

Contrast-enhanced US. After microbubble injection, intratumoral vessels are visualized in the majority of hepatocellular carcinomas during the arterial phase (Dill-Macky et al. 2002; Feruse et al. 2003; Isozaki et al. 2003; Wang et al. 2003; Cosgrove and Blomley 2004; Koda et al. 2004). The classic hemodynamics of hepatocellular carcinoma are characterized by evidence of tumor vessels and a hypervascular appearance during the arterial phase and by the absence of portal blood flow (Koda et al. 2004). Contrast-enhanced US has been shown to display tumor vessels during the first 15–20 s of the arterial phase (Fig. 11 27), with better accuracy than color Doppler US owing to the avoidance of motion and blooming artifacts (Koda et al. 2004).

Following the injection of microbubble-based agents, diffuse homogeneous or heterogeneous contrast enhancement (Figs. 11.28–11.31) is typically observed during the arterial phase (Choi et al. 2002; K.W. Kim et al. 2003), revealing the characteristic hypervascular nature of hepatocellular carcinoma. From 45 to 70 s after injection up to the late phase, hepatocellular carcinomas (whether smaller or larger than 3 cm) display a hypovascular (Figs. 11.28, 11.30) or isovascular (Figs. 11.29, 11.31) appearance compared to the adjacent liver, with or without evidence of peripheral hyperechoic rim-like enhancement.

The isovascular appearance of some hepatocellular carcinomas during the late phase is similar to that of benign focal liver lesions (Quaia et al. 2004). The reason for this atypical behavior is unclear. Possibly, the isoechoic appearance is caused by the recirculation of low levels of microbubbles, but further studies are necessary to determine whether histological or vascular differences exist in these cases. Some studies have correlated the appearance of hepatocellular carcinomas during the late phase with tumoral differentiation and identified better differentiation in hepatocellular carcinomas which appear isoechoic to the adjacent liver in the late phase (Nicolau et al. 2004).

Less frequently, hepatocellular carcinomas display persistent dotted contrast enhancement with either an initial hypovascular and late isovascular appearance (Quaia et al. 2004) or a persistent hypovascular appearance compared to the adjacent liver (Giorgio et al. 2004). This pattern resembles the hypovascular pattern described on CT (Hayashi et al. 2002) after the injection of iodinated agents.

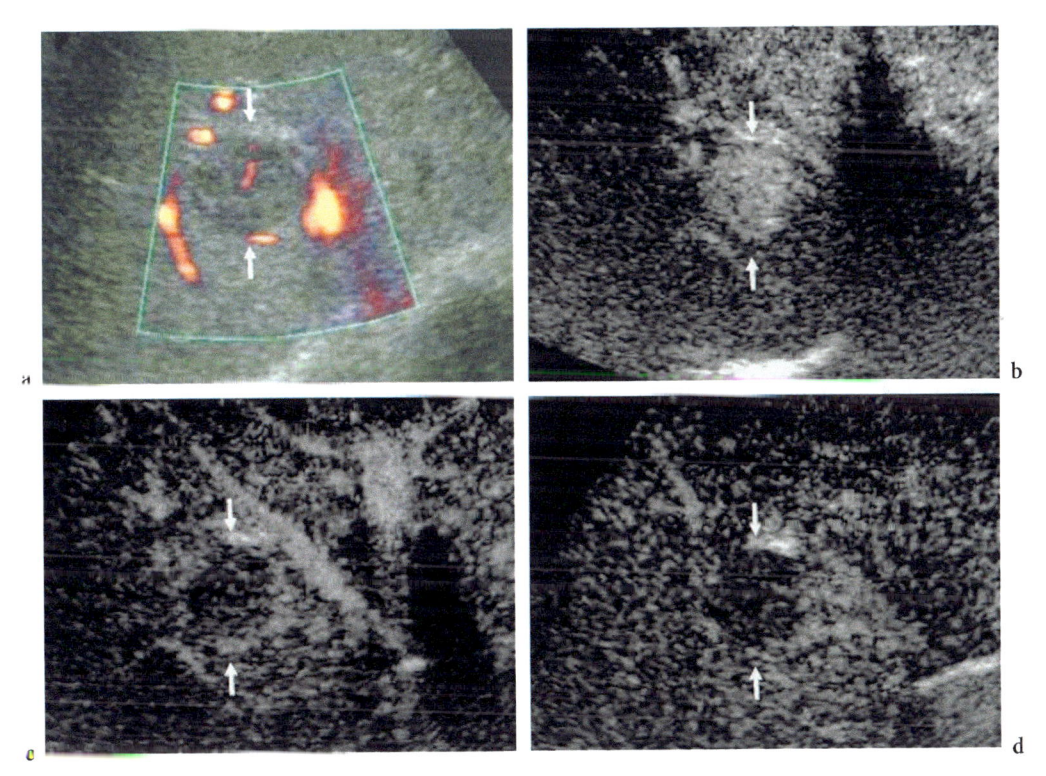

Fig. 11.28a–d. The most frequent and typical appearance of small hepatocellular carcinoma on contrast-enhanced US. Axial plane. a Baseline power Doppler US. The tumor (*arrows*) appears hypoechoic, with peripheral and intratumoral vessels. b–d Contrast-specific mode: Contrast Tuned Imaging (Esaote, Italy) with low acoustic power after the injection of sulfur hexafluoride-filled microbubbles. The hepatocellular carcinoma (*arrows*) presents diffuse homogeneous contrast enhancement with rapid microbubble washout and a hypovascular appearance during the portal (c) and late (d) phases, compared to the adjacent liver.

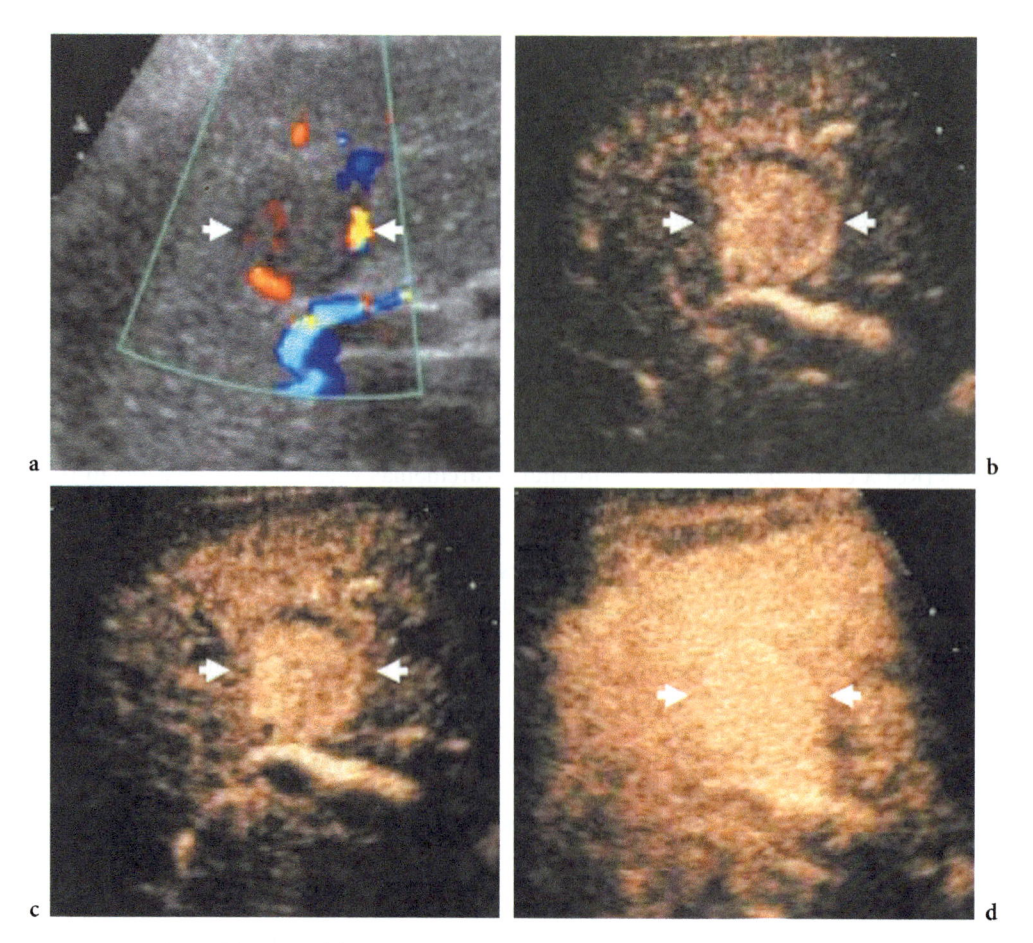

Fig. 11.29a-d. Small hepatocellular carcinoma with an isovascular appearance during the late phase on contrast-enhanced US. Longitudinal plane. a Baseline color doppler US. The tumour (*arrows*) presents prevalently peripheral vossels. b-d Contrast-specific mode: Cadence Contrast Pulse Sequence (Siemens-Acuson, CA, USA) with low acoustic power after the injection of sulfur hexafluoride-filled microbubbles. b Arterial phase (22 s after SonoVue injection). The hepatocellular carcinoma (*arrows*) presents diffuse and heterogeneous contrast enhancement. The tumor (*arrows*) appears isovascular to the adjacent liver during the portal phase (c=65 s after SonoVue injection) and the late phase (d=100 s after SonoVue injection).

Fibrolamellar hepatocellular carcinoma. The fibrolamellar type is a rare form (2%) of hepatocellular carcinoma occurring in younger females without coexisting liver disease and has a better prognosis than the common variety. It is typically large with a central stellate scar (Ichikawa et al. 1999, McLarney et al. 1999). Although it is important to distinguish fibrolamellar hepatocellular carcinoma from conventional hepatocellular carcinoma, it is equally important to distinguish it from certain benign liver lesions with a central scar, especially focal nodular hyperplasia, large hemangiomas (Blachar et al. 2002), and, rarely, hepatocellular adenomas. Calcifications are present in 40–68% of tumors, and areas of hypervascularity are heterogeneous in all cases. After the injection of iodinated or paramagnetic contrast agents for CT and MR imaging, respectively, a heterogeneous appearance was described during the arterial and portal phases, with evidence of a central scar, while a progressively homogeneous appearance was observed in the late phase (Ichikawa et al. 1999; McLarney et al. 1999). Fibrolamellar type hepatocellular carcinoma has been reported to present persistent rim-like or heterogeneous contrast enhancement with a hypoechoic appearance during the late phase (Quaia et al. 2004).

11.4.2
Metastases

Epidemiology and histopathologic features. Metastases are the more common malignant lesions of the liver in Europe and United States, in particular from tumors of the gastrointestinal tract (Ferrucci

Characterization of Focal Liver Lesions

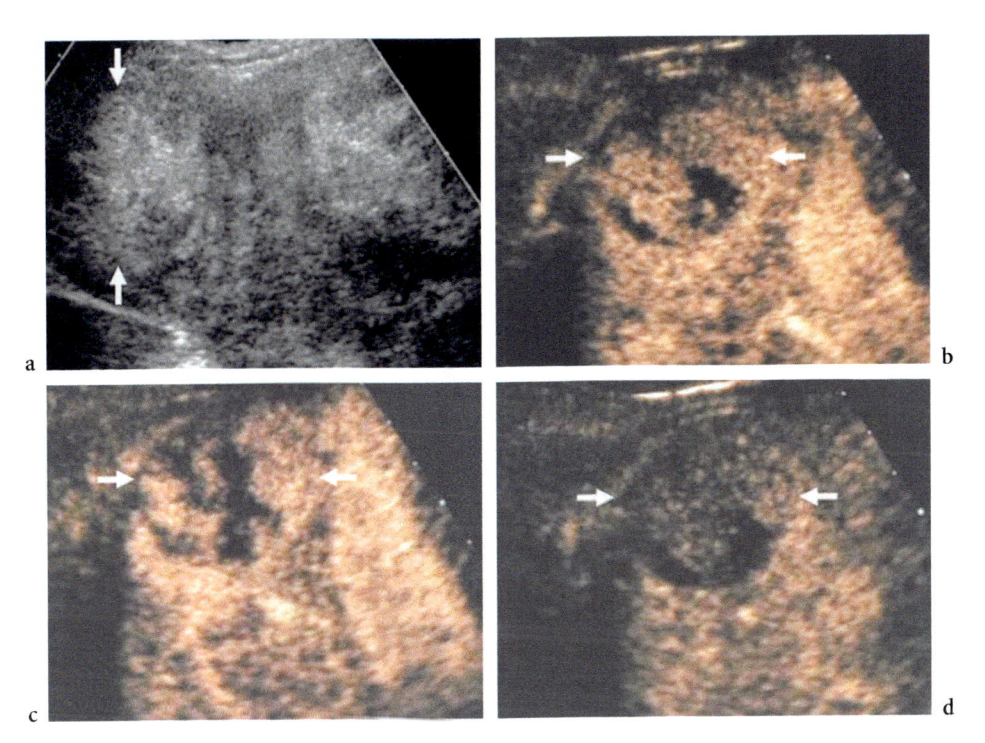

Fig. 11.30a–d. Large hepatocellular carcinoma that has a heterogeneous appearance on contrast-enhanced US and is hypoechoic during the late phase. Axial plane. **a** Baseline US. A heterogeneous lesion is identified. **b–d** Contrast-specific mode: Cadence Contrast Pulse Sequence (Siemens-Acuson, CA, USA) with low acoustic power after injection of sulfur hexafluoride-filled microbubbles. The carcinoma (*arrows*) presents diffuse and heterogeneous contrast enhancement during the arterial (**b**, 22 s after SonoVue injection) and the portal (**c**) phase and has a hypovascular appearance during the late phase (**d**) as compared to the adjacent liver parenchyma.

1994). Among nongastrointestinal malignancies, breast and lung cancers and melanoma are most likely to develop hepatic metastases. In comparison with the adjacent liver, metastases may present a hypovascular or, less frequently, a hypervascular pattern.

Multimodality imaging – US and color Doppler US. Metastases may display a variety of patterns on baseline US. Lesions may appear solid or cystic, with a hyper-, iso-, or hypoechoic pattern in comparison to the adjacent liver. Calcifications with posterior acoustic shadowing are typically observed in metastases from colorectal carcinoma. The peripheral hypoechoic halo, caused by the adjacent compressed liver parenchyma, is the most typical feature on baseline US, allowing characterization of metastases in most cases. On baseline color Doppler US, hypervascular metastases show a similar degree of hypervascularity to fibrous nodular hyperplasia and hepatocellular carcinoma (Harvey and Albrecht 2001).

Multimodality imaging – CT. Metastases typically appear hypodense on nonenhanced scan and present a persistent hypodense appearance on arterial, portal, and late phase scans (Nino-Murcia et al. 2000). After the injection of iodinated contrast agents, hypervascular metastases usually appear hyperdense (Oliver et al. 1997) compared to the adjacent liver in the arterial phase and hypodense in the late phase.

Multimodality imaging – RM. The most typical pattern is hypointensity on T1-weighted images and hyperintensity on T2-weighted images. Metastases appear hypointense on late phase images 1 h after the injection of liver-specific Gd-BOPTA.

Contrast-enhanced US. After microbubble agent administration, hypovascular metastases display absent (Figs. 11.32, 11.33) or dotted enhancement. Evidence of peripheral rim-like enhancement may be obtained during the arterial phase (Fig. 11.33), and fades at the beginning of the portal phase.

Diffusely enhancing hypervascular metastases appear hyperechoic (Harvey and Albrecht 2001; Quaia et al. 2004) from 20 to 30 s after microbubble injection (Figs. 11.34, 11.35), with evidence of a

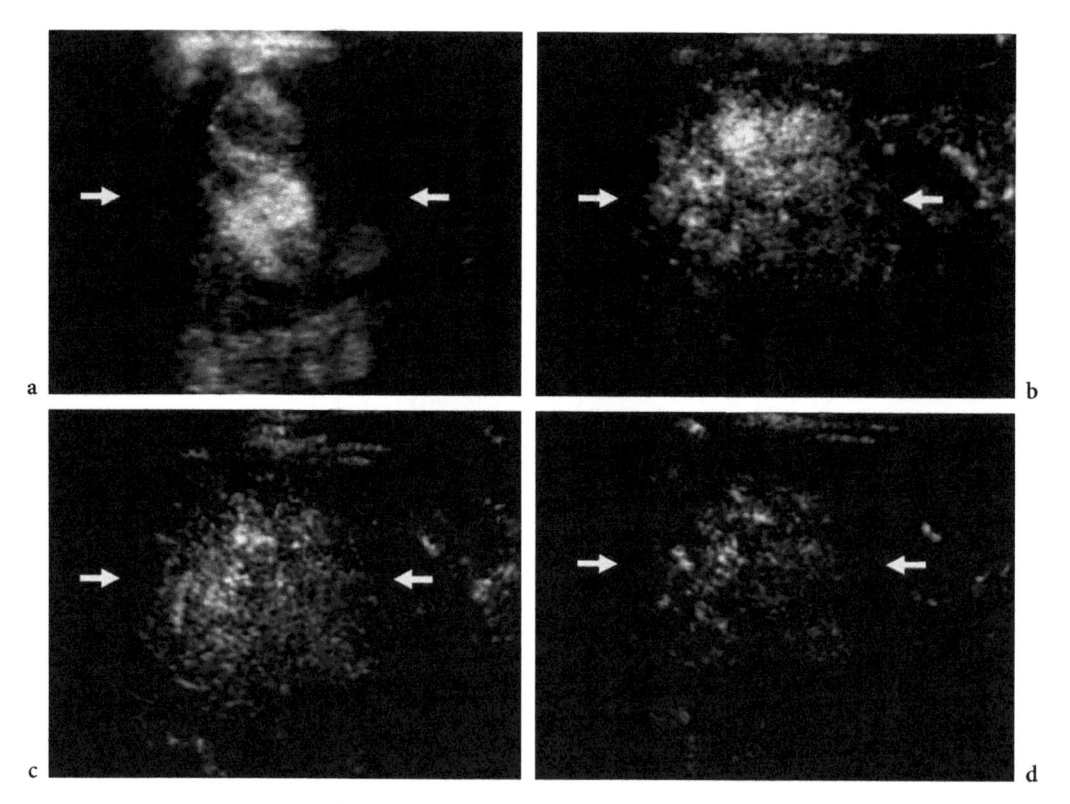

Fig. 11.31a-d. Large hepatocellular carcinoma that has a heterogeneous appearance on contrast-enhanced US and is isoechoic during the late phase. Axial plane. **a** Baseline US. A heterogeneous lesion is identified. **b-d** Contrast-specific mode: Pulse Inversion Mode (Philips-ATL, WA, USA) with low acoustic power after the injection of sulfur hexafluoride-filled microbubbles. The carcinoma (*arrows*) presents diffuse and heterogeneous contrast enhancement during the arterial (**b**, 22 s after SonoVue injection) and portal (**c**) phases and has an isovascular appearance in the late phase (**d**) as compared to the adjacent liver parenchyma.

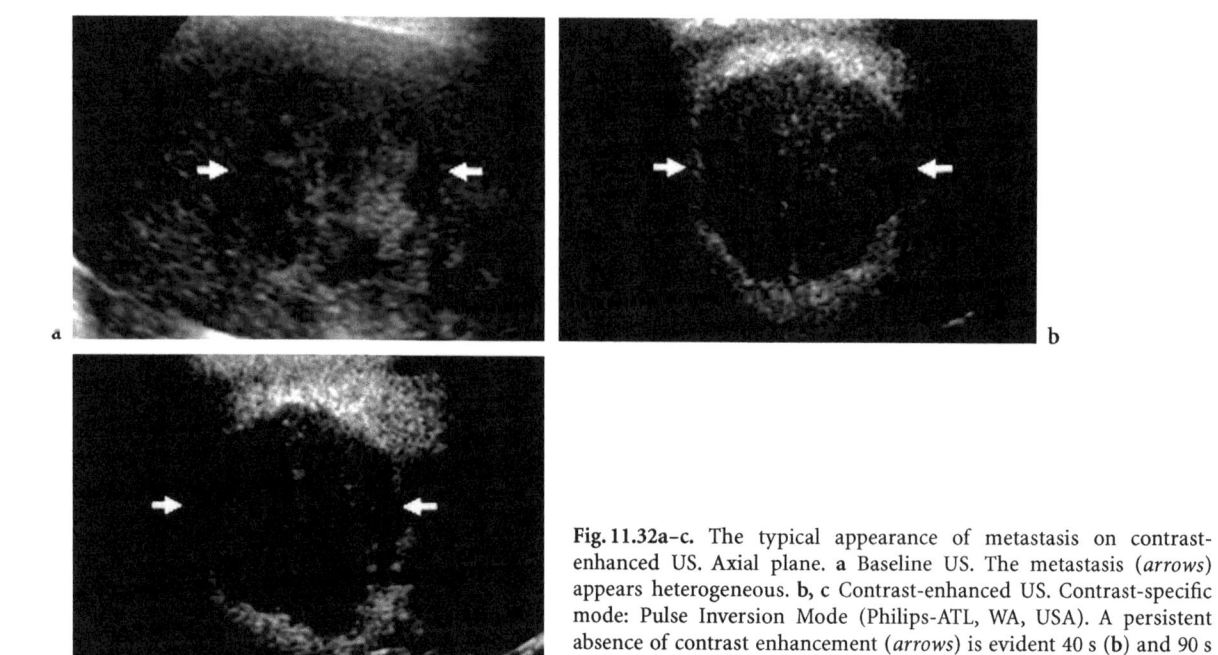

Fig. 11.32a-c. The typical appearance of metastasis on contrast-enhanced US. Axial plane. **a** Baseline US. The metastasis (*arrows*) appears heterogeneous. **b, c** Contrast-enhanced US. Contrast-specific mode: Pulse Inversion Mode (Philips-ATL, WA, USA). A persistent absence of contrast enhancement (*arrows*) is evident 40 s (**b**) and 90 s (**c**) after the injection of sulfur hexafluoride-filled microbubbles.

Characterization of Focal Liver Lesions

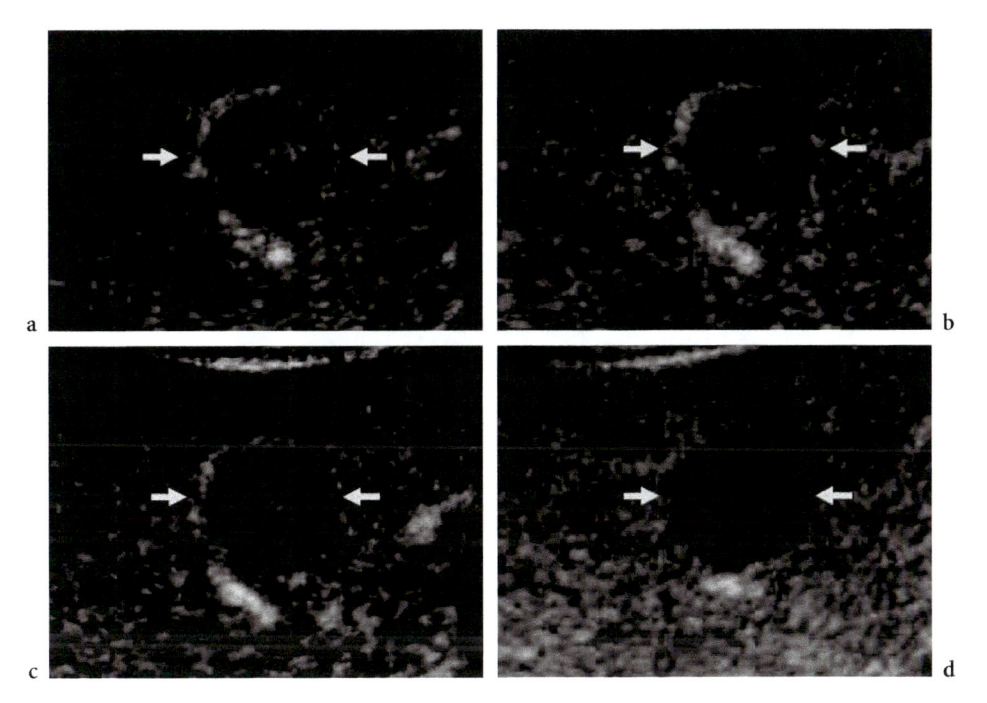

Fig. 11.33a–d. The typical appearance of metastasis on contrast-enhanced US. Axial plane. Contrast-enhanced US. Contrast-specific mode: Contrast Tuned Imaging (Esaote, Genoa, Italy) after the injection of sulfur hexafluoride-filled microbubbles. Persistent peripheral rim-like contrast enhancement (*arrows*) is evident during the arterial (**a**) and the portal phase (**b, c**), with a hypoechoic appearance in the late phase (**d**).

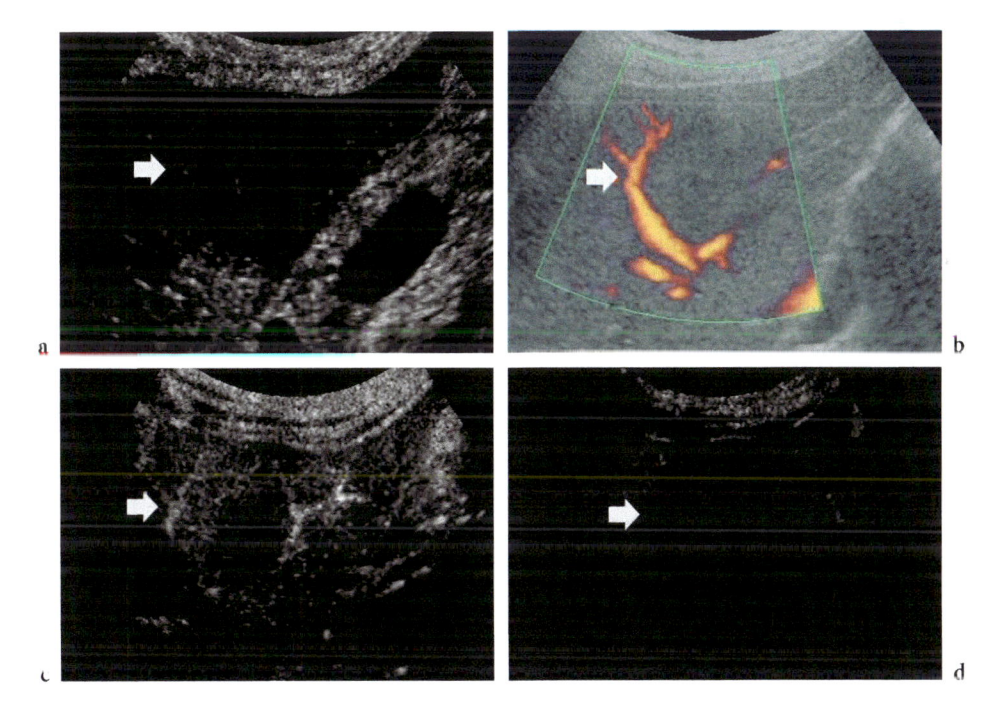

Fig. 11.34a–d. The typical appearance of metastasis on contrast-enhanced US. Axial plane. Baseline US (**a**) reveals a heterogeneous lesion (*arrow*) with a hypovascular appearance on power Doppler (**b**). **c, d** Contrast-enhanced US. Contrast-specific mode: Pulse Inversion Mode (Philips-ATL, WA, USA) with low acoustic power after the injection of sulfur hexafluoride-filled microbubbles. Persistent peripheral contrast enhancement (*arrow*) is identified during the arterial phase, with evidence of diffuse contrast enhancement sparing a peripheral portion of the lesion during the portal phase (**c**). The lesion appears hypoechoic (*arrow*) in the late phase (**d**).

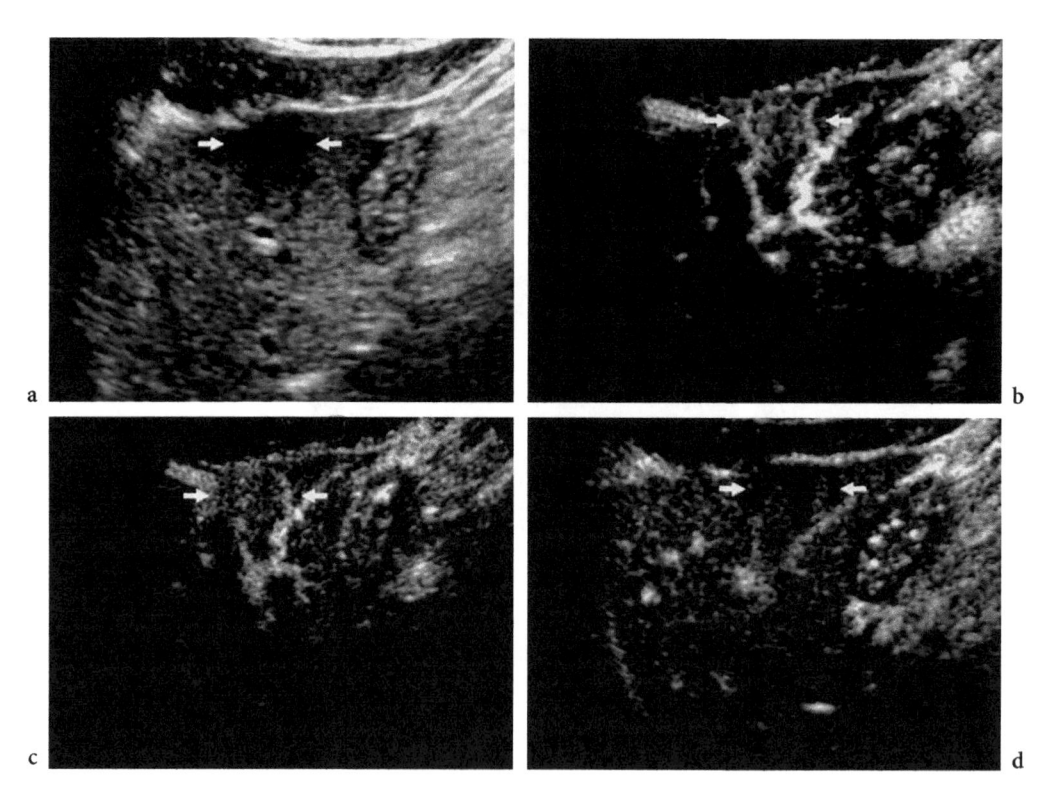

Fig. 11.35a-d. Metastasis. Diffuse contrast enhancement on contrast-enhanced US. Axial plane. a Baseline US. A hypoechoic lesion (*arrows*) with smooth margins is identified in the left lobe of the liver. b-d Contrast-enhanced US. Contrast-specific mode: Pulse Inversion Mode (Philips-ATL, WA, USA) after the injection of sulfur hexafluoride-filled microbubbles. Diffuse contrast enhancement is evident during the arterial (b) and the portal (c) with a hypoechoic appearance in the late phase (d).

peripheral hyperechoic rim in the majority of cases from 40 to 60 s after injection.

During the portal and late phases all metastases appear as hypoechoic defects in the liver with indistinct margins and improved conspicuity in comparison to the baseline scan (HECKEMANN et al. 2000; MEUWLY et al. 2003); as a consequence, detectability is enhanced.

11.4.3
Intrahepatic Cholangiocellular Carcinoma

Epidemiology and histopathologic features. Cholangiocellular carcinoma is the most common tumor of the bile ducts and its incidence is increasing. Predisposing factors include sclerosing cholangitis, ulcerative colitis, choledochal cysts, Caroli's disease, parasitic infections (*Clonorchis sinensis*), and chemicals.

Multimodality imaging. Intrahepatic (or peripheral) cholangiocellular carcinoma demonstrates typically heterogeneous contrast enhancement at different dynamic phases. Rim-like contrast enhancement around the tumor during the arterial phase, and centripetal filling of contrast material during the equilibrium phase, due to the leak in the fibrous stroma of the tumour, are characteristic appearances on contrast-enhanced CT (BERLAND et al. 1989; LEE et al. 2001).

Contrast-enhanced US. Intrahepatic cholangiocellular carcinoma displays a persistent heterogeneous hypoechoic appearance (KHALILI et al. 2003) (Fig. 11.36). In the arterial phase, ring enhancement appears in the periphery of the tumor and lasts until the portal phase in the majority of cholangiocellular carcinomas. In the late phase, absence of contrast enhancement has been observed (TANAKA et al. 2001). The absence of centripetal filling is due to the pure intravascular permanence of microbubbles.

11.4.4
Other Malignant Focal Liver Lesions

Other malignant focal liver lesions may be identified and scanned after the injection of microbubble-based agents, such as epithelioid hemangioendothelioma (GHEKIERE et al. 2004), hepatic lymphoma.

Characterization of Focal Liver Lesions

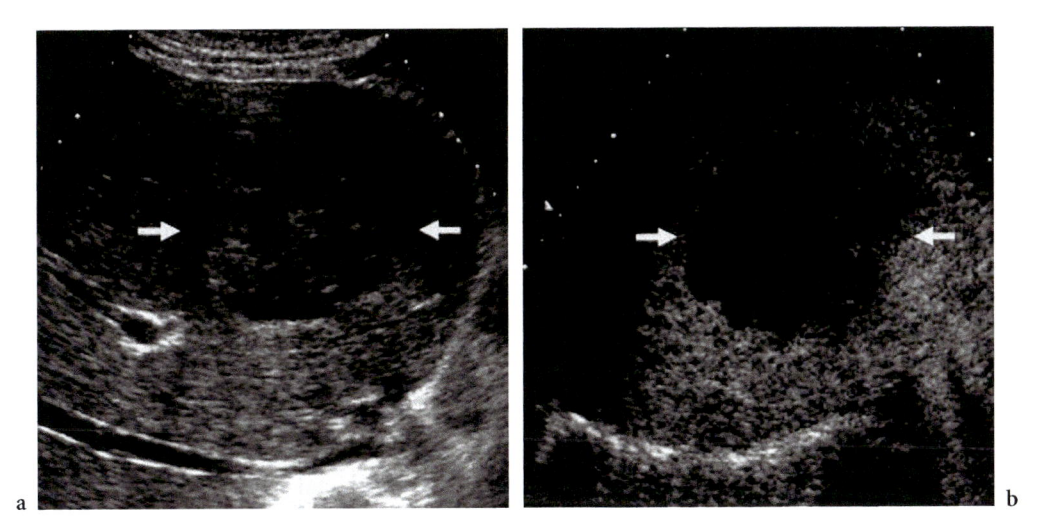

Fig. 11.36a,b. The typical appearance of cholangiocellular carcinoma on contrast-enhanced US. **a** At baseline US a heterogeneous hypoechoic lesion (*arrows*) is identified in the liver. **b** After microbubble injection, during the late phase the lesion appears hypoechoic compared to the adjacent liver.

The appearance of epithelioid hemangioendothelioma on contrast-enhanced US has recently been described (QUAIA et al. 2004). Epithelioid hemangioendothelioma is a rare, low-grade malignant neoplasm of vascular origin composed of epithelioid-appearing endothelial cells. It should not be confused with infantile hemangioendothelioma, which regresses spontaneously. The tumor is characteristically composed of a fibrotic hypovascular central core, a peripheral hyperemic rim, and a further peripheral nonenhancing rim corresponding to a vascular zone between the lesion and the adjacent liver (GHEKIERE et al. 2004). After microbubble injection it displays persistent diffuse contrast enhancement, with a hyperechoic appearance (Fig. 11.37), including during the late phase.

Hepatic lymphoma reveals hypovascular appearance at late phase (VON HERSAY 2004a,b).

11.5
Clinical Results

The development and clinical introduction of microbubble contrast agents has had a particular impact on the detection and differential diagnosis of liver tumors (COSGROVE and BLOMLEY 2004). Malig-

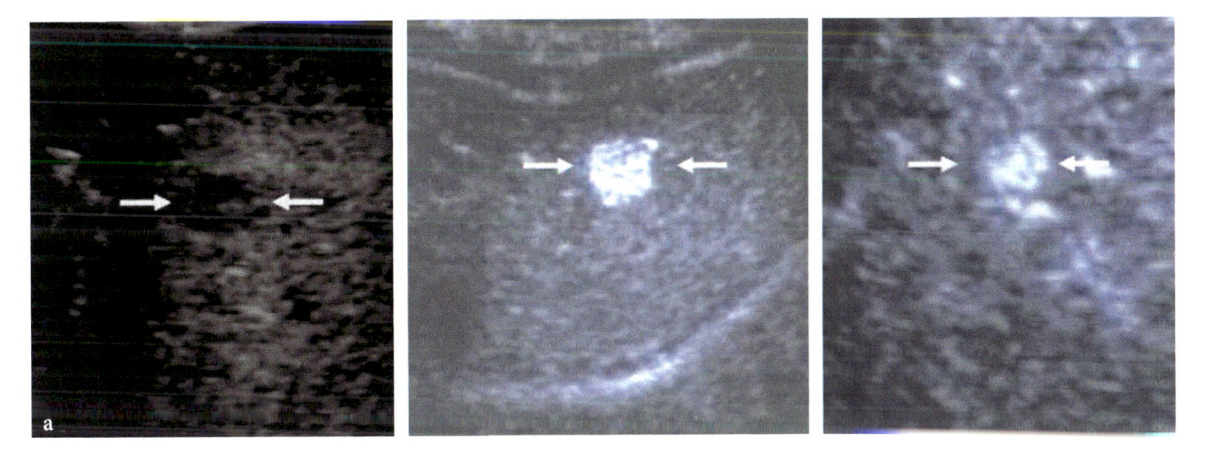

Fig. 11.37a–c. Epithelioid hemangioendothelioma on contrast-enhanced US. **a** On baseline US a hypoechoic lesion (*arrows*) is identified in the liver. **b, c** Contrast-specific mode: Pure Harmonic Detection (Aloka, Tokyo, Japan) with low acoustic power after the injection of sulfur hexafluoride-filled microbubbles. After microbubble injection, during the arterial phase (**b**) the lesion presents diffuse contrast enhancement (*arrows*) that persists into the late phase (**c**).

nancies typically show a low echo signal intensity during the late phase, regardless of whether they are hyper- or hypovascular in terms of their arterial supply. In addition, the arterial supply can be depicted in real time by using the low acoustic power mode, which allows differentiation of most benign masses from each other and from malignancies, and thus improves specificity.

Tanaka et al. (2001) reported that when a diffuse or heterogeneous mosaic enhancement pattern (arterial phase) and/or reticular enhancement (late phase) was regarded as indicative of hepatocellular carcinoma after Levovist injection, the sensitivity, specificity, and positive predictive value of contrast-enhanced US were 92%, 96%, and 96%, respectively. If peripheral rim-like enhancement (arterial to portal phase) or absence of enhancement (late phase) or both were regarded as positive findings for cholangiocellular carcinoma or metastasis, the sensitivity, specificity, and positive predictive value were 90%, 95%, and 88%, respectively. If peripheral nodular enhancement (portal phase) was regarded as a positive finding for hemangioma, the sensitivity, specificity, and positive predictive value were 60%, 100%, and 100%, respectively.

A recent study (von Herbay et al. 2002) found that, compared with baseline US, contrast-enhanced US after Levovist injection improved the sensitivity for the discrimination of malignant versus benign liver lesions from 85% to 100%, and the specificity from 30% to 63%. Receiver operating characteristic analysis revealed a significant improvement in this discrimination [area under curve (A_z)=0.692±0.065 on baseline US, A_z=0.947±0.037 on contrast-enhanced US, $p<0.001$]. All lesions that had homogeneous enhancement in the late phase of Levovist enhancement were benign.

By classifying focal liver lesions with an isoechoic or hyperechoic appearance relative to the adjacent liver during the late phase as suggestive of benignity and hypoechoic lesions as suggestive of malignancy, Nicolau et al. (2003b) were able to differentiate between malignant and benign focal liver lesions with an accuracy of 86.5%.

Quaia et al. (2004) found similar results in the discrimination of benign from malignant lesions by using contrast-enhanced US after SonoVue injection: the hypoechoic appearance in the late phase was found to be the most typical feature of malignancies. Benign lesions display persistent microbubble uptake while malignant lesions show microbubble washout and lower microbubble uptake compared to the adjacent liver during the late phase (Blomley et al. 2001; Albrecht et al. 2003; Nicolau et al. 2003a,b; Quaia et al. 2004). In the same study by Quaia et al. (2004), two off-site readers retrospectively assessed each focal liver lesion and reached a conclusion as to its malignant or benign nature based on the appearance of the lesion before and after microbubble injection. After the additional review of contrast-enhanced scans, diagnostic performance was improved for both readers in about two-thirds of lesions, through the achievement of either correct diagnosis or greater diagnostic confidence. After microbubble injection about 7% of the lesions remained indeterminate and were characterized by histologic analysis of the biopsy or surgical specimen (Quaia et al. 2004).

The two other principal imaging modalities for the evaluation of focal liver lesions are CT and MR imaging. The more suitable imaging procedure for characterization of focal liver lesions that remain indeterminate after microbubble injection is probably contrast-enhanced MR with gadolinium chelates, iron oxide compounds, or manganese chelates. This allows both dynamic and tissue-specific characterization with a better diagnostic performance (85–95%: Grazioli et al. 2001a,b; Oudkerk et al. 2002; Kim et al. 2004b) than multiphase contrast-enhanced CT (68–91%: van Leeuwen et al. 1996; Oudkerk et al. 2002; Kamel et al. 2003).

11.6
When Should Microbubble-Based Agents Be Employed?

Baseline US and color Doppler US are effective in characterizing incidental focal liver lesions as benign or malignant in the normal liver in about 40–50% of cases (Nino-Murcia et al. 1992; Reinhold et al. 1995; Lee et al. 1996). This is because typical hemangiomas, focal nodular hyperplasias, and metastases often display a typical appearance on gray-scale US or characteristic vessel architecture on color Doppler US. In the remaining 50–60% of cases, microbubble-based agents should be employed to improve the characterization of focal liver lesions through the identification of typical contrast enhancement patterns (Tables 11.1 and 11.2). In about 10% of cases, focal liver lesions remain indeterminate even after microbubble injection; contrast-enhanced MR imaging should then be employed, followed when necessary by US-guided biopsy.

The possible diagnosis of hepatocellular carcinoma should be considered for each incidental focal liver lesion identified in the cirrhotic liver. Baseline

Table 11.1. Benign Lesion Summary of the baseline gray-scale and color Doppler US findings and of contrast enhancement patterns after microbubbles injection

Baseline		Contrast Enhancement patterns *		
Gray scale US	color Doppler US	Arterial phase	Portal phase	Late phase
Typical hemangioma Hyperechoic, homogenous, sharp margins and possible posterior enhancement. Frequent sub-caspular location. Multiple in 10% of cases	Extralesional feeding vessels	Peripheral nodular enhancement	Slow centripetal progression of the enhancement leading to an iso- or hyperechoic appearance	Complete fill-in and hyperechoic or sometimes isoechoic appearance.
Atypical hemangioma Hyper-, iso-, hypoechoic or heterogeneous echogenicity with larger hypoechoic areas related to hemorrhage, thrombosis or necrosis.		No enhancement in case of completed thrombosis Diffuse enhancement (rapid fill-in) during arterial phase with hyperechoic appearance		Fill-in may be incomplete in case of thrombosis
Focal nodular hyperplasia Variable echogenicity (iso-, hypo-, hyperechoic or heterogeneious). Central scar may be visible as hypoechoic central area. Multiple in 20% of cases.	Spoke-whell shaped pattern consisting in central and radiating arterial vessels with high diastolic component compared to the systolic component. Large vessels may be present in the lesion periphery. Feeding artery may be present especially in small lesions	Spoke-whell shaped central enhancement. Radial vascular branches and peripheral vessel can be delineated. Diffuse contrast enhancement.	Iso- or hyperechoic	Iso- or hyperechoic. Evidence of the central scar with hypoechoic appearance
Hepatocellular adenomas Variable echogenicity (iso-, hypo-, hyperechoic; heterogeneous in larger lesions secondary to necrosis, hemorrhage or fibrosis). Pseudo-halo possible due to compression of adjacent parenchyma. Rarely isolated calcifications.	Large peripheral arteries and veins; prevalently venous vessels in the lesion center Feeding artery may be identified	Diffuse enhancement with homogeneous or heterogeneous appearance.	Homogeneous or heterogeneous appearance with hypoechoic areas in case of hemorrhage, necrosis or fibrosis	Homogeneous or heterogeneous appearance with hypoechoic areas in case of hemorrhage, necrosis or fibrosis
Macroregenerative or dysplastic nodule Predominantly hypoechoic but also hyperechoic or heterogeneous. Presence of liver cirrhosis as under-lying diseases.	No intralesional vessels	Absent or Dotted enhancement with hypoechoic or isoechoic appearance. Diffuse enhancement possible in dysplastic lesions	Isoechoic	Isoechoic
Focal fatty changes Often geometric/polygonal with sharp margins Hyperechoic with normal surrounding liver tissue Typically located near falciform ligament / antero-medial portion of Segment IV / hilar side of Segment IV / anterolateral portion of Segment III and/ or hepatic hilum.	No vascular abnormalities	Isoechoic	Isoechoic	Isoechoic
Focal fatty sparings Often geometric/polygonal with sharp margins Hypoechoic (surrounding liver tissue hyperechoic [fatty liver]) Typically located along the hepatic hilum and/or around the gallbladder and Segment IV.	No vascular abnormalities	Isoechoic	Isoechoic	Isoechoic

Table 11.2. Malignant Lesions

Baseline		Contrast enhancement patterns *		
Gray scale US	**color Doppler US**	**Arterial phase**	**Portal phase**	**Late phase**
Hepatocellular carcinomas Small lesions (< 3cm): prevalently hypoechoic. Sometimes hyperechoic depending on fat content. Isoechoic appearance is rare Large lesions (>3cm): heterogeneous. Sometimes evidence of hypoechoic rim	Intratumoral arterial vessels depending on degree of differentiation with irregular tortous tumor vessels. I rregular tortous peritumoral vessels. Basket pattern consisting in irregular peripheral arterial vessels with centripetal intratumoral branches	Diffuse homogeneous or heterogeneous enhancement, often with delineation of feeding peripheral and intratumoral vessels. Dotted enhancement. Heterogeneous appearance in large lesions, if necrotic or hemorrhagic areas are present	Iso- or hypoechoic; generally contrast washout begins. Heterogeneous appearance possible	Prevalently hypoechoic Isoechoic appearance.
Intrahepatic cholangiocarcinoma Heterogeneous with diffuse and infiltrating margins Segmental biliary dilatation	Intratumoral vessels often at the edge of the tumor Poorly vascularized lesion	Heterogeneous enhancement Peripheral rim-like enhancement	Heterogeneous enhancement	Hypoechoic
Hypervascular Metastases Variable echogenicity: prevalently hypoechoic (sometimes cystic). frequently isoechoic and hyperechoic. Intratumoral calcifications are possible. Presence of a peripheral hypoechoic halo	Tumor vessels are often restricted to the periphery of the lesion	Diffuse Heterogeneous appearance especially in large lesions and if necrotic areas are present	Iso- or hypoechoic due to rapid contrast washout. Rim-like peripheral enhancement may persist.	Hypoechoic
Hypovascular Metastases Variable echogenicity: prevalently hypoechoic (sometimes cystic). frequently isoechoic and hyperechoic. Presence of a peripheral hypoechoic halo.	Peripheral vessels	Absent or dotted contrast enhancement with hypoechoic appearance	Hypoechoic	Hypoechoic

Note: Different baseline appearance and contrast enhancement patterns of benign and malignant focal liver lesions.
* Echogenicity is compared to the adjacent liver parenchyma.
hyperechoic = hypervascular
hypoechoic = hypovascular
isoechoic = isovascular

US and color Doppler US have a very low diagnostic accuracy with respect to focal liver lesions in the cirrhotic liver (NINO-MURCIA et al. 1992), and microbubble-based agents have to be employed in all cases except those in which a large lesion has an overtly malignant appearance on the baseline scan. Approximately 40-50% of lesions in the cirrhotic liver remain indeterminate or present an atypical appearance after microbubble injection (QUAIA et al. 2004), and contrast-enhanced CT or MR imaging should then be employed. Differentiation of high-grade dysplastic nodules from hepatocellular carcinoma is often not possible using imaging modalities, necessitating US-guided biopsy.

The Efsumb Study Group (2004) recently proposed guide-lines for the employment of microbubbles in liver tumors.

References

Albrecht T, Oldenburg A, Hohmann J et al (2003) Imaging of liver metastases with contrast-specific low-MI real time ultrasound and SonoVue. Eur Radiol 13 [Suppl 3]:N79-N86

Alpers DH, Isselbacher KJ (1975) Fatty liver: biochemical and clinical aspects. In: Schieff L (ed) Diseases of the liver. Lippincott, Philadelphia, pp 815-832

Baker MK, Wenker JC, Cockerill EM, Ellis JH (1985) Focal fatty infiltration of the liver: diagnostic imaging. RadioGraphics 5:923-929

Baron RL, Peterson MS (2001) Screening the cirrhotic liver for hepatocellular carcinoma with CT and MR imaging: opportunities and pitfalls. Radiographics 21:S117-S132

Bartolozzi C, Lencioni R, Paolicchi A et al (1997) Differentiation of hepatocellular adenoma and focal nodular hyperplasia of the liver: comparison of power Doppler imaging and conventional color Doppler sonography. Eur Radiol 7:1410-1415

Berland L, Lee JKT, Stanley RJ (1989) Liver and biliary tract. In: Lee JKT, Sagel SS, Stanley RJ (eds) Computed body tomography with MRI correlation, 2nd edn. Raven, New York, pp 593-659

Bertolotto M, Dalla Palma L, Quaia E, Locatelli M (2000) Characterization of unifocal liver lesions with pulse inversion harmonic imaging after Levovist injection: preliminary results. Eur Radiol 9:1369-1376

Blachar A, Federle MP, Ferris JV et al (2002) Radiologists' performance in the diagnosis of liver tumors with central scars by using specific CT criteria. Radiology 223:532-539

Blomley MJK, Albrecht T, Cosgrove DO et al (1998) Stimulated acoustic emission in liver parenchyma with Levovist. Lancet 351:568-569

Blomley MJ, Albrecht TA, Cosgrove DO et al (1999) Improved detection of liver metastases with stimulated acoustic emission in late phase of enhancement with the US contrast agent SH U 508: early experience. Radiology 210:409-416

Blomley MJK, Sidhu PL, Cosgrove DO et al (2001) Do different types of liver lesions differ in their uptake of the microbubble contrast agent SH U 508A in the late liver phase? Early experience. Radiology 220:661-667

Bluemke D, Weber TM, Rubin D et al (2003) Hepatic MR imaging with ferumoxides: multicenter study of safety and effectiveness of direct injection protocol. Radiology 228:457-464

Brancatelli G, Federle MP, Blachar A, Grazioli L (2001a) Hemangioma in the cirrhotic liver: diagnosis and natural history. Radiology 219:69-74

Brancatelli G, Federle MP, Grazioli L et al (2001b) Focal nodular hyperplasia: CT findings with emphasis on multiphasic helical CT in 78 patients. Radiology 219:61-68

Brancatelli G, Federle MP, Grazioli L, Carr BI (2002a) Hepatocellular carcinoma in noncirrhotic liver: CT, clinical, and pathologic findings in 39 US residents. Radiology 222:89-94

Brancatelli G, Federle MP, Grazioli L et al (2002b) Benign regenerative nodules in Budd-Chiari syndrome and other vascular disorders of the liver: radiologic-pathologic and clinical correlation. Radiographics 22:847-862

Brannigan M, Burns PN, Wilson SR (2004) Blood flow patterns in focal liver lesions at microbubble-enhanced US. Radiographics 24:921-935

Brawer MK, Austin GE, Lewin JK (1980) Focal fatty change of the liver, a hitherto poorly recognized entity. Gastroenterology 78:247-252

Bryant TH, Blomley MJ, Albrecht T et al (2004) Improved characterization of liver lesions with liver-phase uptake of liver specific microbubbles: prospective multicenter trials. Radiology 232:799-809

Burns PN, Powers JE, Simpson DH et al (1996) Harmonic imaging: principles and preliminary results. Clin Radiol 51(Suppl):50-55

Burns P, Wilson S, Simpson D (2000) Pulse inversion imaging of liver blood flow. Improved method for characterization focal masses with microbubble contrast. Invest Radiol 35:58-71

Chen RC, Chen WT, Tu HY et al (2002) Assessment of vascularity in hepatic tumours. Comparison of power Doppler sonography and intraarterial CO2-enhanced sonography. Am J Roentgenol 178:67-73

Chen WP, Chen JH, Hwang JI et al (1999) Spectrum of transient hepatic attenuation differences in biphasic helical CT. AJR Am J Roentgenol 172:419-424

Choi BI, Kim AY, Lee JY et al (2002) Hepatocellular carcinoma: contrast enhancement with Levovist. J Ultrasound Med 21:77-84

Claudon M, Tranquart F, Evans DH et al (2002) Advances in ultrasound. Eur Radiol 12:7-18

Colagrande S, Politi LS, Messerini L et al (2003) Solitary necrotic nodule of the liver: imaging and correlation with pathologic features. Abdom Imaging 28:41-44

Correas JM, Burns PN, Lai X, Qi X (2000) Infusion versus bolus of an ultrasound contrast agent: in vivo dose-response measurements of BR1. Invest Radiol 35:72-79

Correas JM, Bridal L, Lesavre A et al (2001) Ultrasound contrast agents: properties, principles of action, tolerance, and artifacts. Eur Radiol 11:1316-1328

Cosgrove DO, Blomley MJK (2004) Liver tumors: Evaluation with contrast-enhanced ultrasound. Abdom Imaging 29:446-454

Cosgrove DO, Blomley MJK, Eckersley RJ, Harvey C (2002) Innovative contrast specific imaging with ultrasound. Electromedica 70:147-149

De Luca M, Luigi B, Formisano C et al (2000) Solitary necrotic nodule of the liver misinterpreted as malignant lesion: considerations on two cases. J Surg Oncol 74:219-222

Dill-Macky M, Burns P, Khalili K, Wilson S (2002) Focal hepatic masses: enhancement patterns with SH U 508 A and pulse inversion US. Radiology 222:95-102

Ebara M, Ohto M, Shinagawa T et al (1986) Natural history of minute hepatocellular carcinoma smaller than three centimetres complicating cirrhosis. A study of 22 patients. Gastroenterology 90:289-298

Edmondson HA (1958) Tumors of the liver and intrahepatic bile ducts. Atlas of tumor pathology. Armed Forces Institute of Pathology, Washington DC

Efsumb Study Group (2004) Guidelines for the use of contrast agents in ultrasound. Ultraschall Med 25:249–256

Ferrucci JT (1994) Liver tumour imaging. Current concepts. Radiol Clin North Am 32:39-54

Furuse J, Nagase M, Ishii H, Yoshino M (2003) Contrast enhancement patterns of hepatic tumours during the vascular phase using coded harmonic imaging and Levovist to differentiate hepatocellular carcinoma from other focal lesions. Br J Radiol 76:385-392

Gatenby JC, Hoddinott JC, Leeman S (1989) Phasing out speckle. Phys Med Biol 34:1683-1689

Ghekiere O, Weynand B, Pieters T, Coche E (2004) Epithelioid haemangioendothelioma. Eur Radiol 14:1134-1137

Giorgio A, Ferraioli G, Tarantino L et al (2004) Contrast-enhanced sonographic appearance of hepatocellular carcinoma in patients with cirrhosis: comparison with contrast-enhanced helical CT appearance. AJR Am J Roentgenol 183:1319-1326

Golli M, van Nhieu JT, Mathieu D et al (1994) Hepatocellular adenoma: color Doppler US and pathologic correlations. Radiology 190:741-744

Gonzàlez-Anòn M, Cervera-Deval J, Garcia-Vila JH et al (1999) Characterization of solid liver lesions with color and pulsed Doppler imaging. Abdom Imaging 24:137-143

Gramiak R, Shah PM (1968) Echocardiography of the aortic root. Invest Radiol 3:356-366

Grazioli L, Federle MP, Brancatelli G (2001a) Hepatic adenomas: imaging and pathologic findings. Radiographics 21:877-892

Grazioli L, Morana G, Federle MP et al (2001b) Focal nodular hyperplasia: morphologic and functional information from MR imaging with gadobenate dimeglumine. Radiology 221:731-739

Halvorsen RA, Korobkin M, Ram PC, Thompson WM (1982) CT appearance of focal fatty infiltration of the liver. Am J Roentgenol 139:277-281

Harvey CJ, Albrecht T (2001) Ultrasound of focal liver lesions. Eur Radiol 11:1578-1593

Hayashi M, Matsui O, Ueda K et al (1999) Correlation between the blood supply and grade of malignancy of hepatocellular nodules associated with liver cirrhosis: evaluation by CT during intraarterial injection of contrast medium. AJR Am J Roentgenol 172:969-976

Hayashi M, Matsui O, Ueda K et al (2002) Progression to hypervascular hepatocellular carcinoma: correlation with intranodular blood supply evaluated with CT during intraarterial injection of contrast material. Radiology 225:143-149

Hauff P, Fritsch T, Reinhardt M et al (1997) Delineation of experimental liver tumors in rabbits by a new ultrasound contrast agent and stimulated acoustic emission. Invest Radiol 32:94-99

Heckemann R, Cosgrove DO, Blomley MJK et al (2000) Liver lesions: intermittent second-harmonic gray-scale US can increase conspicuity with microbubble contrast material-early experience. Radiology 216:592-596

Hirohashi S, Ueda K, Uchida H et al (2000) Nondiffuse fatty change of the liver: discerning pseudotumor on MR images enhanced with ferumoxides - initial observations. Radiology 217:415-420

Hohmann J, Skrok J, Puls R, Albrecth T (2003) Characterization of focal liver lesions with contrast-enhanced low MI real time ultrasound and SonoVue. Rofo Rontgenstr Fortschr 176:835-843

Hosten N, Puls R, Bechstein WO, Felix R (1999a) Focal liver lesions: Doppler ultrasound. Eur Radiol 9:428-435

Hosten N, Puls R, Lemke AJ et al (1999b) Contrast enhanced power Doppler sonography: improved detection of characteristic flow patterns in focal liver lesion. J Clin Ultrasound 27:107-115

Hussain SH, Zondervan PE, IJzermans JNM et al (2002) Benign versus malignant hepatic nodules: MR imaging findings with pathologic correlation. Radiographics 22:1023-1036

Ichikawa T, Federle MP, Grazioli L et al (1999) Fibrolamellar hepatocellular carcinoma: imaging and pathologic findings in 31 recent cases. Radiology 213:352-361

Ichikawa T, Federle MP, Grazioli L, Nalesnik M (2000) Hepatocellular adenoma: multiphasic CT and histopathologic findings in 25 patients. Radiology 214:861-868

Isozaki T, Numata K, Kiba T (2003) Differential diagnosis of hepatic tumors by using contrast enhancement patterns at US. Radiology 229:798-805

Jespersen SK, Wilhjelm JE, Sillesen H (1998) Multiangle compound imaging. Ultrason Imaging 20:81-102

Leen E, Angerson WJ, Yarmenitis S et al (2002) Multi-centre study evaluating the efficacy of SonoVue (BR1), a new ultrasound contrast agent in Doppler investigation of focal hepatic lesions. Eur J Radiol 41:200-206

Kamel IR, Choti MA, Horton KM et al (2003) Surgically staged focal liver lesions: accuracy and reproducibility of dual-phase helical CT for detection and characterization. Radiology 227:752-757

Kane AG, Redwine MD, Cossi AF (1993) Characterization of focal fatty change in the liver with a fat-enhanced inversion recovery sequence. J Magn Reson Imaging 3:581-586

Karhunen PJ (1986) Benign hepatic tumors and tumor-like conditions in men. J Clin Pathol 39:183-188

Khalili K, Metser U, Wilson SR (2003) Hilar biliary obstruction: preliminary results with Levovist-enhanced sonography. Am J Roentgenol 180:687-693

Kim EA, Yoon KH, MD, Lee YH (2003) Focal hepatic lesions: contrast-enhancement patterns at pulse-inversion harmonic US using a microbubble contrast agent. Korean J Radiol 4:224-233

Kim HC, Kim TK, Sung KB et al (2002) CT during hepatic arteriography and portography: an illustrative review. Radiographics 22:1041-1051

Kim MG, Kim JH, Chung JJ (2003) Focal hepatic lesions: detection and characterization with combination Gadolinium- and Superparamagnetic iron oxide-enhanced MR imaging. Radiology 228:719-726

Kim TK, Han JK, Kim AY, Choi BI (1999) Limitations of characterization of hepatic hemangiomas using an ultrasound contrast agent (Levovist) and power Doppler ultrasound. J Ultrasound Med 18:737-743

Kim TK, Choi BI, Han JK et al (2000) Hepatic tumours: contrast agent-enhancement patterns with pulse inversion harmonic US. Radiology 216:411-417

Kim KW, Choi BI, Park SH et al (2003) Hepatocellular carcinoma: assessment of vascularity with single-level dynamic ultrasonography during the arterial phase. J Ultrasound Med 22:887-896

Kim KW, Choi BI, Park SH et al (2004a) Pyogenic hepatic abscesses: distinctive features from hypovascular hepatic malignancies on contrast-enhanced ultrasound with SH U 508A; early experience. Ultrasound Med Biol 30:725-733

Kim KW, Kim AY, Kim TK et al (2004b) Small (≤2 cm) hepatic lesions in colorectal cancer patients: detection and characterization on mangafodipir trisodium-enhanced MRI. AJR Am J Roentgenol 182:1233-1240

Kindberg GM, Tolleshaug H, Roos N, Skotland T (2003) Hepatic clearance of Sonazoid perfluorobutane microbubbles by Kupffer cells does not reduce the ability of liver to phagocytose or degrade albumin microspheres. Cell Tissue Res 312:49-54

Kirchin MA, Pirovano GP, Spinazzi A (1998) Gadobenate dimeglumine (Gd-BOPTA): an overview. Invest Radiol 33:798-809

Kissin CM, Bellamy EA, Cosgrove DO et al (1986) Focal sparing in fatty infiltration of the liver. Br J Radiol 59:25-28

Koda M, Matsunaga Y, Ueki M et al (2004) Qualitative assessment of tumour vascularity in hepatocellular carcinoma by contrast-enhanced coded ultrasound: comparison with arterial phase of dynamic CT and conventional color/power Doppler ultrasound. Eur Radiol 14:1100-1108

Koea J, Taylor G, Miller M et al (2003) Solitary necrotic nodule of the liver: a riddle that is difficult to answer. J Gastroint Surg 7:627-630

Kudo M, Tomita S, Tochio H et al (1992) Small hepatocellular carcinoma: diagnosis with US angiography with intraarterial CO2 microbubbles. Radiology 182:155-160

Larcos G, Sorokopud H, Berry G, Farrell GC (1998) Sonographic screening for hepatocellular carcinoma in patients with chronic hepatitis or cirrhosis: an evaluation. Am J Roentgenol 171:433-435

Lee MG, Auh YH, Cho KS et al (1996) Color Doppler flow imaging of hepatocellular carcinomas. Comparison with metastatic tumors and hemangiomas by three step grading color hues. Clin Imaging 20:199-203

Lee JY, Choi BI, Han JK et al (2002) Improved sonographic imaging of hepatic hemangioma with contrast-enhanced coded harmonic angiography: comparison with MR imaging. Ultrasound Med Biol 28:287-295

Lee KH, Choi BI, Kim KW et al (2003) Contrast-enhanced dynamic ultrasonography of the liver: optimization of hepatic arterial phase in normal volunteers. Abdom Imaging 28:652-656

Lee WJ, Lim HK, Jang KM (2001) Radiologic spectrum of cholangiocarcinoma: emphasis on unusual manifestations and differential diagnoses. Radiographics 21:S97-S116

Lencioni R, Pinto F, Armillotta N, Bartolozzi C (1996) Assessment of tumor vascularity in hepatocellular carcinoma: comparison of power Doppler US and color Doppler US. Radiology 201:353-358

Lim JH, Cho JM, Kim EY, Park CK (2000) Dysplastic nodules in liver cirrhosis: evaluation of hemodynamics with CT during arterial portography and CT hepatic arteriography. Radiology 214:869-874

Longchampt E, Patriarche C, Fabre M (2000) Accuracy of cytology vs microbiopsy for the diagnosis of well-differentiated hepatocellular carcinoma and macroregenerative nodule. Definition of standardized criteria from a study of 100 cases. Acta Cytol 44:515-523

Mathieu D, Bruneton JN, Drouillard J et al (1986) Hepatic adenomas and focal nodular hyperplasia: dynamic CT study. Radiology 160:53-58

Matsui O, Kadoya M, Kameyama T et al (1991) Benign and malignant nodules in cirrhotic liver: distinction based on blood supply. Radiology 178:493-497

McLarney JK, Rucker PT, Bender GN et al (1999) Fibrolamellar carcinoma of the liver: radiologic-pathologic correlation. Radiographics 19:453-471

Merritt CR, Forsberg F, Shi WT et al (2000) The mechanical index: an inappropriate and misleading indicator for destruction of ultrasound microbubble contrast agents. Radiology 217:395

Meuwly JY, Schnyder P, Gudinchet F, Denys AL (2003) Pulse-inversion harmonic imaging improves lesion conspicuity during US-guided biopsy. J Vasc Interv Radiol 14:335-341

Migaleddu V, Virgilio G, Turilli D et al (2004) Characterization of focal liver lesions in real time using harmonic imaging with high mechanical index and contrast agent Levovist. Am J Roentgenol 182:1505-1512

Mitchell DG, Rubin R, Siegelman ES et al (1991) Hepatocellular carcinoma within siderotic regenerative nodules: appearance as a nodule within a nodule on MR images. Radiology 178:101-103

Morel DR, Schwieger I, Hohn L et al (2000) Human pharmacokinetics and safety evaluation of SonoVue™, a new contrast agent for ultrasound imaging. Invest Radiol 35:80-85

Nicolau C, Catalá V, Brú C (2003a) Characterization of focal liver lesions with contrast-enhanced ultrasound. Eur Radiol 13 [Suppl 3]:N70-N78

Nicolau C, Catalá V, Vilana R (2003b) Is contrast-enhanced ultrasound late vascular phase evaluation enough to differentiate between benign and malignant focal liver lesions? (Abstract.) RSNA 2003, Scientific assembly and annual meeting program

Nicolau C, Catalá V, Vilana R et al (2004) Evaluation of hepatocellular carcinoma using SonoVue, a second generation ultrasound contrast agent: correlation with cellular differentiation. Eur Radiol 14:1092-1099

Nino-Murcia M, Ralls PW, Jeffrey RB Jr, Johnson M (1992) Color flow Doppler characterization of focal hepatic lesions. Am J Roentgenol 159:1195-1197

Nino-Murcia M, Olcott EW, Jeffrey RB et al (2000) Focal liver lesions: pattern-based classification scheme for enhancement at arterial phase. Radiology 215:746-751

Nomura Y, Matsuda Y, Yabuuchi I et al (1993) Hepatocellular carcinoma in adenomatous hyperplasia: detection with contrast-enhanced US with carbon dioxide microbubbles. Radiology 187:353-356

Numata K, Tanaka K, Mitsui K et al (1993) Flow characteristics of hepatic tumors at color Doppler sonography: correlation with arteriographic findings. Am J Roentgenol 160:515-521

Numata K, Tanaka K, Kiba T et al (2001) Contrast-enhanced wide-band harmonic gray-scale imaging of hepatocellular carcinoma: correlation with helical computed tomographic findings. J Ultrasound Med 20:89-98

Oliver JH III, Baron RL, Federle MP et al (1997) Hypervascular liver metastases: Do unenhanced CT and hepatic arterial phase CT images affect tumor detection? Radiology 205:709-715

Oudkerk M, Torres CG, Song B et al (2002) Characterization of liver lesions with mangafodipir trisodium-enhanced MR imaging: multicenter study comparing MR and dualphase spiral CT. Radiology 223:517-524

Peterson MS, Baron RL, Marsh JW et al (2000) Pretransplantation surveillance for possible hepatocellular carcinoma in patients with cirrhosis: epidemiology and CT-based tumor detection rate in 430 cases with surgical pathologic correlation. Radiology 217:743-749

Quaia E, Bertolotto M, Dalla Palma L (2002a) Characterization of liver hemangiomas with pulse inversion harmonic imaging. Eur Radiol 12:537-544

Quaia E, Blomley MJK, Patel S et al (2002b) Initial observations on the effect of irradiation on the liver-specific uptake of Levovist. Eur J Radiol 41:192-199

Quaia E, Forgács B, Calderan L et al (2002c) Characterization of focal hepatic lesions in cirrhotic patients by pulse inversion harmonic imaging US contrast specific technique with levovist. Radiol Med 104:285-294

Quaia E, Bertolotto M, Calderan L et al (2003) US characterization of focal hepatic lesions with intermittent high acoustic power mode and contrast material. Acad Radiol 10:739-750

Quaia E, Calliada F, Bertolotto M et al (2004) Characterization of focal liver lesions by contrast-specific US modes and a sulfur hexafluoride-filled microbubble contrast agent: diagnostic performance and confidence. Radiology 232:420-430

Quiroga S, Sebastià C, Pallisa E et al (2001) Improved diagnosis of hepatic perfusion disorders: value of hepatic arterial phase imaging during helical CT. Radiographics 21:65-81

Reinhold C, Hammers L, Taylor CR et al (1995) Characterization of focal hepatic lesions with duplex sonography: findings in 198 patients. AJR Am J Roentgenol 164:1131-1135

Ros PR (1990) Computed tomography-pathologic correlations in hepatic tumors. In: Ferrucci JT, Mathiew DG (eds) Advances in hepatobiliary radiology. Mosby, St Louis, pp 75-108

Sandler MA, Petrocelli RD, Marks DS, Lopez R (1980) Ultrasonic features and radionuclide correlation in liver cell adenoma and focal nodular hyperplasia. Radiology 135:393

Schneider M, Arditi M, Barrau MB et al (1995) BR1: a new ultrasonographic contrast agent based on sulphur hexafluoride-filled microbubbles. Invest Radiol 30:451-457

Spinazzi A, Lorusso V, Pirovano G, Kirchin M (1999) Safety, tolerance, biodistribution, and MR imaging enhancement of the liver with gadobenate dimeglumine: results of clinical pharmacologic and pilot imaging studies in nonpatient and patient volunteers. Acad Radiol 6:282-291

Stevens WR, Gulino SP, Batts KP et al (1996) Mosaic pattern of hepatocellular carcinoma: histologic basis for a characteristic CT appearance. J Comput Assist Tomogr 20:337-342

Tanaka S, Kitamura T, Fujita M et al (1990) Color Doppler flow imaging of liver tumors. AJR Am J Roentgenol 154:509-514

Tanaka S, Kitamura T, Fujita M et al (1992) Small hepatocellular carcinoma: differentiation from adenomatous hyperplastic nodule with color Doppler flow imaging. Radiology 182:161-165

Tanaka S, Ioka T, Oshikawa O et al (2001) Dynamic sonography of hepatic tumors. Am J Roentgenol 177:799-805

Taylor KJ, Ramos I, Morse SS et al (1987) Focal liver masses: differential diagnosis with pulsed Doppler US. Radiology 164:643-647

Van Leeuwen MS, Noordzij J, Feldberg MA et al (1996) Focal liver lesions: characterization with triphasic spiral CT. Radiology 201:327-336

Vilgrain V, Boulos L, Vullierme MP et al (2000) Imaging of atypical hemangiomas of the liver with pathologic correlation. Radiographics 20:379-397

Vilgrain V, Uzan F, Brancatelli G et al (2003) Prevalence of hepatic hemangioma in patients with focal nodular hyperplasia: MR imaging analysis. Radiology 229:75-79

Von Herbay A, Vogt C, Häussinger D (2002) Late-phase pulse-inversion sonography using the contrast agent levovist: differentiation between benign and malignant focal lesions of the liver. Am J Roentgenol 179:1273-1279

Von Herbay A, Vogt C, Willers R, Haussinger D (2004b) Real time imaging with the sonographic contrast agent SonoVue: Differentiation between benign and malignant hepatic lesions. J Ultrasound Med 23(12):1557–1568

Von Herbay A, Vogt C, Haussinger D (2004a) Differentiation between benign and malignant hepatic lesions: Utility of color stimulated acoustic emission with the microbubble contrast agent levovist. J Ultrasound Med 23(2):207–215

Wang JH, Lu SN, Changchien CS, Huang WS et al (2003) Flash-echo gray-scale imaging in the subtraction mode for assessing perfusion of small hepatocellular carcinoma. J Clin Ultrasound 31:451-456

Wang LY, Wang JH, Lin ZY et al (1997) Hepatic focal nodular hyperplasia: findings on color Doppler ultrasound. Abdom Imaging 22:178-181

Wanless IR, Mawdsley C, Adams R (1985) On the pathogenesis of focal nodular hyperplasia of the liver. Hepatology 5:1194-1200

Wang LY, Wang JH, Lin ZY et al (1997) Hepatic focal nodular hyperplasia: findings on color Doppler ultrasound. Abdom Imaging 22:178-181

Ward B, Baker AC, Humphrey WF (1997) Nonlinear propagation applied to the improvement of resolution in diagnostic medical ultrasound. J Acoust Soc Am 101:143-154

Welch TJ, Sheedy PF, Johnson CM et al (1985) Radiologic characteristics of benign liver tumors: focal nodular hyperplasia and hepatic adenoma. Radiographics 5:673-682

Wen YL, Kudo M, Zheng RQ et al (2004) Characterization of hepatic tumors: value of contrast-enhanced coded phase-inversion harmonic angio. Am J Roentgenology 182:1019-1026

Wilson SR, Burns PN, Murdali D et al (2000) Harmonic hepatic ultrasound with microbubble contrast agent: initial experience showing improved characterization of haemangioma, hepatocellular carcinoma and metastasis. Radiology 215:153-161

Yoshikawa J, Matsui O, Takashima T (1988) Fatty metamorphosis in hepatocellular carcinoma: radiological features in 10 cases. AJR Am J Roentgenol 151:717-720

12 Detection of Focal Liver Lesions

Emilio Quaia, Maja Ukmar, and Maria Cova

CONTENTS

12.1 Detection of Liver Metastases 167
12.1.1 Introduction 167
12.1.2 Scanning Modes 168
12.1.3 Clinical Results 169
12.2 Detection of Hepatocellular Carcinoma 178
12.3 When Should Microbubble-Based Agents Be Employed? 182
References 183

12.1 Detection of Liver Metastases

12.1.1 Introduction

The liver is one of the most common sites for metastatic spread of most malignancies, and the accurate assessment of liver metastatic disease is important for the planning of surgical, interventional, and medical therapy. Baseline gray-scale ultrasound (US) is routinely used as the first imaging technique in the detection of liver metastases, even though its accuracy is related to operator experience. Moreover, the general sensitivity of baseline US in the detection of liver metastases ranges between 53% and 84% (Cosgrove and Bolondi 1993; Carter et al. 1996), while US sensitivity for metastatic lesions smaller than 1 cm has been found to be as low as 20% (Wernecke et al. 1991). Most metastatic lesions missed on baseline US are either smaller than 1 cm or isoechoic relative to adjacent liver parenchyma.

The best available reference standards for imaging diagnosis of liver metastases are computed tomography (CT) and magnetic resonance (MR) imaging with agents targeted to Kupffer cells [superparamagnetic iron oxide (SPIO)] or hepatocytes [gadobenate dimeglumine (Gd-BOPTA)] (Del Frate et al. 2002), CT arterial portography, and surgical exploration with intraoperative US (Robinson 2001). SPIO-enhanced MR imaging shows a higher sensitivity than iodinated contrast material-enhanced CT (99% vs 94%; Ward et al. 1999) in the detection of metastatic lesions larger than 1 cm, but its sensitivity has been reported to be much lower in lesions smaller than 1 cm (Bellin et al. 1994; Haspigel et al. 1995; Ward et al. 1999, 2000a, 2003). Del Frate et al. (2002) found the sensitivity of SPIO-enhanced MR imaging to be superior to that of Gd-BOPTA-enhanced MR imaging for the detection of liver metastases. CT arterial portography is more sensitive than iodinated contrast-enhanced CT and SPIO-enhanced MR imaging in detecting metastases smaller than 1 cm, but it is an invasive imaging technique and produces more false positive lesions (Soyer et al. 1992; Seneterre et al. 1996; Valls et al. 1998). Like CT arterial portography, intraoperative US has been shown to be very sensitive but not specific in the detection of liver metastases (Robinson 2001).

Dedicated US contrast-specific techniques have shown good accuracy in the detection of liver metastases after microbubble injection (Dalla Palma et al. 1999; Harvey et al. 2000a,b; Albrecht et al. 2001a, 2003a,b; Del Frate et al. 2003; Quaia et al. 2003). The first such agents to be employed for this purpose were air-filled microbubbles, such as Levovist and Sonavist (Schering AG, Berlin, Germany). After blood pool clearance, air-filled microbubbles were shown to have a late liver-specific parenchymal phase from 3 to 5 min after injection. During this time microbubbles are stationary in liver and are probably pooling in sinusoids or phagocytosed by Kupffer cells of the reticuloendothelial system (Hauff et al. 1997; Blomley et al. 1998; Bauer et al. 1999; Forsberg et al. 1999, 2000a,b, 2002, Quaia et al. 2002a). The highest microbubble detectability was achieved when the acoustic power of the US beam was high enough (mechanical index = 1.0–1.2) to destroy microbubbles, producing a transient high

---

E. Quaia, MD, Assistant Professor of Radiology;
M. Ukmar, MD; M. Cova, MD, Professor of Radiology
Department of Radiology, Cattinara Hospital, University of Trieste, Strada di Fiume 447, 34149 Trieste, Italy

intensity wideband frequency signal (DALLA PALMA et al. 1999a; QUAIA et al. 2003). During the late phase the normal liver parenchyma displays clear uptake of air-filled microbubbles, while metastatic lesions, which are devoid of liver sinusoids and Kupffer cells, appear as hypoechoic and hypovascular defects compared to the adjacent liver.

New generation sulfur hexafluoride-filled microbubbles (ALBRECHT et al. 2003b) without proven liver-specific properties (LIM et al. 2004), such as SonoVue (Bracco, Milan, Italy), or perfluorocarbon-filled microbubbles with proven liver-specific properties, such as Sonazoid (Amersham Health, Oslo, Norway) (NEEDLMAN et al. 1998; ALBRECHT et al. 2001b; FORSBERG et al. 2002b; LESAVRE et al. 2003; KINDBERG et al. 2003; WATANABE et al. 2003), have shown promise for the detection of liver metastases. In particular, the liver specificity of Sonazoid is similar to that of Levovist, but it shows stronger and more prolonged liver enhancement, which has obvious advantages in terms of both longer scanning opportunity and performance of US-guided biopsy of detected lesions (ALBRECHT et al. 2003a).

12.1.2
Scanning Modes

a) High acoustic power mode. High acoustic power insonation was the first mode employed to detect liver metastases after microbubble-based agent injection.

Dedicated contrast-specific US techniques are employed from 3 to 5 min after the injection of air-filled microbubbles during the liver-specific late phase (BLOMLEY et al. 1998, 1999; DALLA PALMA et al. 1999; HOPE SIMPSON et al. 1999; HARVEY et al. 2000a,b; ALBRECHT et al. 2001a,b, 2003a,b; DEL FRATE et al. 2003; LESAVRE et al. 2003; QUAIA et al. 2003). The aim of high acoustic power insonation is to cause extensive microbubble rupture throughout the liver parenchyma, with production of a wide-band frequency signal. Because of the transience of contrast enhancement due to microbubble destruction (ALBRECHT et al. 2000), the scanning technique has to be optimized to image fresh, undestroyed microbubbles with each new frame (ALBRECHT et al. 2003a). Moreover, since the whole liver parenchyma has to be assessed when investigating the possible presence of liver metastases, the insonation has to be continuous instead of intermittent, as in the characterization of focal liver lesions. For these reasons it is appropriate to transmit the maximal acoustic power (mechanical index >1), switching off the signal persistence and employing the lowest possible frame rate (8–10 Hz) and a single focal zone positioned in the deep third of the field of view (8–10 cm from abdominal surface) in order to minimize and to render more homogeneous the rupture of microbubbles.

Scanning is started from 3 to 5 min after microbubble bolus injection by using a dedicated contrast-specific mode (e.g., Pulse Inversion Mode from Philips-ATL, WA, USA or Agent Detection Imaging from Siemens-Acuson, CA, USA). Scanning of the liver parenchyma is performed, during breath-hold, by one or two transverse sweeps throughout the right liver lobe, and with one longitudinal sweep on the left lobe (Fig. 12.1). Microbubble rupture may produce heterogeneous contrast enhancement in the case of irregular free-hand scanning, with evidence of artifacts which may simulate focal liver lesions. After the sweeps have been completed, each stored digital cine-clip has to be reviewed to detect liver metastases appearing as hypovascular focal liver lesions against the background of enhancing normal liver parenchyma.

b) Low acoustic power mode. The low acoustic power insonation mode is employed with new-generation microbubble-based agents. Since microbubble rupture is minimized with low acoustic power insonation, the liver parenchyma may be scanned

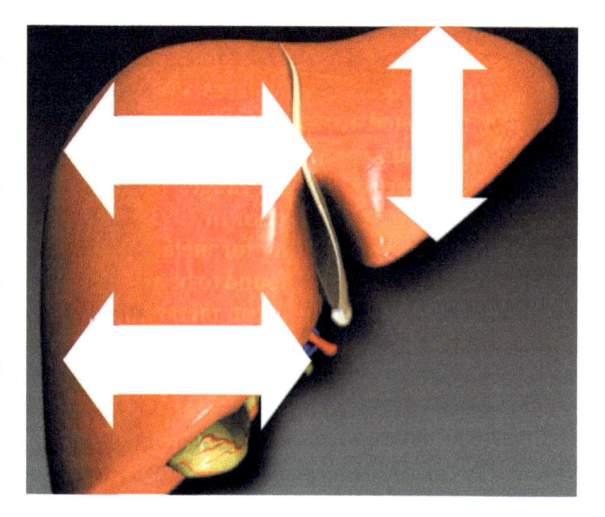

Fig. 12.1. Suggested scanning planes of the liver using the high acoustic power mode to detect focal liver lesions. The right liver is scanned in the transverse plane by one or two continuous sweeps, while the left liver is scanned in the longitudinal plane by one continuous sweep. If low acoustic power insonation is employed, the liver may be scanned on every plane since microbubble rupture is minimized.

continuously during the arterial (10–35 s), portal (40–90 s), and late (95–120 s from injection) phases, with multiple sweeps.

The low acoustic power mode presents several advantages in comparison with high acoustic power. First, it is easier to perform since the same region of the liver may be scanned more times due to the minimization of microbubble rupture. Second, more acoustic views (i.e., intercostal views) may be employed without evidence of significant artifacts, except for posterior acoustic shadowing of ribs. Third, the suppression of background signal from native stationary tissues is complete and the harmonic signal is produced almost completely from microbubble resonance.

12.1.3
Clinical Results

a) Comparison with baseline gray-scale US. In the comparative series with the largest patient numbers (ALBRECHT et al. 2001a, 2003a; QUAIA et al. 2003), high acoustic power insonation was employed after air-filled microbubble injection. In these studies, contrast-enhanced US significantly improved (Figs. 12.2–12.4) the detection of liver metastases (from 47% to 56%) in comparison with baseline scan, and there was an improvement in sensitivity from 63–71% to 87–91%.

These results were achieved through the improved conspicuity (visibility) of metastatic lesions (Figs. 12.5, 12.6). In fact, during the late liver-specific phase, microbubbles spare metastases, which appear as hypovascular defects, while being selectively taken up by the adjacent liver parenchyma (Figs. 12.7, 12.8).

In livers containing metastases and appearing heterogeneous on baseline US, contrast-enhanced US reveals multiple (>5) metastatic lesions (Fig. 12.9). This is because even in the presence of extensive metastatic liver involvement, microbubbles accumulate in the interposed normal liver parenchyma, thereby increasing the visibility of metastases.

Additional metastatic liver lesions, identified after the injection of microbubble-based agents (Figs. 12.2–12.4, 12.8), usually measure less than 1 cm in diameter and are localized in the middle or anterior segment of the liver.

Contrast-enhanced US is most effective in detecting liver metastases in patients in whom metastases have already been identified on baseline US. On the other hand, in a study by QUAIA et al. (2003), a small number of patients without evidence of metastatic liver lesions on the baseline scan were found to have one or more metastatic lesions after microbubble injection. Based on these results it seems reasonable to propose the employment of baseline US in patient follow-up after surgery, since state of the art US equipment with wideband transducers is sufficiently accurate in detecting liver metastases at the screening level. Contrast-enhanced US should be proposed in patients who show from one to five focal liver lesions suspected of being metastases on baseline US, the aim being to reveal additional metastatic lesions and to permit selection of the most suitable therapeutic approach (surgery, radiofrequency or palliative treatment if more than five metastatic lesions are identified; ROBINSON 2001).

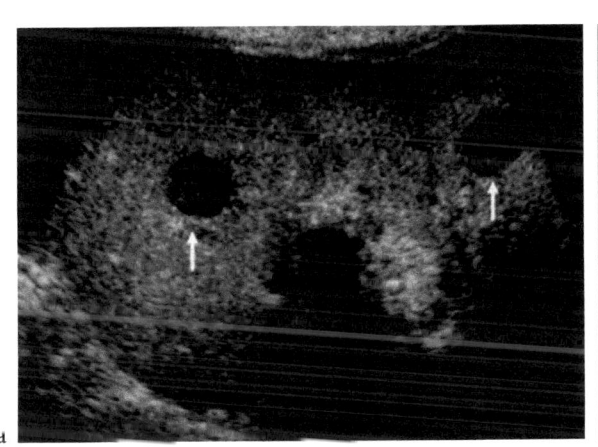

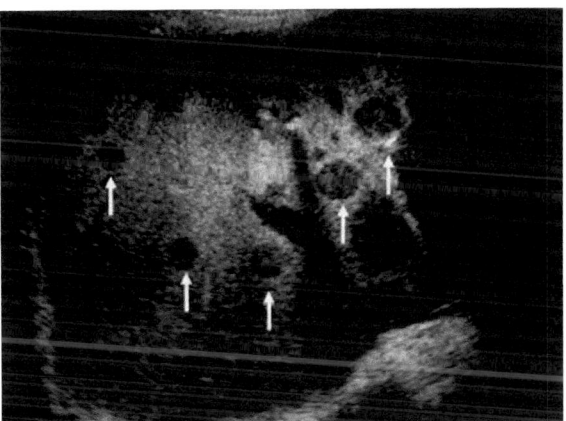

Fig. 12.2a,b. Appearance of metastatic lesions in the late phase, 4 min after the injection of air-filled microbubbles, with high acoustic power insonation. The metastases appear as hypoechoic defects (*arrows*) in the enhancing liver.

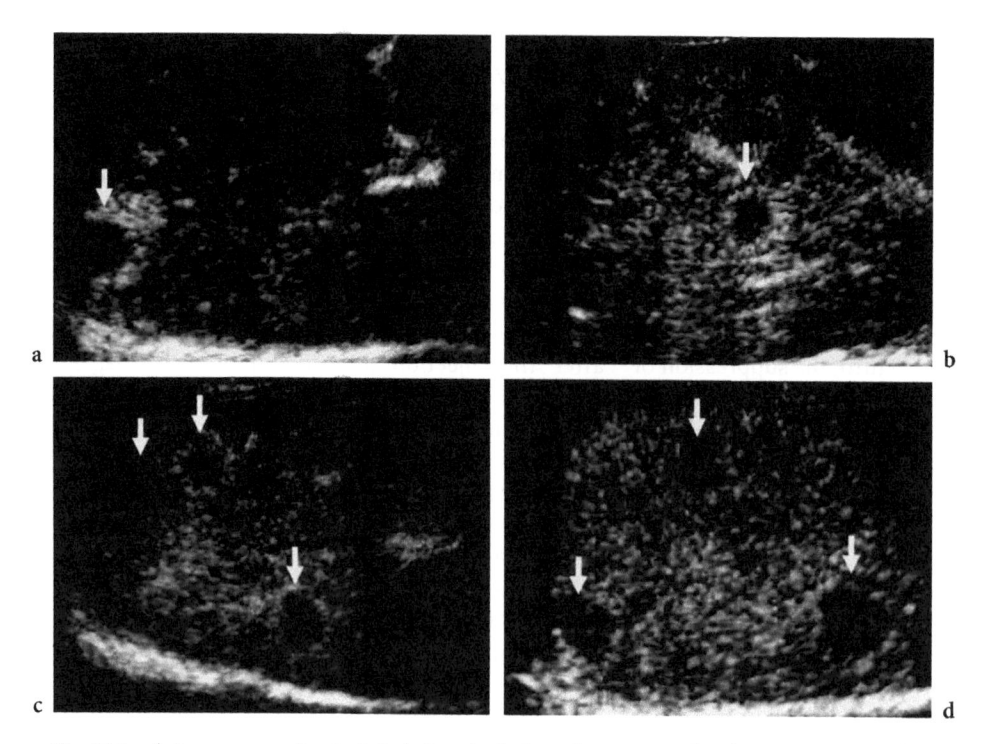

Fig. 12.3a–d. Appearance of metastatic lesions in the late phase, 110 s after the injection of sulfur hexafluoride-filled microbubbles, with low acoustic power insonation. The metastases appear as hypoechoic, hypovascular defects (*arrows*) in the normally enhancing adjacent liver.

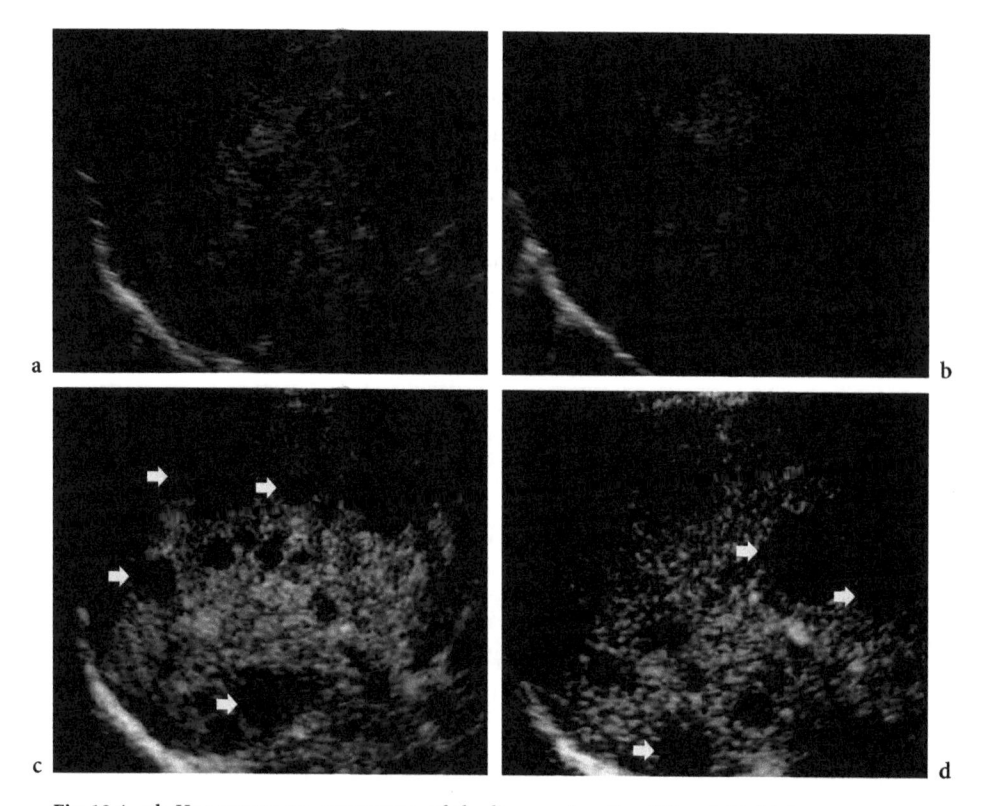

Fig. 12.4. a,b Heterogeneous appearance of the liver on baseline US. **c,d** Multiple metastases appear as hypoechoic defects (*arrows*) in the normally enhancing adjacent liver on contrast-enhanced US, 120 s after the injection of sulfur hexafluoride-filled microbubbles, with low acoustic power insonation.

Detection of Focal Liver Lesions

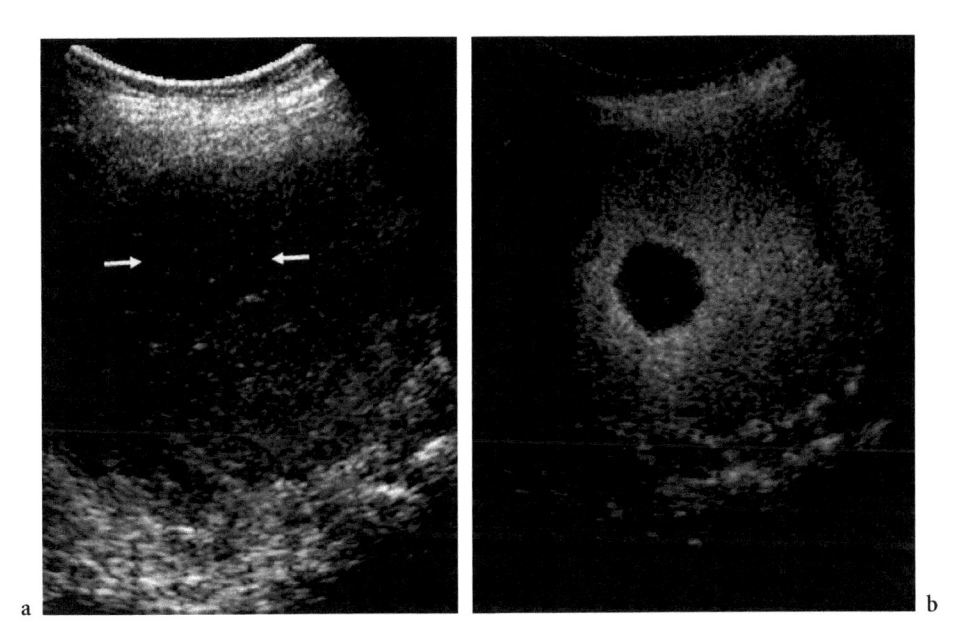

Fig. 12.5a,b. Improved metastatic lesion conspicuity on contrast-enhanced US in comparison with the baseline scan. High acoustic power mode after the injection of air-filled microbubbles. On baseline US (**a**) the metastatic lesion (*arrows*) is barely visible. The contrast between the metastatic lesion and the adjacent liver was clearly improved after microbubble injection (**b**).

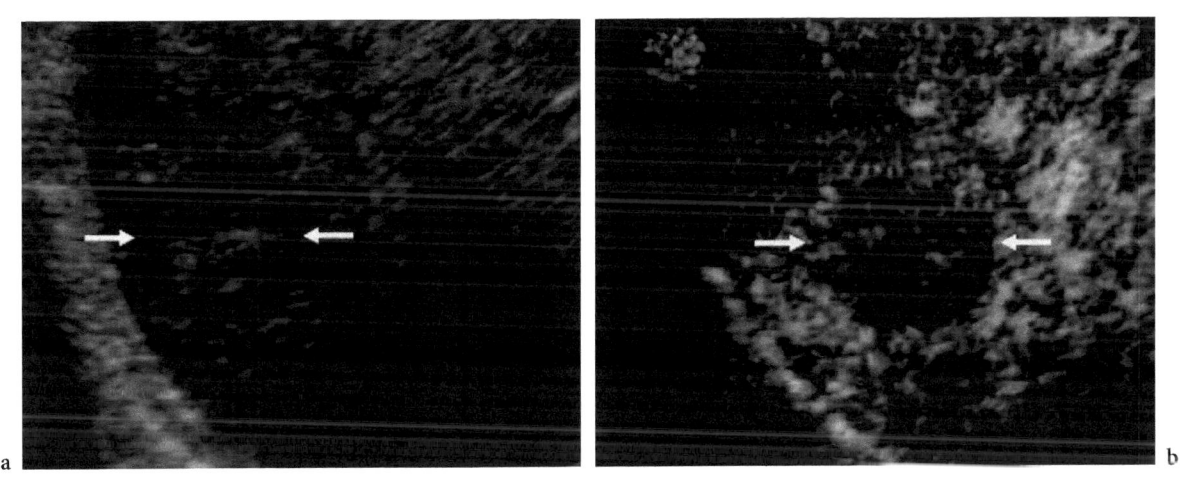

Fig. 12.6a,b. Improved metastatic lesion conspicuity on contrast-enhanced US (**b**) in comparison with the baseline scan (**a**). Low acoustic power mode after sulfur hexafluoride-filled microbubble injection. On baseline US (**a**) the metastatic lesion (*arrows*) presents a peripheral hypoechoic halo. The contrast between the metastatic lesion and the adjacent liver was clearly improved after microbubble injection (**b**).

b) Comparison with contrast-enhanced CT. Contrast-enhanced CT has been considered the reference standard in most of the published series (QUAIA et al. 2003), sometimes with the addition of gadolinium enhanced MR imaging (ALBRECHT et al. 2001a, 2003a). Nevertheless, contrast-enhanced CT cannot be considered a perfect tool for the detection of liver metastases (ROBINSON 2001).

Contrast-enhanced US shows a similar accuracy to contrast-enhanced CT in the detection of liver metastases (Fig. 12.10). A more important finding is that the additional metastatic lesions identified by contrast-enhanced US are predominantly less than a centimeter in diameter (Fig. 12.11) (DALLA PALMA et al. 1999; HARVEY et al. 2000a,b; ALBRECHT et al. 2001a; DEL FRATE et al. 2003; QUAIA et al. 2003). Moreover, the additionally detected liver metastases are mainly located in the middle and anterior segments of the liver (Fig. 12.12), since the contrast enhancement after the injection of microbubble-based agents is

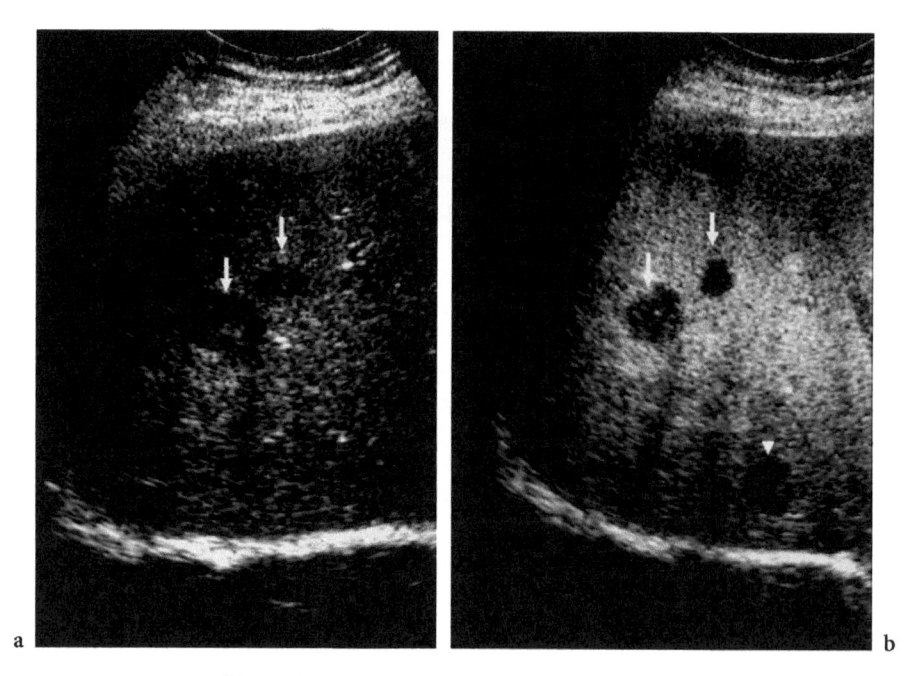

Fig. 12.7a,b. Improved lesion detection by contrast-enhanced US in comparison with the baseline scan. High acoustic power mode after the injection of air-filled microbubbles. Two focal liver lesions (*arrows*) are identified on the baseline scan (a). An additional focal liver lesion (*arrowhead*) is identified in the liver segment close to the diaphragm after microbubble injection (b).

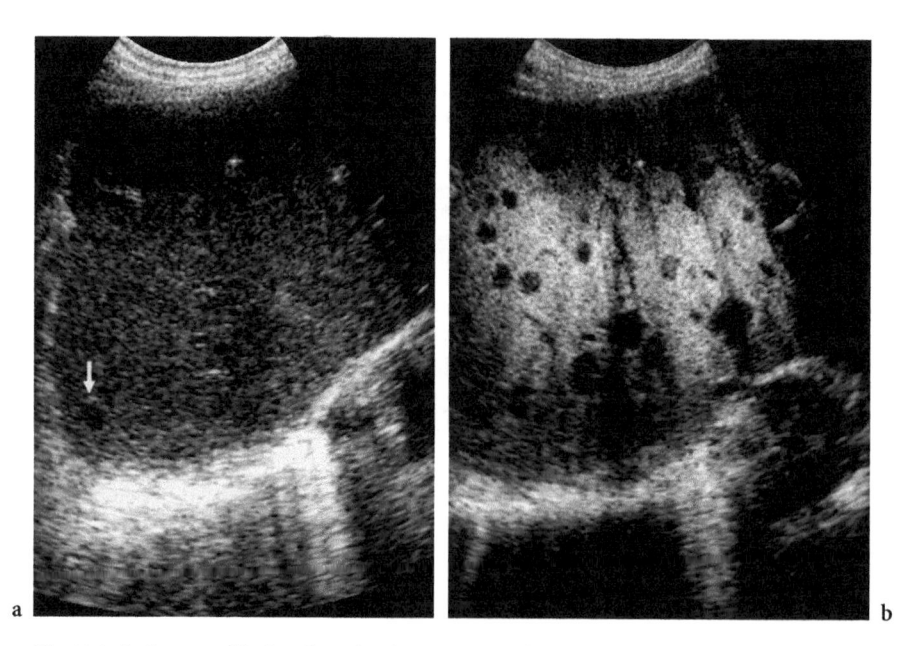

Fig. 12.8a,b. Improved lesion detection by contrast-enhanced US in comparison with the baseline scan. High acoustic power mode after air-filled microbubble injection. Only one metastatic lesion (*arrow*) can be identified on the baseline scan (a), while contrast-enhanced US (b) reveals multiple metastatic lesions.

Detection of Focal Liver Lesions

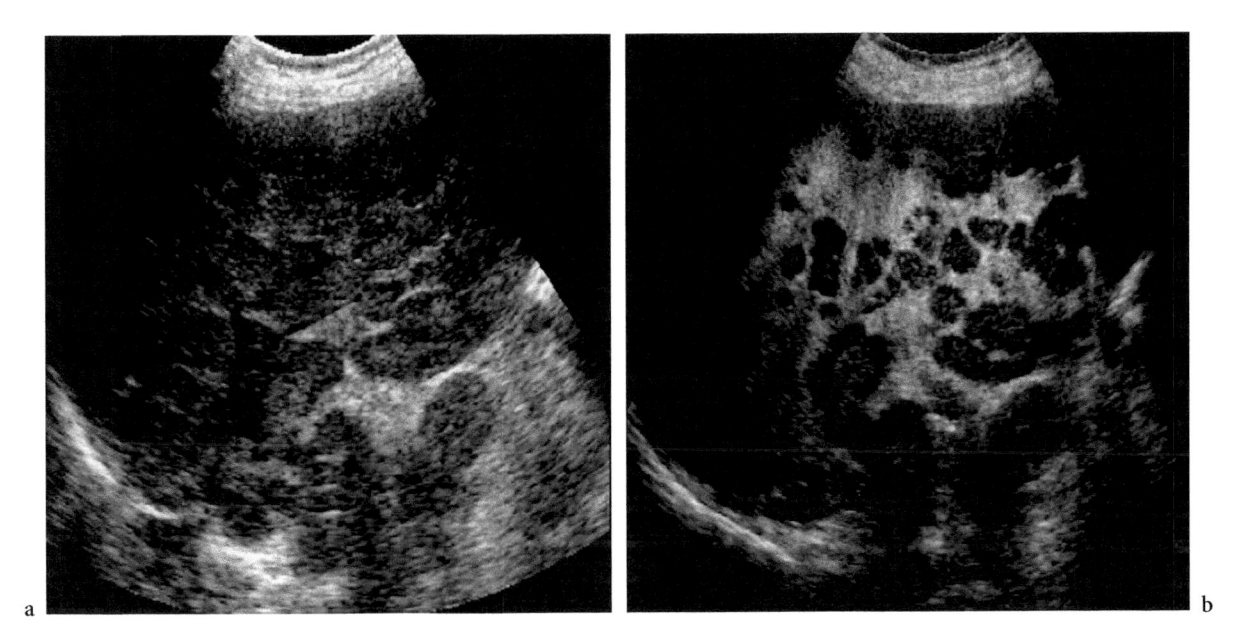

Fig. 12.9a,b. Improved detection of metastatic lesions by contrast-enhanced US (**b**) in comparison with baseline US (**a**). High acoustic power mode after air-filled microbubble injection. A heterogeneous appearance of liver parenchyma is identified on the baseline scan (**a**). Multiple metastatic lesions are identified after microbubble injection in the late phase (**b**).

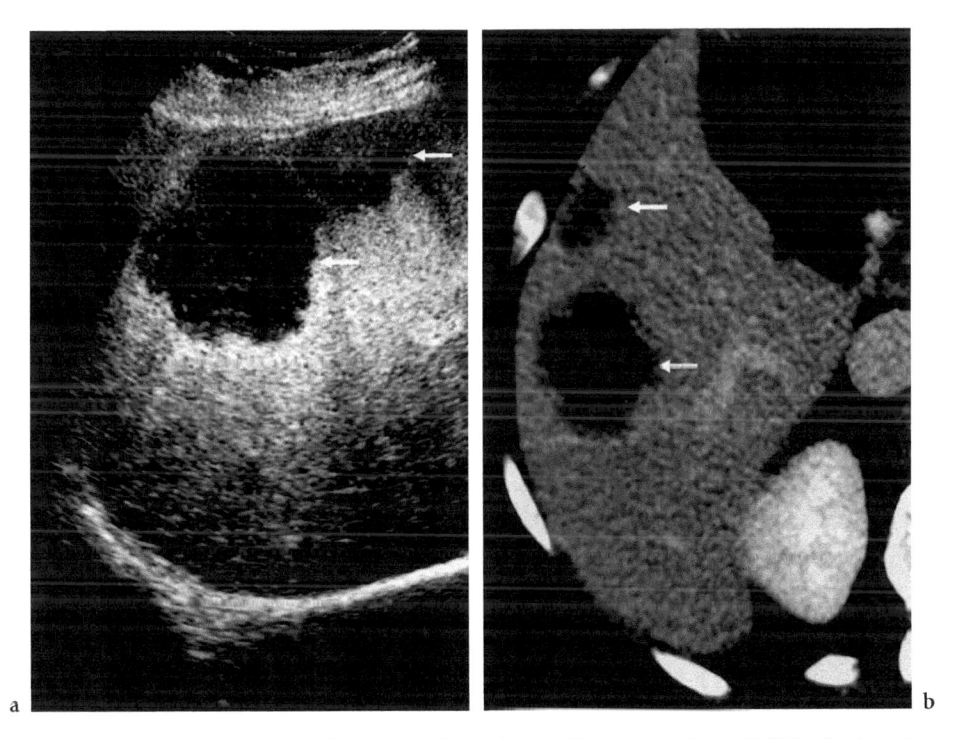

Fig. 12.10a,b. Similar accuracy of contrast-enhanced US and contrast-enhanced CT in the detection of metastatic lesions. Two liver metastases (*arrows*) are identified on contrast-enhanced US (**a**) and confirmed on contrast-enhanced CT (**b**). High acoustic power mode after air-filled microbubble injection.

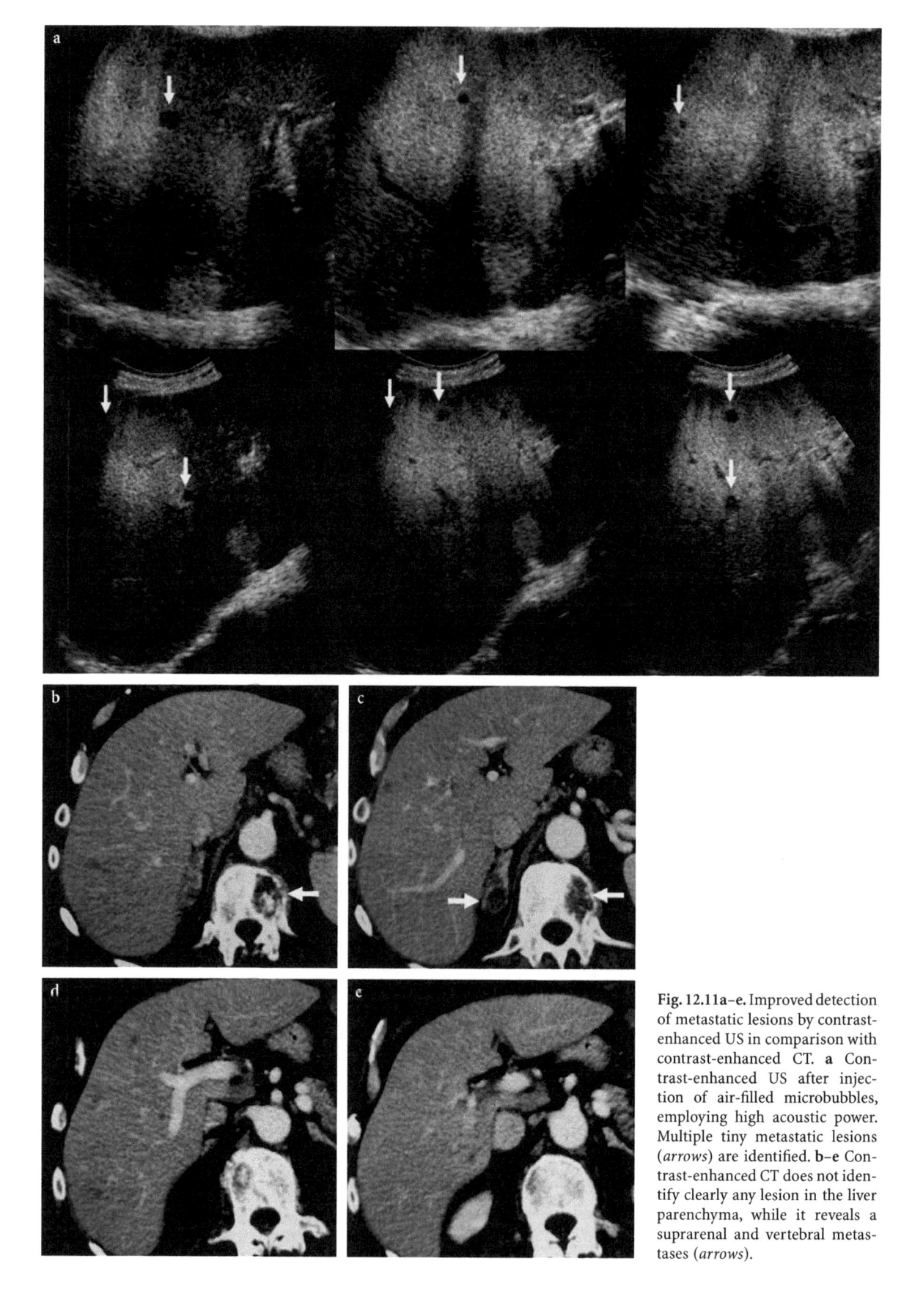

Fig. 12.11a–e. Improved detection of metastatic lesions by contrast-enhanced US in comparison with contrast-enhanced CT. a Contrast-enhanced US after injection of air-filled microbubbles, employing high acoustic power. Multiple tiny metastatic lesions (*arrows*) are identified. b–e Contrast-enhanced CT does not identify clearly any lesion in the liver parenchyma, while it reveals a suprarenal and vertebral metastases (*arrows*).

Detection of Focal Liver Lesions

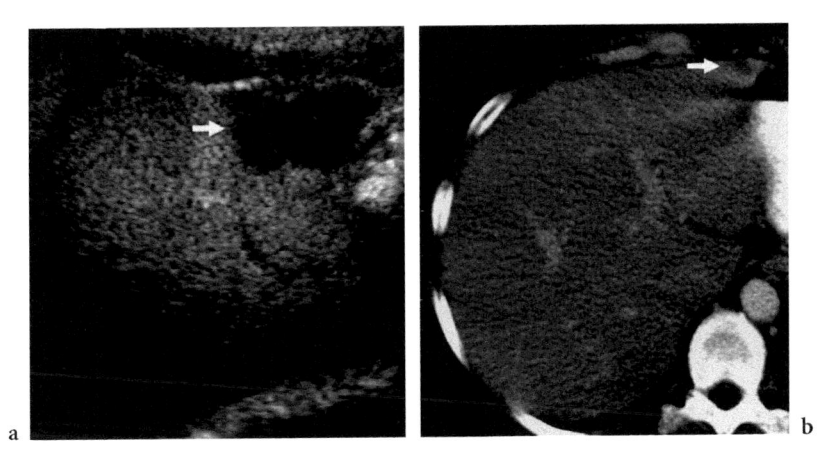

Fig. 12.12a,b. Improved detection of metastatic lesions by contrast-enhanced US in comparison with contrast-enhanced CT. Contrast-enhanced US (a) after the injection of air-filled microbubbles, with high acoustic power. A single metastasis is identified in the anterior region of the left liver lobe. This lesion (*arrow*) was identified only retrospectively on contrast material-enhanced CT (b).

most intense above the focal zone (ALBRECHT et al. 2000), where the intensity of the beam is higher and the microbubble destruction more extensive.

Contrast-enhanced US does, however, have clear limitations in the detection of liver metastases in liver segments close to the diaphragm and inferior vena cava (Fig. 12.13) (QUAIA et al. 2003) and in liver regions hidden by the posterior acoustic shadowing from the bowel gas (Fig. 12.14). The limited value of contrast-enhanced US in the assessment of deep liver segments is principally due to the deep position of the focal zone, which prevents homogeneous and effective bubble rupture throughout liver parenchyma. In fact, even though the deep liver segments are near the focal zone, these segments are the most difficult to assess by contrast-enhanced US since the broadband signal from microbubble destruction is extensively attenuated by superficial planes.

c) Comparison with Gd-enhanced or SPIO-enhanced MR. MR imaging has become an important tool in clinical liver imaging thanks to the introduction of faster imaging techniques. The advent of liver-specific MR imaging contrast materials, which are

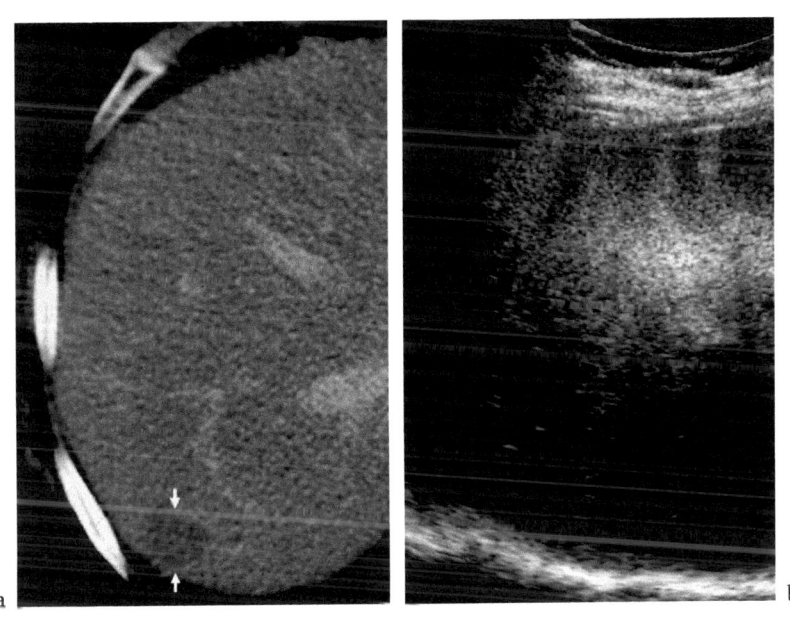

Fig. 12.13a,b. Improved lesion detection on contrast-enhanced CT in comparison with contrast-enhanced US. A single, very deeply located metastatic lesion (*arrows*) is seen on contrast-enhanced CT (a), while contrast-enhanced US (high acoustic power mode after air-filled microbubble injection) (b) does not identify any lesion.

agents targeted at the enhancement of hepatocytes or Kupffer cells, has facilitated an increase in the accuracy of MR imaging in liver metastasis detection (DEL FRATE et al. 2002). In series with Gd-BOPTA- (MOSCONI et al. 2003) or SPIO-enhanced MR (DEL FRATE et al. 2003) as the reference standards, similar results were observed to those using CT as the reference standard, with similar limitations for contrast-enhanced US (Figs. 12.15–12.18).

d) Contrast-enhanced intraoperative US. Dedicated intraoperative US transducers equipped with contrast-specific US modes are available and may be employed after microbubble injection to improve the

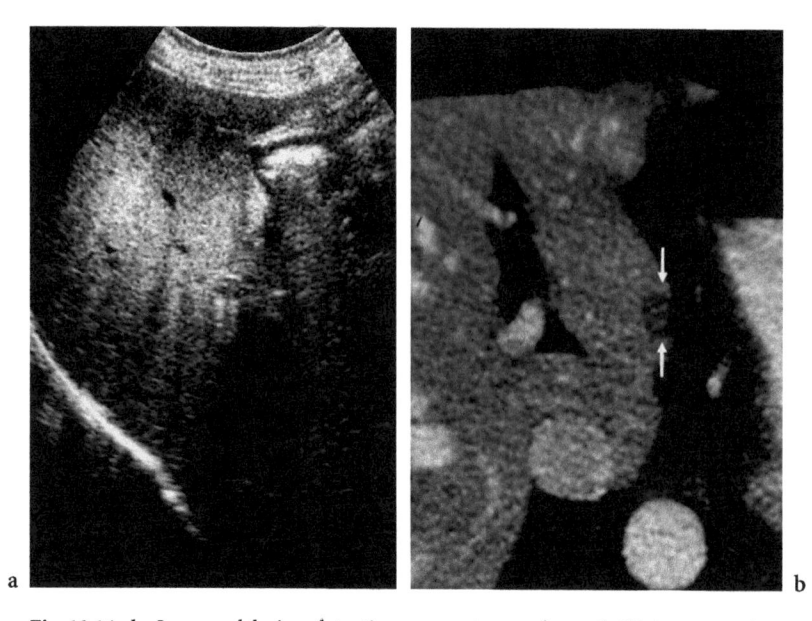

Fig. 12.14a,b. Improved lesion detection on contrast-enhanced CT in comparison with contrast-enhanced US. **a** Contrast-enhanced US was performed employing the high acoustic power mode after air-filled microbubble injection. No lesion is identified in the liver. **b** Contrast-enhanced CT during the portal phase. A single metastatic lesion (*arrows*) is identified behind the stomach.

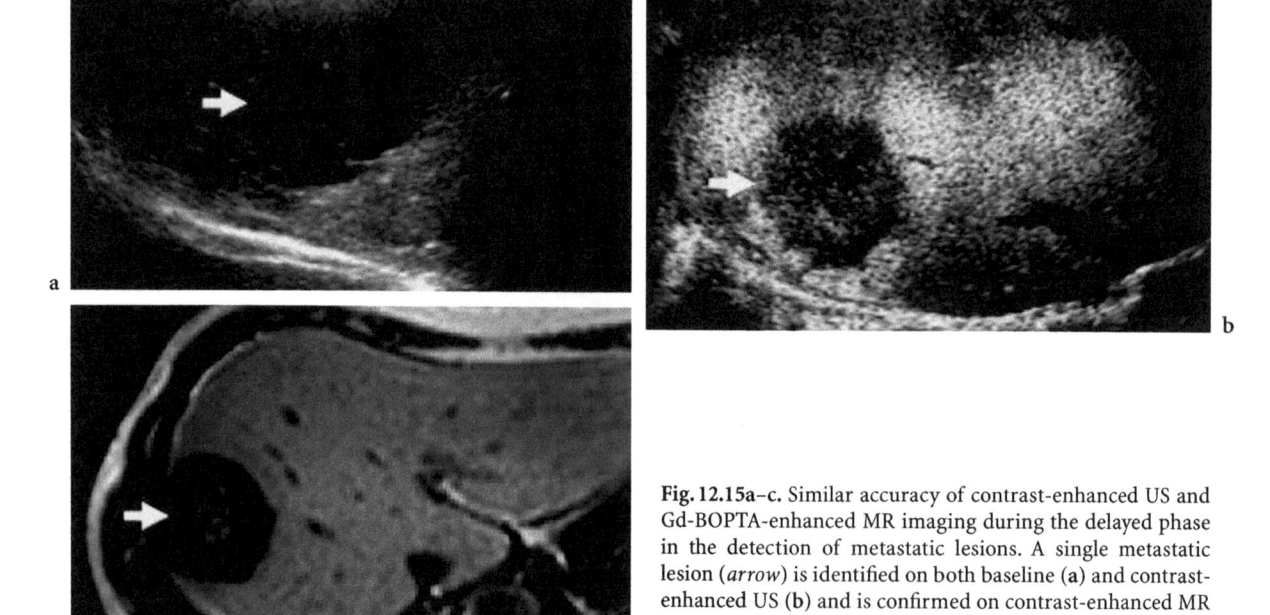

Fig. 12.15a–c. Similar accuracy of contrast-enhanced US and Gd-BOPTA-enhanced MR imaging during the delayed phase in the detection of metastatic lesions. A single metastatic lesion (*arrow*) is identified on both baseline (**a**) and contrast-enhanced US (**b**) and is confirmed on contrast-enhanced MR imaging (**c**) 1 h after Gd-BOPTA injection.

Detection of Focal Liver Lesions

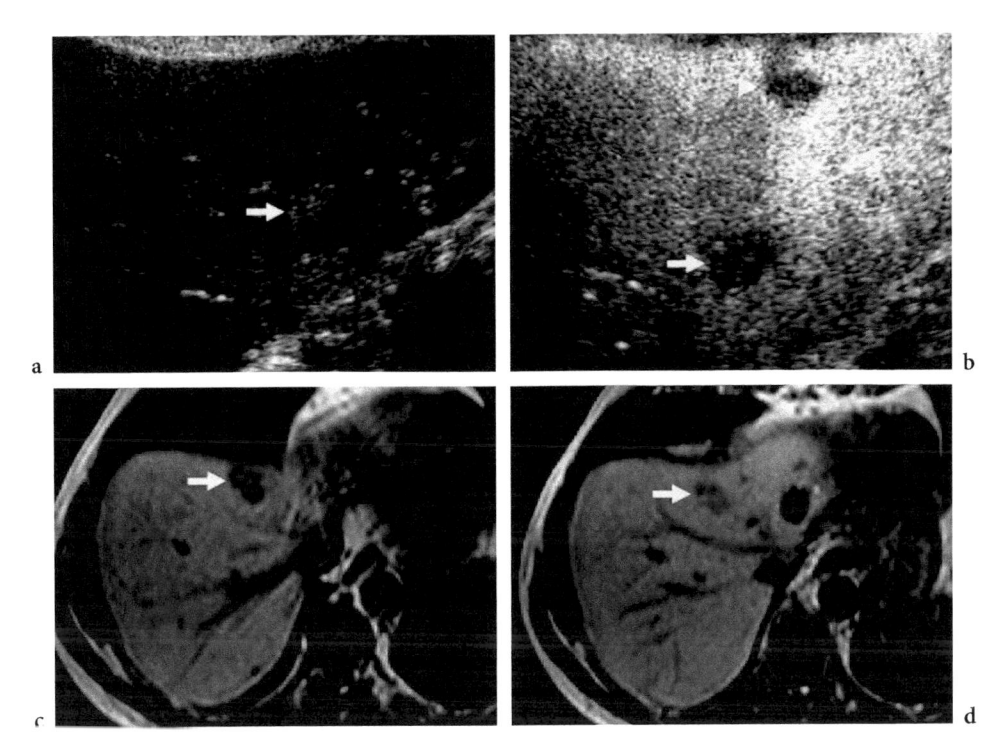

Fig. 12.16a–d. Improved lesion detection by contrast-enhanced US in comparison with Gd-BOPTA-enhanced MR imaging in the delayed phase. **a, b** A single metastatic lesion (*arrow*) is identified by baseline US (**a**), while contrast-enhanced US (high acoustic power mode after air-filled microbubble injection) (**b**) identifies one additional lesion. **c, d** Contrast-enhanced MR imaging performed 1 h after Gd-BOPTA injection confirms only the first lesion (*arrow*).

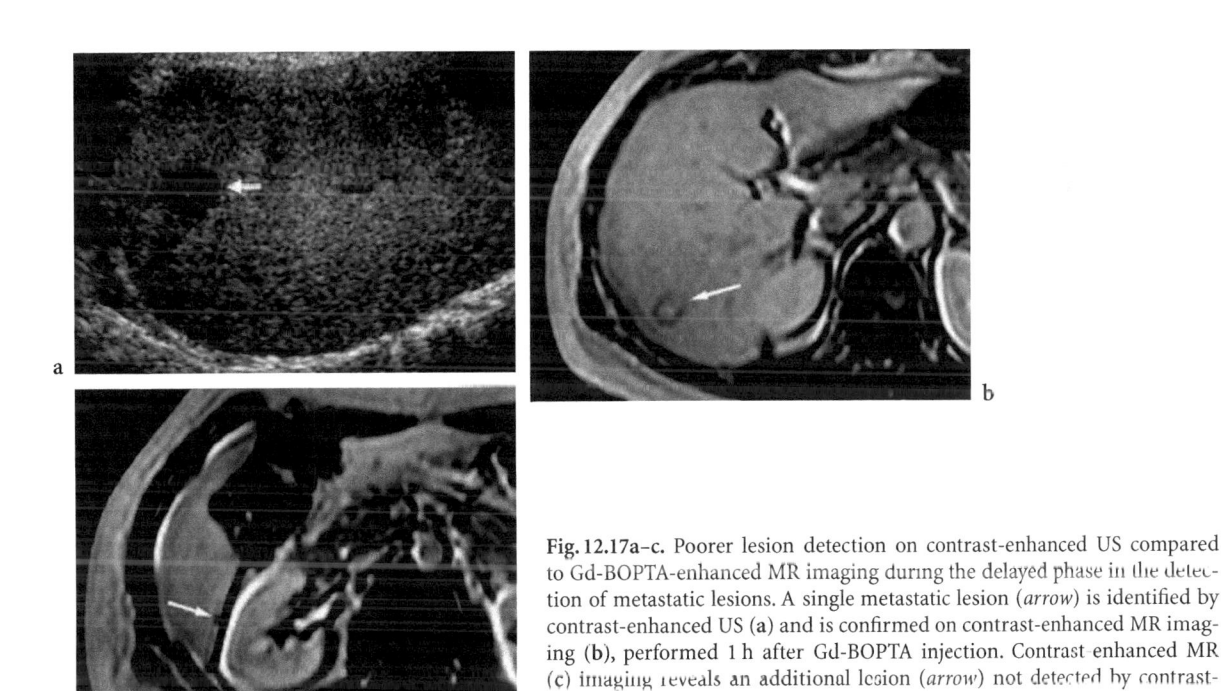

Fig. 12.17a–c. Poorer lesion detection on contrast-enhanced US compared to Gd-BOPTA-enhanced MR imaging during the delayed phase in the detection of metastatic lesions. A single metastatic lesion (*arrow*) is identified by contrast-enhanced US (**a**) and is confirmed on contrast-enhanced MR imaging (**b**), performed 1 h after Gd-BOPTA injection. Contrast-enhanced MR (**c**) imaging reveals an additional lesion (*arrow*) not detected by contrast-enhanced US.

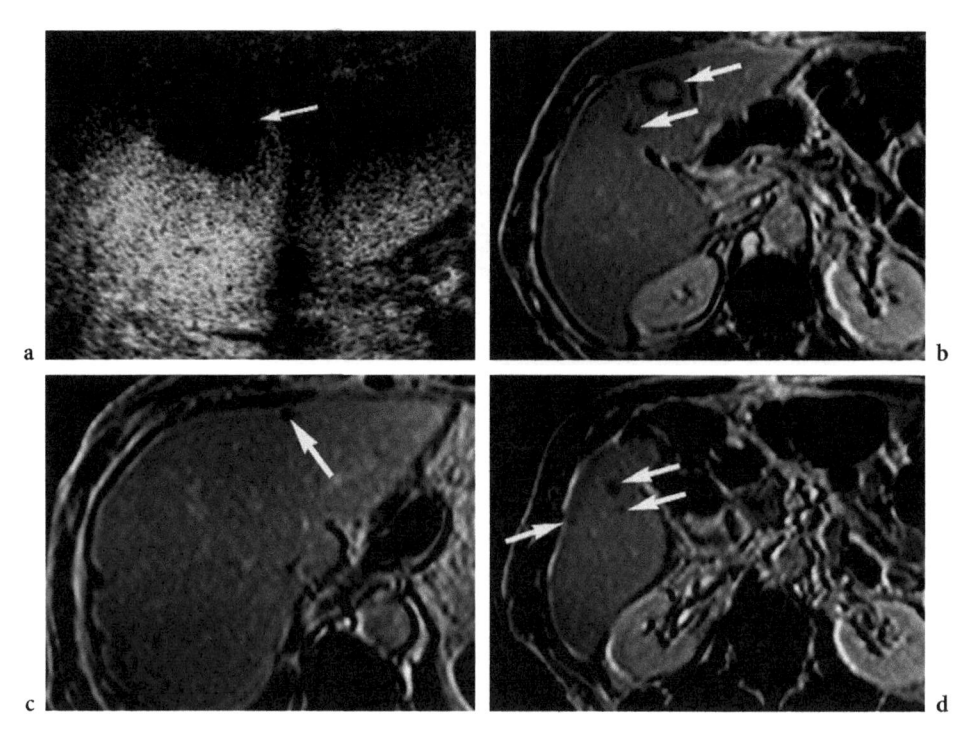

Fig. 12.18a–d. Poorer lesion detection on contrast-enhanced US in comparison with Gd-BOPTA-enhanced MR in the delayed phase. A single metastatic lesion (*arrow*) is identified by contrast-enhanced US in the high acoustic power mode after air-filled microbubble injection (**a**), while contrast-enhanced MR, performed 1 h after Gd-BOPTA injection, confirms the previous lesion (**b**) and reveals multiple additional tiny lesions (**c, d**; *arrows*)

detection of liver metastases (Fig. 12.19). Intraoperative US allows placement of the transducer directly at the liver surface, avoiding the limitations due to bowel gas interposition or a large body habitus. This further improves liver metastasis detection as compared to transabdominal contrast-enhanced US.

e) Limitations of contrast-enhanced US. The real advantage of contrast-enhanced US in the detection of liver metastases is evident in patients with optimal visibility of the liver parenchyma. Contrast-enhanced US has the same limitations as conventional US when there is bowel gas interposition or when the patient has a large body habitus (QUAIA et al. 2003). The effectiveness of contrast-enhanced US is also limited in patients with steatotic or cirrhotic liver parenchyma: it is in such patients that the lowest liver parenchyma enhancement and the poorest visibility of metastases has been observed (QUAIA et al. 2003). This is because in such patients the liver parenchyma appears diffusely hyperechoic even on baseline US and contrast enhancement is difficult to visualize. This limitation is overcome by low acoustic power insonation with new-generation perfluorocarbon- or sulfur hexafluoride-filled microbubbles, which allow good suppression of the background from stationary tissues.

The second important limitation of contrast-enhanced US is the possibility of false positive findings, corresponding to lesions which are not actually present and not confirmed by the reference standards (QUAIA et al. 2003). Moreover, some benign focal liver lesions, such as atypical sclerotic liver hemangioma and focal fatty changes, may simulate liver metastases on contrast-enhanced US (Fig. 12.20) since they sometimes appear as hypovascular defects in the liver-specific late phase (BERTOLOTTO et al. 2000; QUAIA et al. 2002a, 2003); this is especially true for hemangiomas that present a thrombotic pattern or focal fatty changes with a predominant fat component. In addition, artifacts from heterogeneous microbubble rupture appear as hypovascular echoic focal zones and may simulate focal liver lesions on contrast-enhanced US (Fig. 12.21) (QUAIA et al. 2003).

12.2
Detection of Hepatocellular Carcinoma

In chronic diffuse liver disease, macroregenerative nodules and hepatocellular carcinomas are the most characteristic and frequently observed focal liver

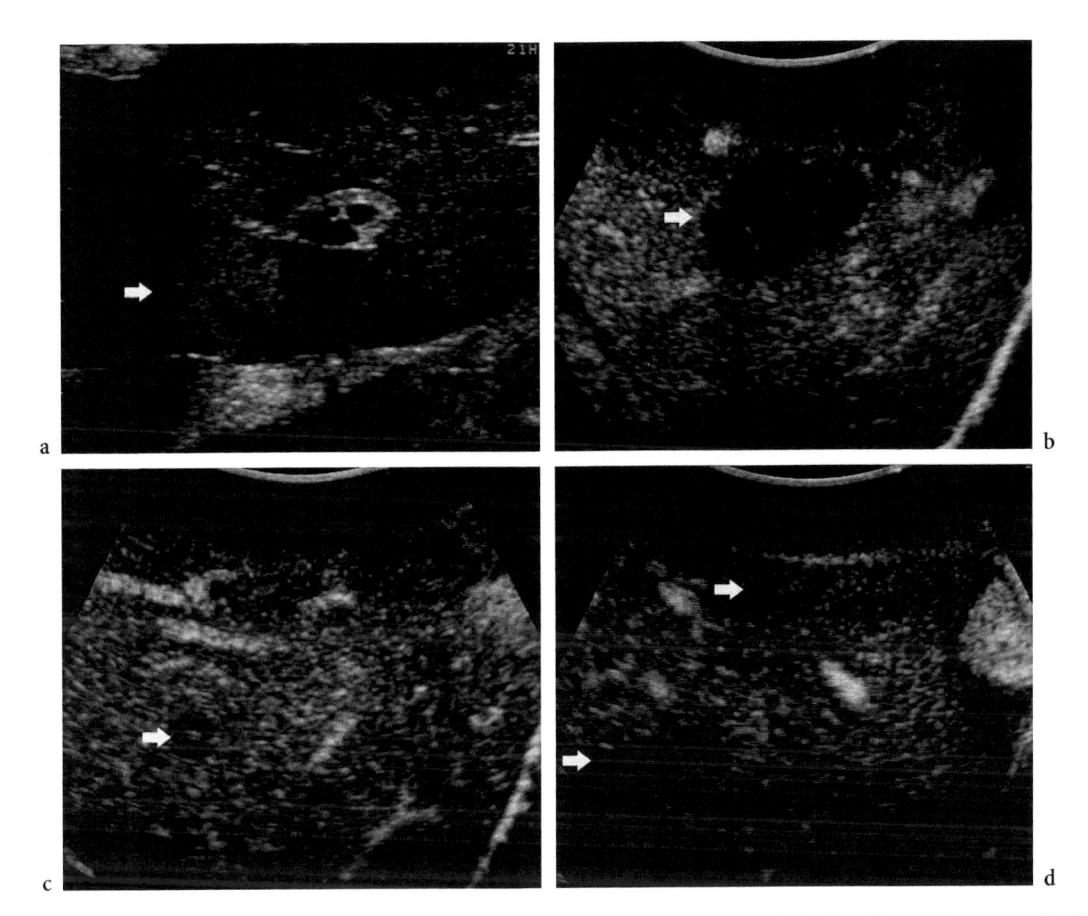

Fig. 12.19. a Baseline intraoperative US identifies one liver metastasis (*arrow*). **b–d** Dedicated intraoperative US transducer equipped with contrast-specific modes; images obtained 90 s after microbubble-based agent injection. The liver metastatic lesion (*arrow*) identified by baseline US is confirmed after microbubble-based agent injection (**b**). Further subcentimeter metastatic lesions (*arrows*) are identified after microbubble injection (**c, d**). Courtesy of Dr. Roberta Padovan, Aloka, Japan.

lesions (BARON and PETERSON 2001), while hemangiomas and focal nodular hyperplasia are occasionally observed. Each focal liver lesion identified in a cirrhotic patient has to be considered a hepatocellular carcinoma until proven otherwise. The detection of hepatocellular carcinoma in patients with cirrhosis has been considered a technical challenge (LAGHI et al. 2003) because cirrhosis alters both liver parenchymal characteristics (through fibrosis, the development of regenerative nodules, and fatty infiltration) and vascularization (through portal hypertension and the creation of arterial–portal venous shunts).

a) Detection by baseline US. The detection of hepatocellular carcinoma by baseline US is related to the size, echogenicity, and location of lesions and to the experience of the sonologist. Baseline US has a detection rate from 46% to 95% for lesions smaller than 2 cm (TAKAYASU et al. 1990, HARVEY and ALBRECHT 2001a; SOLBIATI et al. 2001) and from 13% to 37% for lesions smaller than 1 cm (SOLBIATI et al. 2001). The highest detection rates are achieved for hypoechoic lesions with a peripheral halo and the lowest rates for hyperechoic lesions without a peripheral halo. Multifocality is very frequent in hepatocellular carcinoma, occurring in about 80% of patients (SOLBIATI et al. 2001). The low sensitivity of baseline US is principally caused by the presence of heterogeneous and attenuating liver echotexture due to cirrhotic distortion and focal fibrosis.

b) Detection by cross-sectional imaging techniques. The reported sensitivity in the detection of hepatocellular carcinomas smaller than 3 cm is 46–88% for contrast-enhanced multiphase CT, 61–81% for angiography, 86–91% for CT arterial portography, 71–96% for iodized oil CT, and 94–96% for intraoperative US (CHOI et al. 1989, 1991; TAKAYASU et al. 1990; SOLBIATI et al. 2001; LAGHI et al. 2003).

The principal reason for the limited sensitivity of CT is the presence of cirrhotic distortion and focal

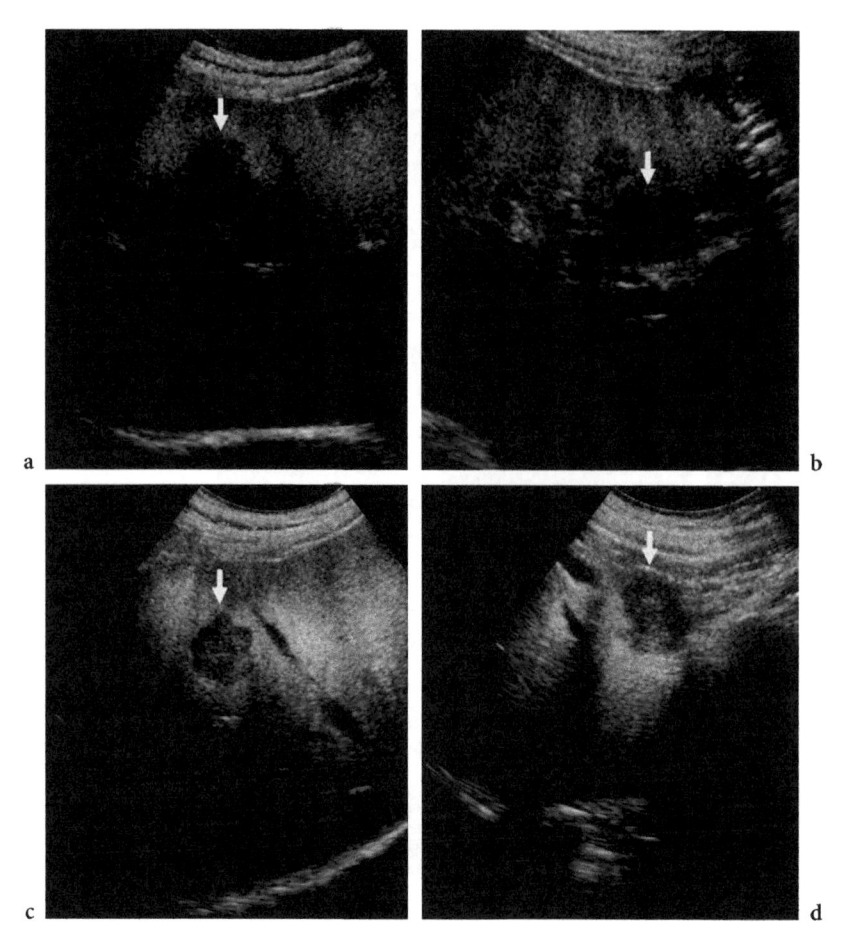

Fig. 12.20a-d. False positive findings of contrast-enhanced US. High acoustic power mode after air-filled microbubble injection. A focal liver lesion (*arrow*) appears hypoechoic on contrast-enhanced US during the late phase (a, b) and was considered to be a metastasis. US-guided biopsy revealed a sclerotic hemangioma which appeared unchanged at follow-up, also performed by contrast-enhanced US (c, d).

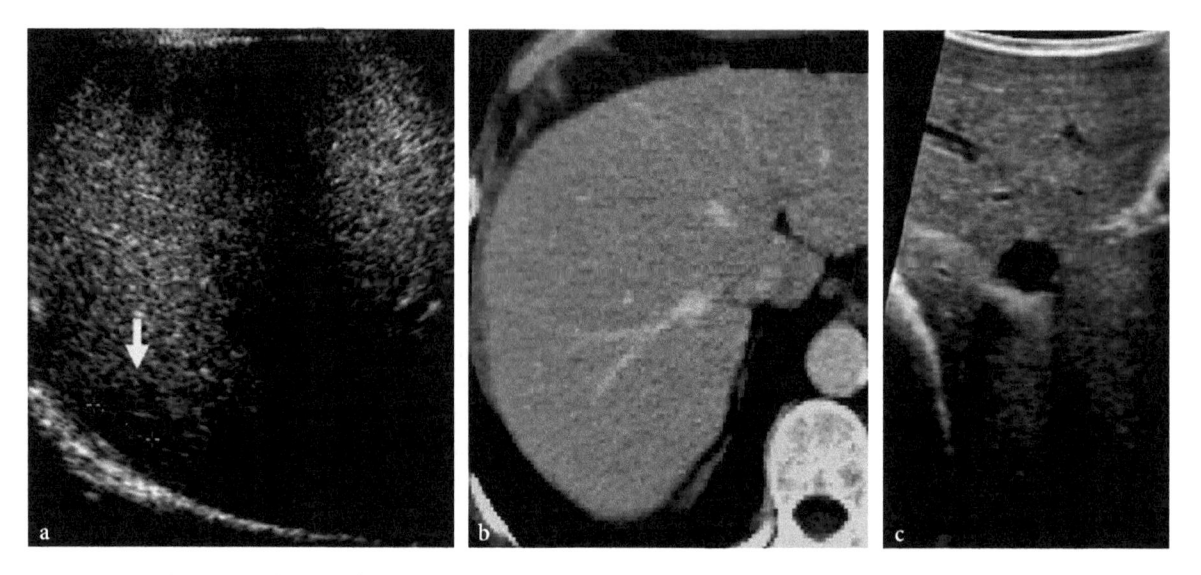

Fig. 12.21a-c. False positive findings of contrast-enhanced US. A focal liver lesion (*arrow*) that was deeply located and hypoechoic on contrast (Levovist)-enhanced US during the late phase (a) was considered to represent a metastasis. Contrast-enhanced CT (b) and intraoperative US (c) did not confirm this finding, which was considered an artifact due to heterogeneous microbubble rupture.

fibrosis, leading to heterogeneous contrast enhancement in the liver parenchyma. Focal liver lesions may be simulated by wedge-shaped areas that are widest at the capsular surface and are frequently associated with liver parenchymal atrophy and capsular retraction. The differentiation from real focal liver lesions is further hindered by the fact that focal liver fibrosis may display enhancement on contrast-enhanced CT (BARON and PETERSON 2001). Moreover, besides cirrhotic distortion of liver parenchyma and focal fibrosis, other types of focal liver parenchymal or vascular abnormalities may simulate focal liver lesions. In fact, it was shown that approximately one-third of the false positive diagnoses of hepatocellular carcinoma made with screening contrast-enhanced CT in a large transplantation series were due to enhancing vascular lesions, such as hemangioma, small arteriovenous shunts, and pseudoaneurysms (BARON and PETERSON 2001).

New diagnostic procedures, such as single- or double-contrast, Gd- and/or SPIO-enhanced MR imaging, have been reported to offer good diagnostic confidence and sensitivity in the detection of hepatocellular carcinoma (YAMASHITA et al. 1996; WARD et al. 2000a,b, 2003; PAULEIT et al. 2002; KANG et al. 2003; TEEFEY et al. 2003), with a lower percentage of false positive findings.

c) Detection by contrast-enhanced US. Since cirrhotic liver parenchyma shows diffusely heterogeneous contrast enhancement after microbubble injection due to the fibrotic component (QUAIA et al. 2002c), contrast-enhanced US cannot be considered a reliable method for the detection of focal liver lesions in cirrhotic patients. The heterogeneous contrast enhancement due to fibrotic changes may simulate multiple focal liver lesions (Fig. 12.22). Persistent microbubble uptake during the late phase in some hepatocellular carcinoma nodules makes detection even more difficult (QUAIA et al. 2002c, 2004). The performance of contrast-enhanced US is better in hepatocellular carcinoma nodules with a hypovascular appearance in the late phase (Figs. 12.23, 12.24).

The low acoustic power mode with new-generation microbubble-based contrast agents seems to

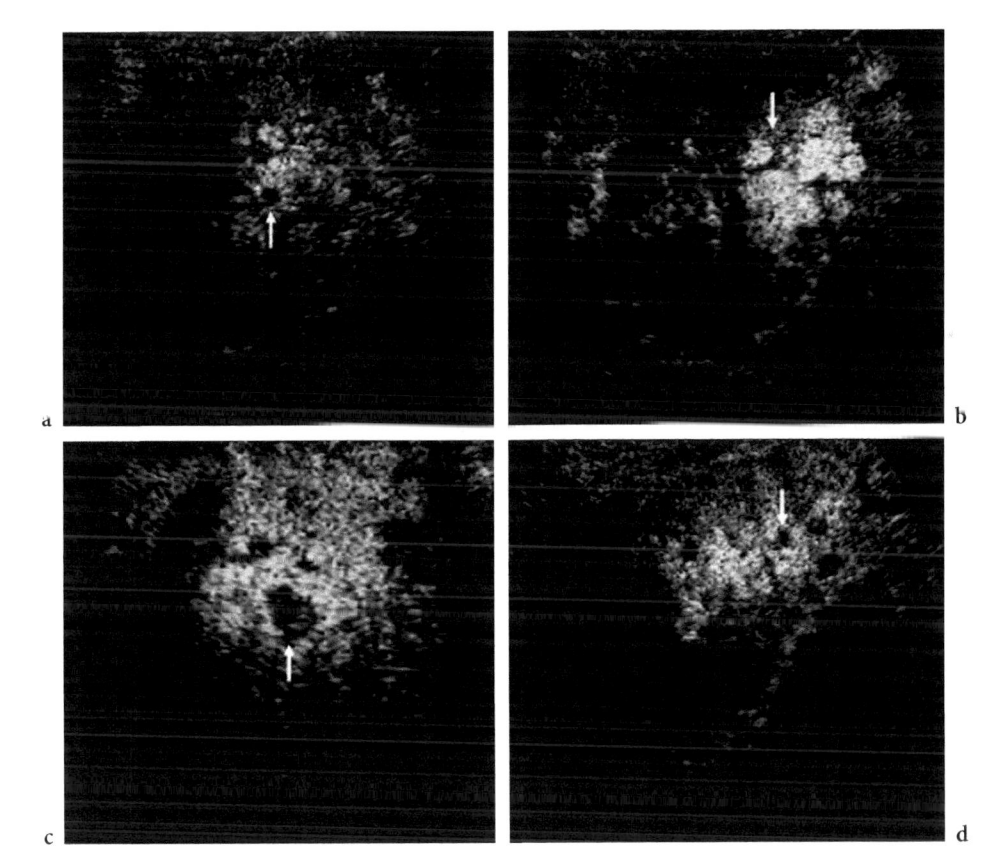

Fig. 12.22a–d. False positive findings of contrast-enhanced US in the cirrhotic liver during the late phase following air-filled microbubble injection. The diffusely heterogeneous contrast enhancement in the cirrhotic liver parenchyma simulates multiple focal liver lesions (*arrows*). The hypoechoic regions in the liver parenchyma are instead due to focal fibrotic changes.

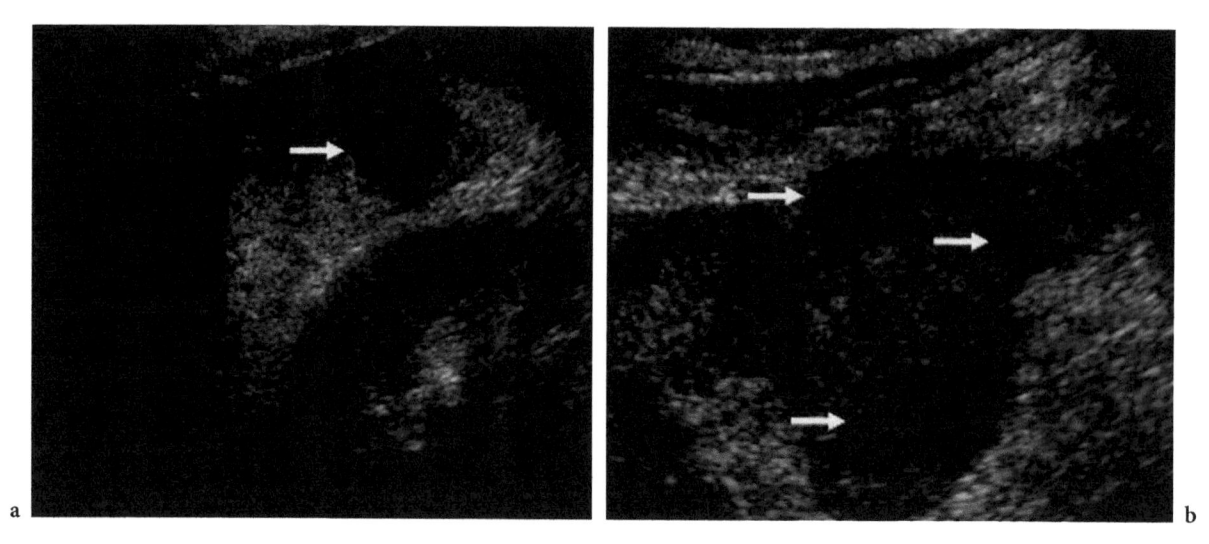

Fig. 12.23a,b. Improved hepatocellular carcinoma detection by contrast-enhanced US in comparison with the baseline US scan. High acoustic power mode after air-filled microbubble injection. One focal liver lesion (*arrows*) is identified on the baseline scan (**a**). Two additional tiny focal liver lesions (*arrowheads*) are identified in the liver after microbubble injection (**b**).

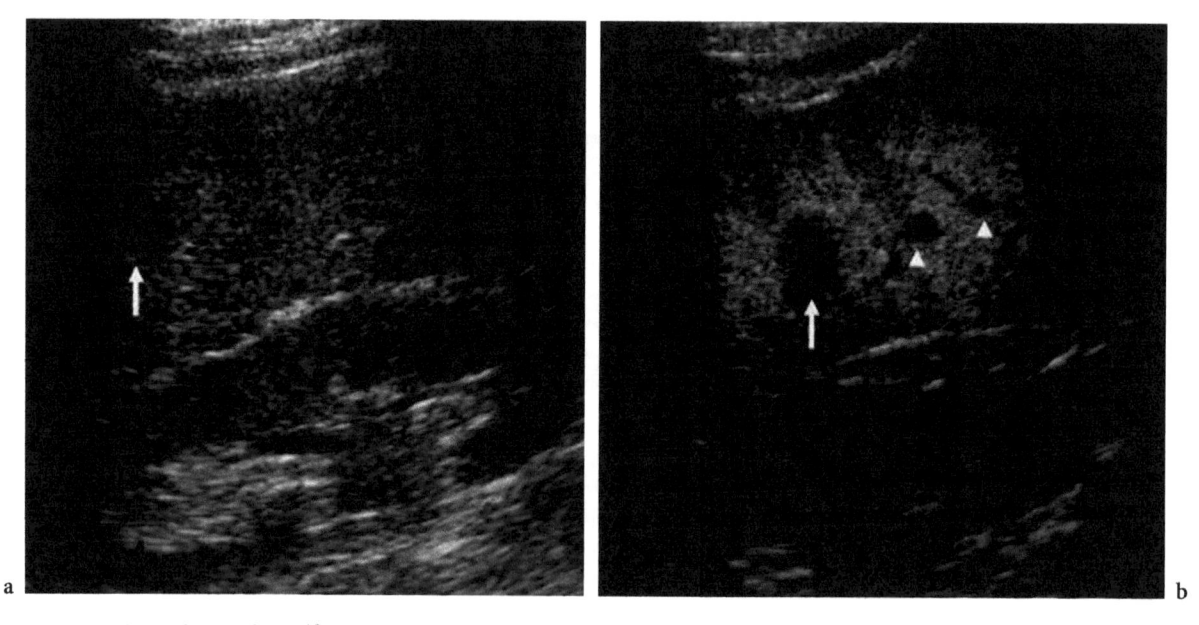

Fig. 12.24a,b. Evidence of multifocal hepatocellular carcinoma in the late phase, 4 min after air-filled microbubble injection and high acoustic power insonation. Multiple hypovascular lesions (*arrows*) are identified in the liver parenchyma. . Courtesy of Prof. M.J.K. Blomley, London, UK.

have improved the detection of hepatocellular carcinomas, primarily because it allows assessment of the liver parenchyma during each dynamic phase (SOLBIATI et al. 2000, 2001). Assessment should be performed both during the arterial phase to improve the detection of hypervascular lesions and during the late phase to enhance the detection of hepatocellular carcinomas that have a hypoechoic appearance in this phase (Fig. 12.25).

12.3
When Should Microbubble-Based Agents Be Employed?

Microbubble-based agents have been found to be very effective in facilitating the detection of liver metastases, especially subcentimeter lesions (DALLA PALMA et al. 1999; HARVEY et al. 2000a,b; ALBRECHT et al. 2001a; DEL FRATE et al. 2003; QUAIA et al.

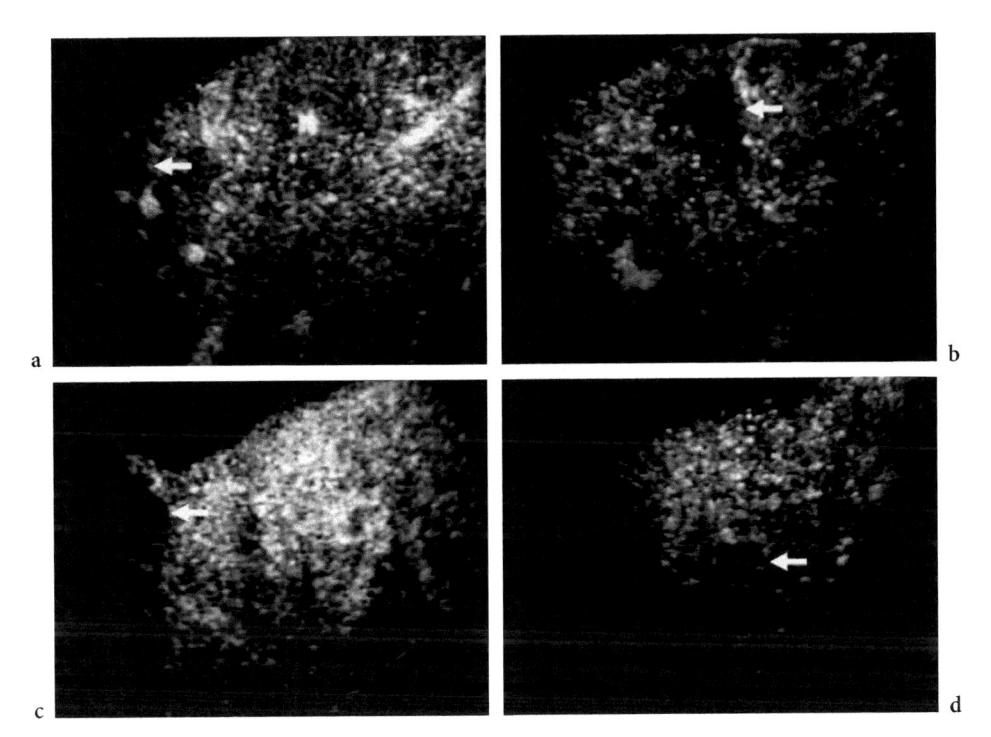

Fig. 12.25a-d. Evidence of multifocal hepatocellular carcinoma in the late phase, 90 s after the injection of sulfur hexafluoride-filled microbubbles, with low acoustic power insonation. Single hepatocellular carcinoma nodules appear as hypoechoic defects (*arrows*) in the enhancing adjacent cirrhotic liver parenchyma.

2003). Nevertheless, contrast-enhanced US has the same limitations as baseline US for the evaluation of liver parenchyma in patients with high-grade liver steatosis, a large body habitus, or interposing bowel gas. For these reasons, microbubble-based agents should be employed only in patients with a satisfactory liver parenchyma assessment at baseline US.

Moreover, since contrast-enhanced US has been found useful in identifying additional liver metastases in patients with one to three lesions, suspicious lesions, or heterogeneous liver parenchyma on baseline US (QUAIA et al. 2003), microbubbles should not be employed in patients with a normal liver parenchyma on baseline US. Nowadays, state of the art US equipment allows reliable assessment of liver parenchyma on the baseline scan, including with the aid of speckle-reducing techniques such as tissue harmonic and compound imaging. Patients who are positive for or are suspected of having liver metastases at baseline US can be accurately assessed after microbubble injection. This technique can assist in the decision on whether to employ conservative or palliative treatment, depending on whether fewer or more than five metastases are detected.

References

Albrecht T, Hoffmann CW, Schettler S et al (2000) B-mode enhancement using phase inversion US with air-based microbubble contrast agent: initial experience in humans. Radiology 216:273-278

Albrecht T, Hoffmann CW, Schmitz SA et al (2001a) Phase inversion sonography during the liver specific late phase of contrast enhancement: improved detection of liver metastases. Am J Roentgenol 176:1191-1198

Albrecht T, Needleman L, Blomley MJ et al (2001b) Detection of focal liver lesions with the new US contrast agent NC100100: results of an exploratory multicentre study. Eur Radiol 11 [Suppl 1]:213

Albrecht T, Blomley MJK, Burns P et al (2003a) Improved detection of hepatic metastases with Pulse-Inversion US during the liver-specific phase of SHU 508A: multicenter study. Radiology 227:361-370

Albrecht T, Oldenburg A, Hohmann J et al (2003b) Imaging of liver metastases with contrast-specific low-MI real time ultrasound and SonoVue. Eur Radiol 13 [Suppl 3]:N79-N86

Baron RL, Peterson MS (2001) Screening the cirrhotic liver for hepatocellular carcinoma with CT and MR imaging: opportunities and pitfalls. Radiographics 21:S117-S132

Bauer A, Blomley MJK, Leen E et al (1999) Liver-specific imaging with SH U563A: Diagnostic potential of a new class of ultrasound contrast media. EUR Radiol 9 [Suppl 3]: S349-S352

Bellin MF, Zaim S, Auberton E (1994) Liver metastases: safety and efficacy of detection with superparamagnetic iron oxide in MR imaging. Radiology 193:657-663

Bertolotto M, Dalla Palma L, Quaia E, Locatelli M (2000) Characterization of unifocal liver lesions with pulse inversion harmonic imaging after Levovist injection: preliminary results. Eur Radiol 10:1369-1376

Blomley MJK, Albrecht T, Cosgrove DO et al (1998) Stimulated acoustic emission in liver parenchyma with Levovist. Lancet 351:568-569

Blomley MJ, Albrecth TA, Cosgrove DO et al (1999) Improved detection of liver metastases with stimulated acoustic emission in late phase of enhancement with the US contrast agent SH U 508: early experience. Radiology 210:409-416

Carter R, Hemingway D, Pickard R et al (1996) A prospective study of six method for detection of hepatic colorectal metastases. Ann Royal Coll Surg Engl 78:27-30

Choi BI, Park JH, Kim BH et al (1989) Small hepatocellular carcinoma: detection with sonography, computed tomography (CT), angiography and lipiodol CT. Br J Radiol 62:897-903

Choi BI, Han JH, Song IS et al (1991) Intraoperative sonography of hepatocellular carcinoma: detection of lesions and validity in surgical resection. Gastrointest Radiol 16:329-333

Cosgrove DO, Bolondi L (1993) Malignant liver disease. In: Cosgrove D, Meire H, Dewbury K (eds) Abdominal and general ultrasound. Churchill Livingstone, Edinburgh, Scotland, pp 271-293

Dalla Palma L, Bertolotto M, Quaia E, Locatelli M (1999) Detection of liver metastases with pulse inversion harmonic imaging: preliminary results. Eur Radiol 9 [Suppl 3]:S382-S387

Del Frate C, Bazzocchi M, Mortele KJ et al (2002) Detection of liver metastases: comparison of gadobenate dimeglumine-enhanced and ferumoxides-enhanced MR imaging examinations. Radiology 225:766-772

Del Frate C, Zuiani C, LonderoV et al (2003) Comparing Levovist-enhanced pulse inversion harmonic imaging and ferumoxides-enhanced MR imaging of hepatic metastases. Am J Roentgenol 180:1339-1346

Forsberg F, Goldberg BB, Liu JB et al (1999) Tissue specific US contrast agent for evaluation of hepatic and splenic parenchyma. Radiology 209:125-132

Forsberg F, Liu JB, Chiou HJ et al (2000a) Comparison of fundamental and wideband harmonic contrast imaging of liver tumors. Ultrasonics 38:110-113

Forsberg F, Liu JB, Merton DA et al (2000b) Grayscale second harmonic imaging of acoustic emission signals improves detection of liver tumors in rabbits. J Ultrasound Med 19:557-563

Forsberg F, Piccoli CW, Liu JB et al (2002) Hepatic tumor detection: MR imaging and conventional US versus pulse-inversion harmonic US of NC100100 during its reticuloendothelial system-specific phase. Radiology 222:824-829

Harvey CJ, Albrecht T (2001) Ultrasound of focal liver lesions. Eur Radiol 11:1578-1593

Harvey CJ, Blomley MJ, Eckersley RJ et al (2000a) Pulse inversion mode imaging of liver specific microbubbles: improved detection of subcentimeter metastases. Lancet 355:807-808

Harvey CJ, Blomley MJ, Eckersley RJ et al (2000b) Hepatic malignancies: improved detection with pulse inversion US in late phase of enhancement with SH U 508 A - early experience. Radiology 216:903-908

Haspigel KD, Neidl KFW, Eichenberger AC et al (1995) Detection of liver metastases. Comparison of superparamagnetic iron oxide-enhanced and unenhanced MR imaging at 1.5 T with dynamic CT, intraoperative US and percutaneous US. Radiology 196:471-478

Hauff P, Fritsch T, Reinhardt M et al (1997) Delineation of experimental liver tumors in rabbits by a new ultrasound contrast agent and stimulated acoustic emission. Invest Radiol 32:94-99

Hope Simpson D, Chin CT, Burns PN (1999) Pulse inversion Doppler: a new method for detecting non-linear echoes from microbubble contrast agents. IEEE Trans Ultrason Ferroelectr Freq Contr 46:372-382

Kang BK, Lim JH, Kim SH et al (2003) Preoperative depiction of hepatocellular carcinoma: ferumoxides-enhanced MR imaging versus triple-phase helical CT. Radiology 226:79-85

Kindberg GM, Tolleshaug H, Roos N, Skotland T (2003) Hepatic clearance of Sonazoid perfluorobutane microbubbles by Kupffer cells does not reduce the ability of liver to phagocytose or degrade albumin microspheres. Cell Tissue Res 312:49-54

Laghi A, Iannaccone R, Rossi P et al (2003) Hepatocellular carcinoma: detection with triple-phase multi-detector row helical CT in patients with chronic hepatitis. Radiology 226:543-549

Lesavre A, Correas JM, Bridal L et al (2003) Efficacy of a specific ultrasound contrast agent in the detection of liver masses: quantitative evaluation and comparison to other US modalities (abstract). RSNA 2003

Lim AK, Patel N, Eckersley RJ et al (2004) Evidence of splenic-specific uptake of a microbubble contrast agent: a quantitative study in healthy volunteers. Radiology 231:785-788

Mosconi E, Quaia E, Bertolotto M et al (2003) Detection of liver metastases by pulse inversion harmonic imaging with Levovist in comparison to conventional ultrasound and with magnetic resonance imaging (MRI) with Gd-BOPTA as reference procedure. Eur Radiol 13 [Suppl 1]:365

Needleman L, Leen E, Kyriakkopoulou K et al (1998) NC100100: a new US contrast agent for fundamental and harmonic imaging of hepatic lesions (abstract). Radiology 209:189

Pauleit D, Textor J, Bachmann R (2002) Hepatocellular carcinoma: detection with gadolinium- and ferumoxides-enhanced MR imaging of the liver. Radiology 222:73-80

Quaia E, Bertolotto M, Ukmar M et al (2002a) Characterization of liver hemangiomas by pulse inversion harmonic imaging. Eur Radiol 12:537-544

Quaia E, Blomley MJK, Patel S et al (2002b) Initial observations on the effect of irradiation on the liver-specific uptake of Levovist. Eur J Radiol 41:192-199

Quaia E, Harvey CJ, Blomley MJK et al (2002c) Study of pulse inversion mode with the late phase of Levovist to detect hepatocellular carcinoma (HCC) in cirrhotic liver (abstract). ECR 2002

Quaia E, Bertolotto M, Forgács B et al (2003) Detection of liver metastases by pulse inversion harmonic imaging during Levovist late phase: comparison to conventional ultrasound and helical CT in 160 patients. Eur Radiol 13:475-483

Quaia E, Calliada F, Bertolotto M et al (2004) Characterization of focal liver lesions by contrast-specific US modes and a sulfur hexafluoride-filled microbubble contrast agent: diagnostic performance and confidence. Radiology 232:420-430

Robinson PJA (2001) Imaging liver metastases: current limitations and future prospects. Br J Radiol 73:234-241

Seneterre E, Taourel P, Bouvier Y et al (1996) Detection of hepatic metastases: ferumoxides-enhanced MR imaging versus unenhanced MR imaging and CT during arterial portography. Radiology 200:785-792

Solbiati L, Cova L, Ierace T et al (2000) The importance of arterial phase imaging for wideband harmonic sonography for the characterization of focal liver lesions in liver cirrhosis using a second generation contrast agent (abstract). Radiology 217:305

Solbiati L, Tonolini M, Cova L, Goldberg N (2001) The role of contrast-enhanced ultrasound in the detection of focal liver lesions. Eur Radiol 11 [Suppl 3]:E15-E26

Soyer P, Lacheheb D, Levesque M (1992) False positive diagnosis based on CT portography: correlation with pathologic findings. Am J Roentgoenol 160:285-289

Takayasu K, Moriyama N, Muramatsu Y et al (1990) The diagnosis of small hepatocellular carcinoma: efficacy of various imaging procedures in 100 patients. Am J Roentgenol 155:49-54

Teefey SA, Hildeboldt CC, Dehdashti F et al (2003) Detection of primary hepatic malignancies in liver transplant candidates: prospective comparison of CT, MR imaging, US and PET. Radiology 226:533-542

Valls C, Lopez E, Guma A et al (1998) Helical CT versus CT arterial portography in the detection of hepatic metastases from colorectal carcinoma. Am J Roentgenol 170:1341-1347

Ward J, Naik KS, Guthrie JA et al (1999) Hepatic lesion detection: comparison of MR imaging after the administration of superparamagnetic iron oxide with dual phase CT by using alternative-free response receiver operating characteristic analysis. Radiology 210:459-466

Ward J, Cheng F, Guthrie JA et al (2000a) Hepatic lesion detection after superparamagnetic Iron oxide enhancement: comparison of five T2-weighted sequences at 1.0 T by using alternative-free response receiver operating characteristic analysis. Radiology 214:159-166

Ward J, Guthrie JA, Scott DJ et al (2000b) Hepatocellular carcinoma in the cirrhotic liver: double-contrast MR imaging for diagnosis. Radiology 216:154-162

Ward J, Guthrie JA, Wilson D et al (2003) Colorectal hepatic metastases: detection with SPIO-enhanced breath-hold MR imaging - comparison of optimized sequences. Radiology 228:709-718

Watanabe R, Matsumura M, Chen CJ et al (2003) Gray-scale liver enhancement with Sonazoid (NC100100), a novel ultrasound contrast agent; detection of hepatic tumors in a rabbit model. Biol Pharm Bull 26:1272-1277

Wernecke K, Rummeny E, Bongartz G et al (1991) Detection of hepatic masses in patients with carcinoma: comparative sensitivities of sonography, CT and MR imaging. AJR 157:731-739

Yamashita Y, Mitsuzaki K, Yi T et al (1996) Small hepatocellular carcinoma in patients with chronic liver damage: prospective comparison of detection with dynamic MR imaging and helical CT of the whole liver. Radiology 200:79-84

13 Guidance and Assessment of Interventional Therapy in Liver

RICCARDO LENCIONI and DANIA CIONI

CONTENTS

13.1 Introduction 187
13.2 General Eligibility Criteria for Percutaneous Ablation Treatment 188
13.3 Percutaneous Ethanol Injection 188
13.4 Radiofrequency Ablation 189
13.4.1 Hepatocellular Carcinoma 189
13.4.2 Hepatic Metastases 191
13.5 Guidance and Assessment of Percutaneous Ablation Treatment 194
13.5.1 Contrast-Enhanced CT and Contrast-Enhanced MR Imaging 194
13.5.2 Contrast-Enhanced US 195
13.5.3 Multimodality Navigation Tool "Navigator" 199
13.6 Conclusions 200
References 201

13.1 Introduction

Hepatocellular carcinoma is the fifth most common cancer, and its incidence is increasing worldwide because of the dissemination of hepatitis B and C virus infection (LLOVET et al. 2003). Patients with cirrhosis are at the highest risk of developing hepatocellular carcinoma. Currently, hepatocellular carcinoma is the leading cause of death among cirrhotic patients. Surveillance can lead to diagnosis at an early stage, when the tumor may be curable by resection, liver transplantation, or percutaneous ablation (BRUIX and LLOVET 2002; BRUIX et al. 2001).

Resection is currently indicated in patients with single asymptomatic hepatocellular carcinoma and extremely well preserved liver function who have neither clinically significant portal hypertension nor abnormal bilirubin (BRUIX and LLOVET 2002; LLOVET et al. 2003). However, less than 5% of cir-

R. LENCIONI, MD, Associate Professor of Radiology;
D. CIONI, MD, Assistant Professor of Radiology
Division of Diagnostic and Interventional Radiology, Department of Oncology, Transplants and Advanced Technologies in Medicine, University of Pisa, Via Roma 67, 56126 Pisa, Italy

rhotic patients with hepatocellular carcinoma fit these criteria (LLOVET et al. 1999). Liver transplantation benefits patients who have decompensated cirrhosis and one tumor smaller than 5 cm or up to three nodules smaller than 3 cm, but donor shortage greatly limits its applicability (BRUIX and LLOVET 2002; LLOVET et al. 2003). This difficulty might be overcome by living donation, which, however, is still at an early stage of clinical application.

Hepatic metastases are a frequent event in the natural history of colorectal cancer. Twenty percent of patients with colorectal cancer have evidence of hepatic metastases at diagnosis, and 50% will develop metachronous metastatic disease (JESSUP et al. 1996). Of the patients who develop hepatic metastases, nearly 25% will have disease isolated to the liver (JESSUP et al. 1996).

Surgery is established as the standard of care for hepatic colorectal metastases. The 5-year overall survival rate after hepatic resection ranges from 27% to 58%, with the higher figures having been obtained recently as a result of improvements in patient selection and peri- and postoperative care, multidisciplinary treatment, and an appropriately aggressive approach to safe hepatic resection (SCHEELE et al. 1995; JAMISON et al. 1997; FONG et al. 1999a; CHOTI et al. 2002; VAUTHEY et al. 2004). Nevertheless, only 10–25% of patients with colorectal metastases isolated to the liver are eligible for surgical resection, because of the extent and location of the disease or concurrent medical conditions (SILEN 1989). Unfortunately, conventional treatment of inoperable or nonresectable patients with systemic or intra-arterial chemotherapy protocols is not entirely satisfactory in terms of survival outcome (JONKER et al. 2000).

As a result, image-guided techniques for percutaneous tumor ablation play a major role in the therapeutic management of these patients. While percutaneous ethanol injection (PEI) is a well-established technique for percutaneous treatment of hepatocellular carcinoma, several newer methods of tumor destruction have been developed and clinically tested over the past few years (LENCIONI et al. 2004a; LIVRAGHI et al. 1991). Among these methods, radiofrequency (RF) ablation has emerged as the most powerful technique for tumor destruction and is nowadays established as the primary ablative modality at most institutions (GALANDI and ANTES 2004 pp. 10–20; GOLDBERG et al. 1998b; VOLG et al. 1999; MCGAHAN and DODD 2000; MORITA et al. 2004; MALA et al. 2004; SHIBATA et al. 2002; GOLDBERG 2002; BERBER et al. 2004).

13.2
General Eligibility Criteria for Percutaneous Ablation Treatment

A careful clinical, laboratory, and imaging assessment has to be performed by a multidisciplinary team to evaluate eligibility for percutaneous tumor ablation (LENCIONI et al. 2001).

In the case of cirrhotic patients with hepatocellular carcinoma, those classified as stage 0 (very early stage) or stage A (early stage) according to the Barcelona Clinic Liver Cancer staging classification for treatment schedule may qualify for percutaneous ablation if surgical resection and liver transplantation are not suitable options (LLOVET et al. 2003). Patients are required to have (a) either a single tumor smaller than 5 cm or as many as three nodules smaller than 3 cm each, in the absence of vascular involvement and extrahepatic spread, (b) a performance status test of 0, and (c) liver cirrhosis in Child-Pugh class A or B.

In the case of patients with hepatic colorectal metastases, inclusion criteria for RF ablation require the patient not to be a surgical candidate. However, all the negative prognostic factors affecting the results of surgery, such as stage III colorectal cancer and metastases to the portal, hepatic, or celiac lymph nodes, also affect the outcome of RF ablation (FONG et al. 1999a; IWATSUKI et al. 1999; SASSON and SIGURDSON 2002; AUGUST et al. 1985; MURATA et al. 1998; HEADRICK et al. 2001; MINEO et al. 2003; PATEL et al. 2003). Patients are required to have four or fewer lesions not exceeding 3.5 cm in the longest axis in order to obtain a safety margin of 1 cm all around the lesion (BERBER et al. 2004; GOLDBERG et al. 2003).

Pretreatment imaging planning must carefully define the size, shape, and location of each lesion.

Lesions located along the surface of the liver can be considered for percutaneous ablation, although their treatment requires adequate expertise and may be associated with a higher risk of complications. RF ablation of superficial lesions that are adjacent to any part of the gastrointestinal tract must be avoided because of the risk of thermal injury of the gastric or bowel wall (RHIM et al. 2004; LIVRAGHI et al. 2003a; BUSCARINI and BUSCARINI 2004). The colon appears to be at greater risk than the stomach or small bowel for thermally mediated perforation (RHIM et al. 2004). Gastric complications are rare, likely owing to the relatively greater wall thickness of the stomach or the rarity of surgical adhesions along the gastrohepatic ligament. The mobility of the small bowel may also provide the bowel with greater protection compared with the relatively fixed colon. Treatment of lesions adjacent to the gallbladder or to the hepatic hilum entails the risk of thermal injury of the biliary tract. In experienced hands, RF ablation of tumors located in the vicinity of the gallbladder has been shown to be feasible, although associated in most cases with self-limited iatrogenic cholecystitis (CHOPRA et al. 2003). In contrast, RF ablation of lesions adjacent to hepatic vessels is possible, since flowing blood usually protects the vascular wall from thermal injury; in these cases, however, the risk of incomplete treatment of the neoplastic tissue close to the vessel may increase because of the heat loss. The potential risk of RF damage to critical structures should be weighed against benefits on a case-by-case basis.

Laboratory tests should include measurement of serum tumor markers, such as alpha-fetoprotein (AFP) in cirrhotic patients and carcinoembryonic antigen (CEA) in patients with hepatic colorectal metastases, and a full evaluation of coagulation status. A prothrombin time ratio (normal time/patient's time) greater than 50% and a platelet count higher than 50,000/µl are required to keep the risk of bleeding at an acceptable low level.

13.3
Percutaneous Ethanol Injection

Percutaneous ethanol injection (PEI) is a well-established technique for tumor ablation (BARTOLOZZI and LENCIONI 1996). Several studies have shown that PEI is an effective treatment for small, nodular-type hepatocellular carcinoma. Hepatocellular carcinoma nodules have a soft consistency and are surrounded by a firm cirrhotic liver. Consequently, injected ethanol diffuses within them easily and selectively, leading to complete tumor necrosis in about 70% of the cases (SHIINA et al. 1991). Although there have not been any prospective randomized trials comparing PEI and best supportive care or PEI and surgical resection, several series have provided indirect evidence that PEI improves the natural history of hepatocellular carcinoma: the long-term outcome of patients with early stage tumors who were treated with PEI was shown to be similar to that of patients who had undergone resection, with 5-year survival rates ranging from 32% to 52% (CASTELLS et al. 1993; LENCIONI et al. 1995, 1997; LIVRAGHI et al. 1995; SHIINA et al. 1993). In a recent prospective comparative study, the 1-, 3-, and 5-year survival rates were almost identical between two cohorts of patients who underwent surgical resection (97%, 84%, and 61%, respectively) or PEI (100%, 82%, and 59%, respectively) (YAMAMOTO et al. 2001).

Although PEI is a low-risk procedure, severe complications have been reported. In a multicenter survey including 1,066 patients (8,118 PEI sessions), one death (0.1%) and 34 complications (3.2%), including seven cases of tumor seeding (0.7%), were reported (DI STASI et al. 1997). The major limitation of PEI, besides the uncertainty of tumor ablation and the long treatment times, is the high local recurrence rate, which may reach 33% in lesions smaller than 3 cm and 43% in lesions exceeding 3 cm (KHAN et al. 2000; KODA et al. 2000). The injected ethanol does not always accomplish complete tumor necrosis because of its inhomogeneous distribution within the lesion, especially in the presence of intratumoral septa, and the limited effect on extracapsular cancerous spread. Also, PEI is unable to create a safety margin of ablation in the liver parenchyma surrounding the nodule, and therefore may not destroy tiny satellite nodules that, even in small tumors, may be located in close proximity to the main lesion (OKUSAKA et al. 2002) (Table 13.1).

13.4
Radiofrequency Ablation

13.4.1
Hepatocellular Carcinoma

Early clinical experiences with RF ablation were conducted in the framework of feasibility studies (CURLEY et al. 1999; ROSSI et al. 2000). These investigations had merit in showing the efficacy and safety of the procedure. However, the data were heterogeneous and unsystematically presented (GALANDI

Table 13.1. Survival outcomes of patients with early-stage hepatocellular carcinoma receiving percutaneous ablation

Treatment	No. of patients	Survival rate (%) 1year	3year	5year
Percutaneous ethanol injection				
CASTELLS et al. (1993)	30	83	55	N/A
SHIINA et al. (1993)	98	85	62	52
LENCIONI et al. (1995)	105	96	68	32
LIVRAGHI et al. (1995)				
Child class A, single HCC	293	98	79	47
Child class B, single HCC	149	93	63	29
Radiofrequency ablation				
LENCIONI et al. (2005)				
Child class A	144	100	76	51
Child class A, single HCC	116	100	89	61
Child class B	43	89	46	31
Microwave coagulation				
SHIINA et al. (2002)	122	90	68	N/A

N/A not available, HCC hepatocellular carcinoma.

and ANTES 2004). Moreover, RF treatment was not compared to any established treatment for hepatocellular carcinoma. The European Association for the Study of the Liver has recommended comparison of newer methods of tumor destruction, such as RF ablation, with the well-established and accepted PEI through randomized trials (BRUIX et al. 2001). In fact, methodological research has yielded convincing evidence that less rigorous study designs are likely to produce biased results and to exaggerate the estimated effect of a new therapy (GALANDI and ANTES 2004).

One randomized study compared RF ablation versus PEI for the treatment of early stage hepatocellular carcinoma (LENCIONI et al. 2003). In this trial, 104 patients with 144 hepatocellular carcinoma lesions were randomly assigned to receive RF ablation or PEI. No statistically significant differences between RF ablation and PEI groups were observed with respect to baseline characteristics, except for patient age and albumin concentration. At the time of the analysis, the mean follow-up was 22 months. The overall survival rates at 1 and 2 years were 100% and 98%, respectively, in the RF group, and 96% and 88%, respectively, in the PEI group. Despite the tendency favoring RF ablation, the observed difference did not reach statistical significance (hazard ratio, 0.20; 95% confidence interval, 0.02–1.69; $p=0.138$). However, 1- and 2-year recurrence-free survival rates were clearly higher in RF-treated patients than in PEI-treated patients (86% and 64%, respectively, in the RF ablation group versus 77% and 43%, respectively, in the PEI group; hazard ratio, 0.48; 95% confidence interval, 0.27–0.85; $p=0.012$). RF treatment was confirmed as an independent prognostic factor for local recurrence-free survival by multivariate analysis. This trial suggested that RF ablation can achieve higher recurrence-free survival rates than PEI, thereby confirming findings in two previous comparative studies, in which higher complete tumor response rates were observed in tumors treated with RF ablation than in those submitted to PEI (IKEDA et al. 2001; LIVRAGHI et al. 1999). However, likely because of the short follow-up period and the limited sample size, no difference was found with respect to overall survival.

Recently, a prospective intention-to-treat clinical trial reported the long-term survival outcomes of RF ablation-treated patients (LENCIONI et al. 2005b). In this study, 206 patients with early stage hepatocellular carcinoma who were not candidates for resection or transplantation were enrolled. RF ablation was considered as the first-line nonsurgical treatment and was actually performed in 187 (91%) of the 206 patients. The remaining 19 (9%) had to be excluded from RF treatment because of the unfavorable location of the tumor. Noncompliant patients were treated with either PEI or segmental transcatheter arterial chemoembolization. The overall survival rates in the intention-to-treat analysis including all 206 patients enrolled in the study (67% at 3 years and 41% at 5 years) were not significantly different from those achieved in the 187 compliant patients who received RF ablation (71% at 3 years and 48% at 5 years; $p=0.5094$). In patients who underwent RF ablation, survival depended on the severity of the underlying cirrhosis and the tumor multiplicity. Patients in Child class A had 3- and 5-year survival rates of 76% and 51%, respectively. These figures were significantly higher than those obtained in Child class B patients (46% at 3 years and 31% at 5 years; $p=0.0006$). Patients with a solitary hepatocellular carcinoma had 3- and 5-year survival rates of 75% and 50%, respectively, while those with multiple tumors had 3- and 5-year survival rates of 51% and 34%, respectively; again, this difference was statistically significant ($p=0.0133$). Of interest, a subgroup of 116 patients in Child class A who had a solitary hepatocellular carcinoma showed 3- and 5-year survival rates of 89% and 61%, respectively. In this series, recurrence of the tumor treated by RF ablation occurred in 10 of 187 patients. Despite the absence of viable neoplastic tissue on post-treatment spiral CT images, residual microscopic nests of tumor or small undetected satellite nodules led to local tumor progression. The actuarial 5-year local tumor progression rate was 10%. However, new hepatocellular carcinoma tumors developed in 93 patients during the follow-up. The rate of recurrence with new tumors reached 81% at 5 years. Such a high rate of new tumors is an expression of the inherent multicentric nature of hepatocellular carcinoma in cirrhosis and does not seem to represent a drawback of RF ablation, being found also in cirrhotic hepatocellular carcinoma patients treated with either percutaneous therapies or surgical resection.

The data on long-term outcome of RF ablation must be compared with those obtained in patients with early stage tumors who received other potentially curative treatments. Liver transplantation was shown to be the only treatment option that consistently provided 5-year survival rates in the range of 71–75% (BISMUTH et al. 1999; JONAS et al. 2001; LLOVET et al. 1999; MAZZAFERRO et al. 1996). Surgical resection of early stage hepatocellular carcinoma resulted in 5-year survival rates in the range of 41–51% (FONG et al. 1999b; JONAS et al. 2001; LLOVET et al. 1999; WAYNE et al. 2002). Resection achieved substantially higher survival rates only when patients with a solitary tumor and extremely well preserved liver function, who had neither clinically significant portal hypertension nor abnormal bilirubin, were selected (LLOVET et al. 1999). In large series, PEI achieved 5-year survival rates ranging from 32% to 52%. In a multicenter study, survival of 293 patients with Child class A cirrhosis and a solitary tumor smaller than 5 cm who received PEI was 47% at 5 years (LIVRAGHI et al. 1995). Comparison of results obtained with RF ablation with those achieved in the past by using PEI, however, may be biased by the ability to better select patients with early stage tumors owing to the improvement in imaging techniques.

In most of the reported series, RF ablation was associated with acceptable morbidity. In a multicenter survey in which 2,320 patients with 3,554 lesions were included, six deaths (mortality, 0.3%) were noted, including two caused by multiorgan failure following intestinal perforation, one case each of septic shock following *Staphylococcus aureus*-caused peritonitis, massive hemorrhage following tumor rupture, and liver failure following stenosis of the right bile duct, and one sudden death of unknown cause 3 days after the procedure. Fifty (2.2%) patients had additional major complications. Tumor seeding, in particular, occurred in only 12 (0.5%) of 2,320 patients (LIVRAGHI et al. 2003a). However, lesions with a subcapsular location or an invasive tumoral pattern, as shown by a poor differentiation degree, may be at risk for such a complication (LLOVET et al. 2001).

Recently, following advances in RF technology, RF ablation has also been used to treat patients with intermediate stage tumors. However, results obtained by RF ablation alone were not entirely satisfactory. LIVRAGHI et al. (2000) treated 114 patients with 126 hepatocellular carcinoma lesions greater than 3 cm in diameter. Complete necrosis (on imaging) was attained in only 60 lesions (47.6%), nearly complete (90–99%) necrosis in 40 lesions (31.7%), and partial (50–89%) necrosis in the remaining 26 lesions (20.6%). Therefore, there is currently a focus on a multimodality strategy in attempts to ensure more effective percutaneous ablation of large hepatocellular carcinoma tumors.

Of interest, recent studies have proved the influence of perfusion-mediated tissue cooling on the area of RF necrosis achievable with RF treatment. GOLDBERG et al. (1998a) applied RF in vivo to normal porcine liver without and with balloon occlusion of the portal vein, celiac artery, or hepatic artery, and to ex vivo calf liver. RF application during vascular occlusion produced larger areas of RF necrosis than RF with unaltered blood flow. LEES et al. (2000) showed that hypotensive anesthesia improved the effectiveness of liver RF ablation in a human study. Assuming that the volume of RF necrosis produced by RF treatment is strongly dependent on blood flow, and considering that in hepatocellular carcinoma blood flow is mainly sustained by the hepatic artery, we performed a multicenter clinical trial aimed at investigating whether interruption of the tumor arterial blood supply by means of occlusion of either the hepatic artery with a balloon catheter or the feeding arteries with gelatin sponge particles could increase the extent of RF-induced coagulation necrosis (ROSSI et al. 2000). A series of 62 consecutive patients with a single, large hepatocellular carcinoma ranging from 3.5 to 8.5 cm in diameter (mean 4.7 cm) accompanying cirrhosis underwent RF ablation after occlusion of the tumor arterial supply. The RF energy was delivered by using an expandable electrode needle at the time of balloon catheter occlusion of the hepatic artery ($n=40$), at the time of occlusion of the hepatocellular carcinoma feeding arteries with gelatin sponge particles ($n=13$), or 2–5 days thereafter ($n=9$). Two patients underwent liver resection after the RF ablation; the remaining 60 patients were followed up for a mean of 12.1 months (range 3–26 months). During the follow-up, 49 (82%) of the 60 treated hepatocellular carcinoma nodules showed a stable complete response, while the remaining 11 (18%) nodules showed local progression. Histopathologic analysis of one autopsy and the two surgical specimens revealed more than 90% necrosis in one specimen and 100% necrosis in two. No fatal or major complications related to the treatment occurred, despite the more aggressive RF treatment protocol. The results of this study provide evidence that areas of RF necrosis that are much larger than those previously reported can be created if RF ablation is performed in hepatocellular carcinoma nodules after occlusion of their arterial supply.

The results achieved with this technique were confirmed by two recent studies. YAMASAKI et al. (2002) compared the necrosis diameters obtained with balloon-occluded RF and standard RF in 31 patients with 42 hepatocellular carcinoma lesions measuring less than 4 cm in the greatest dimension. There were no significant differences between the groups in terms of the ablation conditions, such as the frequency of a fully expanded electrode, the number of needle insertions, the application cycles, or the treatment times. However, the greatest dimension of the area coagulated by balloon-occluded RF ablation was significantly larger than that coagulated by standard RF ablation. YAMAKADO et al. (2002) evaluated the local therapeutic efficacy of RF ablation after transarterial chemoembolization in 64 patients with 108 lesions. Sixty-five lesions were small (3 cm or less), 32 were intermediate in size (3.1–5 cm), and 11 were large (5.1–12 cm). Complete necrosis was achieved in all lesions, and there were no local recurrences in small or intermediate-sized lesions during a mean follow-up of 12.5 months (Table 13.1).

Despite these encouraging preliminary results, there are no reports showing that RF ablation, performed alone or in combination with intra-arterial procedures, results in improved survival in patients with intermediate stage hepatocellular carcinoma. A randomized trial comparing an optimized RF technology with chemoembolization would be needed to establish the potential role of the technique in this patient population.

13.4.2
Hepatic Metastases

In two pioneering studies published in 1997–1998 by SOLBIATI et al. (1997) and LENCIONI et al. (1998), patients with limited hepatic metastatic disease, who were excluded from surgery, were submitted to RF ablation. In the first series, 29 patients with 44 hepatic metastases ranging from 1.3 to 5.1 cm in diameter were treated. Each tumor was treated in one or two sessions, and technical success – defined as lack of residual unablated tumor on CT or MR imaging obtained 7–14 days after completion of treatment – was achieved in 40 of 44 lesions. However, follow-up imaging studies confirmed complete necrosis of the entire metastasis in only 66% of the cases, while local tumor progression was observed in the remaining 34%. Only one complication, self-limited hemorrhage, was seen. One-year survival was 94%. In the study by LENCIONI et al. (1998), 29 patients with 53 hepatic metastases ranging from 1.1 to 4.8 cm in diameter were enrolled. A total of 127 insertions were performed (mean, 2.4 insertions/lesion) during 84 treatment sessions (mean, 1.6 sessions/lesion) in the absence of complications. Complete tumor response – defined as the presence of a nonenhancing ablation zone larger than the treated tumor on post-treatment spiral CT – was seen in 41 (77%) of the 53 lesions. After a mean follow-up period of 6.5 months (range 3–9 months), local tumor progression was seen in 12% of cases. One-year survival was 93%.

In 2000–2001, owing to the advances in RF techniques, reported rates of successful RF ablation increased substantially. DE BAERE et al. (2000) treated 68 patients with 121 hepatic metastases, mainly of colorectal origin, with 76 sessions, either percutaneously (47 patients with 88 metastases, 10–42 mm in diameter) or intraoperatively (21 patients with 33 metastases, 5–20 mm in diameter). Procedure efficacy was evaluated with CT and MR imaging performed 2, 4, and 6 months after treatment and then every 3 months. RF ablation allowed eradication of 91% of the 100 treated metastases that were followed up for 4–23 months (mean, 13.7 months). The rate was similar for percutaneous RF ablation (90%) and intraoperative RF ablation (94%). One bile leakage in peritoneum and two abscesses were the major complications encountered after treatment. HELMBERGER et al. (2001) reported a similar technical success rate of RF ablation (97%) in a series of 37 patients with 74 metastases. In this study, four cases of hematoma of the liver capsule occurred. During the limited follow-up period of 9 months, no case of local tumor progression was seen.

Recently, data on long-term survival rates of patients treated by RF ablation have been reported. In the series of GILLIAMS and LEES (2000), the impact of RF ablation on survival in 69 patients with colorectal metastases – with an average number of 2.9 lesions with a mean diameter of 3.9 cm – was analyzed. All patients had been excluded from surgery. Eighteen (26%) patients had undergone previous hepatic resection and 62 (93%) received chemotherapy at some stage. One-, 2-, 3-, and 4-year survival rates were 90%, 60%, 34%, and 22%, respectively. In the study of SOLBIATI et al. (2001), 117 patients with 179 metachronous colorectal hepatic metastases were treated. Estimated median survival was 36 months, and 1, 2, and 3-year survival rates were 93%, 69%, and 46%, respectively. In 77 (66%) of the 117 patients, new metastases were observed at follow-up. Seventy (39%) of 179 lesions developed local recurrence after treatment. The same authors performed an update of their series (2003): in a group of 166 patients with 378 metastases ranging from 0.7 to 5.2 cm in diameter, local tumor control (absence of tumor regrowth at the site of ablation during the follow-up) was achieved in 78% of lesions smaller than 2.5 cm, and in 17% of metastases larger than 4 cm. Only two major complications related to RF ablation occurred. The overall survival rates were 96%, 64%, 45%, 36%, and 22% at 1, 2, 3, 4, and 5 years, respectively.

LENCIONI et al. (2004b) recently analyzed the long-term results of RF ablation in the treatment of hepatic colorectal metastases in a series of 423 patients collected in a multicenter trial. All patients had four or fewer metachronous metastases (overall number of lesions, 615; mean number of lesions per patient, 1.4±0.7), each 5 cm or less in greatest dimension (range, 0.5–5 cm; mean, 2.7±0.9 cm), and were free from extrahepatic disease. The surgical option had been excluded or been refused by the patient. The participating centers shared diagnostic, staging, and follow-up protocols, and performed RF ablation by using the same technology (expandable multitined electrodes by RITA Medical Systems). The follow-up period ranged from 1 to 78 months (mean, 19±15 months). The primary effectiveness rate (percentage of tumors successfully eradicated following the planned treatment schedule) was 85.4% (525 of 615 lesions). During the follow-up, local tumor progression was observed in 132 (25.1%) of 525 lesions. The overall survival by the Kaplan-Meier method was 86% at 1 year, 63% at 2 years, 47% at 3 years, 29% at 4 years, and 24% at 5 years. Survival rates were significantly higher in patients with a single lesion 2.5 cm or less in diameter (56% at 5 years) than in patients with a single lesion larger than 2.5 cm (13% at 5 years) or multiple lesions (11% at 5 years) ($p=0.0002$, log-rank test).

The long-term survival figures obtained in nonsurgical patients who received RF ablation are substantially higher than those obtained with any chemotherapy regimens and provide indirect evidence that RF ablation therapy improves survival in patients with limited hepatic metastatic disease. In fact, in a meta-analysis of the results of chemotherapy in metastatic colorectal cancer, in which trials using fluoropyrimidine-based treatment schedules were included, mortality at 2 years was not significantly different from that observed with supportive care alone (JONKER et al. 2000). With the latest advances in chemotherapy strategies and the use of combination protocols with fluorouracil-leucovorin, irinotecan, and oxaliplatin, initial promising results have been reported. However, data from seven recently published phase III trials showed that the improvement in median survival did not exceed 3.5 months (GROTHEY et al. 2004).

Recent studies analyzed the role of RF ablation with respect to surgical resection. ABDALLA et al. (2004) examined the survival of 418 patients with colorectal metastases isolated to the liver who were treated with hepatic resection ($n=190$), RF ablation plus resection ($n=101$), RF ablation only ($n=57$), or chemotherapy only ($n=70$). Overall survival for patients treated with RF ablation plus resection or RF ablation only was greater than for those who received chemotherapy only ($p=0.0017$). However, overall survival was highest after resection: 4-year survival rates after resection, RF ablation plus resection, and RF ablation only were 65%, 36%, and 22%, respectively ($p<0.0001$). In contrast, in the series of OSHOWO et al. (2003), survival outcome of patients with solitary colorectal liver metastases treated by surgery ($n=20$) or by RF ablation ($n=25$) did not differ. In this study, the survival rate at 3 years was 55% for patients treated with surgery and 52% for those who underwent RF ablation, suggesting that the survival after resection and RF ablation is comparable.

ELIAS et al. (2002) used RF ablation instead of repeated resection for the treatment of liver tumor recurrence after partial hepatectomy in 47 patients. A retrospective study of the authors' database over two similar consecutive periods showed that RF ablation increased the percentage of curative local treatments for liver recurrence after hepatectomy from 17% to 26% and decreased the proportion of repeat hepatectomies from 100% to 39%. LIVRAGHI et al. (2003b) evaluated the potential role of performing RF ablation during the interval between diagnosis and resection as part of a "test-of-time" management approach. Eighty-eight consecutive patients with 134 colorectal liver metastases who were potential candidates for surgery were treated with RF ablation. Among the 53 patients in whom complete tumor ablation was achieved after RF treatment, 52 (98%) were spared surgical resection: in 23 cases (44%) because they remained free of disease and in 29 cases (56%) because they developed additional metastases leading to irresectability. No patient in whom RF treatment did not achieve complete tumor ablation became unresectable due to the growth of the treated metastases.

A general assessment of complications following RF ablation of liver malignancies has been recently performed by LIVRAGHI et al. (2003a). In this study 2,320 patients with 3,554 lesions were included. Six deaths (0.3%) were noted, including two caused by multiorgan failure following intestinal perforation, one case each of septic shock following *Staphylococcus aureus*-caused peritonitis, massive hemorrhage following tumor rupture, and liver failure following stenosis of right bile duct, and one sudden death of unknown cause 3 days after the procedure. Fifty (2.2%) patients had additional major complications, defined as those that, if left untreated, might threaten the patient's life, lead to substantial morbidity and disability, or result in hospital admission or substantially lengthened hospital stay (GOLDBERG et al. 2003). In the large single-institution series of DE BAERE et al. (2003), 312 patients underwent 350 sessions of RF ablation (124 intraoperative and 226 percutaneous) for treatment of 582 liver tumors (115 hepatocellular carcinomas and 467 metastatic tumors) over a 5-year period. Five (1.4%) deaths were related to RF treatment. The deaths were caused by liver insufficiency ($n=1$), colon perforation ($n=1$), and portal vein thrombosis ($n=3$). Portal vein thrombosis was significantly ($p<0.00001$) more frequent in cirrhotic livers than in noncirrhotic livers after RF radiofrequency ablation performed during a Pringle maneuver. Liver abscess ($n=7$) was the most common complication. Abscess occurred significantly ($p<0.00001$) more frequently in patients bearing a bilioenteric anastomosis than in other patients. The authors encountered five pleural effusions, five skin burns, four cases of hypoxemia, three pneumothoraces, two small subcapsular hematomas, one case of acute renal insufficiency, one hemoperitoneum, and one instance of needle tract seeding. Among the 5.7% major complications, 3.7% required less than 5 days of hospitalization for treatment or surveillance and 2% required more than 5 days for treatment. While these data indicate that RF ablation is a relatively safe procedure and suggest that with increased expertise and knowledge in regard to the use of the technique it could become even safer, caution should be exercised in patients presenting with risk factors, and a careful assessment of the risks and benefits associated with RF ablation has to be made in each individual patient by a multidisciplinary team (Table 13.2).

13.5
Guidance and Assessment of Percutaneous Ablation Treatment

Image-guided tumor ablation aims at tumor eradication or substantial tumor destruction using the direct application of chemical (such as ethanol) or thermal (such as RF ablation) therapies. The region or zone of induced treatment effect (corresponding to the area of gross tumor destruction) as demonstrated by radiologic studies is termed the "ablation zone." Due to the actual limitations in contrast and spatial resolution of imaging studies, the extent of the ablation zone is only an approximation to the zone of "coagulation necrosis," which means cell death at pathologic examination (GOLDBERG et al. 2003).

13.5.1
Contrast-Enhanced CT and Contrast-Enhanced MR Imaging

Contrast-enhanced CT and contrast-enhanced dynamic MR imaging are considered the gold standard techniques for pretreatment staging of liver tumors and for the immediate and long-term assessment of treatment outcome (McGAHAN and DODD 2000).

In the setting of evaluation of treatment outcome, successfully ablated lesions appear on CT as hypoattenuating areas which fail to enhance in both the arterial and the portal venous phase. With MR imaging, necrosis induced by PEI and RF ablation is depicted as a low-intensity area on T2-weighted images. The change from hyperintensity on T2-weighted images of the native tumor to hypointensity of the lesion after the procedure is usually associated with tumor necrosis. However, unenhanced MR imaging has some limitations, with a non-negligible rate of false negative and false positive results. False negative results are caused by the difficulty in detecting small areas of residual viable tumor, espe-

Table 13.2. Survival outcomes of patients with hepatic colorectal metastases treated with radiofrequency ablation.

Study	Year	No. of patients	Survival rate (%) 1year	3year	5year
SOLBIATI et al.	1997	29	94	N/A	N/A
LENCIONI et al.	1998	29	93	N/A	N/A
GILLAMS and LEES	2000	69	90	34	N/A
SOLBIATI et al.	2001	117	93	46	N/A
SOLBIATI et al.	2003	166	96	45	22
OSHOWO et al.	2003	25	100	52	N/A
ABDALLA et al.	2004	57	92	37	N/A
LENCIONI et al.	2004b	423	86	47	24

N/A not available.

cially along the periphery of the treated lesion. On the other hand, the appearance of lesions ablated by RF ablation may not be consistent on unenhanced MR imaging – especially when the examination is performed shortly after the procedure –, with mixed hyperintense and hypointense areas reflecting the complexity of the necrotic phenomena induced by the treatment. This appearance may cause false positive results and greatly reduces the radiologist's confidence in evaluating tumor response. Therefore, the use of a dynamic, contrast-enhanced study is to be recommended as a mandatory part of the MR imaging examination aimed at assessing the therapeutic effect of the procedure. Necrotic tumor will show absence of enhancement throughout the contrast-enhanced dynamic MR imaging study (LENCIONI et al. 2001).

In the case of hepatocellular carcinoma, the areas of residual viable neoplastic tissue can be easily recognized with both CT and MR imaging as they stand out in the arterial phase against the faintly enhanced normal liver parenchyma and the unenhanced areas of necrosis. In the case of hepatic metastases, a confident diagnosis of successful ablation is obtained when an area of necrosis volume exceeding that of the original lesion, with a safety margin of necrosis in the liver parenchyma all around the tumor, is depicted.

If the imaging assessment of the outcome of therapy is performed shortly after the RF treatment, contrast-enhanced CT and contrast-enhanced dynamic MR imaging may show the presence of a peripheral enhancing halo surrounding the treated lesion. This halo, which may be irregular in shape and thickness, enhances predominantly in the arterial phase and is due to the hyperemia and the inflammatory reaction along the periphery of the area of necrosis. It is usually more pronounced in hepatic metastases than in hepatocellular carcinoma since metastases produce greater injury in the adjacent liver parenchyma, and the lack of a clear border between tumor and normal liver and the higher conductivity of noncirrhotic tissue facilitate progression of RF waves into the noncancerous parenchyma. The enhancing halo is depicted for a few days after treatment, and usually disappears at later follow-up studies. Awareness of this feature is, of course, of utmost importance in order to prevent misinterpretation of a peripheral inflammatory reaction associated with successful ablation as tumor progression. However, the risk of overestimation of the therapeutic effect of the procedure – with peripheral persistence of tumor – also should not be disregarded.

To make a reliable assessment, it is crucial to compare pretreatment and post-treatment studies performed by using the same technical examination protocol, and in the event of inconclusive findings to schedule close follow-up of the patient. Alternatively, when questionable enhancing areas are observed at the periphery of a treated tumor, additional information can be obtained with the use of tissue-specific MR contrast agents, such as hepatobiliary and reticuloendothelial system-targeted agents (LENCIONI et al. 2001).

13.5.2
Contrast-Enhanced US

Conventional US examination is often insufficient in the detection of liver tumors and the accurate evaluation of their burden in patients with liver cirrhosis or oncology patients (LENCIONI et al. 2002). Among the limitations of conventional US, one of the most important is its inaccuracy in patients with inhomogeneity of the liver parenchyma due to cirrhosis, fatty disease, previous chemotherapy, or local treatments. Conventional US examination is also often insufficient in the characterization of liver tumors due to their nonspecific US appearance (LENCIONI et al. 2002).

On conventional US examination after PEI, a hyperechoic zone appears within the tumor due to ethanol deposition. During RF ablation, a zone of increased echogenicity progressively develops around the distal electrode, within and surrounding the treated tumor. This transient finding, previously known by the jargon term "cloud," lasts up to 30–90 min and corresponds to microbubbles of water vapor and other tissue products that form as a result of tissue vaporization during active heating.

This US structural change is relatively independent of the tumor histotype. At the end of the treatment, the US pattern of the lesion is usually modified, and the hyperechoic zone replaces the original lesion. This US feature, however, is unreliable for assessing the outcome of PEI and RF treatment since it does not provide adequate demonstration of the areas of necrosis and residual viable tumor tissue. Moreover, US examination, even when combined with contrast-enhanced color and power Doppler US techniques, does not provide any reliable information in the pre- and post-treatment evaluation of liver tumors due to its low sensitivity in the assessment of tumor vascularity (LENCIONI et al. 2002). Conventional US examination, on the other hand, is the most commonly used imaging modality for the guidance of percutaneous ablation treatments because of its availability, rapidity, and ease of use; the same procedure is more technically challenging and lengthy in CT and MR environments.

The introduction of microbubble-based US contrast agents and, more recently, the development of contrast-specific techniques that display microbubble enhancement in gray scale have substantially improved the ability of US studies to assess liver tumor macro- and microvascularity. With the advent of new-generation sulfur hexafluoride- or perfluorocarbon-filled microbubbles and low mechanical index real-time scanning techniques, contrast-enhanced US has made a significant comeback in the fields of liver tumor detection and characterization and liver tumor ablation. This is because it is an easy-to-perform and reproducible examination that appears to be ready for routine clinical application (LENCIONI et al. 2002).

These developments prompted the European Federation of Societies for Ultrasound in Medicine and Biology to organize a Consensus Conference on the use of microbubble-based contrast agents in liver US. During the meeting, a multidisciplinary panel of international experts met to prepare a document giving updated guidelines on US practice. The guidelines define the indications and provide recommendations for the use of microbubble-based contrast agents in the detection and characterization of focal liver lesions and in the pre- and post-treatment evaluation of liver tumors (EFSUMB STUDY GROUP 2004).

Currently, contrast-enhanced US examination of liver parenchyma is performed by using a new-generation microbubble-based contrast agent in association with a low mechanical index real-time scanning technique. This technique allows study of the enhancement pattern of each liver tumor throughout the vascular phases of hepatic parenchyma in real time. In fact, due to the dual blood supply of hepatic parenchyma by the hepatic artery (25–30%) and the portal vein (70–75%), three vascular phases can be visualized during contrast-enhanced US study of hepatic parenchyma. Hepatic parenchyma enhancement resulting exclusively from the hepatic artery supply usually starts at 10–20 s after injection of the US contrast agent and lasts approximately 10–15 s. This is followed by the tissue enhancement resulting from the portal vein supply, which usually lasts until 2 min after injection of the US contrast agent. The delayed enhancement of hepatic parenchyma persists until 4–6 min after US contrast injection. Most hypervascular hepatic tumor lesions, such as hepatocellular carcinoma, are hyperenhancing during the arterial phase, while the majority of hypovascular hepatic tumor lesions, such as hepatic metastases, are hypoenhancing during the portal and delayed phases. This approach has resulted in improved lesion detection and characterization (EFSUMB STUDY GROUP 2004).

Contrast-enhanced US examination is also highly valuable in all phases of percutaneous tumor ablation, such as treatment planning, targeting of lesions and treatment guidance, and immediate and long-term assessment of treatment outcome. Contrast-enhanced US examination allows (a) better delineation of lesions poorly visualized on conventional US, (b) guidance of the ablation needle into tumors not visualized or not well delineated with conventional US, (c) pretreatment assessment of tumor vascularity as a basis for comparison of pre- and post-treatment patterns at the end of tumor ablation, (d) immediate assessment of the treatment outcome in order to detect residual viable tumor tissue, and (e) post-treatment follow-up in order to assess locally recurrent tumor tissue or new tumor lesions (EFSUMB STUDY GROUP 2004).

Treatment planning. In the setting of patient evaluation for eligibility for percutaneous ablation treatment of liver tumors, digital storage of images and/or movie clips of contrast-enhanced US studies is employed to permit careful comparison of US contrast-enhanced findings with those of contrast-enhanced CT or contrast-enhanced dynamic MR imaging in order to maximize lesion detection. Precise knowledge of lesion number, dimensions, and localization is essential for correct judgment as to the feasibility of treatment. Tumor diameters are very important in treatment planning since the choice of ablation modality (PEI vs RF) and of RF procedure modality varies depending on the actual size and whether there is a capsulated or an infiltrating pattern.

Lesion(s) Targeting. In the setting of lesion targeting for percutaneous ablation of liver tumors, contrast-enhanced US study is performed as the initial step in the PEI or RF session, during the induction of anesthesia, in order to reproduce mapping of lesions as shown on the pretreatment CT or MR imaging study. Images and/or movie clips are again digitally stored for comparison with the immediate postablation study. The continuous contrast-enhanced US technique allows real-time targeting of the lesion(s), allowing precise needle insertion during the specific phase of maximum lesion detectability: this is the arterial phase for highly vascularized lesions such as hepatocellular carcinoma, and the portal or delayed phase for hypovascular lesions such as hepatic metastases. Real-time guidance of needle positioning during contrast-enhanced US study does not significantly prolong the total duration of the PEI or RF session. The use of contrast-enhanced US guidance is mandatory for small hepatocellular carcinomas detected by CT or MR imaging but not visible on conventional US. These lesions may only be reached during the transient arterial phase of contrast-enhanced study, during which they appear as hyperenhancing areas. The use of contrast-enhanced US guidance is also mandatory in the case of small hepatic metastases detected by CT or MR imaging but barely or not perceptible on conventional US. These lesions appear as hypoenhancing areas in the portal or delayed phase of the contrast-enhanced US study. Finally, the use of contrast-enhanced US guidance is mandatory in the context of areas of residual untreated or locally recurrent tumor, whether primary or metastatic. While conventional US almost always cannot differentiate between necrosis and viable tumor, during contrast-enhanced US study viable tumor tissue shows its native, characteristic enhancement pattern.

Assessment of Treatment Outcome. For assessment of the immediate post-treatment outcome, a contrast-enhanced US study is performed 5–10 min after completion of the PEI or RF session, with the patient still under anesthesia. Conventional US findings observed after PEI and during the RF session, represented by a zone of increased echogenicity, in fact offer only a rough estimate of the extent of induced tumor necrosis and therefore do not permit reliable assessment of

Guidance and Assessment of Interventional Therapy in Liver

treatment outcome. Comparison of immediate post-treatment images with stored pretreatment images is necessary to assess the diameter of the induced ablation zone in relation to the diameter of the treated lesion (Fig. 13.1). In the case of the RF procedure, as with CT and MR imaging, a benign periablational area of enhancement can be seen on contrast-enhanced US studies. A thin, relatively concentric and uniform enhancing rim (usually 1–2 mm thick, and no more than 5 mm) surrounding the ablation zone corresponds to a physiologic response to RF damage characterized mainly by reactive hyperemia. Residual

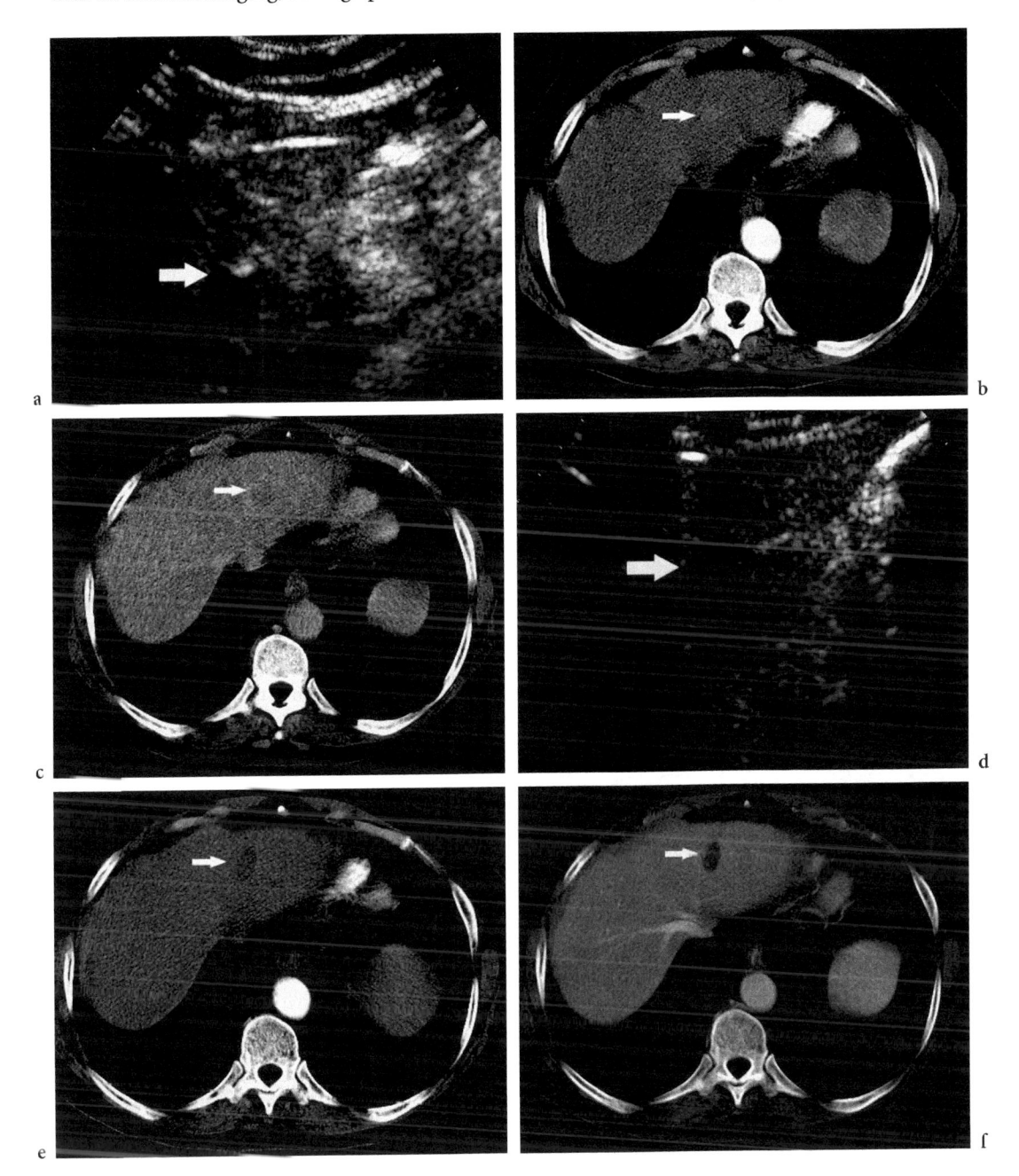

Fig. 13.1a–f. Small hepatocellular carcinoma before and after RF thermal ablation. a Contrast-enhanced US examination shows the lesion as a homogeneous hyperenhancing area (*arrow*), 25–35 s after the administration of US contrast agent before the procedure. b, c Contrast-enhanced spiral CT confirms the presence of the small hypervascular hepatocellular carcinoma (*arrow*). d Immediately after the procedure, contrast-enhanced US examination shows the lesion as a hypoenhancing area (*arrow*) throughout the study, suggesting complete tumor ablation. e, f Contrast-enhanced spiral CT, obtained 1 week after the procedure, confirms complete tumor ablation (*arrow*).

viable tumor tissue, usually recognized at the periphery of the treated lesion, maintains the enhancement behavior characteristics of native tumor as depicted on pretreatment studies. As on CT and MR imaging, residual unablated tumor tissue usually shows irregular, eccentric, or nodular peripheral enhancement. In patients with hepatocellular carcinoma, partial tumor necrosis may be confidently diagnosed when hypervascularity is maintained in a portion of the original lesion in the arterial phase (Fig. 13.2). Residual untreated hepatic metastases sometimes appear indistinguishable from tumor necrosis in the portal and delayed phases. With contrast-enhanced US, evaluation of the arterial phase is important since viable tumor tissue shows weak but perceptible enhancement. A CT and/or an MR imaging study may be performed on the first day after the procedure, mainly to check for possible complications related to the treatment and to confirm the results of the early post-treatment contrast-enhanced US study.

Long-term Follow-up. In the setting of long-term follow-up, contrast-enhanced CT and contrast-enhanced dynamic MR imaging remain the gold standard techniques. The main advantages of these modalities that render them preferable to contrast-enhanced US are their reproducibility and their panoramic quality, i.e. they offer easy coverage of the entire abdomen and extension to the lungs when indicated. Involution of tumor necrosis causes the ablation zones usually to show slow, progressive shrinkage over months and years of follow-up. Benign periablational areas of enhancement may, however, persist for a few months, and zones of altered vascularity such as arterioportal shunt tend to remain stable over time. In this setting, contrast-enhanced US study is of proven value, and is currently used to confirm or exclude doubtful or suspicious local recurrences or new metachronous lesions detected by CT and MR imaging, and to assess the possibility of retreating them under contrast-enhanced US guidance (Fig. 13.3).

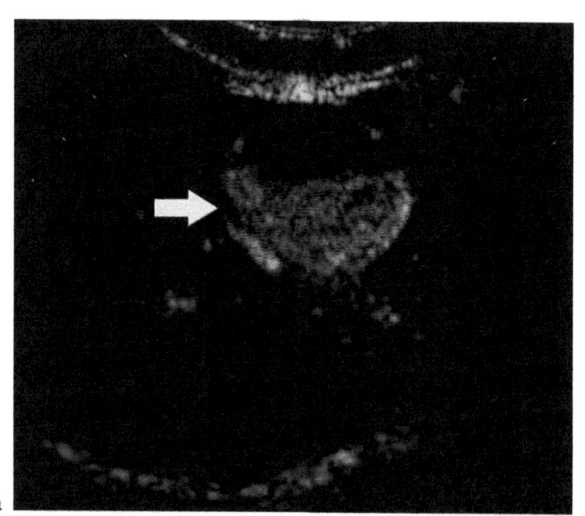

Fig. 13.2a–c. Large hepatocellular carcinoma after RF thermal ablation. **a** Contrast-enhanced US examination, performed immediately after the procedure, shows peripheral residual viable tumor tissue (*arrow*) as an arterial hyperenhancing area. **b** Arterial phase CT image, obtained 1 week after the procedure, confirms the presence of residual viable tumor tissue (*arrow*) as a hyperattenuating area in the anterior aspect of the lesion. **c** The portal venous phase image better visualizes the necrotic portion of the tumor as a hypoattenuating area (*arrow*) in the posterior aspect of the lesion.

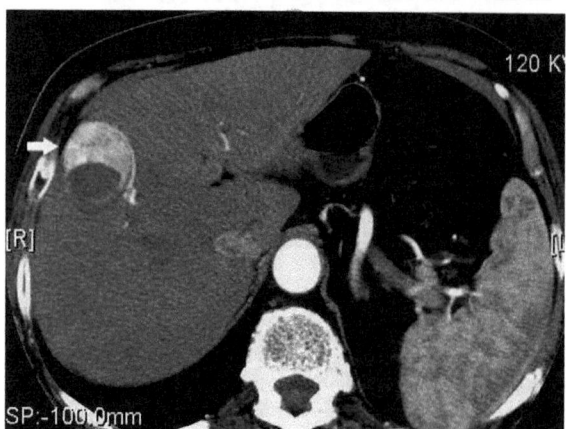

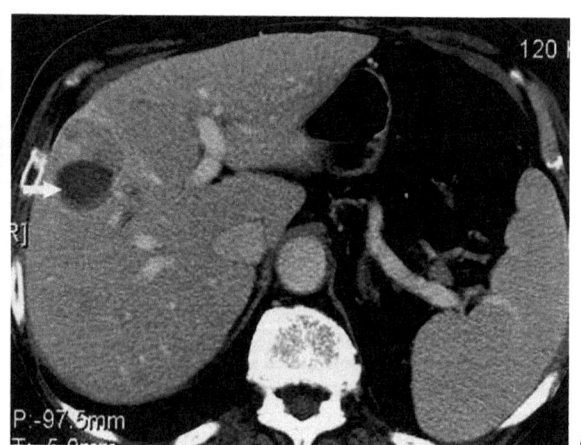

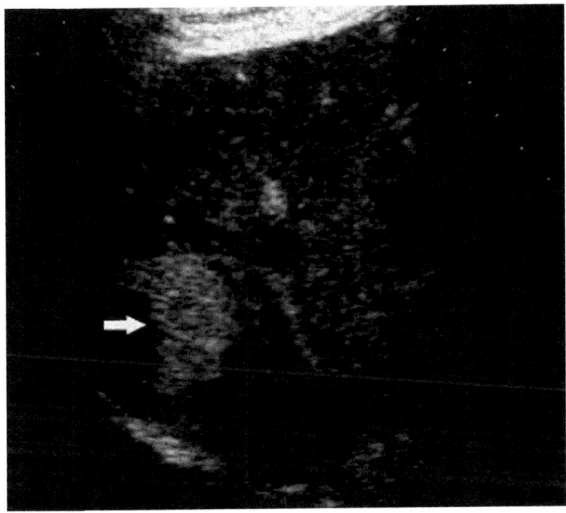

Guidance and Assessment of Interventional Therapy in Liver

Fig. 13.3a–c. Locally recurrent small hepatocellular carcinoma 6 months after RF thermal ablation. **a** Contrast-enhanced US examination, performed during the follow-up, shows a small peripheral arterial hyperenhancing area (*arrow*) suspicious for local recurrence. **b, c** Contrast-enhanced dynamic MR imaging confirms the presence of locally recurrent tumor tissue in the anterior aspect of the lesion (**b**, *arrow*), with evidence of the necrotic portion in the posterior aspect of the lesion (**c**, *arrow*).

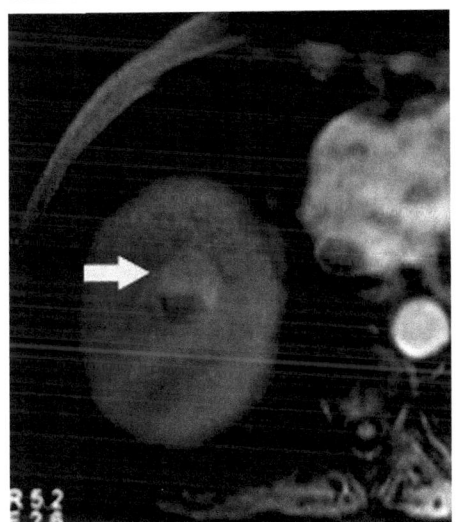

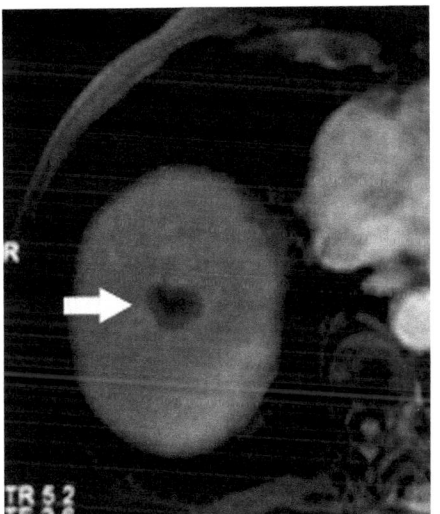

13.5.3
Multimodality Navigation Tool "Navigator"

The Navigator (Esaote SpA and MedCom GmbH) enhances the images produced by a US scanner by combining them with a second modality (such as CT or MR imaging) in real time. The system consists of a US scanner (Technos ^{MPX} Esaote SpA) connected to the Navigation units (Fig. 13.4).

The connection between the two devices consists of a video cable (to grab the US screen image) and a network cable (to query the current scan geometry of the US scanner). The US system provides the US image together with its characteristics, such as the spatial dimensions, the orientation of the probe, and the field of view. Access to the US geometry is

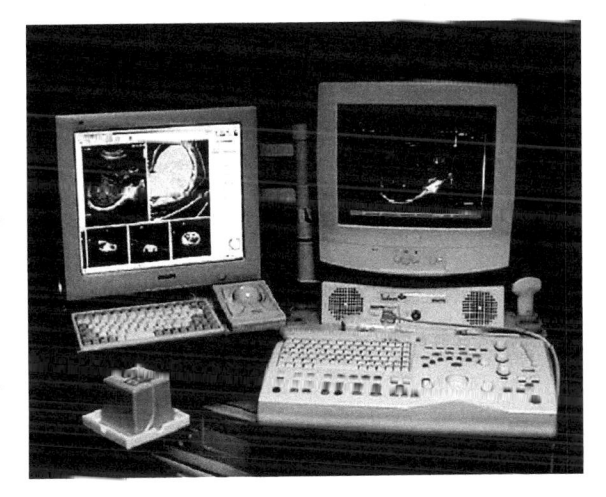

Fig. 13.4. Navigation units.

mandatory in order to be able to compute the correct size and orientation of the virtual slice from the second modality dataset. These data are provided by the US scanner by the network connection and are automatically updated at every change on the console of the scanner. The US image is provided trough the video cable and is digitized by a standard frame grabber for presentation beside the virtual slice. An electromagnetic tracking system, composed of a transmitter and a small receiver (mounted on the US probe), provides the position and orientation of the US probe in relation to the transmitter. For this kind of application the use of an electromagnetic tracker (as opposed to an optical system) is particularly appropriate, since no special accuracy is required by the body regions under examination; the operative field is sufficiently extended and the system is not affected by tools or bodies located between the transmitter and the receiver. It can thus be easily placed in any environment and, furthermore, it has an acceptable cost. Of course, the big disadvantage of the magnetic principle is the sensitivity to metallic objects near to the receiver or transmitter. Thus, any ferromagnetic material that may disturb the field between the transmitter and the receiver must be avoided. Since neither the probe nor the biopsy needles influence the accuracy, it has been found during clinical tests that this requirement can be achieved without affecting clinical routine use in any noticeable way.

In order to start a multimodality examination, it is necessary to scan the patient with the second modality, applying at least three skin markers on the area of interest. The slices will be imported into the Navigation unit in DICOM format through PACS or data CD. The Navigation system processes every slice and, by taking into account the slice to slice distance and dimensions, generates a surface volume.

Once the patient has been positioned on the treatment couch and the transmitter fixed in a suitable position, the registration phase is commenced. The registration procedure combines the patient coordinate system, the probe position, and the 3D dataset in a known and fixed coordinate system; this is mandatory in order to compute a correct virtual slice at the current probe position. To this end it is necessary to select the same markers in the volume and on the patient skin and to register the marker position with the tracking device. During this registration step and also during the subsequent treatment, it is important to keep the patient and the transmitter in a fixed position. Once all markers have been registered, a registration matrix is computed by the software in order to correlate the probe spatial position with the second modality volume, which, after this procedure, fits with the patient body. For any probe position and, of course, for any US image, the system gives the related reference modality slice obtained by virtually cutting the volume according to the probe spatial coordinates.

At our Institution, the system is currently under investigation for the detection and characterization of liver tumors in patients with liver cirrhosis and oncology patients, and as a tool for image-guided tumor ablation. The system shows real advantages deriving from the merging of a real-time modality such as US with a static second modality such as CT or MR imaging that provides a whole organ scan. The major benefit, also due to the combination with use of a US contrast agent, lies in the ease of liver tumor detection and characterization, particularly when a tumor is hardly or not visible on conventional US. The system is also helpful in all phases of image-guided tumor ablation such as treatment planning, targeting of lesions and treatment guidance, and immediate and long-term assessment of treatment outcome. The system increases the precision of target lesion localization when the US image is not clear. A volumetric reference modality dataset allows the analysis of different planes, thereby permitting better understanding of the morphology of the target lesion and the anatomical structures that surround the target.

13.6
Conclusions

According to the EFSUMB guidelines for the use of microbubble-based contrast agents in US in the setting of percutaneous tumor ablation, contrast-enhanced US is complementary to CT and/or MR imaging for pretreatment staging and assessment of target lesion vascularity. Pretreatment optimized CT and/or MR imaging, however, is still recommended. Contrast-enhanced US facilitates needle positioning in cases of incomplete or insufficient lesion delineation on conventional US. It also allows evaluation of the immediate treatment effect after the ablation and assessment of locally recurrent tumor tissue during the follow-up when CT and/or MR imaging is contraindicated or inconclusive. Although CT and MR imaging are considered the gold standard techniques for the assessment of treatment outcome, contrast-enhanced US may be used in the follow-up protocols.

More recently, the introduction of the Navigator system increases the precision of target lesion localization when the US image is unclear. A volumetric reference modality dataset elucidates the morphology of the target lesion and the anatomical structures surrounding the target.

References

Abdalla EK, Vauthey JN, Ellis LM et al (2004) Recurrence and outcomes following hepatic resection, radiofrequency ablation, and combined resection/ablation for colorectal liver metastases. Ann Surg 239:818-825

August DA, Sugarbaker PH, Schneider PD (1985) Lymphatic dissemination of hepatic metastases. Implications for the follow-up and treatment of patients with colorectal cancer. Cancer 55:1490-1494

Bartolozzi C, Lencioni R (1996) Ethanol injection for the treatment of hepatic tumours. Eur Radiol 6:682-696

Berber E, Herceg NL, Casto KJ, Siperstein AE (2004) Laparoscopic radiofrequency ablation of hepatic tumors: prospective clinical evaluation of ablation size comparing two treatment algorithms. Surg Endosc 18:390-396

Bismuth H, Majno PE, Adam R (1999) Liver transplantation for hepatocellular carcinoma. Semin Liver Dis 19:311-322

Bruix J, Llovet JM (2002) Prognostic prediction and treatment strategy in hepatocellular carcinoma. Hepatology 35:519-524

Bruix J, Sherman M, Llovet JM (2001) EASL Panel of Experts on HCC. Clinical management of hepatocellular carcinoma. Conclusions of the Barcelona-2000 EASL conference. European Association for the Study of the Liver. J Hepatol 35:421-430

Buscarini E, Buscarini L (2004) Radiofrequency thermal ablation with expandable needle of focal liver malignancies: complication report. Eur Radiol 14:31-37

Castells A, Bruix J, Bru C et al (1993) Treatment of small hepatocellular carcinoma in cirrhotic patients: a cohort study comparing surgical resection and percutaneous ethanol injection. Hepatology 18:1121-1126

Chopra S, Dodd GD 3rd, Chanin MP et al (2003) Radiofrequency ablation of hepatic tumors adjacent to the gallbladder: feasibility and safety. AJR Am J Roentgenol 180:697-701

Choti MA, Sitzmann JV, Tiburi MF et al (2002) Trends in long-term survival following liver resection for hepatic colorectal metastases. Ann Surg 235:759-765

Curley SA, Izzo F, Delrio P et al (1999) Radiofrequency ablation of unresectable primary and metastatic malignancies: results in 123 patients. Ann Surg 230:1-8

De Baere T, Elias D, Dromain C et al (2000) Radiofrequency ablation of 100 hepatic metastases with a mean follow-up of more than 1 year. AJR Am J Roentgenol 175:1619-1625

De Baere T, Risse O, Kuoch V et al (2003) Adverse events during radiofrequency treatment of 582 hepatic tumors. AJR Am J Roentgenol 181:695-700

Di Stasi M, Buscarini L, Livraghi T et al (1997) Percutaneous ethanol injection in the treatment of hepatocellular carcinoma. A multicenter survey of evaluation practices and complication rates. Scand J Gastroenterol 32:1168-1173

EFSUMB Study Group (2004) Guidelines for the use of contrast agents in ultrasound. Ultraschall Med 25:249-256

Elias D, de Baere T, Smayra T et al (2002) Percutaneous radiofrequency thermoablation as an alternative to surgery for treatment of liver tumour recurrence after hepatectomy. Br J Surg 89:752-756

Fong Y, Fortner J, Sun RL et al (1999a) Clinical score for predicting recurrence after hepatic resection for metastatic colorectal cancer: analysis of 1001 consecutive cases. Ann Surg 230:309-318

Fong Y, Sun RL, Jarnagin W et al (1999b) An analysis of 412 cases of hepatocellular carcinoma at a Western center. Ann Surg 229:790-800

Galandi D, Antes G (2004) Radiofrequency thermal ablation versus other interventions for hepatocellular carcinoma (Cochrane Review). The Cochrane Library, issue 2. Wiley, Chichester, UK

Gillams AR, Lees WR (2000) Survival after percutaneous, image-guided, thermal ablation of hepatic metastases from colorectal cancer. Dis Colon Rectum 43:656-666

Goldberg SN (2002) Comparison of techniques for image-guided ablation of focal liver tumors. Radiology 223:304-307

Goldberg SN, Hahn PF, Tanabe KK et al (1998a) Percutaneous radiofrequency tissue ablation: does perfusion-mediated tissue cooling limit coagulation necrosis? J Vasc Interv Radiol 9:101-115

Goldberg SN, Solbiati L, Hahn PF et al (1998b) Large volume tissue ablation with radiofrequency by using a clustered, internally cooled electrode technique: laboratory and clinical experience in liver metastases. Radiology 209:371-379

Goldberg SN, Charboneau JW, Dodd GD III et al for the International Working Group on Image-Guided Tumor Ablation (2003) Image-guided tumor ablation: proposal for standardization of terms and reporting criteria. Radiology 228:335-345

Grothey A, Sargent D, Goldberg RM, Schmoll HJ (2004) Survival of patients with advanced colorectal cancer improves with the availability of flurouracil-leucovirin, irinotecan, and oxaliplatin in the course of treatment. J Clin Oncol 22:1209-1214

Headrick JR, Miller DL, Nagorney DM et al (2001) Surgical treatment of hepatic and pulmonary metastases from colon cancer. Ann Thorac Surg 71:975-979

Helmberger T, Holzknecht N, Schopf U et al (2001) Radiofrequency ablation of liver metastases. Technique and initial results. Radiologe 41:69-76

Ikeda M, Okada S, Ueno H et al (2001) Radiofrequency ablation and percutaneous ethanol injection in patients with small hepatocellular carcinoma: a comparative study. Jpn J Clin Oncol 31:322-326

Iwatsuki S, Dvorchik I, Madariaga JR et al (1999) Hepatic resection for metastatic colorectal adenocarcinoma: a proposal of a prognostic scoring system. J Am Coll Surg 189:291-299

Jamison RL, Donohue JH, Nagorney DM et al (1997) Hepatic resection for metastatic colorectal cancer results in cure for some patients. Arch Surg 132:505-510

Jessup JM, McGinnis LS, Steele GD Jr et al (1996) Report on colon cancer. The National Cancer Data Base. Cancer 78:918-926

Jonas S, Bechstein WO, Steinmuller T et al (2001) Vascular invasion and histopathologic grading determine outcome after liver transplantion for hepatocellular carcinoma in cirrhosis. Hepatology 33:1080-1086

Jonker DJ, Maroun JA, Kocha W (2000) Survival benefit of chemotherapy in metastatic colorectal cancer: a meta-analysis of randomized controlled trials. Br J Cancer 82:1789-1794

Khan KN, Yatsuhashi H, Yamasaki K et al (2000) Prospective analysis of risk factors for early intrahepatic recurrence of hepatocellular carcinoma following ethanol injection. J Hepatol 32:269-278

Koda M, Murawaki Y, Mitsuda A et al (2000) Predictive factors for intrahepatic recurrence after percutaneous ethanol injection therapy for small hepatocellular carcinoma. Cancer 88:529-537

Lees WR, Schumillian C, Gillams AR (2000) Hypotensive anesthesia improves the effectiveness of radiofrequency ablation in the liver. Radiology 217:228

Lencioni R, Bartolozzi C, Caramella D et al (1995) Treatment of small hepatocellular carcinoma with percutaneous ethanol injection. Analysis of prognostic factors in 105 Western patients. Cancer 76:1737-1746

Lencioni R, Pinto F, Armillotta N et al (1997) Long-term results of percutaneous ethanol injection therapy for hepatocellular carcinoma in cirrhosis: a European experience. Eur Radiol 7:514-519

Lencioni R, Goletti O, Armillotta N et al (1998) Radio-frequency thermal ablation of liver metastases with a cooled-tip electrode needle: results of a pilot clinical trial. Eur Radiol 8:1205-1211

Lencioni R, Cioni D, Bartolozzi C (2001) Percutaneous radio-frequency thermal ablation of liver malignancies: techniques, indications, imaging findings, and clinical results. Abdom Imaging 26:345-360

Lencioni R, Cioni D, Bartolozzi C (2002) Tissue harmonic and contrast-specific imaging: back to gray scale in ultrasound. Eur Radiol 12:151-165

Lencioni R, Allgaier HP, Cioni D et al (2003) Small hepatocellular carcinoma in cirrhosis: randomized comparison of radiofrequency thermal ablation versus percutaneous ethanol injection. Radiology 228:235-240

Lencioni R, Cioni D, Crocetti L et al (2004a) Percutaneous ablation of hepatocellular carcinoma: state-of-the-art. Liver Transplant 10:S91-S97

Lencioni R, Cioni D, Crocetti L et al (2005) Early-stage hepatocellular carcinoma in cirrhosis: long-term results of percutaneous image-guided radiofrequency ablation. Radiology (in press)

Lencioni R (2004b) Tumor Radiofrequency Ablation Italian Network (TRAIN): Long-term results in hepatic colorectal cancer metastases [Abstract] RSNA meeting 2004

Livraghi T, Vettori C, Lazzaroni S (1991) Liver metastases: results of percutaneous ethanol injection in 14 patients. Radiology 179:709-712

Livraghi T, Giorgio A, Marin G et al (1995) Hepatocellular carcinoma and cirrhosis in 746 patients: long-term results of percutaneous ethanol injection. Radiology 197:101-108

Livraghi T, Goldberg SN, Lazzaroni S et al (1999) Small hepatocellular carcinoma: treatment with radio-frequency ablation versus ethanol injection. Radiology 210:655-661

Livraghi T, Goldberg SN, Lazzaroni S et al (2000) Hepatocellular carcinoma: radio-frequency ablation of medium and large lesions. Radiology 214:761-768

Livraghi T, Solbiati L, Meloni MF et al (2003a) Treatment of focal liver tumors with percutaneous radio-frequency ablation: complications encountered in a multicenter study. Radiology 226:441-451

Livraghi T, Solbiati L, Meloni F et al (2003b) Percutaneous radiofrequency ablation of liver metastases in potential candidates for resection: the "test-of-time approach". Cancer 97:3027-3035

Llovet JM, Fuster J, Bruix J (1999) Intention-to-treat analysis of surgical treatment for early hepatocellular carcinoma: resection versus transplantation. Hepatology 30:1434-1440

Llovet JM, Vilana R, Bru C et al (2001) Barcelona Clinic Liver Cancer (BCLC) Group. Increased risk of tumor seeding after percutaneous radiofrequency ablation for single hepatocellular carcinoma. Hepatology 33:1124-1129

Llovet JM, Burroughs A, Bruix J (2003) Hepatocellular carcinoma. Lancet 362:1907-1917

Mala T, Edwin B, Mathisen O et al (2004) Cryoablation of colorectal liver metastases: minimally invasive tumour control. Scand J Gastroenterol 39:571-578

Mazzaferro V, Regalia E, Doci R et al (1996) Liver transplantation in the treatment of small hepatocellular carcinomas in patients with cirrhosis. N Engl J Med 334:693-699

McGahan JP, Dodd GD III (2000) Radiofrequency ablation of the liver: current status. AJR Am J Roentgenol 176:3-16

Mineo TC, Ambrogi V, Tonini G et al (2003) Long-term results after resection of simultaneous and sequential lung and liver metastases from colorectal carcinoma. J Am Coll Surg 197:386-391

Morita T, Shibata T, Okuyama M et al (2004) Microwave coagulation therapy for liver metastases from colorectal cancer. Gan To Kagaku Ryoho 31:695-699

Murata S, Moriya Y, Akusa T et al (1998) Resection of both hepatic and pulmonary metastases in patients with colorectal carcinoma. Cancer 83:1086-1093

Patel NA, Keenan RJ, Medich DS et al (2003) The presence of colorectal hepatic metastases does not preclude pulmonary metastasectomy. Am Surg 69:1047-1053

Okusaka T, Okada S, Ueno H et al (2002) Satellite lesions in patients with small hepatocellular carcinoma with reference to clinicopathologic features. Cancer 95:1931-1937

Oshowo A, Gillams A, Harrison E et al (2003) Comparison of resection and radiofrequency ablation for treatment of solitary colorectal liver metastases. Br J Surg 90:1240-1243

Rhim H, Dodd GD 3rd, Chintapalli KN et al (2004) Radiofrequency thermal ablation of abdominal tumors: lessons learned from complications. Radiographics 24:41-52

Rossi S, Garbagnati F, Lencioni R et al (2000) Percutaneous radio-frequency thermal ablation of nonresectable hepatocellular carcinoma after occlusion of tumor blood supply. Radiology 217:119-126

Sasson AR, Sigurdson ER (2002) Surgical treatment of liver metastases. Semin Oncol 29:107-118

Scheele J, Stang R, Altendorf-Hofmann A et al (1995) Resection of colorectal liver metastases. World J Surg 19:59-71

Shibata T, Iimuro Y, Yamamoto Y et al (2002) Small hepatocellular carcinoma: comparison of radio-frequency ablation and percutaneous microwave coagulation therapy. Radiology 223:331-337

Shiina S, Tagawa K, Unuma T et al (1991) Percutaneous ethanol injection therapy for hepatocellular carcinoma: a histopathologic study. Cancer 68:1524-1530

Shiina S, Tagawa K, Niwa Y et al (1993) Percutaneous ethanol injection therapy for hepatocellular carcinoma: results in 146 patients. AJR Am J Roentgenol 160:1023-1028

Shiina S, Teratani T, Obi S et al (2002) Nonsurgical treatment of hepatocellular carcinoma: from percutaneous ethanol injection therapy and percutaneous microwave coagulation therapy to radiofrequency ablation. Oncology 62 [Suppl 1]:64-68

Silen W (1989) Hepatic resection for metastases from colorectal carcinoma is of dubious value. Arch Surg 124:1021-1022

Solbiati L, Goldberg SN, Ierace T et al (1997) Hepatic metastases: percutaneous radio-frequency ablation with cooled-tip electrodes. Radiology 205:367-373

Solbiati L, Livraghi T, Goldberg SN et al (2001) Percutaneous radio-frequency ablation of hepatic metastases from colorectal cancer: long-term results in 117 patients. Radiology 221:159-166

Solbiati L, Ierace T, Tonolini M, Bellabuono A, Cova L (2003) Long-term survival of patients treated with radiofrequency ablation for liver colorectal metastases: improved outcome with increasing experience. Radiology 229:411

Vauthey JN, Pawlik TM, Abdalla EK et al (2004) Is extended hepatectomy for hepatobiliary malignancy justified? Ann Surg 239:722-730

Vogl TJ, Muller PK, Mack MG et al (1999) Liver metastases: interventional therapeutic techniques and results, state of the art. Eur Radiol 9:675-684

Wayne JD, Lauwers GY, Ikai I et al (2002) Preoperative predictors of survival after resection of small hepatocellular carcinomas. Ann Surg 235:722-731

Yamakado K, Nakatsuka A, Ohmori S et al (2002) Radiofrequency ablation combined with chemoembolization in hepatocellular carcinoma: treatment response based on tumor size and morphology. J Vasc Interv Radiol 13:1225-1232

Yamamoto J, Okada S, Shimada K et al (2001) Treatment strategy for small hepatocellular carcinoma: comparison of long-term results after percutaneous ethanol injection therapy and surgical resection. Hepatology 34:707-713

Yamasaki T, Kurokawa F, Shirahashi H et al (2002) Percutaneous radiofrequency ablation therapy for patients with hepatocellular carcinoma during occlusion of hepatic blood flow. Comparison with standard percutaneous radiofrequency ablation therapy. Cancer 95:2353-2360

14 Applications of Ultrasound Microbubbles in the Spleen

Christopher J. Harvey, Adrian K.P. Lim, Madeleine Lynch, Martin J.K. Blomley, David O. Cosgrove

CONTENTS

14.1 Introduction 205
14.2 Microbubble Behaviour in the Normal Spleen 205
14.3 Splenic Lesions 207
14.3.1 Congenital Lesions 207
14.3.2 Benign Focal Splenic Lesions 208
14.3.3 Malignant Focal Splenic Lesions 212
14.3.4 Splenic Renal Perfusion Defects - Infarctions 216
14.3.5 Splenic Abscesses 216
14.3.6 Heterogeneous Splenic Echotexture 216
14.4 Summary 216
References 218

14.1 Introduction

Ultrasound (US) is a reliable method of demonstrating and estimating the size of focal splenic abnormalities with the added benefits that there is no risk of ionizing radiation and that it is quick and easy to perform. It is only relatively recently, since the advent of microbubble contrast agents, that US has been able to investigate splenic enhancement patterns and characterize focal lesions. This chapter describes the applications of US microbubbles in the identification and characterization of focal splenic lesions.

14.2 Microbubble Behaviour in the Normal Spleen

Microbubbles were initially thought to be purely vascular agents. However, three agents demonstrate

---

C. J. Harvey, MRCP FRCR, Consultant Radiologist
A. K. P. Lim, MRCP FRCR, Consultant Radiologist
M. Lynch, MSc, Senior Sonographer
M. J. K. Blomley, MD, FRCR, Professor of Radiology
D. O. Cosgrove, FRCP FRCR, Professor of Clinical Ultrasound
Department of Imaging, Imaging Sciences Department, Hammersmith Hospital, Imperial College Faculty of Medicine, 150 Du Cane Road, W12 OH5, London, UK

hepatosplenic-specific uptake after their disappearance from the blood pool phase (Blomley et al. 1999; Forsberg et al. 1999). They are Levovist, Sonavist (both Schering AG, Germany) (Blomley et al. 1999; Forsberg et al. 1999) and Sonazoid (NC100100; Nycomed Amersham, Norway) (Leen et al. 1998), of which only Levovist remains in clinical use. The site of accumulation within these organs is unknown but is thought to be the reticuloendothelial system or sinusoids (Leen et al. 1998; Blomley et al. 1999; Forsberg et al. 1999; Kono et al. 2002). However, there is relatively few published data with regard to microbubbles and their behaviour in the spleen. The most widely used microbubble in Europe, SonoVue (Bracco, Italy), had always been thought to be a purely vascular contrast agent (Schneider et al. 1995; Correas et al. 2001; Harvey et al. 2001).

We investigated the enhancement characteristics of SonoVue in the normal spleen in a cohort of ten healthy volunteers. Using a low acoustic power technique [Cadence Contrast Pulse Sequence (CPS), Sequoia, Acuson-Siemens, USA], the spleen was continuously scanned from 0 to 60 s and then again at 4 min. SonoVue (2.4 ml) was injected intravenously in all volunteers. Early analysis of this unpublished data revealed that in nine out of ten volunteers, there was heterogeneous, patchy enhancement of the spleen from 0 to 20 s (Fig. 14.1), with the spleen then becoming homogeneous throughout by 50 s (Fig. 14.2a). In one volunteer the spleen homogeneously enhanced even in the arterial phase. These enhancement characteristics are similar to those reported with iodinated contrast agents within the spleen on computed tomography (CT) and magnetic resonance (MR) imaging (Glazer et al. 1981; Mirowitz et al. 1991). These imaging characteristics are thought to be due to variable flow rates through the cords and sinuses of the red pulp (Groom 1987). Therefore it is recommended that lesion detection and assessment of the spleen with microbubbles should be in the late phase, at least 60 s post intravenous injection. The images at 4 min revealed that there was still a significant amount of contrast

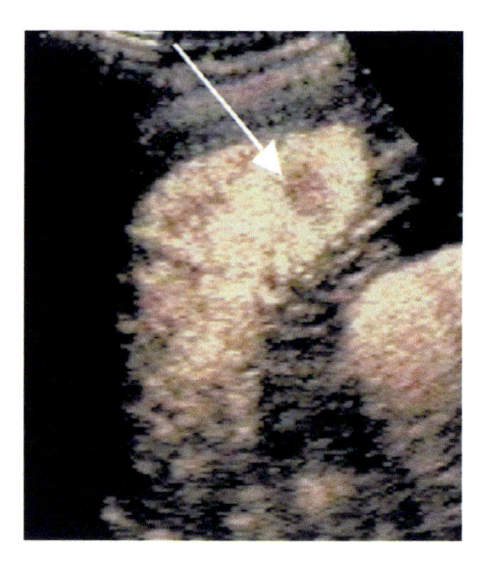

Fig. 14.1. This is a low acoustic power microbubble specific mode (Cadence Contrast Pulse Sequencing, CPS, Sequoia, Acuson-Siemens, USA), which depicts microbubbles in a colour overlay. This is an example of the heterogeneous enhancement of the spleen in the arterial phase. Note the apparent rounded defect, which could be mistaken for a lesion (*arrow*).

agent in the splenic tissue after the normal vascular phase (Fig. 14.2b), suggesting that SonoVue also has splenic specificity.

An expanded study of these normal volunteers confirmed the splenic tropism of SonoVue at least 5 min after the blood pool phase (LIM et al. 2004). Figure 14.3 demonstrates a series of images of the spleen from 0 to 5 min after contrast injection in the same volunteer. The green pixels depict stationary microbubbles using low acoustic power software [Vascular Recognition Imaging (VRI), Aplio, Toshiba, Tokyo, Japan]. Note that the intensity of the green pixels remains relatively unchanged over the 5 min. The percentage of green pixels in a region of interest was used for quantification, and Fig. 14.4 is a graph illustrating the mean quantity of microbubbles within each organ (i.e. liver, spleen and both kidneys) over 5 min in the 20 normal volunteers. These data confirmed specific uptake of SonoVue by the spleen but not the liver.

It is interesting that, of the aforementioned agents, SonoVue demonstrated only splenic-specific uptake without significant liver tropism. Thus the exact mechanism of microbubble uptake in the spleen, which has previously been attributed to phagocytosis by macrophages (this also applies to liver uptake), remains questionable. The behaviour of SonoVue may be analogous to that of the heat-damaged red blood cells used in nuclear medicine, which are highly spleen-specific and are not taken up by the liver, unlike colloid-labelled tracers (MASSEY and STEVENS 1991; PERSON and BENDER 2000). Phase contrast microscopic studies by IIJIMA et al. (2003) with in vitro hepatic macrophages suggested that these cells were selective for microbubble agents that were phagocytosed and that this process was possibly dependent on the structure of the agent.

Though the exact physiology and kinetics of these microbubble agents in the spleen may be unknown, this unique spleen specificity provides a useful alternative method for identifying or confirming splenic tissue, as well as for characterizing focal splenic lesions with an accuracy that rivals that of CT, MR imaging, or nuclear medicine imaging.

Contrast-specific techniques operating at low acoustic power [mechanical index (MI) <0.2 and sometimes as low as 0.02] present the major advantage that tissue harmonics are suppressed, and that bubble destruction is minimised. These technological advances com-

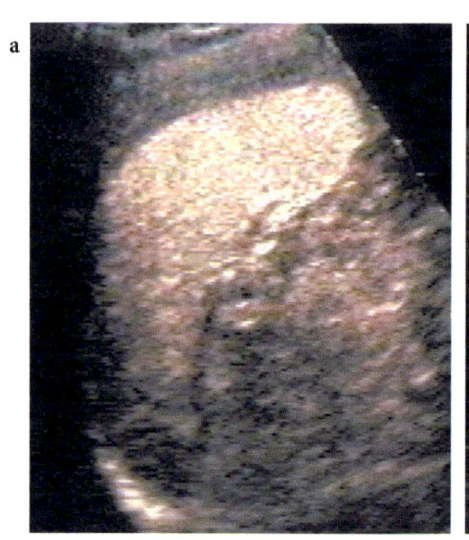

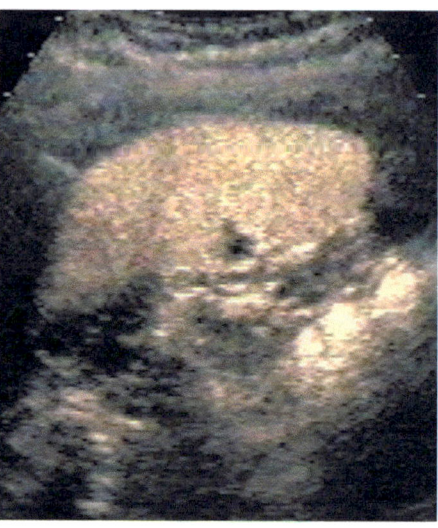

Fig. 14.2. a The spleen in the same volunteer as in Fig. 14.1 now demonstrates homogeneous enhancement at 60 s. The apparent defect in Fig. 14.1 is not visible now. **b** At 4 min there is still microbubble agent within the spleen.

Applications of Ultrasound Microbubbles in the Spleen

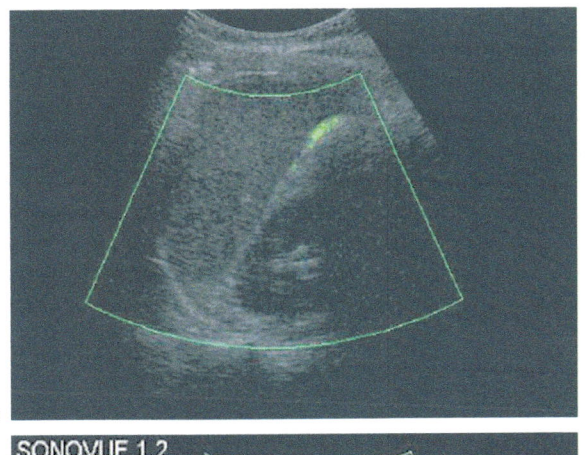

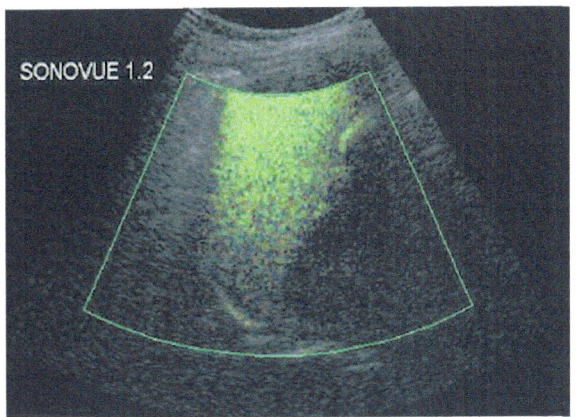

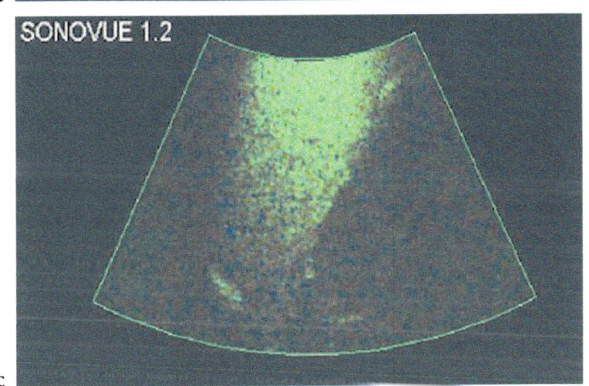

Fig. 14.3a–c. The images are of the same volunteer as in Figs. 14.1 and 14.2, at baseline (**a**), 3 min after contrast injection (**b**) and 5 min after contrast injection (**c**). In this mode, stationary microbubbles are depicted in a green colour (Vascular Recognition Imaging, Aplio, Toshiba, Japan).

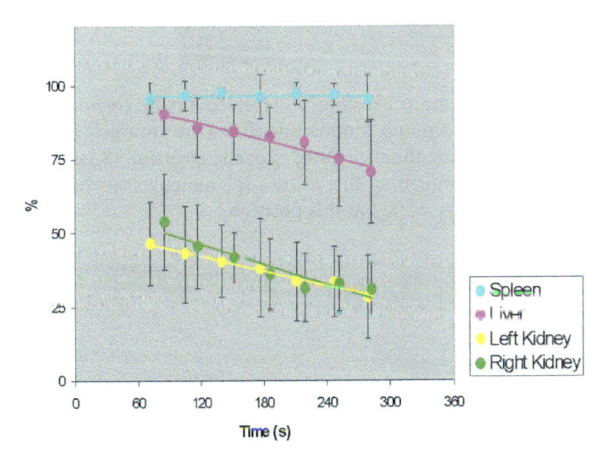

Fig. 14.4 A graph illustrating the mean total microbubble uptake against time (s) in a cohort of 20 volunteers over 5 min. Gradients of best-fit straight lines have been plotted. Note that the line for the spleen is virtually horizontal, while the other organs demonstrate decreases at a similar rate. The elevated values for the liver compared with the kidneys were thought to be due to the larger vascular volume of the liver.

bined with the availability of more stable microbubbles (e.g. SonoVue) have facilitated the development of real-time non-destructive (MI 0.06–0.12) imaging modes that can demonstrate the capillary bed as well as larger vessels (HARVEY and ALBRECHT 2001). Contrast-enhanced imaging of focal splenic lesions may be divided into arterial (20–25 s) and portal (45–90 s) phases and sinusoidal (>90 s). Real-time imaging allows these phases to be followed successively so that the dynamic enhancement pattern and vascular morphology may be assessed. The low acoustic power means that continuous imaging can be performed for as long as the agent persists (5–10 min after a full dose of SonoVue). This technique has replaced the destructive high acoustic power approaches.

14.3
Splenic Lesions

14.3.1
Congenital Lesions

A splenunculus is accessory splenic tissue which is present in 10–30% of the population (GORG 2001; PEDDU et al. 2004). Splenunculi may be single or multiple and most commonly occur at the splenic hilum (75%) (WADHAM et al. 1981). They typically have a round contour and their echogenicity is identical to that of the parent spleen. Any pathological process affecting the spleen may affect the splenunculus. Splenunculi have a vascular hilum with an arterial and venous supply running in opposite directions (BERTOLOTTO et al. 1998). Splenunculi have identical enhancement patterns, with US microbubbles, to the adjacent spleen. Splenunculi and the parent spleen enhance simultaneously in the arterial phase and exhibit a heterogeneous sinusoidal phase. As described above, some agents (Levovist, SonoVue) have a delayed splenic-specific parenchymal phase which is useful in differentiating splenunculi from lymph nodes or pancreatic masses (Figs. 14.5, 14.6).

14.3.2
Benign Focal Splenic Lesions

Cystic Lesions

Cystic splenic lesions may be subdivided into primary cysts, which are either non-parasitic (epithelial) or parasitic (echinococcosis infection), and secondary cysts, which are thought to be traumatic in aetiology (DACHMAN et al. 1986; SINILUOTO et al. 1994; URRUTIA et al. 1996). They contain blood and debris and may exhibit mural calcification.

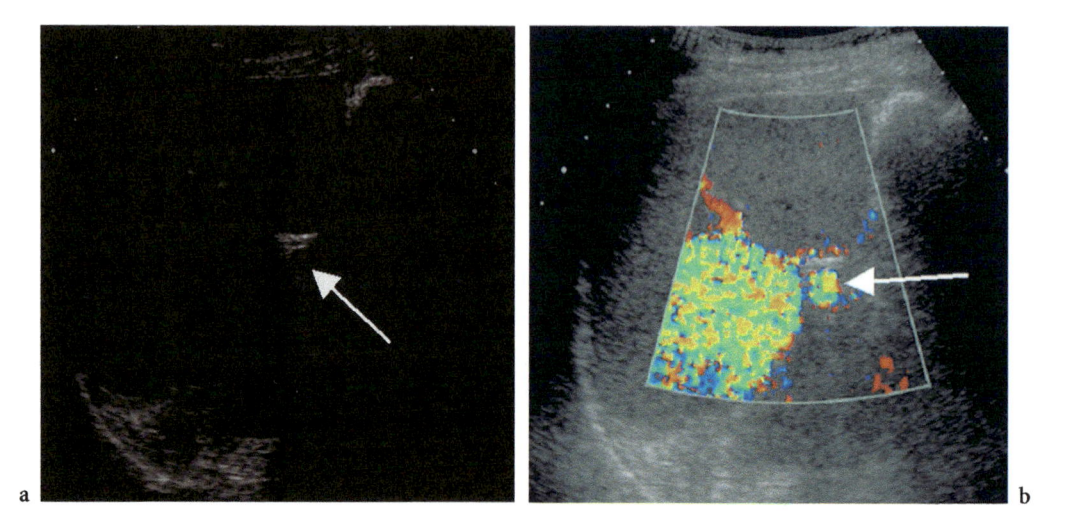

Fig. 14.5a, b. A 56-year-old patient with a past history of pancreatic gastrinoma. **a** Baseline US revealed a mass (*arrow*) at the splenic hilum and a tumour recurrence was queried. Note that the lesion has a smooth contour and shows the same echogenicity as the spleen. **b** Three minutes after an IV bolus injection of 2 g Levovist, using the stimulated acoustic emission (SAE) mode, similar colour phenomena are revealed in the spleen and adjacent lesion, confirming this to be a splenunculus (*arrow*). Note the marked focal zone dependence of this mode as the highest acoustic power occurs at this position.

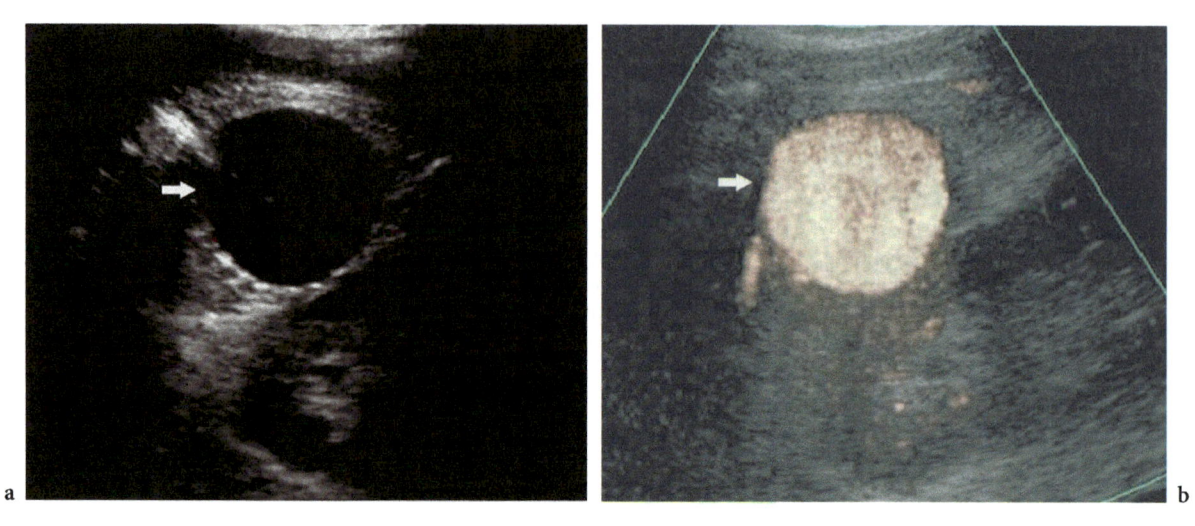

Fig. 14.6a,b. Enlarged accessory spleen in a patient who had undergone splenectomy 5 years previously. Baseline US (**a**) reveals a tumour-like round lesion (*arrow*) at the splenic site. The splenic-specific concentration of sulphur hexafluoride-filled microbubbles 4 min after injection (**b**) proves the splenic nature of the lesion. (From the editor, E. Quaia).

Non-parasitic cysts show the classic US features of anechoic contents, with posterior acoustic enhancement and smooth walls. They are avascular on Doppler imaging (Gorg and Schwerk 1994; Gorg et al. 1991).

Microbubble contrast agents may be helpful in defining the thin wall of the cyst and demonstrating the absence of central enhancement to differentiate benign simple cysts (Fig. 14.7) from infective or neoplastic cystic lesions.

Hydatid cysts are rare in the spleen (less than 5% of *Echinococcus* infections). They may be anechoic or have heterogeneous echogenicity due to scolices (Beggs 1985; Polat et al. 2003). The 'water-lily sign' is characteristic of the condition and is caused by separation of the membranes of the cyst. With IV microbubbles, hydatid cysts show peripheral but not internal enhancement.

Haemangiomas

Haemangiomas are the commonest benign primary splenic neoplasm, with a prevalence of 0.3–14% at autopsy (Ros et al. 1987; Ramani et al. 1997). They are tumours of the epithelium of the vascular sinuses and are more commonly cavernous than capillary in pattern. Cavernous haemangiomas are usually small (<2 cm) and are incidental findings on imaging. They are slow growing. Occasionally haemangiomas may be large and may present as a mass or with rupture and bleeding (Husni 1961). Multiple splenic haemangiomas occur in Klippel-Trenaunay syndrome and may be complicated by rupture, hypersplenism and malignant change.

On US, haemangiomas typically appear as well-defined avascular echogenic lesions (Ros et al. 1987; Urrutia et al. 1996; Wan et al. 2000). Atypical features, which are more commonly present in large cavernous haemangiomas, include cystic change and calcification.

Small haemangiomas uniformly enhance with microbubbles (Fig. 14.8), whereas larger lesions exhibit centripetal filling in on delayed imaging (Fig. 14.9). However, larger lesions with cystic/necrotic/thrombotic components may show heterogeneous enhancement (Fig. 14.10) rather than the centripetal pattern (Abbott et al. 2004). This is due to the fact that cystic spaces (often central) do not possess blood-filled vascular spaces. Also, splenic haemangiomas do not exhibit the well-defined peripheral globular coalescing enhancement pattern seen in hepatic haemangiomas (Urrutia et al. 1996; Ramani et al. 1997; Abbott et al. 2004). This may be due to differences in vascular supply such that peripheral nodules (present in liver haemangiomas on contrast-enhanced US, CT and MR) are less conspicuous in splenic haemangiomas in the arterial phase because splenic enhancement obscures them (Ferrozzi et al. 1996).

Hamartomas

Splenic hamartomas, also known as splenomas, splenadenomas and nodular hyperplasia of the

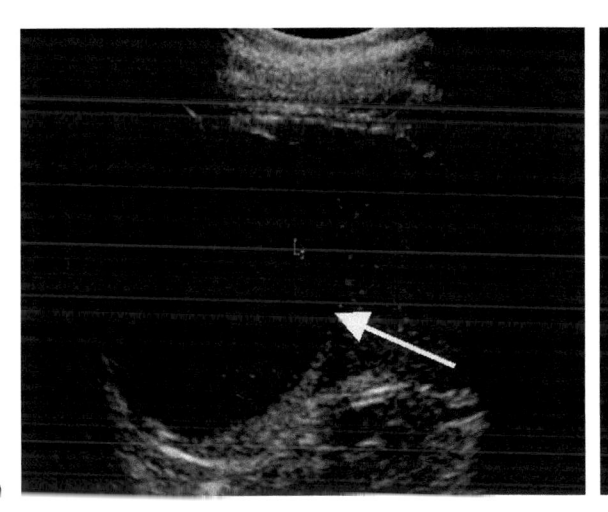

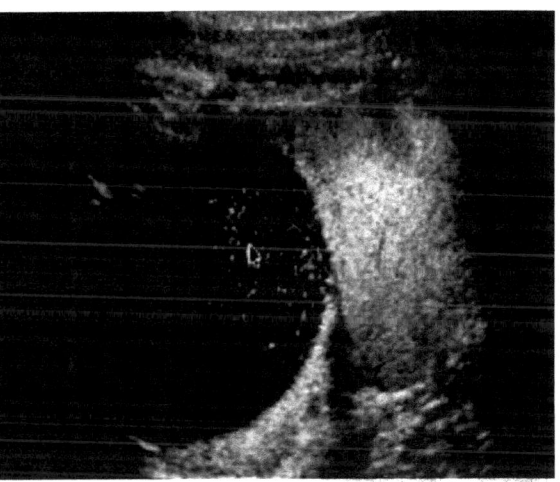

Fig. 14.7a,b. A 40-year-old man who presented with left upper quadrant pain. a Baseline US showed a well-defined, predominantly echo-poor splenic lesion with mobile debris within it, consistent with a complex cyst. b Imaging in the late splenic-specific phase of Levovist using the phase inversion mode (ATL-Philips, USA) showed no microbubble activity in the cyst but demonstrated normal uptake in the adjacent spleen, rendering the cyst more conspicuous. The final diagnosis was thought to be haemorrhage into a simple epithelial cyst as there was no evidence of sepsis.

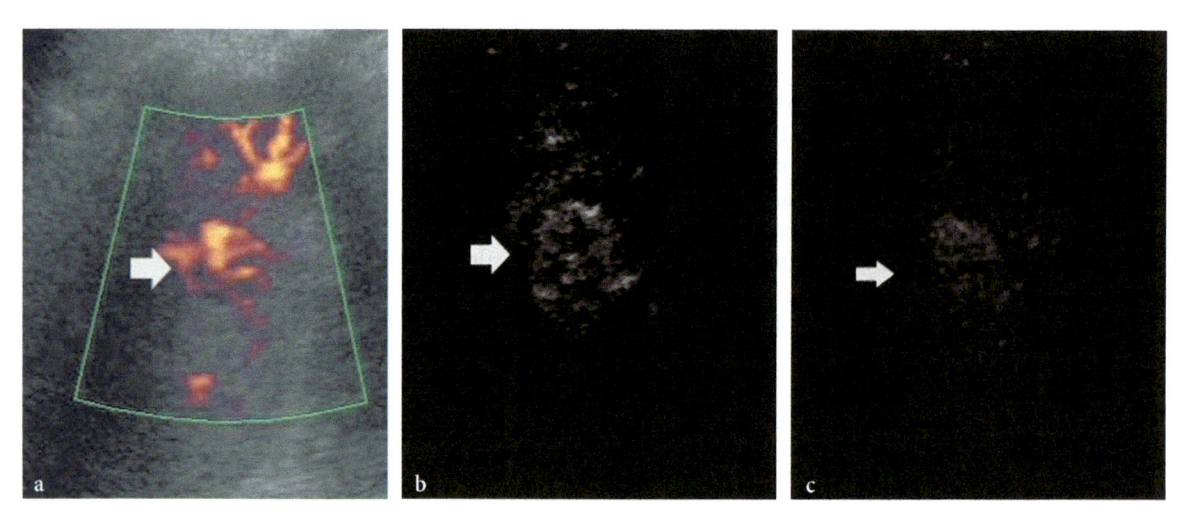

Fig. 14.8a–c. Small splenic haemangioma. The lesion (*arrow*) appears hypervascular with peripheral and central vessels on Power Doppler US (**a**). Diffuse and persistently homogeneous enhancement is evident (*arrow*) at phase inversion more (ATL-Philips, USA) both 25 s (**b**) and 2 min (**c**) after microbubble injection. (From the editor, E. Quaia).

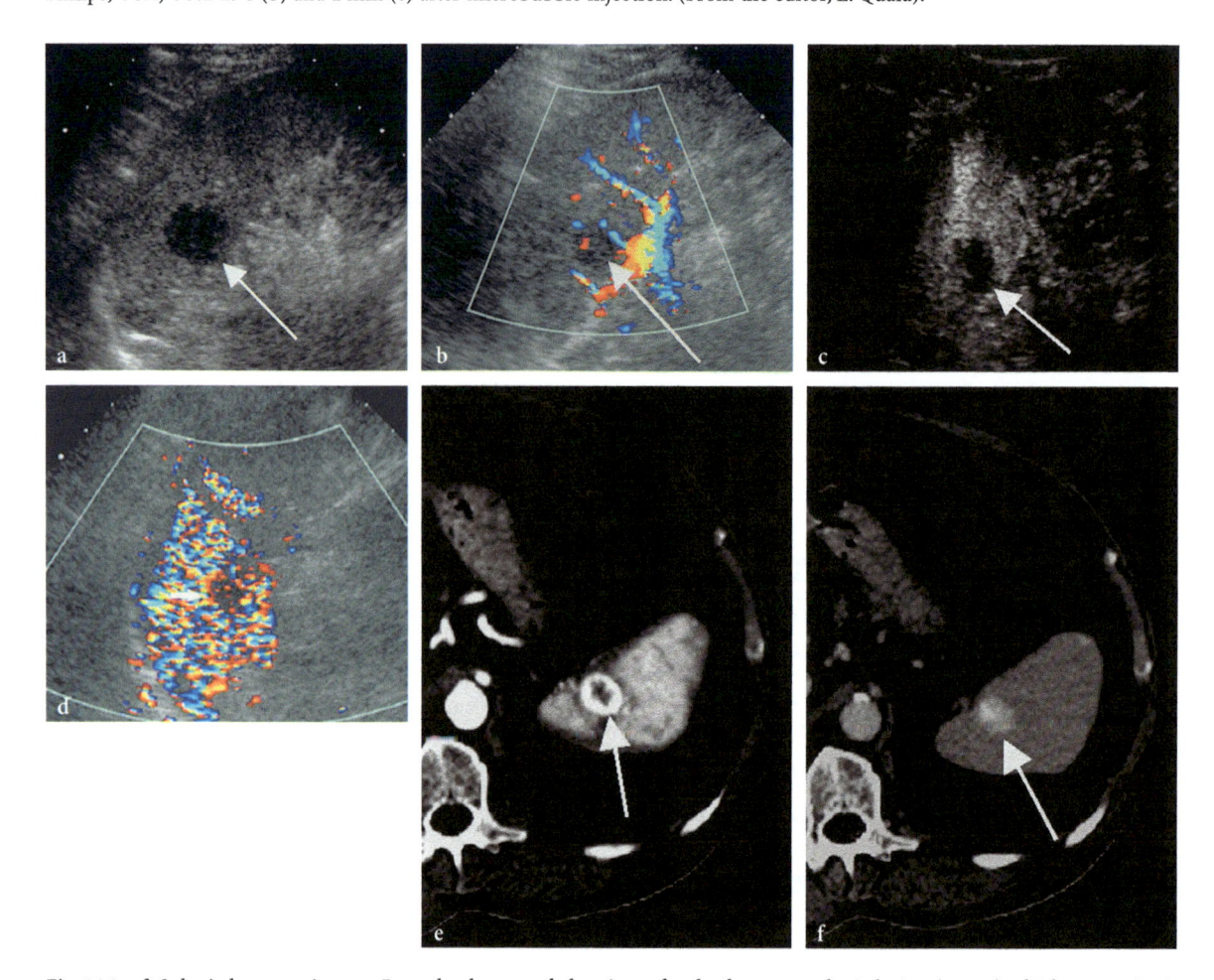

Fig. 14.9a–f. Splenic haemangioma. **a** B-mode ultrasound showing a focal echo-poor splenic lesion (*arrow*) which was an incidental finding. **b** No colour Doppler signal was present in the lesion (*arrow*). **c** Imaging in the late splenic-specific phase of Levovist using the phase inversion mode (ATL-Philips, USA) shows partial centripetal filling-in of the lesion (*arrow*) at 3 min post injection. **d** Imaging using the stimulated acoustic emission (SAE) mode also exhibits filling-in (*arrow*) at 3 min post injection. **e** Arterial phase CT shows intense peripheral enhancement (*arrow*). **f** Delayed phase CT (5 min post contrast) shows that the lesion (*arrow*) has completely filled in. The appearances are consistent with a haemangioma although the echo-poor appearance on B-mode ultrasound is atypical.

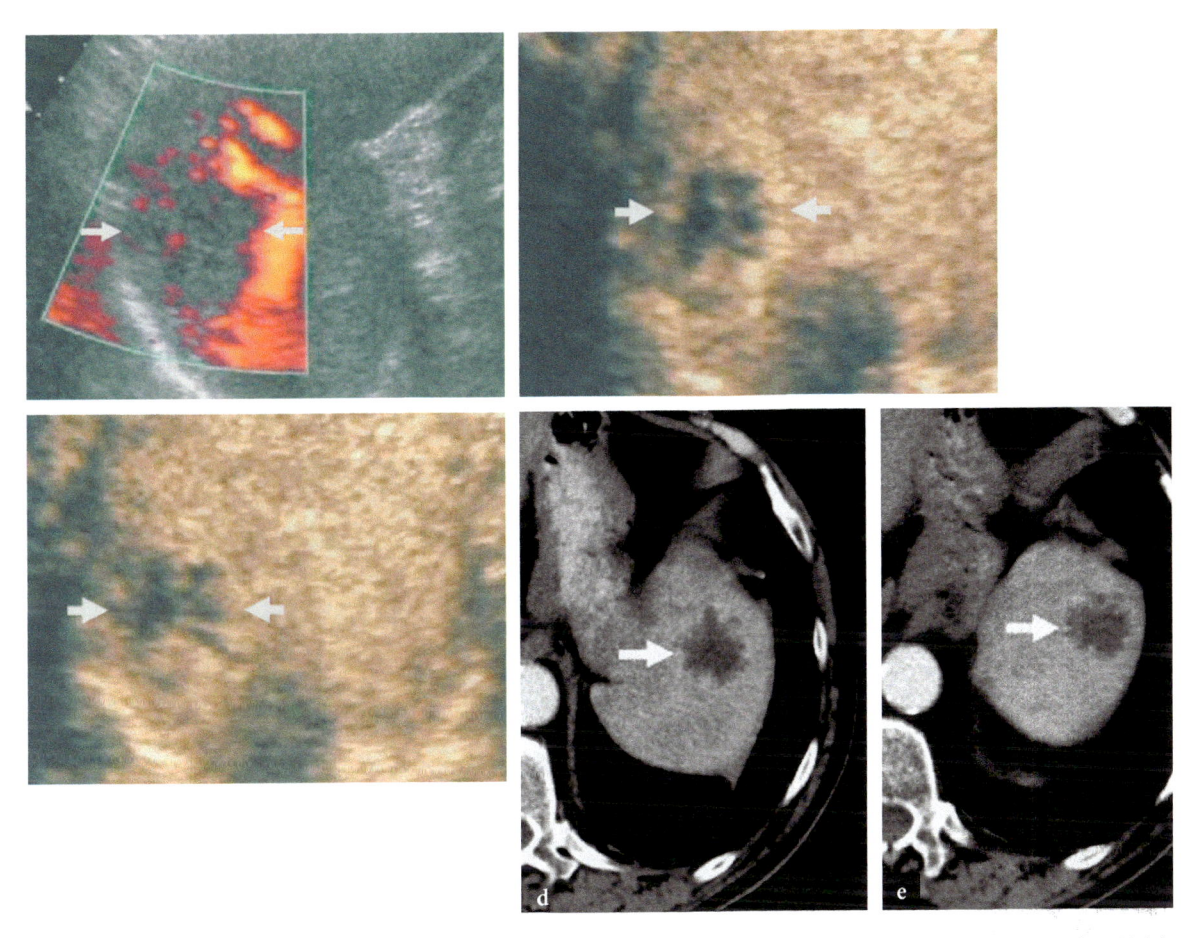

Fig. 14.10a-e. Large splenic haemangioma. The lesion (*arrows*) shows some central vessels on baseline power Doppler US (**a**). Globular peripheral enhancement with centripetal progression is evident (*arrows*) at 30 s (**b**) and 6 min (**c**) after microbubble injection at cadence contrast pulse sequence. The same pattern (*arrow*) is confirmed on contrast-enhanced CT during the arterial (**d**) and late (**e**) phases. (From the editor, E. Quaia).

spleen, are rare benign tumours occurring with an incidence of 0.024–0.13% in autopsies (SILVERMAN and LIVOISI 1978). Splenic hamartomas are usually found incidentally, although rupture has been described (FERGUSON et al. 1993).

On US, splenic hamartomas are usually solid homogeneous masses and hyperechoic relative to the adjacent splenic parenchyma (GORG and SCHWERK 1994; FERGUSON et al. 1993; RAMANI et al. 1997; WAN et al. 2000). However, some may be heterogeneous, with cystic changes and areas of calcification secondary to ischaemia or haemorrhage. They are usually hypervascular on colour Doppler (TANG et al. 2000) (Fig. 14.11). This is thought to reflect the hypervascularity of the red pulp in the hamartoma. Variable enhancement is seen following intravenous microbubble injection.

Lymphangioma

Splenic lymphangioma is a rare slow-growing benign tumour. It is characterized by splenic cysts of varying sizes from a few millimetres to several centimetres (KOMATSUDA et al. 1999). Splenic lymphangiomas may occur in isolation or with multisystem organ involvement (RAO et al. 1981; MORGENSTERN et al. 1992; WADSWORTH et al. 1997; KOMATSUDA et al. 1999). Complications are associated with the more extensive or larger lymphangiomas and include bleeding, hypersplenism, consumptive coagulopathy and portal hypertension. Malignant transformation has been described in one case (FEIGENBERG et al. 1983).

On US, splenic lymphangiomas appear as cystic lesions with septation, echogenic debris and calcification (Fig. 14.12) (BEZZI et al. 2001). Lymphangi-

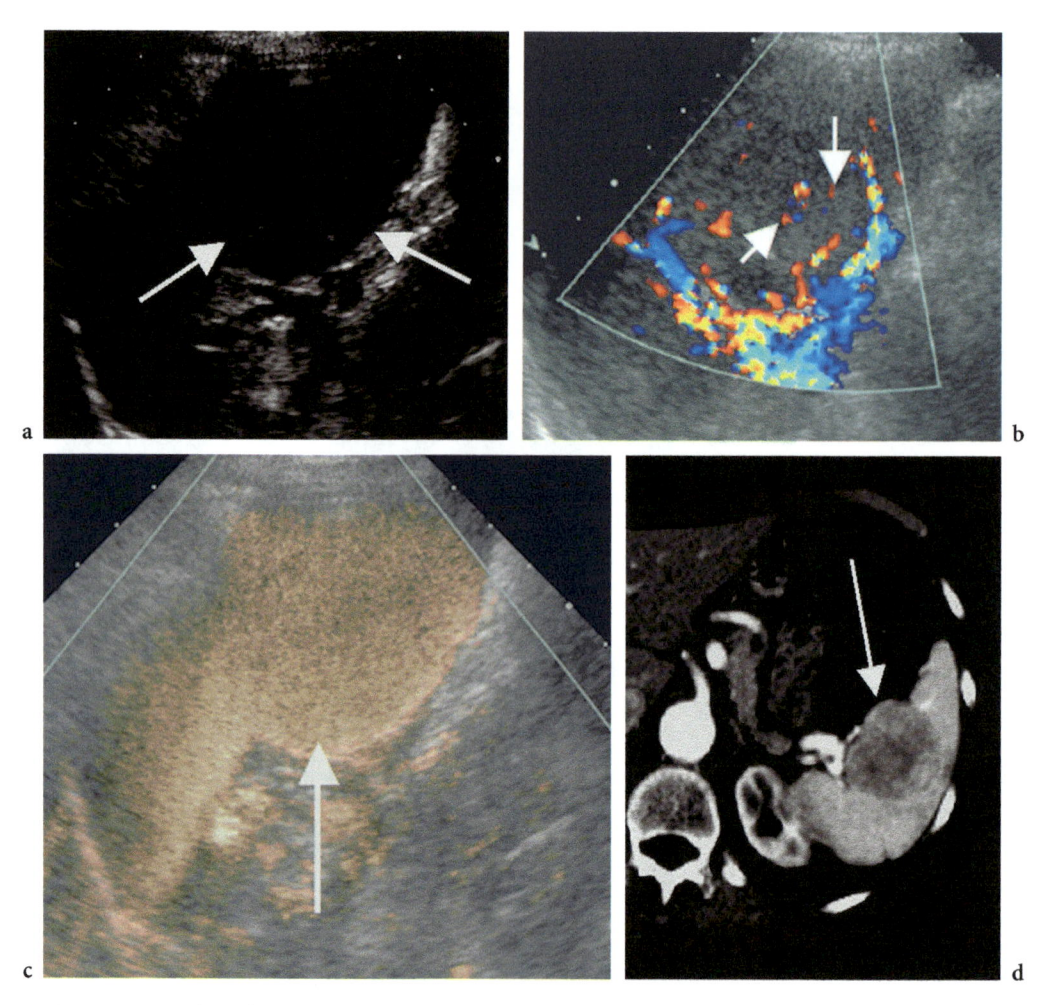

Fig. 14.11. a A splenic hamartoma (*arrows*) is seen as a slightly lower echogenicity focal lesion on B-mode ultrasound. b On colour Doppler imaging, flow is seen in a radial distribution (*arrows*). c Three minutes after Levovist injection, imaging using a late-phase destructive mode (Agent Detection Imaging; ADI, Acuson-Siemens, USA) demonstrates microbubble uptake in the hamartoma (*arrow*). d Contrast-enhanced CT showing a complex lobulated lesion with variable enhancement (*arrow*). Reproduced with permission from PEDDU et al. Clin Rad 2004; 59 777-792.

omas are avascular on colour Doppler and do not enhance with microbubbles. CT demonstrates lymphangiomas as typically subcapsular low-attenuation non enhancing septate lesions. The presence of curvilinear mural calcification is highly suggestive of lymphangioma (PISTOIA and MARKOWITZ 1988).

14.3.3
Malignant Focal Splenic Lesions

Malignant splenic tumours are uncommon. Primary lymphoma and angiosarcoma are well recognized but rare. Metastases most commonly occur from lymphoma, breast, ovary, bronchus and stomach.

Lymphoma

Malignant lymphoma is the most common cause of splenic infiltration. The typical US appearances are of echo-poor focal lesions that may be difficult to distinguish from cysts (WERNECKE et al. 1987; GORG et al. 1990). The borders of the lesions may be poorly defined. 'Target sign' lesions and echogenic lesions have been described (WERNECKE et al. 1987; GORG et al. 1990). Typically Hodgkin's and low-grade non-Hodgkin's lymphomas result in diffuse infiltration or focal lesions less than 3 cm in size (Fig. 14.13). By comparison, high-grade non-Hodgkin's lymphoma causes focal lesions of greater than 3 cm in size (GORG et al. 1990, 1991) (Fig. 14.14). With microbubbles,

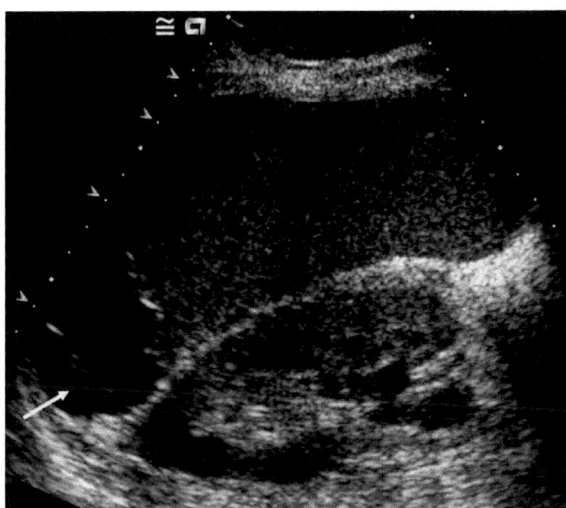

Applications of Ultrasound Microbubbles in the Spleen

Fig. 14.12. a A cystic, septate lesion in the upper aspect of the spleen (*arrow*) demonstrating features of a lymphangioma. **b** Post SonoVue (Bracco, Italy) imaging using a low mechanical index technique (Coherent Contrast Imaging, CCI, Acuson-Siemens, USA) defines the septate cystic lesion. **c** Contrast-enhanced CT of the lymphangioma clearly depicts the septations (*arrows*). Reproduced with permission from PEDDU et al. Clin Rad 2004; 59 777-792.

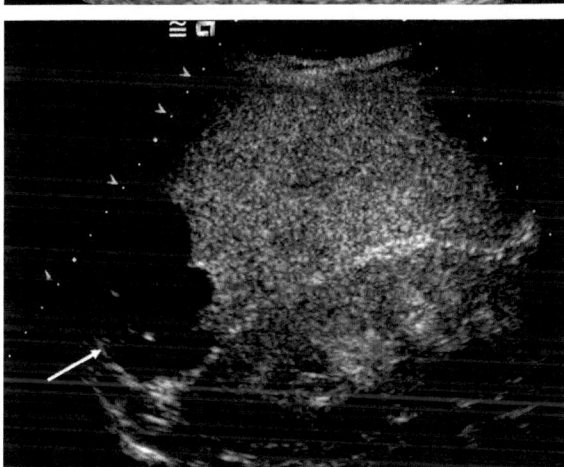

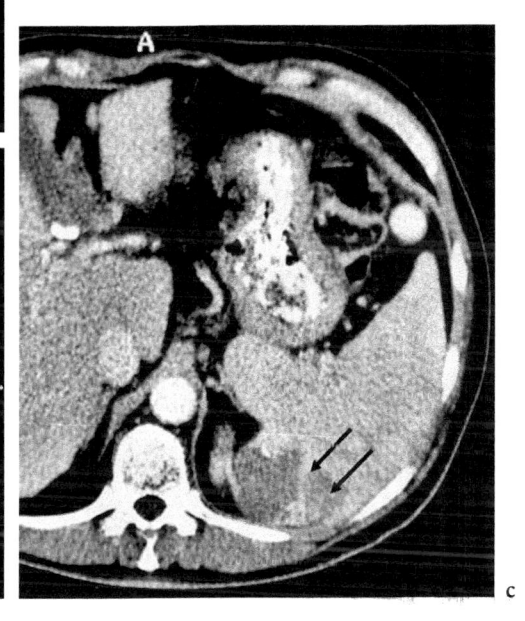

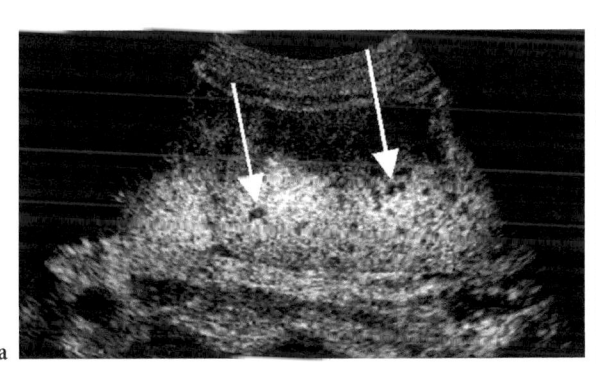

Fig. 14.13a,b. Case of Hodgkin's lymphoma. **a** Imaging in the phase-inversion mode (ATL-Philips, USA) 3 min after Levovist injection, showing multiple subcentimetre splenic lesions (*arrows*). No focal abnormality could be demonstrated on B-mode ultrasound (not shown). **b** Contrast-enhanced CT in the same patient shows no focal splenic lesions.

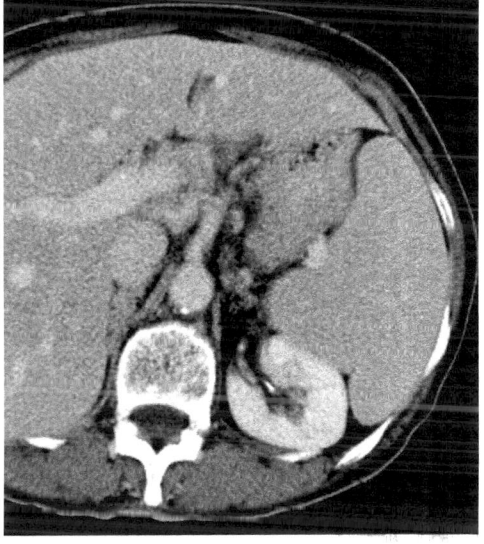

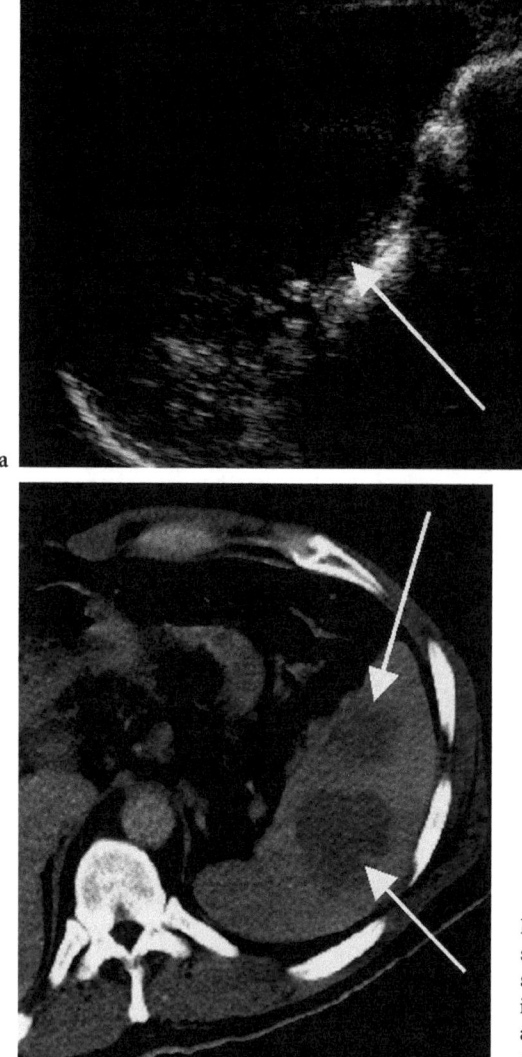

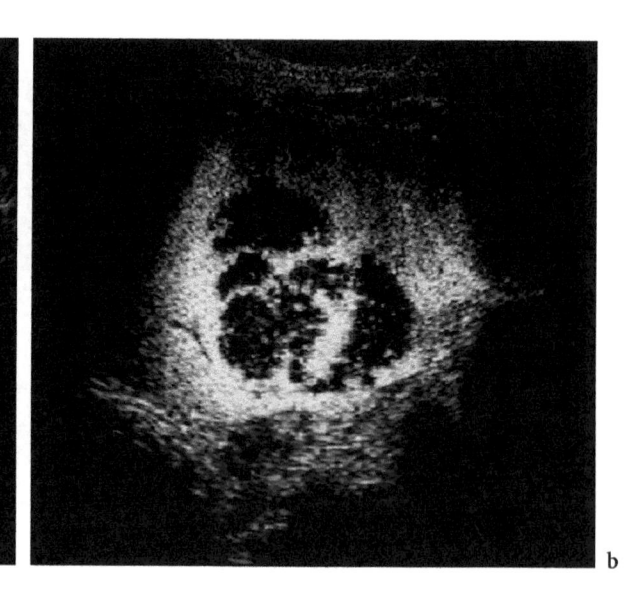

Fig. 14.14a–c. Case of non-Hodgkin's lymphoma. a Baseline B-mode US showing a complex echo-poor lesion (*arrow*). b Imaging in phase-inversion mode (ATL-Philips, USA) 3 min after Levovist injection, showing irregular peripheral microbubble uptake with the lesions appearing as defects that are more conspicuous than on B-mode. c Contrast-enhanced CT in the same patient shows multifocal hypodense splenic lesions (*arrows*).

irregular peripheral enhancement is seen, with the lesions appearing as defects in the late phase.

Metastases

Splenic metastases are rare: they are found in 7% of post-mortems in patients with metastatic carcinomas, and 8% of all splenic lesions were shown to be metastases in one series (Gorg et al. 1991). The spleen may be involved by direct tumour invasion in pancreatic tail, colon, stomach, bronchial and diaphragmatic carcinomas. The US appearances are variable, with echo-poor metastases being the most common (Gorg et al. 1990, 1991, 1994; Solbiati et al. 1983). Echogenic metastases are the least common (Mittelstaed and Partain 1980) and target lesions are less common than in the liver. Serosal metastases from ovarian carcinoma result in scalloping of the splenic margin. On Doppler, metastases are usually avascular. Imaging with microbubbles may show variable peripheral enhancement, with lesions appearing as defects surrounded by normally enhancing splenic parenchyma. Metastases may be revealed that are not seen on baseline B-mode (Harvey et al. 2000) (Figs. 14.15, 14.16) by increasing their conspicuity. This improves detection and facilitates the identification of subcentimetre metastases that would otherwise remain occult.

Applications of Ultrasound Microbubbles in the Spleen

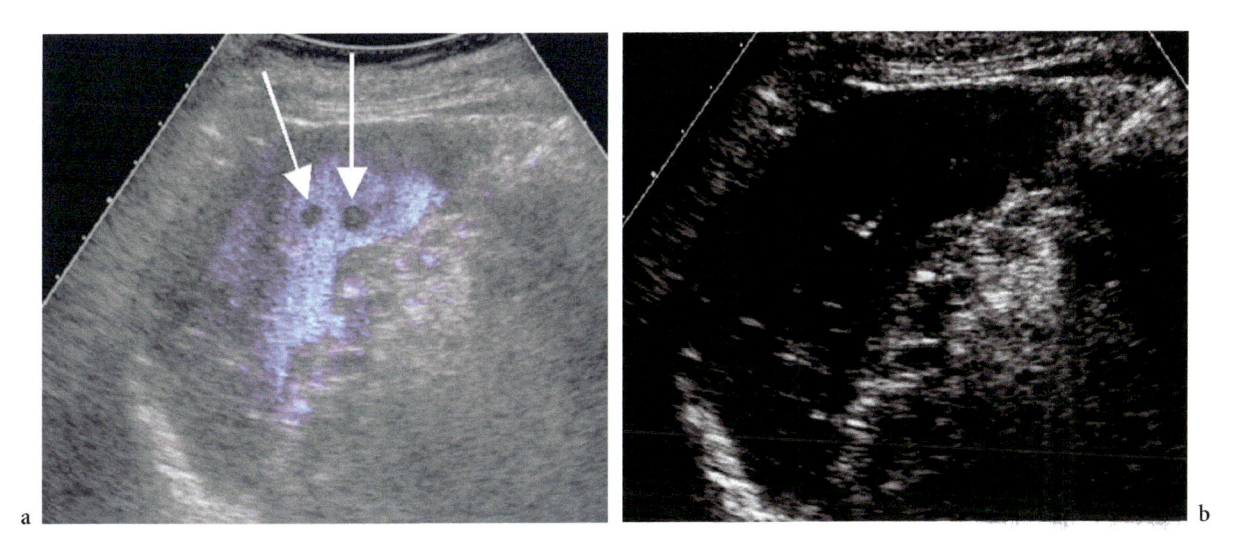

Fig. 14.15a,b. Splenic metastases from melanoma. **a** Three minutes after Levovist injection, imaging using a late-phase destructive mode (Agent Detection Imaging; ADI, Acuson-Siemens, USA) demonstrates two metastases as defects (*arrows*) surrounded by normal splenic microbubble uptake. **b** When the colour overlay is removed, no corresponding B-mode lesions could be identified. This case demonstrates that imaging of the late splenic-specific phase of Levovist improves the detection of occult metastases by increasing their conspicuity.

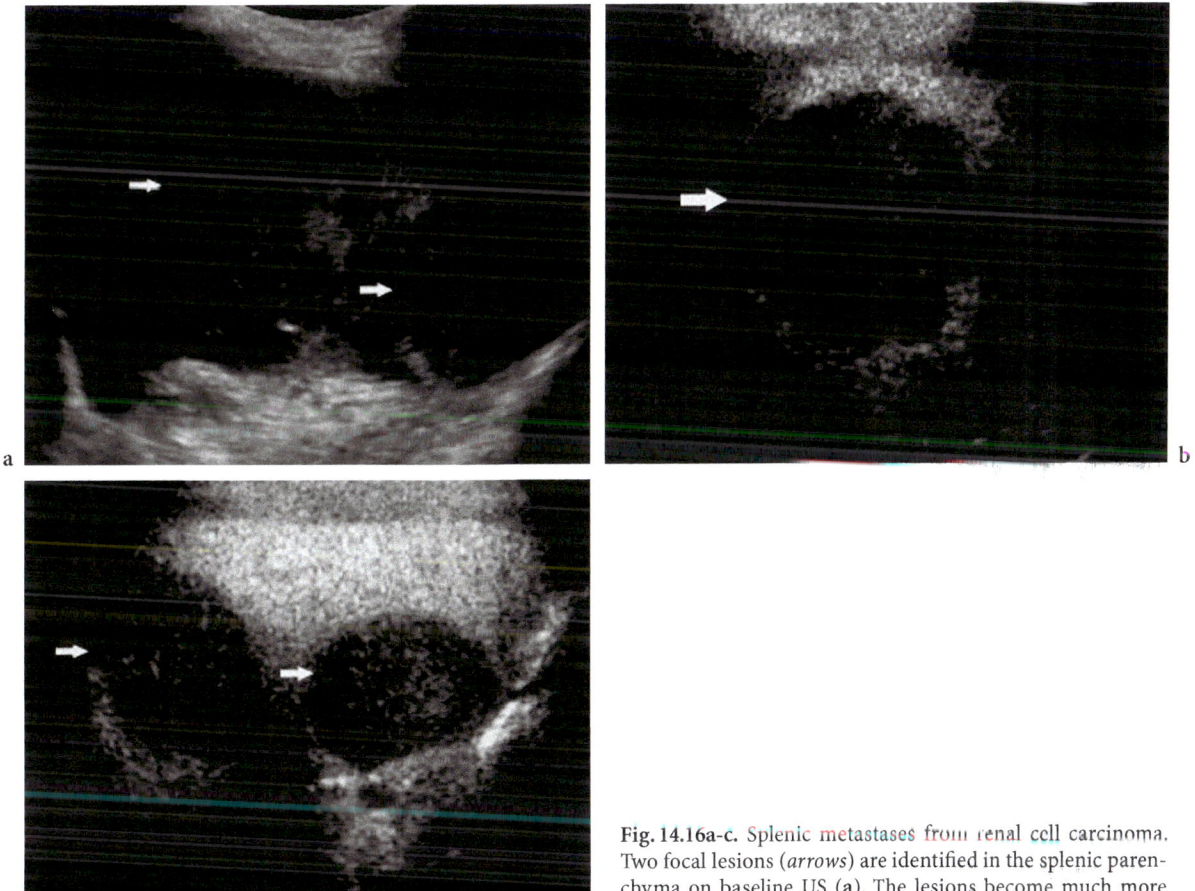

Fig. 14.16a-c. Splenic metastases from renal cell carcinoma. Two focal lesions (*arrows*) are identified in the splenic parenchyma on baseline US (**a**). The lesions become much more conspicuous (*arrows*) 120 s after microbubble injection at phase inversion mode (ATL-Philips, USA) (**b,c**). (From the editor, E. Quaia).

14.3.4
Splenic Infarction

Splenic infarction may result from emboli (endocarditis), hyperviscosity syndromes, sickle cell disease and myeloproliferative disorders. On B-mode, acute infarction is ill-defined, characteristically peripheral, wedge shaped and echo-poor (MARESCA et al. 1986; GORG and SCHWERK 1990; GORG et al. 1990, 1991, 1994; WAN et al. 2000). On colour Doppler, absent signals confirm the diagnosis. Chronic infarction is seen as an echogenic area due to fibrotic change or calcification with overlying cortical retraction secondary to scarring. Microbubbles improve the confidence in diagnosing early infarction with US (Figs. 14.17, 14.18).

14.3.5
Splenic Abscesses

Splenic abscesses on US may be echo-poor, septated and irregularly walled, containing debris and gas (GORG and SCHWERK 1990; GORG et al. 1990, 1991, 1994; WAN et al. 2000). They may have variable peripheral vascularity. Microbubbles may show the vascular rim of the abscesses. Common organisms include *Mycobacterium tuberculosis* (KAPOOR et al. 1991), *Pneumocystis carinii* (HARVEY et al. 1987) and candidiasis. The latter have been described as showing a characteristic 'bull's eye' appearance with multifocal small lesions (0.5–2 cm in size) consisting of echogenic centres surrounded by echo-poor rims (GORG et al. 1994; PORCEL-MARTIN et al. 1998). The detection of these lesions is improved by using a high-frequency linear probe (MURRAY et al. 1995). US contrast improves the detection of microabscesses by improving their conspicuity against the normal splenic parenchyma (Fig. 14.19).

14.3.6
Heterogeneous Splenic Echotexture

This is seen as multiple tiny (2–3 mm) echogenic foci or just a heterogeneous echo pattern on B-mode US. It is a non-specific finding typically seen in previous granulomatous infection such as tuberculosis and fungal disease, as well as sarcoidosis (Fig. 14.20) (KESSLER et al. 1993), Wegener's granulomatosis, amyloidosis and Crohn's disease.

14.4
Summary

US is a reliable method of imaging splenic abnormalities. The introduction of microbubbles has further improved the diagnostic capabilities of US, allowing the investigation of splenic enhancement patterns and characterization of focal lesions. US imaging with contrast is useful in distinguishing splenunculi from lymph nodes, demonstrating the characteristic enhancement patterns in haemangiomas, improving the visualization of splenic infarction and improving the detection of microabscesses and focal malignancies.

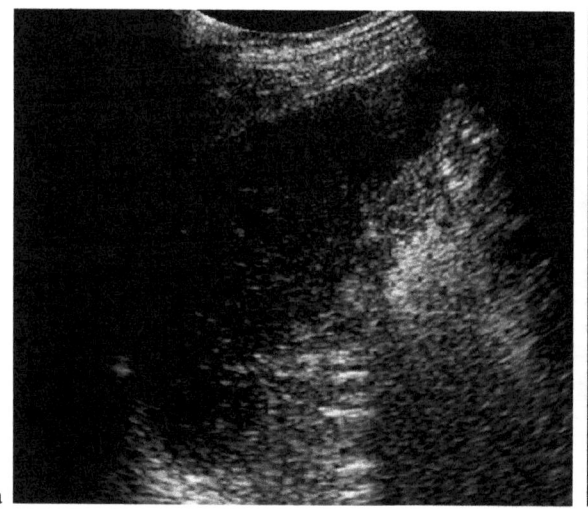

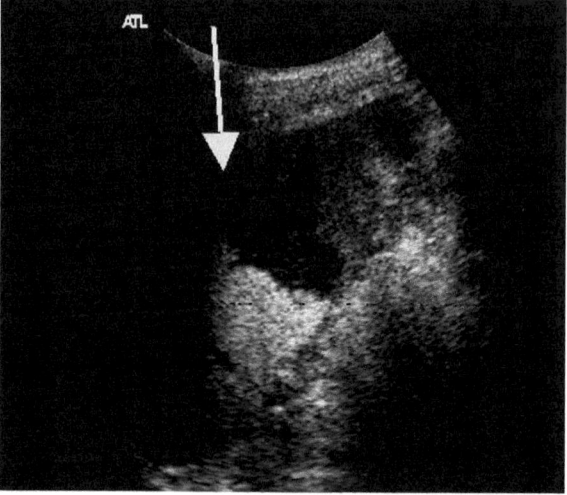

Fig 14.17a,b. This 56-year-old man presented with left upper quadrant pain. a B-mode ultrasound appears normal. b Imaging in phase-inversion mode 3 min after Levovist injection shows a wedge-shaped non-enhancing defect consistent with an infarct (*arrow*), with normal enhancement of the surrounding spleen.

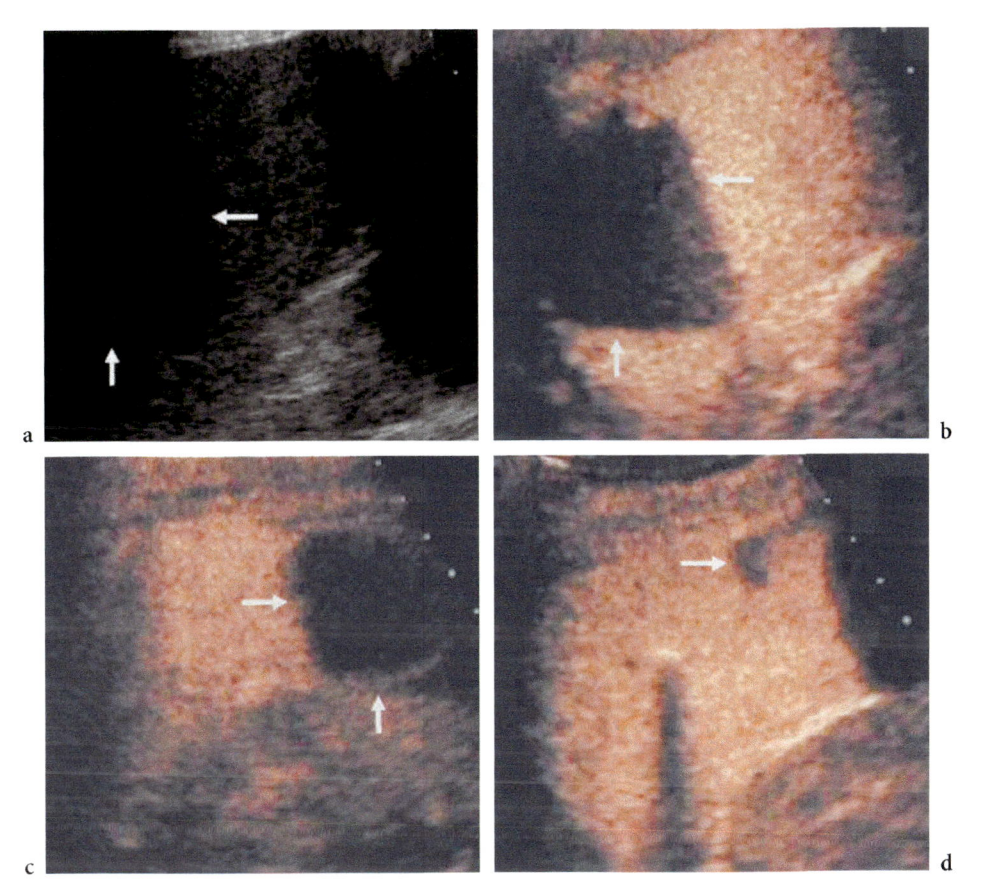

Applications of Ultrasound Microbubbles in the Spleen

Fig. 14.18a–d. Splenic perfusion defects in an enlarged spleen. Baseline US (**a**) reveals an enlarged spleen with one wedge-shaped splenic perfusion defect (*arrows*) with the base on the splenic capsule, which becomes much more conspicuous (*arrows*) 100 s after microbubble injection (**b**). Two further splenic infarcts become evident after microbubble injection, during the late phase at cadence contrast pulse sequence (*arrows* **c, d**). (From the editor, E. Quaia).

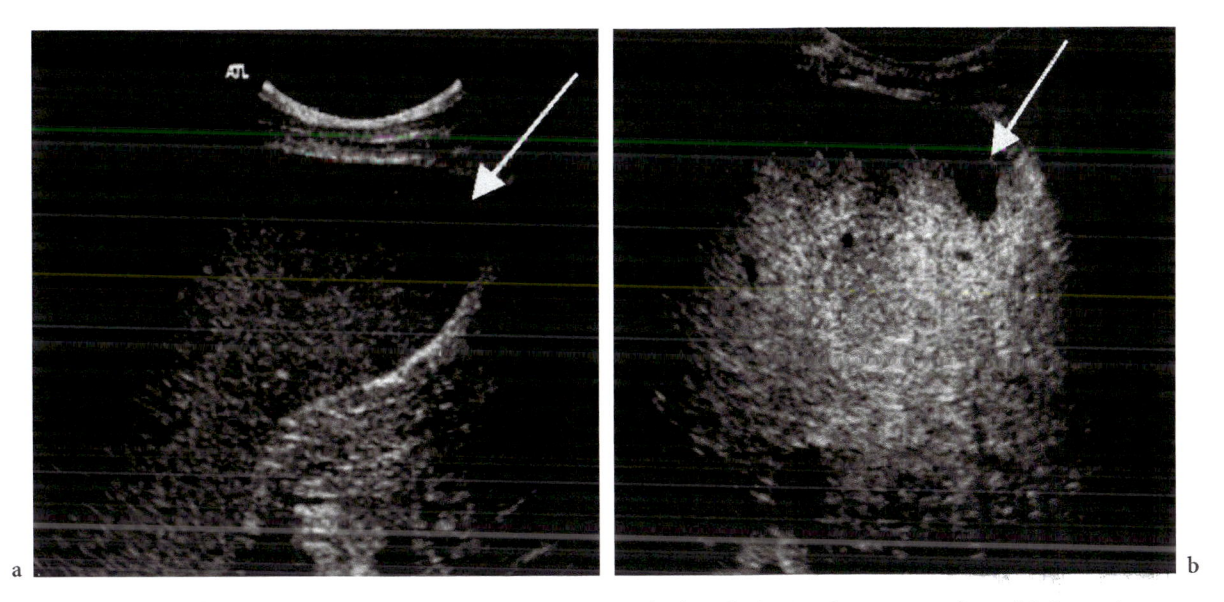

Fig. 14.19. a B-mode US of the spleen in a patient with disseminated tuberculosis. An echo-poor mycobacterial abscess is seen (*arrow*). **b** Post-microbubble contrast media imaging (Levovist) using the phase-inversion mode (ATL-Philips, USA) increases the conspicuity of the lesion (*arrow*), which is surrounded by normally enhancing spleen.

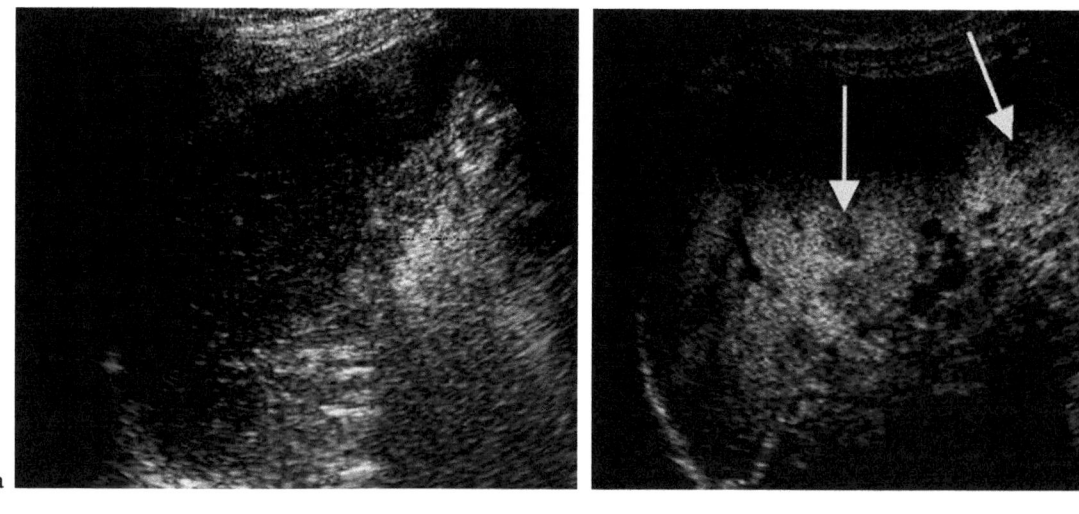

Fig. 14.20a,b. A 43-year-old woman with known sarcoidosis presented with abnormal liver function tests. a B-mode ultrasound of the spleen was normal. b Post-microbubble contrast media imaging (Levovist) using the phase-inversion mode (ATL-Philips, USA) revealed a heterogeneous enhancement pattern with multiple subcentimetre defects (*arrows*) not seen on B-mode and consistent with multifocal granulomatous infiltration. The same pattern was seen in the liver (not shown).

References

Abbott RM, Levy AD, Aguilera NS et al (2004) Primary vascular neoplasms of the spleen: radiologic-pathologic correlation. Radiographics 24:1137-1163

Beggs I (1985) The radiology of hydatid disease. AJR Am J Roentgenol 145:639-648

Bertolotto M, Gioulis E, Ricci C et al (1998) Ultrasound and Doppler features of accessory spleens and grafts. Br J Radiol 71:595-600

Bezzi M, Spinelli A, Pierleoni M, Andreoli G (2001) Cystic lymphangioma of the spleen: US-CT-MR correlation. Eur Radiol 11:1187-1190

Blomley MJK, Albrecht T, Cosgrove DO et al (1999) Stimulated acoustic emission to image a late liver and spleen-specific phase of Levovist in normal volunteers and patients with and without liver disease. Ultrasound Med Biol 25:1341-1352

Correas JM, Bridal L, Lesavre A et al (2001) Ultrasound contrast agents: properties, principles of action, tolerance, and artifacts. Eur Radiol 11:1316-1328

Dachman AH, Ros PR, Murari PJ et al (1986) Nonparasitic splenic cysts: a report of 52 cases with radiologic-pathologic correlation. AJR 147: 537-542

Feigenberg Z, Wysenbeek A, Avidor E, Dintsman M (1983) Malignant lymphangioma of the spleen. Isr J Med Sci 19:202-204

Ferguson ER, Sardi A, Beckman EN (1993) Spontaneous rupture of splenic hamartoma. J La State Med Soc 145:48-52

Ferrozzi F, Bova D, Draghi F, Garlaschi G (1996) CT findings in primary vascular tumors of the spleen. AJR Am J Roentgenol 166:1097-1101

Forsberg F, Goldberg BB, Liu JB et al (1999) Tissue-specific US contrast agent for evaluation of hepatic and splenic parenchyma. Radiology 210:125-132

Glazer GM, Axel L, Goldberg HI, Moss AA (1981) Dynamic CT of the normal spleen. AJR Am J Roentgenol 137:343-346

Gorg C (2001) The spleen. In: Meire H, Cosgrove DO, Dewbury K, Farrant P (eds) Clinical ultrasound (a comprehensive text). Abdominal and general ultrasound, 2nd edn. Churchill-Livingstone, Edinburgh, pp 379-445

Gorg C, Schwerk WB (1990) Splenic infarction: sonographic patterns, diagnosis, follow-up and complications. Radiology 174:803-807

Gorg C, Schwerk WB (1994) Color Doppler imaging of focal splenic masses. Eur J Radiol 18:214-219

Gorg C, Schwerk WB, Gorg K, Havermann K (1990) Sonographic patterns of the affected spleen in malignant lymphoma. J Clin Ultrasound 18:569-574

Gorg C, Schwerk WB, Gorg K (1991) Sonography of focal lesions of the spleen. AJR Am J Roentgenol 156:949-953

Gorg C, Weide R, Schwerk WB et al (1994) Ultrasound evaluation of hepatic and splenic microabscesses in the immunocompromised patient: sonographic patterns, differential diagnosis and follow-up. J Clin Ultrasound 22:525-529

Groom AC (1987) The Microcirculatory Society Eugene M. Landis award lecture. Microcirculation of the spleen: new concepts, new challenges. Microvasc Res 34:269-289

Harvey CJ, Rockall AG, Lees WR, Miller RF (1987) Splenic pneumocystosis in AIDS: unusual ultrasound appearances. Int J STD AIDS 8:342-344

Harvey CJ, Blomley MJK, Eckersley RJ et al (2000) Hepatic malignancies: improved detection with pulse inversion US in late phase of enhancement with SH U 508A - early experience. Radiology 216:903-908

Harvey CJ, Blomley M, Cosgrove DO et al (2000) Characterisation of splenic lesions using pulse inversion mode and stimulated acoustic emission (SAE) imaging with the ultrasound contrast agent Levovist. Eur Radiol 10 (suppl 1):S120

Harvey CJ, Albrecht T (2001) Ultrasound of focal liver lesions. Eur Radiol 11(9):1578-1593

Harvey CJ, Blomley MJ, Eckersley RJ, Cosgrove DO (2001) Developments in ultrasound contrast media. Eur Radiol 11:675-689

Harvey CJ, Pilcher J, Eckerley R, Blomley MJK, Cosgrove DO (2002) Advances in Ultrasound. Clin Rad 57:157-177.

Husni EA (1961) The clinical course of splenic haemangioma with emphasis on spontaneous rupture. Arch Surg 83:681-688

Iijima H, Miyahara T, Suzuki S et al (2003) Sinusoidal endothelium and microbubble: Kupffer imaging and bioeffect. Ultrasound Med Biol 29:S222

Kapoor R, Jain AK, Chatulvedi U, Saha MM (1991) Case report: ultrasound detection of tuberculomas of the spleen. Clin Rad 43:128-129

Kessler A, Mitchell DG, Israel HL, Goldberg BB (1993) Hepatic and splenic sarcoidosis: ultrasound and MR imaging. Abdom Imaging 18:159-163

Komatsuda T, Ishida H, Konno K et al (1999) Splenic lymphangioma: ultrasound and CT diagnosis and clinical manifestations. Abdom Imaging 24:414-417

Kono Y, Steinbach GC, Peterson T et al (2002) Mechanism of parenchymal enhancement of the liver with microbubble-based US contrast medium; an intravital microscopy study in rats. Radiology 224:253-257

Leen E, Ramnarine K, Kyriakopoulou K et al (1998) Improved characterization of focal liver tumors: dynamic doppler imaging using NC100100: a new liver specific echoenhancer. Radiology 209:293

Lim AKP, Patel N, Eckersley RJ et al (2004) Evidence for spleen-specific uptake of a microbubble contrast agent: a quantitative study in healthy volunteers. Radiology 231:785-788

Maresca G, De Gaetano A, Barbaro B, Colagrande C (1986) Sonographic patterns in splenic infarct. J Clin Ultrasound 14:23-28

Massey MD, Stevens JS (1991) Residual spleen found on denatured red blood cell scan following negative colloid scans. J Nucl Med 32:2286-2287

Mirowitz SA, Gutierrez E, Lee JK et al (1991) Normal abdominal enhancement patterns with dynamic gadolinium-enhanced MR imaging. Radiology 180:637-640

Mittelstaed C, Partain L (1980) Ultrasonographic classification of splenic abnormalities gray scale patterns. Radiology 134:697

Morgenstern L, Bello JM, Fisher BL, Verham RP (1992) Clinical spectrum of lymphangiomas and lymphangiomatosis of the spleen. Am Surg 58:599-604

Murray JG, Patel MD, Lee S et al (1995) Microabscesses of the liver and spleen in AIDS: detection with 5-MHz sonography. Radiology 197:723-727

Peddu P, Shah M, Sidhu PS (2004) Splenic abnormalities: a comparative review of ultrasound, microbubble-enhanced ultrasound and computed tomography. Clin Rad 59:777-792

Person RE, Bender JM (2000) Hepatic lesion differentiated from accessory spleen by a heat-damaged red blood cell scan. Clin Nucl Med 25:516-518

Pistoia F, Markowitz SK (1988) Splenic lymphangiomatosis: CT diagnosis. AJR Am J Roentgenol 150:121-122

Polat P, Kantarci M, Alper F et al (2003) Hydatid disease from head to toe. Radiographics 23:475-494

Porcel-Martin A, Rendon-Unceta P, Bascunana-Quirell A et al (1998) Focal splenic lesions in patients with AIDS: sonographic findings. Abdom Imaging 23:196-200

Ramani M, Reinhold C, Semelka R et al (1997) Splenic haemangiomas and hamartomas: MR imaging characteristics of 28 lesions. Radiology 202:166-172

Rao B, AuBuchon J, Lieberman L, Polcyn R (1981) Cystic lymphangiomatosis of the spleen: a radiologic-pathologic correlation. Radiology 141:781-782

Ros P, Moser R Jr, Dachman A et al (1987) Haemangioma of the spleen: radiologic-pathologic correlation in ten cases. Radiology 162:73-77

Schneider M, Arditi M, Barrau MB et al (1995) BR1: a new ultrasonographic contrast agent based on sulfur hexafluoride-filled microbubbles. Invest Radiol 30:451-457

Silverman ML, Livoisi VA (1978) Splenic hamartomas. Am J Clin Pathol 70:224-229

Siniluoto TM, Paivansalo MJ, Lahde ST et al (1994) Nonparasitic splenic cysts: Ultrasound features and follow-up. Acta Radiol 35:447-451

Solbiati L, Bossi MC, Belotti F et al (1983) Focal lesions in the spleen: sonographic patterns and guided biopsy. AJR Am J Roentgenol 140:59-65

Tang S, Shimizu T, Kikuchi Y et al (2000) Colour Doppler sonographic findings in splenic hamartoma. J Clin Ultrasound 28:249-253

Urrutia M, Mergo PJ, Ros LH et al (1996) Cystic masses of the spleen: radiologic-pathologic correlation. Radiographics 16:107-129

Wadham BM, Adams PB, Johnson MA (1981) Incidence and location of accessory spleens. N Engl J Med 304:1111

Wadsworth DT, Newman B, Abramson SJ et al (1997) Splenic lymphangiomatosis in children. Radiology 202:173-176

Wan YL, Cheung YC, Lui KW et al (2000) Ultrasonographic findings and differentiation of benign and malignant focal splenic lesions. Postgraduate Med J 76:488-493

Wernecke K, Peters PE, Kruger KG (1987) Ultrasonographic patterns of focal hepatic and splenic lesions in Hodgkin's and low-grade non-Hodgkin's lymphoma. Br J Radiol 60:655-660

Abdominal Applications: Kidneys

15 Characterization and Detection of Renal Tumors

Emilio Quaia

CONTENTS

15.1 Introduction 223
15.2 Dynamic Phases in Renal Parenchyma Enhancement After Microbubble Injection 224
15.3 Scanning Modes 224
15.4 Contrast Enhancement Patterns in Solid Renal Tumors After Microbubble Injection 225
15.5 Benign Solid Renal Tumors 225
15.5.1 Embryonal Metanephric Adenoma 225
15.5.2 Angiomyolipoma 226
15.5.3 Renal Oncocytoma 227
15.6 Malignant Solid Renal Tumors 229
15.6.1 Solid Renal Cell Carcinoma 229
15.6.2 Renal Metastasis 232
15.7 Contrast Enhancement Patterns in Cystic Renal Tumors After Microbubble Injection 236
15.7.1 Benign Cystic Renal Tumors 237
15.7.2 Malignant Cystic Renal Tumors 237
15.8 Clinical Results 239
15.9 Detection of Renal Tumors 242
15.10 When Should Microbubble-Based Agents Be Employed? 242
References 243

15.1 Introduction

Baseline gray-scale ultrasound (US), which may be supplemented by speckle- and noise-reducing techniques such as tissue harmonic imaging and compound imaging (CLAUDON et al. 2002), is a reliable imaging technique for the early diagnosis of renal tumors (HÉLÉNON et al. 2001).

a) Solid renal tumors. Baseline gray-scale US may reveal various echo patterns which are considered essential in the characterization of solid renal tumors. A hypoechoic appearance, sometimes with evidence of an anechoic rim or small intratumoral cysts, is frequently observed in renal cell carcinoma, while a homogeneously bright and wedge-shaped appearance, with evidence of posterior acoustic shadowing, is considered typical for renal angiomyolipoma (YAMASHITA et al. 1992; HÉLÉNON et al. 1997, 2001; JINZAKI et al. 1997). Some typical US patterns have also been described for renal oncocytoma, such as the presence of a central scar that appears as a stellate hypoechoic area and the absence of hemorrhage and necrosis (HÉLÉNON et al. 2001).

Nevertheless, baseline US has low accuracy in the characterization of renal masses, especially if smaller than 4 cm in diameter, since benign and malignant tumors frequently present a similar appearance (CORREAS et al. 1999). In fact, approximately 30% of small renal cell carcinomas appear as hyperechoic masses (FORMAN et al. 1993), while atypical iso-hypoechoic and slightly hyperechoic angiomyolipomas account for 6% and 29% respectively (HÉLÉNON et al. 2001). Furthermore, even benign and malignant renal masses >4 cm may present a similar appearance, and large renal cell carcinomas can resemble large angiomyolipomas on baseline US (large renal cell carcinomas usually display a heterogeneous appearance due to intratumoral necrosis, calcifications, and hemorrhage, while large angiomyolipomas may also appear heterogeneous owing to solid, adipose, and hemorrhagic components).

Power Doppler and color Doppler US may reveal different vascular patterns in renal tumors. JINZAKI et al. (1998) identified four vascular patterns relevant to lesion characterization. Intratumoral (pattern 1) or penetrating (pattern 2) vessels were described as typical for benign renal tumors, and in particular for angiomyolipoma, while peripheral (patterns 3) or mixed penetrating and peripheral (pattern 4) vessels were considered typical for renal cell carcinomas, even though they could also be observed in 20% of renal angiomyolipomas.

Even though the description of these vascular patterns represents a first endeavor to differentiate the different histotypes of renal tumors using color and power Doppler, this technique does not significantly

---

E. QUAIA, MD
Assistant Professor of Radiology, Department of Radiology, Cattinara Hospital, University of Trieste, Strada di Fiume 447, 34149 Trieste, Italy

improve US capabilities in the characterization of renal tumors (Hélénon et al. 2001) . This is because benign and malignant renal tumors may present a similar vascular architecture on color and power Doppler US (Kier et al. 1990; Correas et al. 1999).

b) Cystic renal tumors. Renal cystic tumors have been classified according to their computed tomography (CT) appearance (Bosniak 1986; Israel and Bosniak 2003a). Type 1 are simple benign cysts containing fluid with the attenuation of water and having thin walls without septa or calcification, while type 2 are minimally complicated cysts. These masses are benign cystic lesions that may contain hairline-thin septa, fine calcification in the walls or septa, or a short segment of slightly thickened calcification. Minimal enhancement of a hairline-thin, smooth septum or wall is sometimes present. Category 2F (F means follow-up) lesions are more complex cysts that cannot be classified either as category 2 or as category 3 cysts. These cysts may contain an increased number of septa and an increased amount of calcifications, which may be thicker and nodular (Israel and Bosniak 2003a).

Type 3 are indeterminate cystic masses since their benignity or malignancy cannot be determined with imaging studies. These lesions have thick peripheral walls or septa, may appear hyperdense, and may contain either small or large amounts of calcification. Enhancement of the wall or septa can be clearly appreciated on contrast material-enhanced CT. If findings are equivocal or suspicious, follow-up in 3–6 months with renal CT is recommended (Zagoria 2000).

Type 4 are cystic renal tumors. Category 4 lesions are malignant cystic masses containing either small or large amounts of calcification within a thick, enhancing irregular wall or septum. Enhancing soft tissue components are present adjacent to or extending from, but are independent of, the wall or septum.

Type 1 or 2 cysts and type 4 cysts, respectively benign and malignant, are characterized by baseline US (Hélénon et al. 2001). When the imaging features on CT are equivocal for benign versus malignant cystic renal masses, US may further show the internal architecture of the cystic renal mass (Zagoria 2000). Calcification in a cystic renal mass is not as important in diagnosis as the presence of associated enhancing soft tissue elements (Israel and Bosniak 2003a). Color signal saturation, motion and blooming artifacts, insensitivity to the flow of capillary vessels, and limited sensitivity to the signal produced by microbubble-based agents represent important limitations of color Doppler US. Microbubble-based contrast agents and dedicated US contrast-specific modes have been introduced to overcome the limitations of baseline gray-scale and color Doppler US.

15.2
Dynamic Phases in Renal Parenchyma Enhancement After Microbubble Injection

The injection of iodinated or paramagnetic contrast agents shows different phases of nephrographic progression, including the vascular (15–25 s), the corticomedullary or cortical nephrographic (25–80 s), the nephrographic or diffuse nephrographic (85–120 s), and the excretory (3–5 min post injection) phases. A hyperattenuating cortical nephrogram with corticomedullary differentiation is obtained during the corticomedullary phase, while a homogeneous nephrogram can be obtained during the nephrographic phase. Unlike contrast agents employed in CT or magnetic resonance (MR) imaging, which present an interstitial phase, microbubbles remain entirely intravascular and may be considered as pure blood pool agents which are not excreted by the kidneys and present neither a nephrographic nor an excretory phase.

Renal cortex rapidly enhances from 15 to 20 s after microbubble injection, while the vessels of the renal medulla are progressively filled from 30 to 35 s and completely filled from 40 to 50 s after microbubble injection. This is because the renal medulla has a lower global perfusion than renal cortex (about 400 vs 190 ml/min per 100 g of renal tissue). For these reasons, it is appropriate to identify, after microbubble injection, an early or arterial corticomedullary phase (from 20 to 40 s) with corticomedullary differentiation and a late corticomedullary phase (from 45 to 120 s) with homogeneous enhancement in both renal cortex and medulla.

15.3
Scanning Modes

Each renal tumor must undergo preliminary scanning by baseline gray-scale and color Doppler US, including with the employment of a speckle-reducing technique such as tissue harmonic imaging or compound imaging (Claudon et al. 2002). Baseline color Doppler US is performed by using slow-flow settings (pulse repetition frequency 800–1,500 Hz, wall filter of 50 Hz, high levels of color versus echo priority, and color persistence). Color gain is varied dynamically during the examination to enhance color signals and avoid excessive noise, with the size of the color box being adjusted to include the entire lesion in the field of view. Spectral analysis of central and peripheral tumoral vessels is performed by pulsed Doppler to reveal continuous venous or pulsatile arterial flows.

After baseline assessment, the employment of contrast-specific US modes with microbubbles may provide important additional findings relevant to renal tumor characterization. As in the scanning of focal liver lesions (HARVEY et al. 2000), high or low acoustic power mode insonation may be employed.

a) Destructive high acoustic power intermittent mode. The high acoustic power mode has to be employed with air-filled microbubble contrast agents. When insonated with a high acoustic power (mechanical index, MI>0.8–1), microbubbles collapse, producing a high-intensity, broadband transient signal which may be detected using dedicated contrast-specific techniques. Before microbubble injection, a suitable acoustic window offering the best visualization of the renal mass on the axial or longitudinal plane has to be identified with one single focus below the tumor. During breath-hold, different high acoustic power trains of four to six US pulses are transmitted intermittently by using manual (every 25–30 s) or ECG-triggered insonation to minimize microbubble rupture. High acoustic power insonation has the advantage of producing high-intensity harmonic signals, though it has several drawbacks, e.g., intermittence of insonation, technical difficulty of performance, and a high incidence of artifacts.

b) Nondestructive low acoustic power continuous mode. Renal masses are insonated continuously during both the early and the late corticomedullary phase in real time by employing a low acoustic power mode to achieve microbubble resonance with production of harmonic frequencies. The low acoustic power mode has to be employed with perfluorocarbon- or sulfur hexafluoride-filled microbubble contrast agents, such as SonoVue (BR1, Bracco, Milan, Italy), Definity (DMP 115, Du Pont Merck, Billerica, USA), and Optison (FS069, developed by Molecular Biosystem Inc., San Diego, CA; distributed by Amersham Health Inc., Princeton, NJ). These agents have been reported to increase diagnostic confidence in the characterization of renal tumors, to improve renal lesion conspicuity, and to effectively delineate tumoral microvessels (BARR et al. 2001; CORREAS et al. 2001).

The low acoustic power mode is technically more simple to perform than the high acoustic power mode since the sonologist may change transducer position during scanning and may perform a real-time sweep without the risk of losing the correct scanning plane. Moreover, the low acoustic power mode allows more effective suppression of the background signal arising from the native tissues and selective visualization of microbubbles with a reduced frequency of artifacts. However, the low acoustic power mode has a lower signal to noise ratio and offers limited visibility of the deep parenchymal regions due to US signal attenuation.

15.4
Contrast Enhancement Patterns in Solid Renal Tumors After Microbubble Injection

Different contrast enhancement patterns may be observed in both solid and cystic renal tumors.

Both in benign and in malignant solid renal tumors, four fundamental patterns of contrast enhancement may be visualized (Fig. 15.1): (a) absent, no difference in renal tumor appearance before and after microbubble injection; (b) dotted, tiny separate spots distributed throughout the lesion; (c) diffuse homogeneous, involving the entire lesion with the same echo intensity throughout the lesion, or (d) diffuse heterogeneous, involving the entire lesion.

The echogenicity of renal tumors on baseline gray-scale US and the tumoral vascularity and staining after microbubble-based contrast agent injection have to be compared with the adjacent kidney. Tumors with a homogeneous or slightly heterogeneous echo intensity distribution are defined as hyper-, iso-, or hypoechoic (or hyper-, iso-, or hypovascular) depending on whether they display similar or lower echogenicity relative to the adjacent renal parenchyma. In the other cases, renal tumors are defined as heterogeneous.

15.5
Benign Solid Renal Tumors

15.5.1
Embryonal Metanephric Adenoma

Embryonal metanephric adenoma is a rare benign renal tumor which shows a heterogeneous appearance

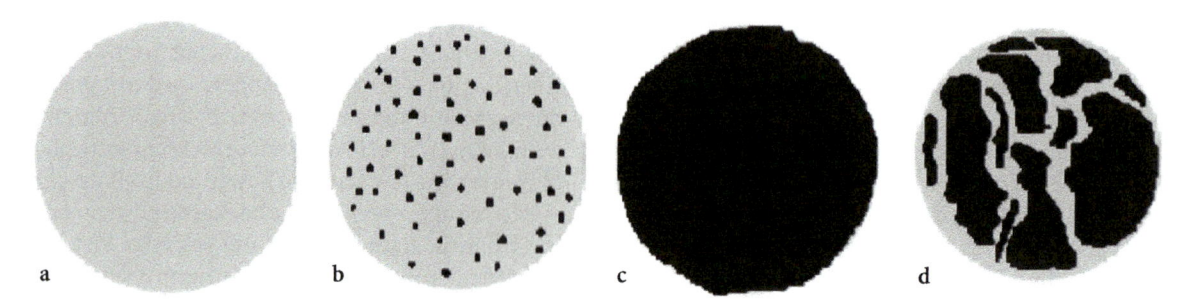

Fig. 15.1a–d. The different patterns of contrast enhancement which may be observed in solid renal tumors after the injection of microbubble-based agents. **a** absent, **b** dotted, **c** diffuse homogeneous, **d** diffuse heterogeneous.

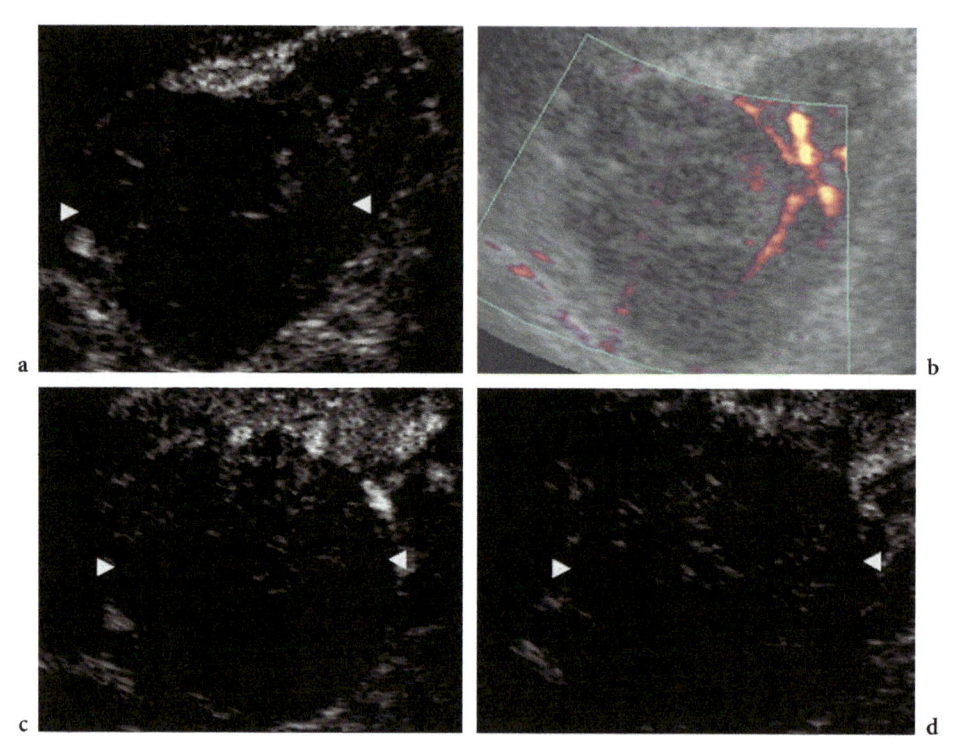

Fig. 15.2a–d Embryonic metanephric adenoma. **a** Baseline US and **b** Power Doppler US. A heterogeneous solid large renal mass (*arrowheads*) is identified at the upper pole of the right kidney with peripheral and penetrating vessels on Power Doppler US. **c, d** Contrast-specific mode: Pulse Inversion Mode (Philips-ATL, WA, USA) with high acoustic power insonation after air-filled microbubble injection. Diffuse heterogeneous contrast enhancement (*arrowheads*) is demonstrated during the arterial phase (**c**) and decreases during the late phase (**d**).

on baseline US (Fig. 15.2a), with a mixed arterial vessel distribution on color Doppler US (Fig. 15.2b). After microbubble injection, embryonal metanephric adenoma demonstrates heterogeneous contrast enhancement during the arterial and late phases (Fig. 15.2c,d).

15.5.2
Angiomyolipoma

Epidemiology and histopathologic features. Angiomyolipoma is a relatively uncommon renal tumor, with a prevalence of 0.3% to 3%, and it occurs more commonly in women than in men (ISRAEL and BOSNIAK 2003b). Angiomyolipoma contains smooth muscle, vascular, lipomatous, and myeloid elements (SHERMAN et al. 1981; WAGNER et al. 1997) in different proportions. It usually appears as an expansive unifocal large tumor which looks yellowish on section when the fat component is predominant, white if the muscular component is predominant, or red when the vascular component is predominant (a hemorrhagic pattern may then be present) (HARTMAN 2001).

Baseline US and color Doppler US. Angiomyolipomas smaller than 3 cm typically appear hyperechoic and homogeneous, with sharp margins (FORMAN et al. 1993; JINZAKI et al. 1998; YAMASHITA et al. 1992; POZZI MUCELLI and LOCATELLI 2002). Large angiomyolipomas may display a heterogeneous appearance due to solid, adipose, and hemorrhagic components. The presence of posterior acoustic shadowing may suggest angiomyolipoma (YAMASHITA et al. 1992; HÉLÉNON et al. 1997; JINZAKI et al. 1997). Color Doppler US reveals penetrating, peripheral, or mixed peripheral and intratumoral distribution, with predominance of the mixed distribution in atypical hypervascular angiomyolipomas.

Multimodality imaging – CT and MR imaging. The CT diagnosis of angiomyolipoma is related to the identification of fat within the lesion (POZZI MUCELLI and LOCATELLI 2002). Angiomyolipomas larger than 3 cm usually demonstrate a predominant hypodense fat component on nonenhanced CT, with low contrast enhancement of the solid peripheral or central component (sparing the fat component) after iodinated contrast agent injection. Angiomyolipomas smaller than 3 cm present low-grade contrast enhancement during the arterial and late phases, appearing hypodense in comparison with the adjacent enhancing renal parenchyma.

Differential diagnosis between atypical angiomyolipomas and nonfatty renal tumors is not always solved even by CT and MR imaging (PRETORIUS et al. 2000). Atypical angiomyolipomas with absence of a fat component account for about 5% of cases (POZZI MUCELLI and LOCATELLI 2002) and usually appear iso- or slightly hyperdense compared to the adjacent kidney on nonenhanced CT. A similar pattern may be observed in complicated benign cysts (hemorrhagic, protein-rich, or gelatinous), renal metastasis, and renal cell carcinoma. Atypical hypervascular angiomyolipomas display diffuse contrast enhancement after the injection of iodinated or paramagnetic contrast agents, and complicated benign cysts may be excluded in this way.

Contrast enhanced US. Typical hyperechoic homogeneous or slightly heterogeneous angiomyolipomas typically display persistent dotted contrast enhancement (Fig. 15.3) (QUAIA et al. 2003a,b), with an isoechoic (isovascular) appearance compared to the adjacent enhancing renal parenchyma, particularly if high acoustic power insonation is employed. Using low acoustic power insonation, more effective suppression of the background hyperechoic appearance is achieved, and angiomyolipomas usually appear hypoechoic compared to the adjacent kidney after microbubble injection (Fig. 15.3).

Atypical angiomyolipomas show diffuse contrast enhancement with a hypervascular appearance during the arterial phase (Figs. 15.4, 15.5), with (Fig. 15.4) or without (Fig. 15.5) progressive reduction of contrast enhancement in the late phase. This contrast enhancement pattern is caused by the hypervascular nature of most atypical angiomyolipomas.

15.5.3
Renal Oncocytoma

Epidemiology and histopathologic features. Renal oncocytomas (2–3% of renal tumors) are benign tumors arising from proximal tubular epithelial cells that can be treated by local excision or heminephrectomy. Their preoperative differentiation from renal cell carcinoma is very important. Oncocytoma is characterized by large cells with small, uniform, round nuclei and an abundant eosinophilic cytoplasm. It appears brown on section owing to the lipochromic pigment of mitochondria, with or without calcifications; usually necrosis and hemorrhage are absent, and there is a fibromyxoid stroma in the central scar (AMIN et al. 1997).

Baseline and color Doppler US. The presence of a central scar appearing as a stellate hypoechoic area and the absence of hemorrhage and necrosis are considered typical in renal oncocytoma (HÉLÉNON et al. 2001). Large oncocytomas with a stellate hypoechoic central area may also display a central spoke-wheel shaped distribution of tumor vessels on color Doppler US (HÉLÉNON et al. 2001).

Multimodality imaging – CT and MR imaging. The classic angiographic findings described for renal oncocytoma, including a spoke-wheel shaped pattern, a homogeneous nephrogram, and a sharp, smooth rim (AMBOS et al. 1978; DE CARLI et al. 2000; HAJRI et al. 2001), may be observed on contrast-enhanced CT. On contrast-enhanced CT scans, diffuse homogeneous contrast enhancement throughout the tumor and a central, sharply marginated, stellate area of low attenuation are found in 70–80% of lesions (DAVIDSON et al. 1993). Nevertheless, areas of decreased attenuation different from the stellate central area, which are usually found in renal cell carcinoma, may be observed in about 20–30% of oncocytomas (DAVIDSON et al. 1993), and particularly those larger than 3 cm. Rarely,

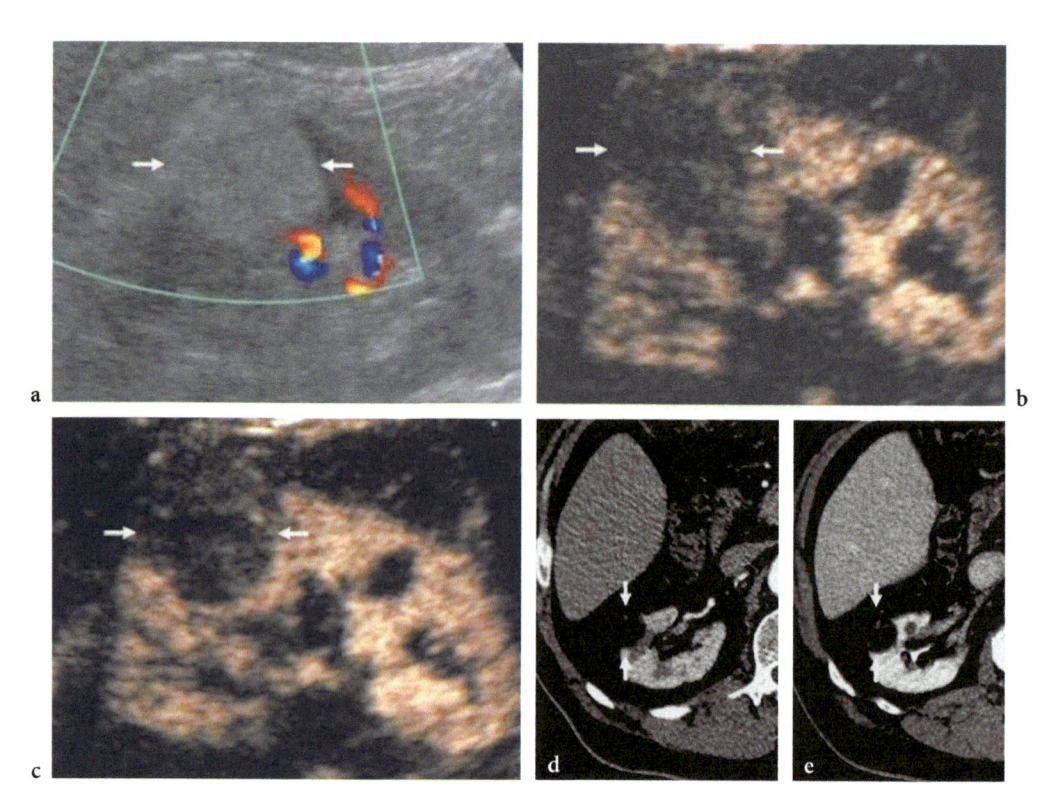

Fig. 15.3a–e Angiomyolipoma with dotted contrast enhancement. **a** Baseline color Doppler US. A hyperechoic and homogeneous large renal mass (*arrows*) with peripheral vessels is identified. **b, c** Contrast-specific mode: Cadence Contrast Pulse Sequence (Siemens-Acuson, CA, USA) with low acoustic power after the injection of sulfur hexafluoride-filled microbubbles. A hypoechoic (hypovascular) appearance with dotted contrast enhancement (*arrows*) is demonstrated during both the arterial (**b**) and the late (**c**) phase. **d, e** Contrast-enhanced CT: persistent hypodense appearance of the tumor in both the corticomedullary (**d**) and the tubular phase (**e**) with a fat density appearance (*arrows*).

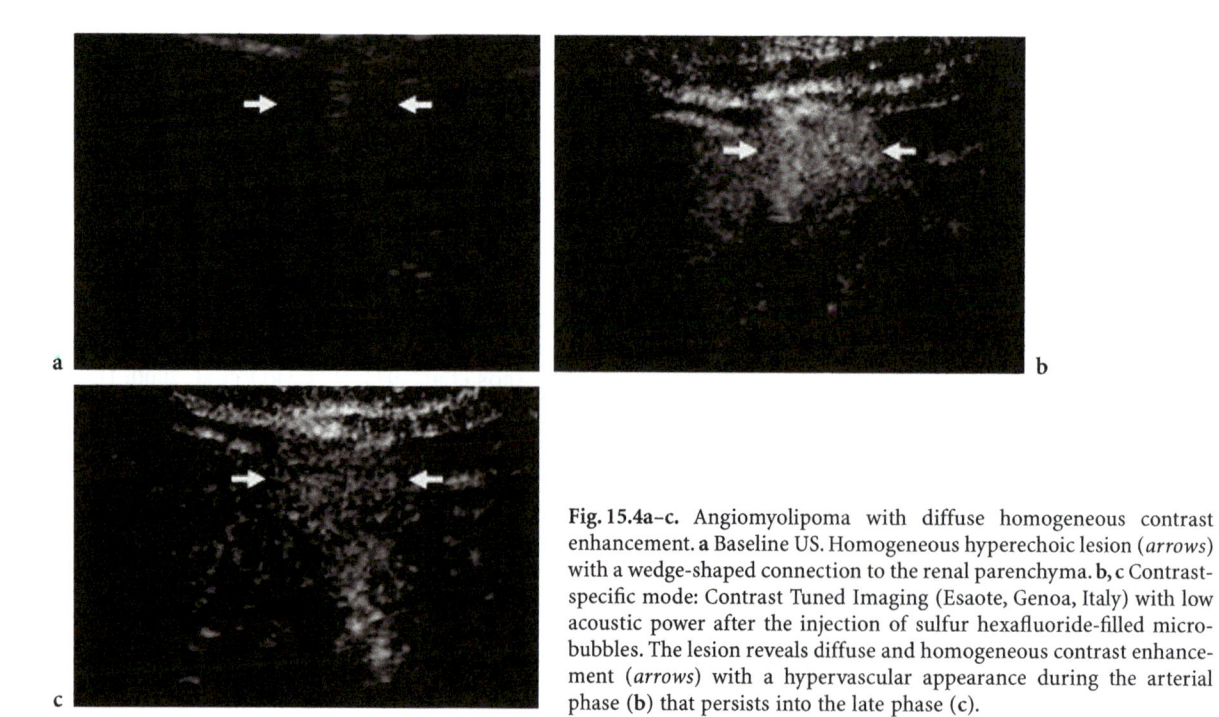

Fig. 15.4a–c. Angiomyolipoma with diffuse homogeneous contrast enhancement. **a** Baseline US. Homogeneous hyperechoic lesion (*arrows*) with a wedge-shaped connection to the renal parenchyma. **b, c** Contrast-specific mode: Contrast Tuned Imaging (Esaote, Genoa, Italy) with low acoustic power after the injection of sulfur hexafluoride-filled microbubbles. The lesion reveals diffuse and homogeneous contrast enhancement (*arrows*) with a hypervascular appearance during the arterial phase (**b**) that persists into the late phase (**c**).

a fat component may be identified (HÉLÉNON et al. 1997). Diffuse homogeneous enhancement has also been described on Gd-DTPA enhanced MR imaging (EILENBERG et al. 1990).

Contrast-enhanced US. After the injection of a microbubble-based contrast agent, renal oncocytoma shows persistent diffuse homogeneous contrast enhancement, with a hypervascular appearance, in the early corticomedullary phase. The enhancement progressively declines during the late corticomedullary phase, resulting in a hypovascular appearance (Fig. 15.6).

15.6
Malignant Solid Renal Tumors

15.6.1
Solid Renal Cell Carcinoma

Epidemiology and histopathologic features. Solid renal cell carcinoma is the most common malignancy of the kidney and accounts for 2% of all cancers (SHETH et al. 2001). Various histopathologic subtypes of malignant solid renal parenchyma tumors have been described: (1) clear cell (70–80%), (2) papillary cell (10–15%), (3) granular cell (5%), (4) chromophobe cell (5%), (5) sarcomatoid cell (1–2%), (6) collecting duct carcinoma, and (7) medullary carcinoma (1–2%). Types 1–4 usually present an expansile growth pattern while types 5–7 usually show an infiltrative pattern (STORKEL et al. 1997; OYEN 1998; OYEN et al. 2001; PICKHARDT et al. 2000).

Baseline US and color Doppler US. Most solid renal cell carcinomas smaller than 3 cm appear hypoechoic on baseline US, with approximately 30% appearing as hyperechoic masses (FORMAN et al. 1993). Presence of an anechoic rim or small intratumoral cysts may suggest renal cell carcinoma (YAMASHITA et al. 1992; HÉLÉNON et al. 1997; JINZAKI et al. 1997). Solid renal cell carcinomas larger than 3 cm usually appear heterogeneous on baseline US. Renal cell carcinomas predominantly present arterial vessels with a mixed distribution on color Doppler US (Fig. 15.7).

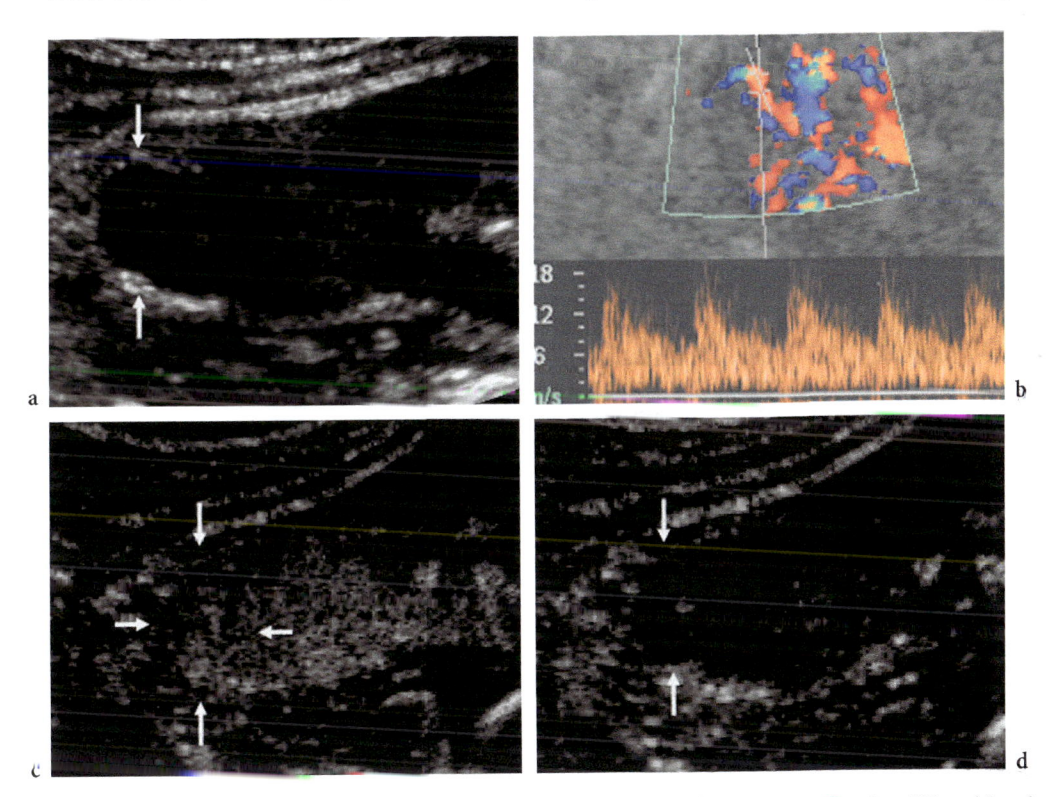

Fig. 15.5a–d. Angiomyolipoma with diffuse homogeneous contrast enhancement. **a** Baseline US and **b** color Doppler US. A hypoechoic exophytic renal mass (*arrows*) is identified at the upper pole of the right kidney. Arterial intratumoral and penetrating vessels are identified on color Doppler US. **c, d** Contrast-specific mode: Pulse Inversion Mode (Philips-ATL, WA, USA) with high acoustic power after the injection of air-filled microbubbles. The renal tumor (*arrows*) shows diffuse and homogeneous contrast enhancement during the arterial phase (**c**), while contrast enhancement progressively decreases in the late phase (**d**). Biopsy revealed angiomyolipoma with a prevalent vascular component.

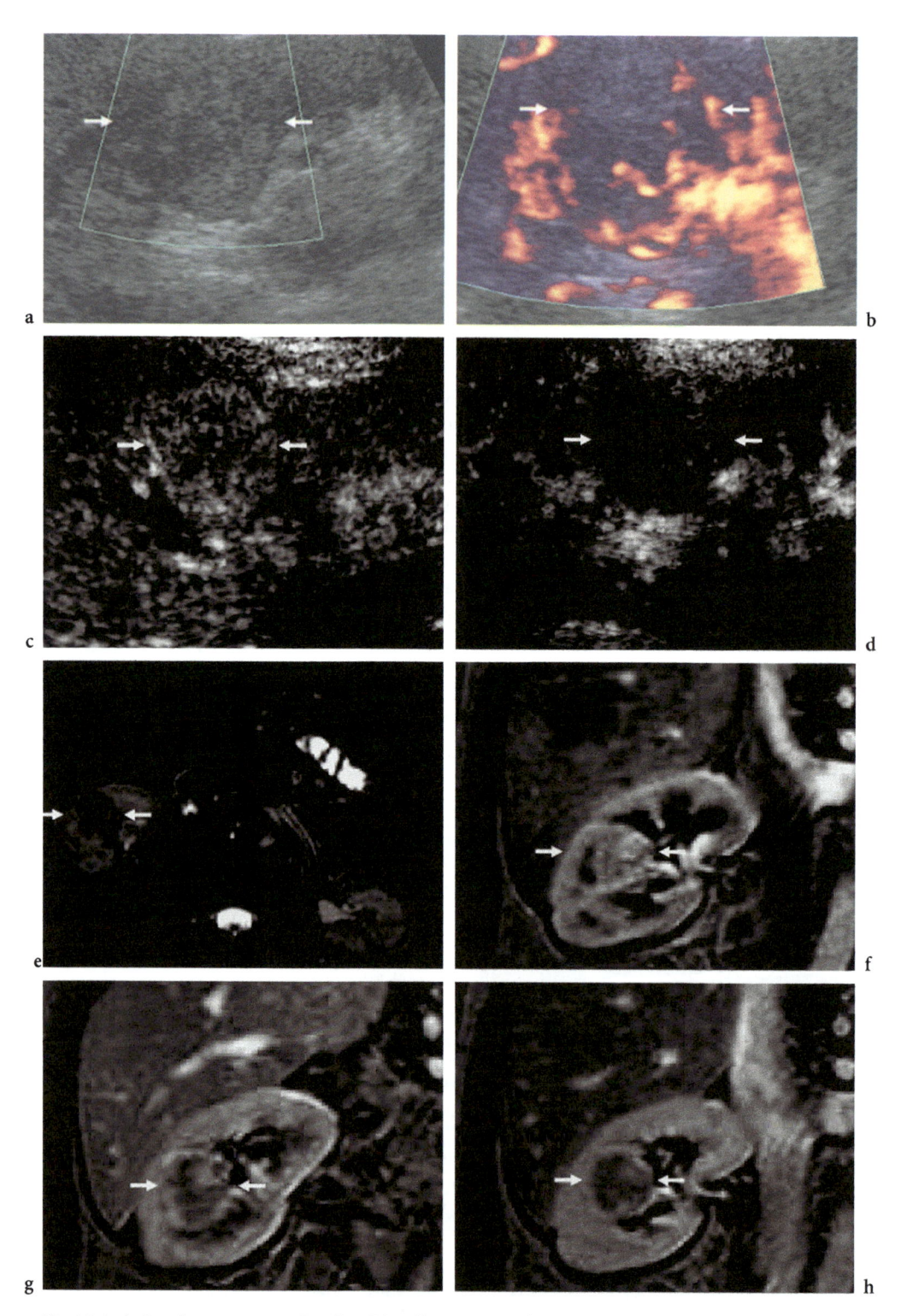

Fig. 15.6a–h. Renal oncocytoma. **a** Baseline US and **b** Power Doppler US. Longitudinal scan shows a heterogeneous and hypoechoic lesion (*arrows*) with peripheral and intratumoral vessels. **c, d** Contrast-specific mode: Contrast Tuned Imaging (Esaote, Genoa, Italy) with low acoustic power after the injection of sulfur hexafluoride-filled microbubbles. Diffuse homogeneous contrast enhancement (*arrows*) with a hypervascular appearance is identified in the arterial phase (**c**); the enhancement decreased during the late phase, with a hypovascular appearance (**d**). **e** T2-weighted and **f–h** Gd-BOPTA-enhanced T1-weighted MR sequences. The renal tumor (*arrows*) appears hypointense on the T2-weighted sequence (**e**). Contrast enhancement is evident during the corticomedullary phase (**f**) and decreases in the tubular (**g**) and excretory (**h**) phases.

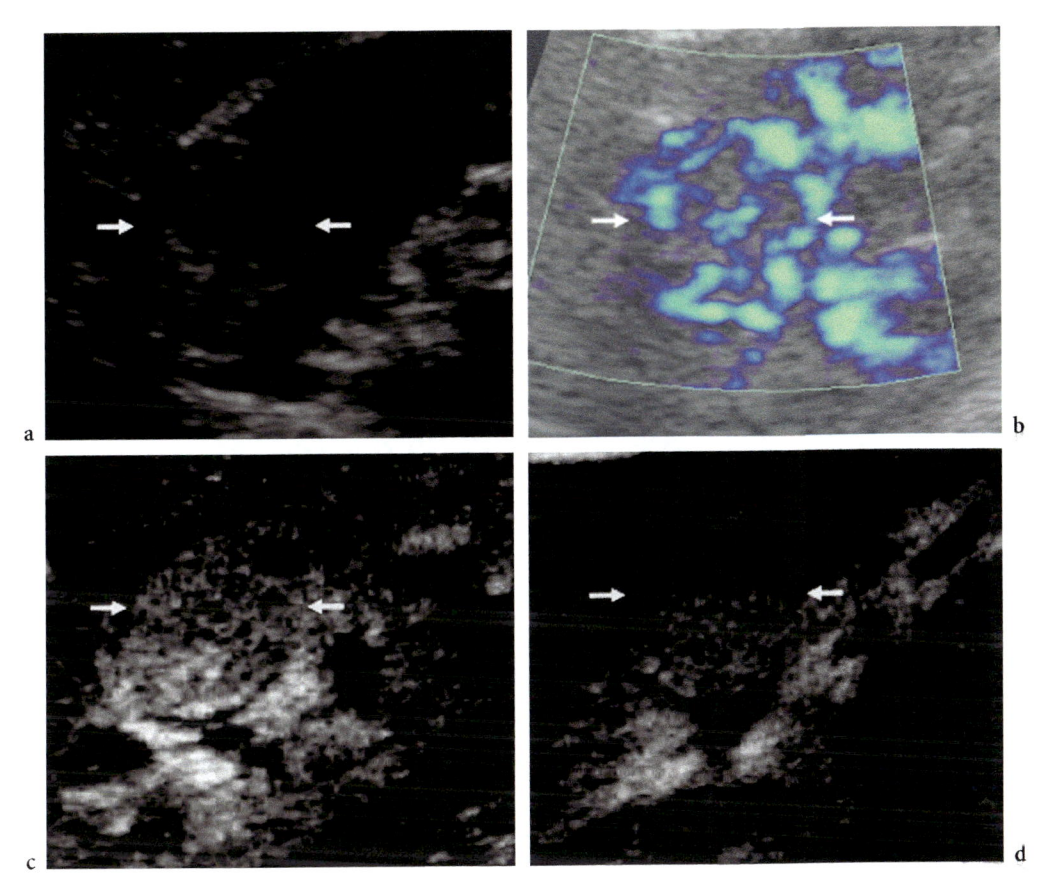

Characterization and Detection of Renal Tumors

Fig. 15.7a–d. Renal cell carcinoma of the clear cell type with diffuse homogeneous contrast enhancement. **a** Baseline US and **b** Power Doppler US. Longitudinal scan shows a hyperechoic and slightly heterogeneous lesion (*arrows*) with peripheral and intratumoral vessels. **c, d** Contrast-specific mode: Contrast Tuned Imaging (Esaote, Genoa, Italy) with low acoustic power after the injection of sulfur hexafluoride-filled microbubbles. Diffuse homogeneous contrast enhancement, with a hypervascular appearance (*arrows*), is identified in the arterial phase (**c**) and is seen to decrease in the late phase (**d**).

Presence of intratumoral arteriovenous shunts is suggestive of renal cell carcinoma (HÉLÉNON et al. 2001), even though angiomyolipomas may reveal the same pattern. Large (>4 cm) renal cell carcinomas typically show a heterogeneous appearance due to intratumoral necrosis, calcifications (HÉLÉNON et al. 2001), and hemorrhage.

Multimodality imaging – CT and MR imaging. Most renal cell carcinomas are solid lesions with attenuation values of 20 HU or greater on nonenhanced CT (SILVERMAN et al. 1994). An increase of 15–20 HU on CT (HARTMANN et al. 1988; MAKI et al. 1999) and of 15% signal intensity on MR imaging (Ho et al. 2002) within a renal lesion after the intravenous administration of contrast agent has generally been accepted as a threshold for contrast enhancement. The demonstration of enhancement is considered a reliable sign of a vascular renal tumor even though it is not considered a sign of malignancy. Nevertheless, in renal cell carcinoma contrast enhancement on CT or MR imaging is usually diffuse and intense, sparing necrotic intratumoral areas (SOYER et al. 1997). An exception is the papillary cell subtype, which appears hypovascular on contrast-enhanced CT or MR imaging (CHOYKE et al. 1997, 2003). Distinct areas of fat may be present as well. Cystic areas may predominate so that the tumor presents a frank cystic appearance.

Contrast-enhanced US. After microbubble injection, solid renal cell carcinomas smaller than 3 cm show diffuse (Fig. 15.7), homogeneous or heterogeneous contrast enhancement (Fig. 15.8) during the early corticomedullary phase, often with a hypervascular appearance. The enhancement is limited to the solid viable regions, sparing intratumoral avascular necrotic, hemorrhagic, or cystic components and thereby increasing their conspicuity (Fig. 15.8). Renal cell carcinomas appear isovascu-

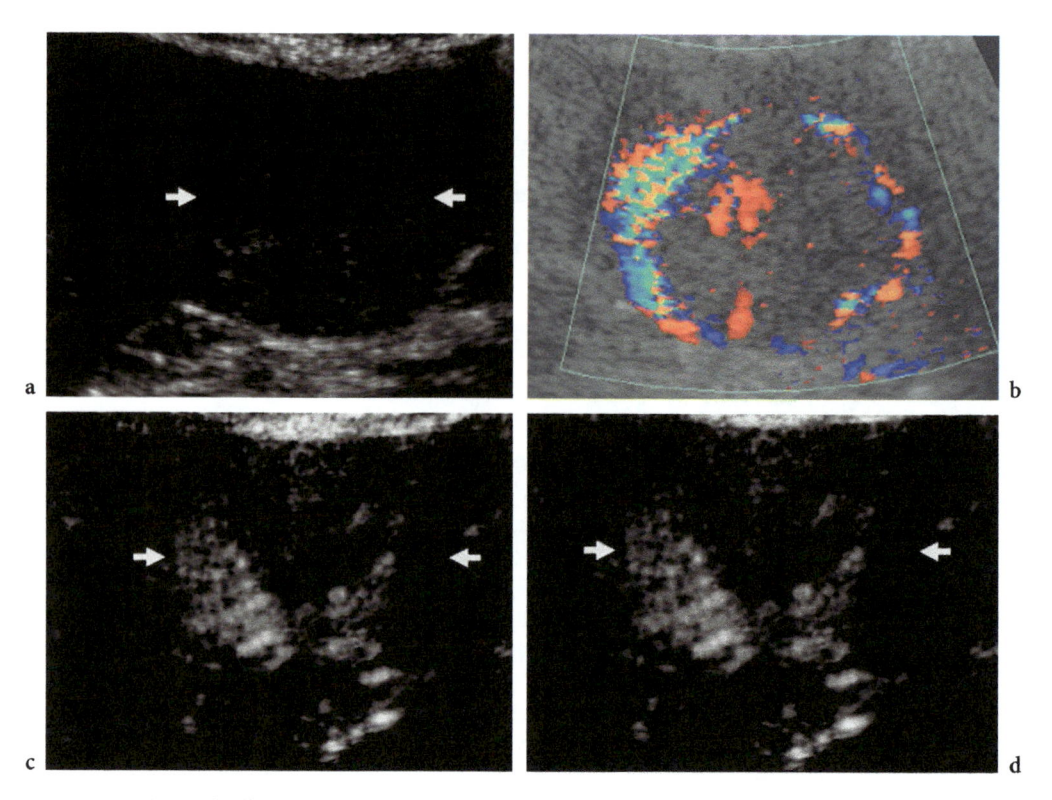

Fig. 15.8a–d. Renal cell carcinoma of the clear cell type with diffuse heterogeneous contrast enhancement. a Baseline US and b color Doppler US. Axial scan shows a heterogeneous lesion (*arrows*) with peripheral and intratumoral vessels. c, d Contrast-specific mode: Contrast Tuned Imaging (Esaote, Genoa, Italy) with low acoustic power after the injection of sulfur hexafluoride-filled microbubbles. Diffuse heterogeneous contrast enhancement (*arrows*) is identified in the arterial phase (c), and decreases during the late phase (d).

lar or slightly hypovascular relative to the adjacent renal parenchyma, with progressive reduction of contrast enhancement in the late corticomedullary phase (Figs. 15.7, 15.8). If tumoral thrombus is present in the renal vein or inferior vena cava, it may show contrast enhancement (Correas et al. 1999, 2003). At objective analysis of contrast enhancement, renal cell carcinomas displayed significantly higher echo intensity enhancement during both the arterial and the late phase compared to benign renal tumors (Quaia et al. 2003a).

Contrast-enhanced US may be even more sensitive than contrast-enhanced CT in showing contrast enhancement in solid renal tumors (Fig. 15.9), due to the high sensitivity of US contrast-specific modes to the harmonic signal produced by microbubble insonation.

Papillary cell-type carcinomas prevalently displays absent or slight contrast enhancement after microbubble injection (Figs. 15.10, 15.11), with a hypovascular appearance relative to the adjacent renal parenchyma, as is also seen on contrast-enhanced CT or MR imaging (Herts et al. 2002). CT may differentiate type 3 hyperdense cysts from hyperdense renal cell carcinoma by demonstrating contrast enhancement after the injection of an iodinated contrast agent, while US may differentiate type 3 hyperdense cysts from iso-hyperdense hypovascular tumors by revealing a cystic anechoic pattern (30–50% of cases) or a solid echoic pattern (Fig. 15. 11).

15.6.2
Renal Metastasis

The frequency of metastases to the kidney in cancer patients is 7–13% in large autopsy series (Bracken et al. 1979; Pickhardt et al. 2000). Renal metastases are usually detected late in the course of the malignancy and are usually multifocal (Choyke et al. 1987). Metastases arising from colon, lung, and breast carcinoma and melanoma may involve the kidney. As with lymphoma, renal metastases can display either an expansile or an infiltrative growth pattern (Choyke et al. 1987; Pickhardt et al. 2000). However, the most frequent pattern is that of multiple discrete bilateral lesions. Solitary exophytic

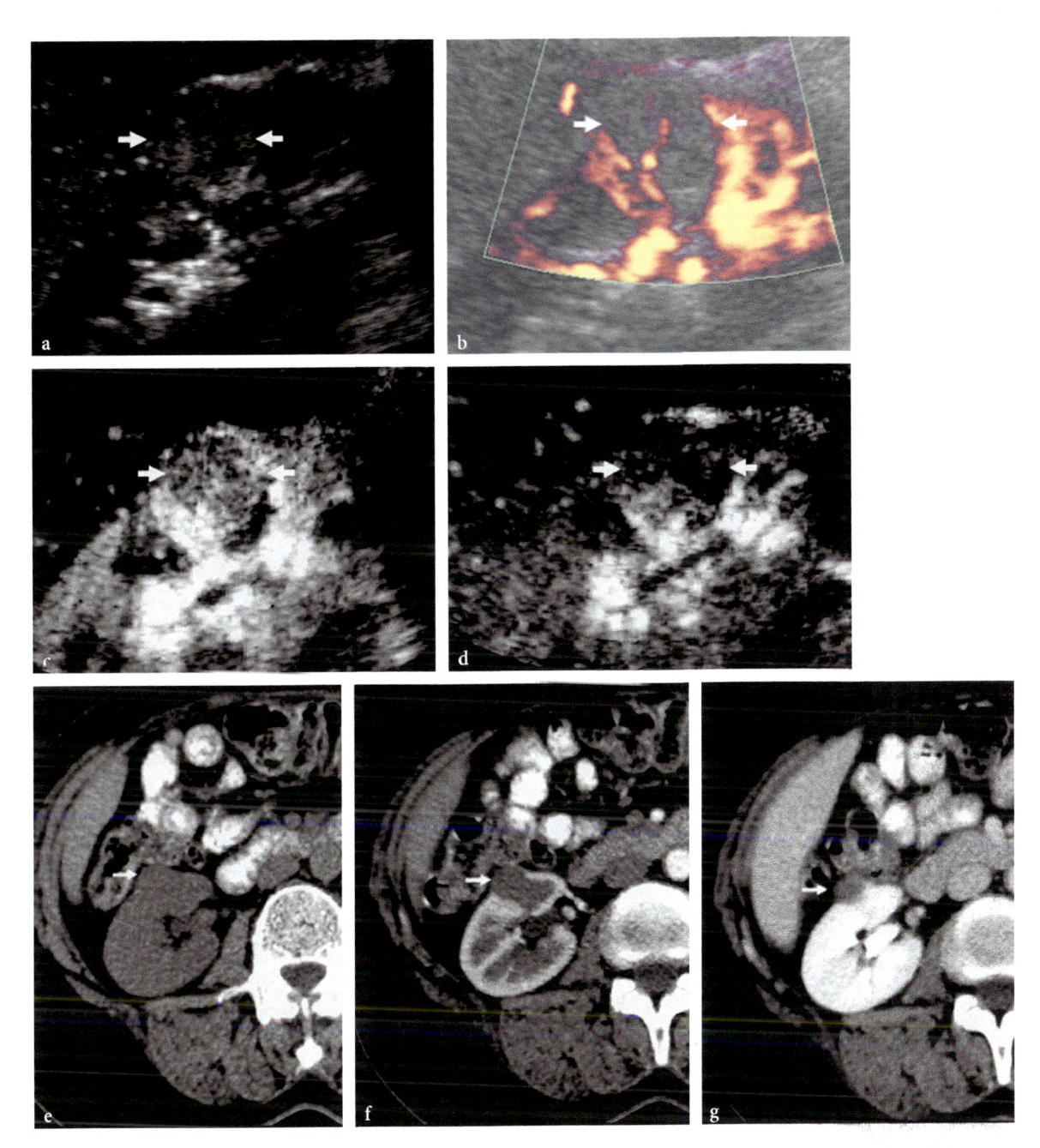

Fig. 15.9a–g. Higher sensitivity of US contrast-specific modes after the injection of microbubble-based agents in the detection of contrast enhancement, in comparison with contrast-enhanced CT. **a** Baseline US and **b** Power Doppler US. Longitudinal scan showing hyperechoic renal mass (*arrows*) with peripheral and intratumoral vessels. **c, d** Contrast specific mode: Contrast Tuned Imaging (Esaote, Genoa, Italy) with low acoustic power after the injection of sulfur hexafluoride-filled microbubbles. Diffuse contrast enhancement (*arrows*) is identified in the early corticomedullary phase (**c**) and decreases during the late corticomedullary phase (**d**), with a consequent hypovascular appearance of the tumor. **e–g** Contrast-enhanced CT. Renal tumor (*arrow*) does not display significant contrast enhancement after iodinated contrast agent injection. Histologic analysis of the surgical specimen revealed a renal cell carcinoma of the clear cell type.

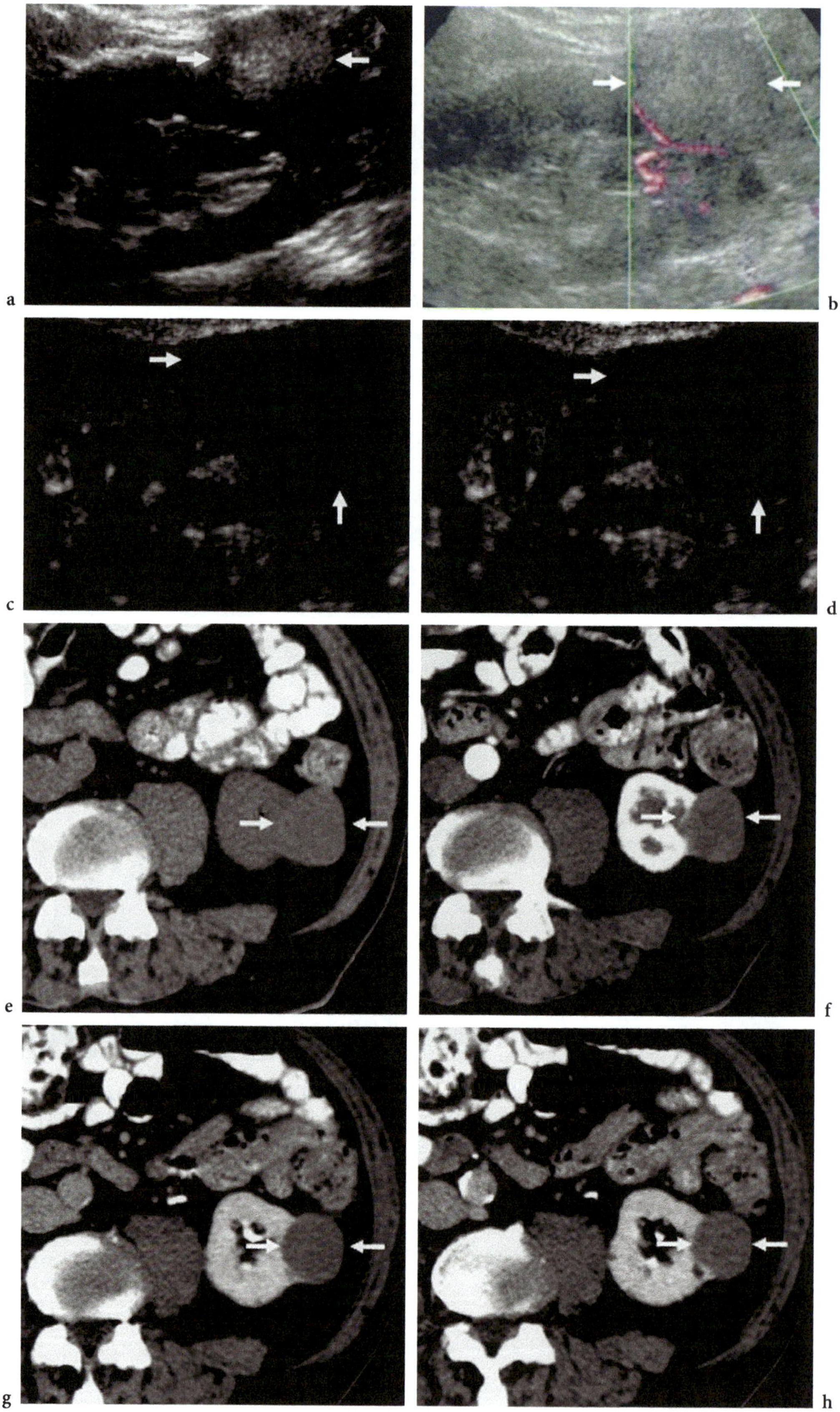
a
b
c
d
e
f
g
h

Characterization and Detection of Renal Tumors 235

Fig. 15.10a–h. Absent enhancement in a solid papillary cell type carcinoma. **a** Baseline US and **b** power Doppler US. A hyperechoic exophytic lesion (*arrows*) is identified in the left kidney with no vascular signal at power Doppler analysis. **c, d** Contrast-specific mode: Contrast Tuned Imaging (Esaote, Genoa, Italy). No contrast enhancement is identified after the injection of sulfur hexafluoride-filled microbubbles at low acoustic power insonation, with a persistent hypovascular appearance (*arrows*). **e–h.** Nonenhanced (**e**) and contrast-enhanced (**f–h**) CT. The renal tumor (*arrows*) shows slight contrast enhancement after iodinated contrast agent injection, with a persistent hypovascular appearance. Solid papillary renal cell carcinoma was revealed after surgical resection.

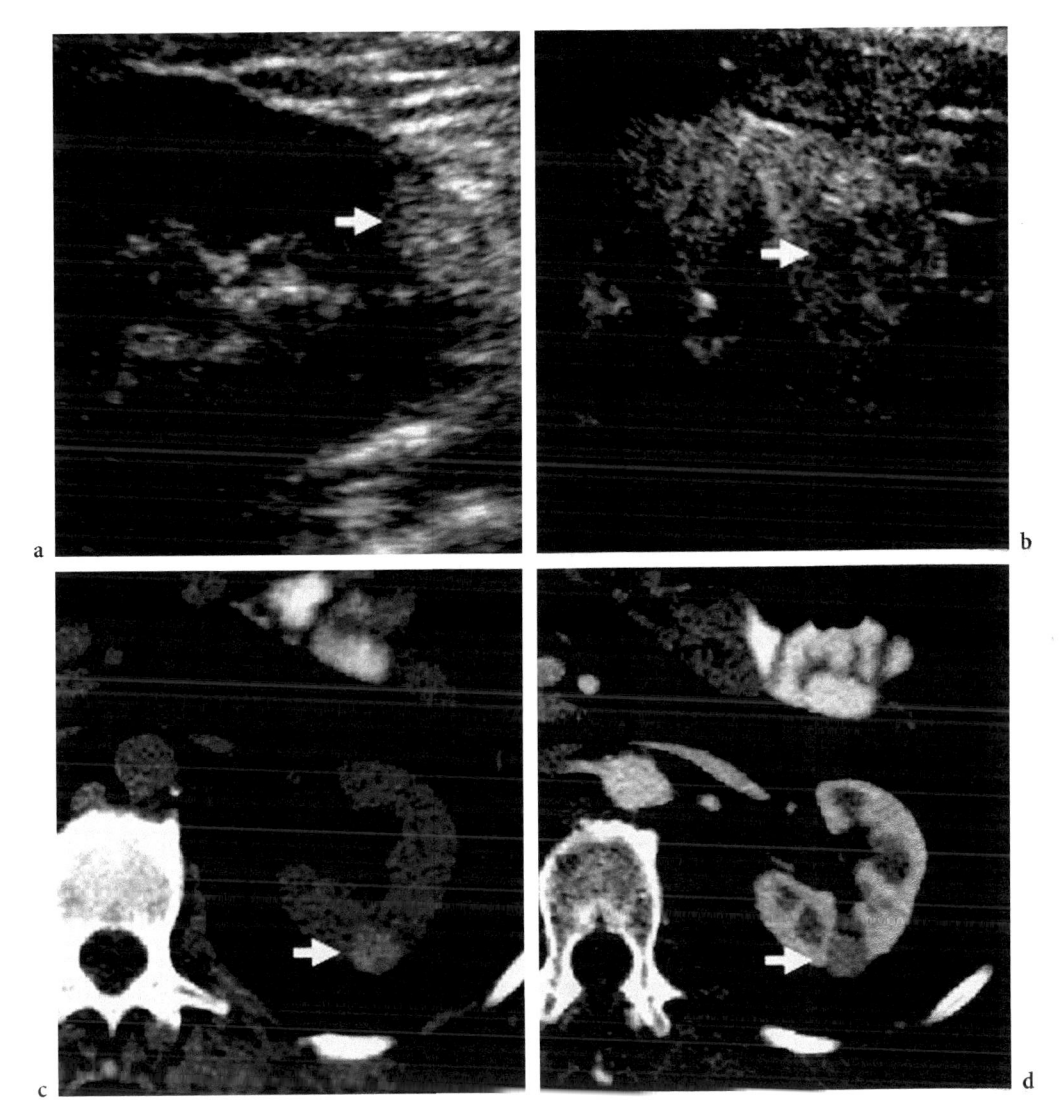

Fig. 15.11a–d. Hypovascular appearance of a small solid papillary cell type carcinoma. **a** Baseline US reveals a small (1.5-cm) hyperechoic tumor (*arrow*) in the left kidney. **b** After injection of the microbubble-based agent, the renal tumor (*arrow*) appears hypovascular compared to the adjacent kidney. **c** Nonenhanced CT displays a hyperdense tumor (*arrow*). **d** The tumor appears hypovascular on contrast-enhanced CT during the corticomedullary phase, after the injection of iodinated contrast agent. Solid papillary renal cell carcinoma was revealed after surgical resection.

metastases are more common in patients with colon cancer, and perinephric tumor extension is typical of melanoma (PICKHARDT et al. 2000). The presence of an associated exophytic component, cystic necrosis, hemorrhage, or calcification on CT depends on the nature of the underlying primary tumor.

Renal metastases do not display contrast enhancement on either contrast-enhanced CT/MR imaging (CHOYKE et al. 1987; PICKHARDT et al. 2000) or contrast-enhanced US (QUAIA et al. 2003b). In particular, after microbubble injection, renal metastases appear persistently hypovascular compared to the adjacent renal parenchyma and their visibility is improved (Fig. 15.12).

15.7
Contrast Enhancement Patterns in Cystic Renal Tumors After Microbubble Injection

Contrast-enhanced US is a valuable tool to identify contrast enhancement in the peripheral wall or intratumoral septa of cystic renal tumors. This is due to the high sensitivity of the contrast-specific mode to the harmonic signals produced by microbubbles. As a result, contrast-enhanced US is probably even more effective than contrast-enhanced CT and MR imaging in the detection of contrast enhancement in cystic renal tumors. Microbubble-based contrast agents have been shown to improve the characterization of renal cysts and atypical cystic renal masses by revealing different enhancement patterns(KIM et al. 1999; QUAIA et al. 2003a,b).

After microbubble injection a variety of contrast enhancement patterns may be observed in cystic renal tumors (Fig. 15.13): (a) absent, no difference before and after microbubble injection; (b) continuous or (c) discontinuous peripheral rim-like enhancement in a cystic lesion with or without intratumoral septa; (d) peripheral nodular enhancement limited to the peripheral wall and to the nodular papillary endocystic components; (e) peripheral wall and septal enhancement; or (f) diffuse nodular and septal enhancement with nodular components both in the peripheral wall and in the intratumoral septa.

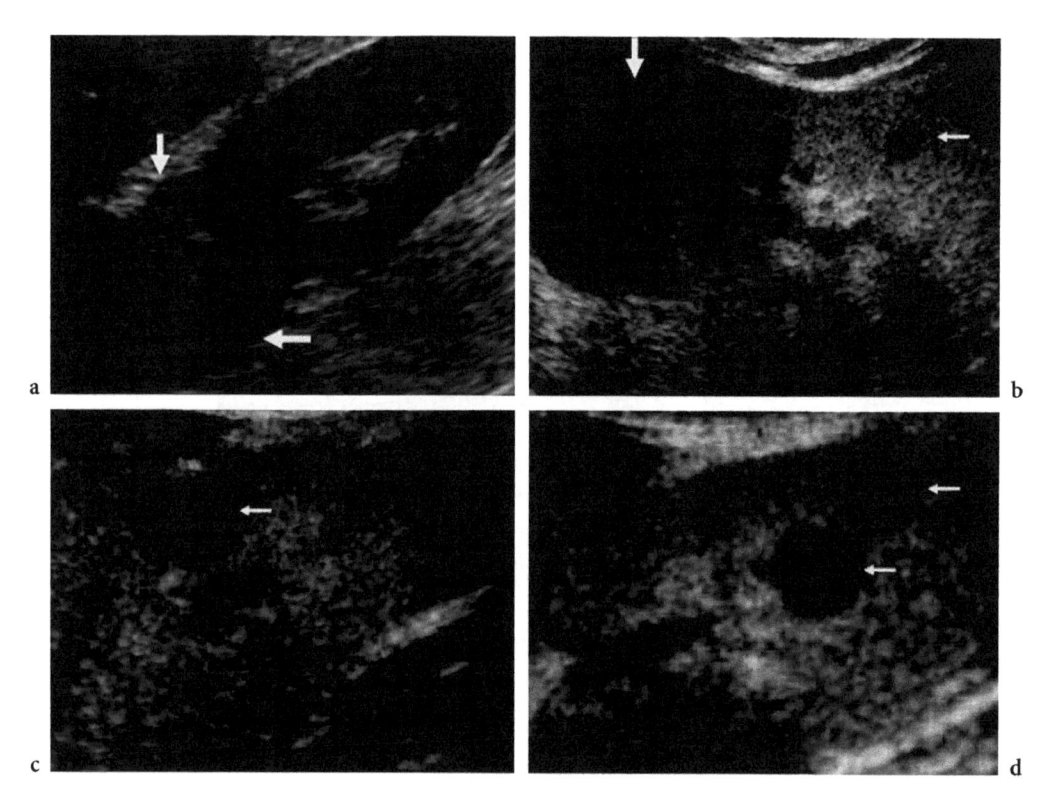

Fig. 15.12a–d. Renal metastasis. a Baseline US. A heterogeneous mass (*arrows*) is identified at the upper right renal pole. b–d Contrast-specific mode: Contrast Tuned Imaging (Esaote, Genoa, Italy) with low acoustic power after the injection of sulfur hexafluoride-filled microbubbles. A persistent absence of contrast enhancement with a hypovascular appearance (*large arrow*) is identified (b), and there is evidence of additional small hypovascular lesions (*small arrows*) in the late corticomedullary phase (c, d).

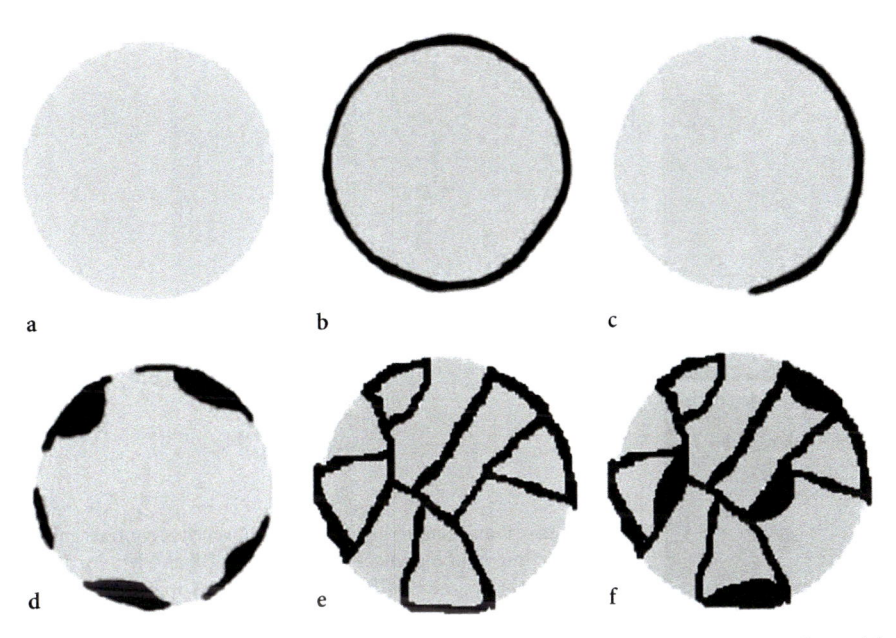

Fig. 15.13a–f. The different patterns of contrast enhancement in cystic renal tumors: **a** absent (observed in simple renal cysts), **b** continuous rim like peripheral enhancement, **c** discontinuous rim-like peripheral enhancement, **d** nodular peripheral enhancement, **e** peripheral wall and septal enhancement, **f** diffuse nodular and septal enhancement.

15.7.1
Benign Cystic Renal Tumors

Complex renal inflammatory or hemorrhagic cysts. Inflammatory or hemorrhagic cysts may show a type 3 pattern according to the BOSNIAK classification (1986), consisting in a thick peripheral wall characterized by absence of vascular signals or by a few spots on baseline color Doppler US or in a corpuscular hyperechoic dense content. After microbubble injection, benign renal cysts with echoic content display absent (Fig. 15.14) or continuous/discontinuous peripheral rim-like (Fig. 15.15) contrast enhancement in both the arterial and the late corticomedullary phase.

Multilocular cystic nephroma. Multilocular cystic nephroma is an uncommon neoplasm composed of multiple, variably sized cysts with prominent septa (HARTMAN 1989). The cysts contain nonhemorrhagic fluid and do not communicate with each other. Calcification is only uncommonly present in the cyst wall and septa. This tumor is characterized by a dense peripheral fibrous capsule. The cysts are lined by cuboidal epithelial cells that project into the cyst lumen. The septal stroma is composed of loose connective tissue with sparse cellularity. Typically, no contrast enhancement is identified in intratumoral septa on contrast-enhanced CT (HARTMAN 1989; DALLA PALMA et al. 1990). Multilocular cystic nephroma may display continuous or discontinuous peripheral rim-like contrast enhancement in the thick peripheral wall (Fig. 15.16) after microbubble-based contrast agent injection.

15.7.2
Malignant Cystic Renal Tumors

Cystic renal cell carcinoma. Clear cell and papillary cell type carcinomas may present a cystic pattern (ROBERTS et al. 1997). Cystic clear cell carcinomas tend to be large, rounded, or polylobular lesions (HARTMAN 1989). Cystic renal cell carcinoma may appear as a cystic lesion with echoic content or a thick peripheral wall or as a pseudocystic tumor with a thick, irregular peripheral wall or peripheral echoic mural nodules. The peripheral wall or the mural nodules usually display some arterial flow signals on color Doppler US. Typically, intense contrast enhancement is identified in intratumoral septa and mural nodules on contrast-enhanced CT (HARTMAN 1989; DALLA PALMA et al. 1990).

After microbubble injection, cystic renal cell carcinoma shows discontinuous peripheral rim-like (Fig. 15.17) or peripheral nodular (Fig. 15.18) or diffuse nodular and septal (Fig. 15.19) contrast enhancement. In pseudocystic renal tumors, better

Fig. 15.14a–c Renal hemorrhagic cyst with absence of contrast enhancement after microbubble injection. **a** Baseline US and **b** color Doppler US. An exophytic lesion with echoic content (*arrow*) is identified in the left kidney on baseline US (**a**); it does not present a vascular signal on color Doppler US (**b**). **c** Contrast-specific mode: Pulse Inversion Mode (Philips-ATL, WA, USA). No contrast enhancement is identified (*arrow*) after the injection of sulfur hexafluoride-filled microbubbles at low acoustic power insonation. This behavior allows differentiation of this corpuscular cyst from solid renal tumor.

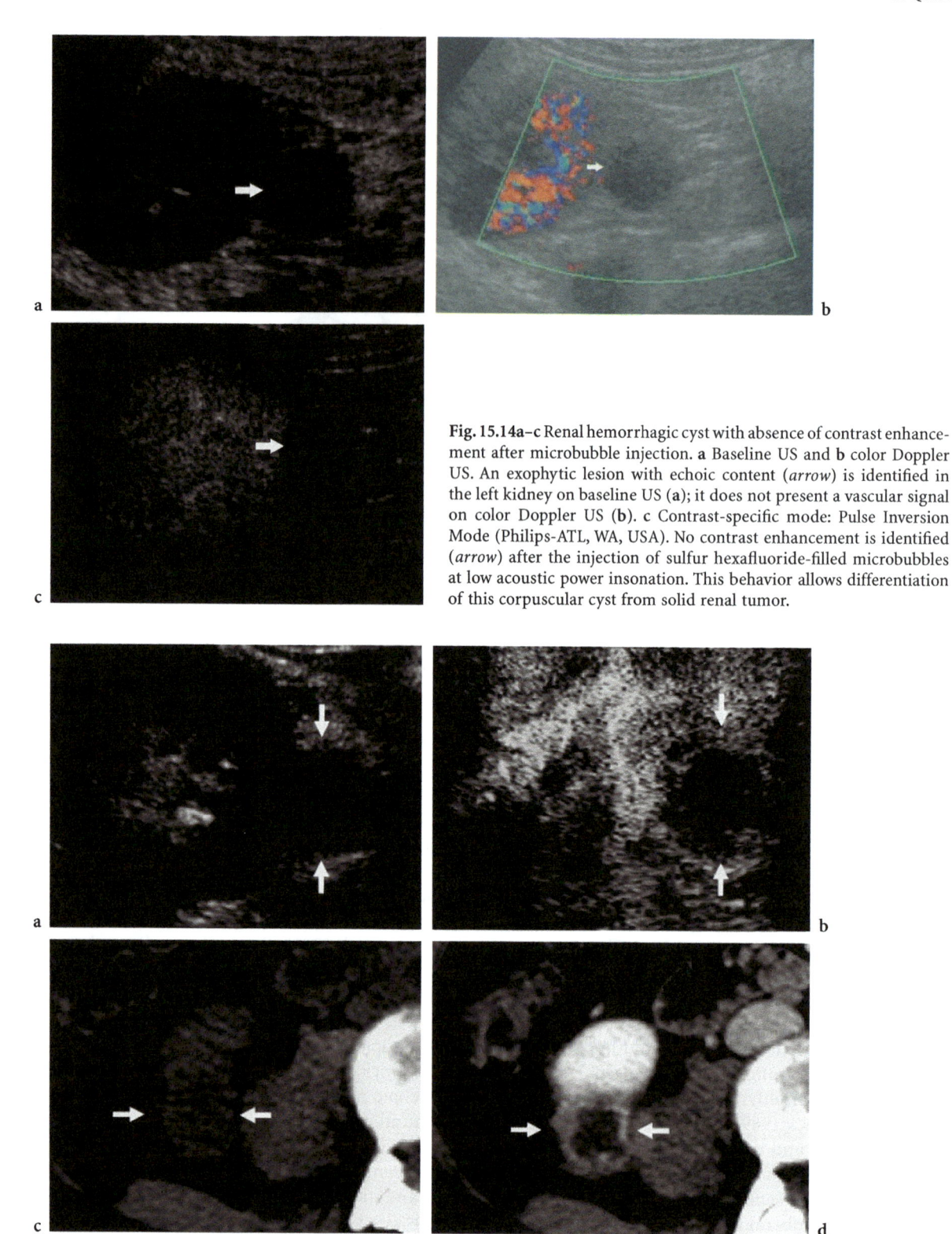

Fig. 15.15a–d. Renal inflammatory cyst with rim-like continuous peripheral enhancement. **a** Baseline US. A hypoechoic exophytic lesion (*arrows*) is identified at the right kidney. **b** Contrast-specific mode: Pulse Inversion Mode (Philips-ATL, WA, USA). Peripheral wall enhancement is identified after the injection of air-filled microbubbles at intermittent high acoustic power insonation. **c** Nonenhanced CT and **d** contrast-enhanced CT. A renal lesion (*arrows*) displays peripheral contrast enhancement after iodinated contrast agent injection. An inflammatory cystic lesion was diagnosed at histologic analysis of the surgical specimen.

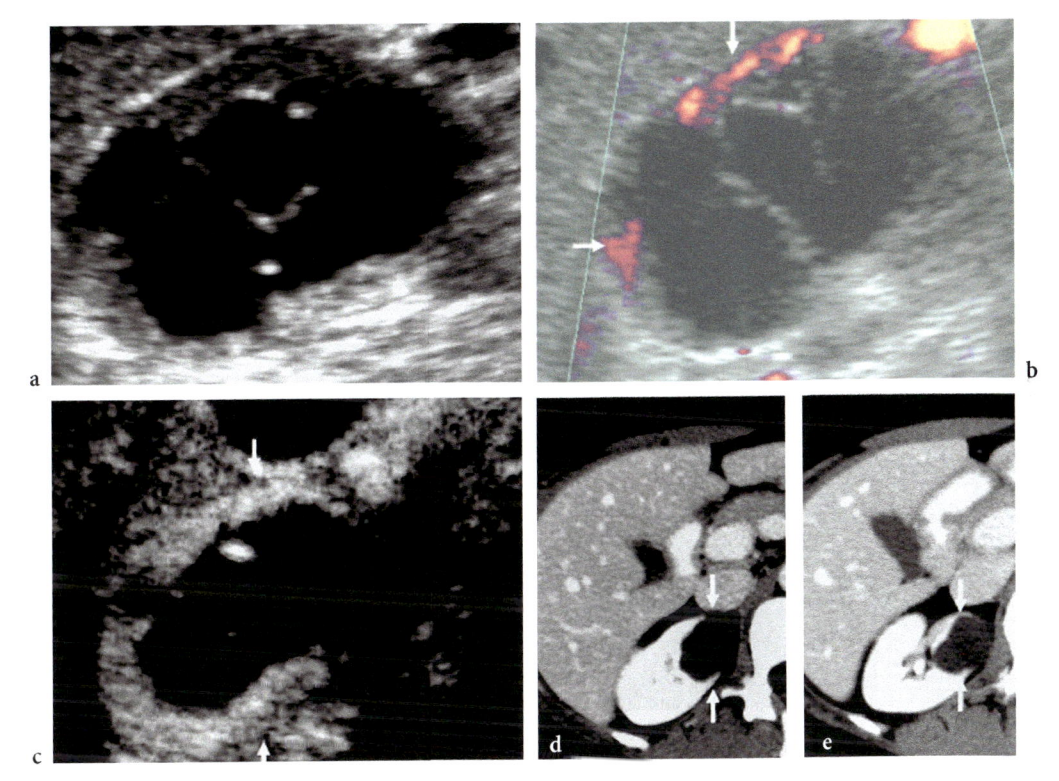

Characterization and Detection of Renal Tumors

Fig. 15.16a–e. Renal multicystic nephroma with continuous rim-like peripheral enhancement. **a** Baseline US and **b** color Doppler US. Longitudinal scan shows a cystic renal mass with intratumoral septa and evidence of vessels (*arrows*) in the peripheral wall. **c** Contrast-specific mode: Contrast Tuned Imaging (Esaote, Genoa, Italy) with low acoustic power after the injection of sulfur hexafluoride-filled microbubbles. Peripheral contrast enhancement is identified in the peripheral wall (*arrows*), without evidence of septal enhancement. **d, e** Contrast-enhanced CT. Peripheral wall contrast enhancement is identified after iodinated contrast agent injection (*arrows*), without evidence of tumoral septa.

delineation between the solid and the liquid intratumoral components is possible after microbubble injection (Fig. 15.20).

15.8
Clinical Results

Varying contrast enhancement patterns may be identified in both malignant and benign renal tumors. Despite this, the diagnostic performance of US in the diagnosis of malignancy has not been shown to increase significantly after microbubble injection (Quaia et al. 2003b). This is because the appearance of renal tumors on baseline US, whether solid or cystic, is often characteristic (Quaia et al. 2003b), as in the case of hyperechoic renal angiomyolipoma, large heterogeneous renal cell carcinoma, multilocular cystic nephroma, and multiseptate cystic renal cell carcinoma with mural nodules (Hélénon et al. 2001). The injection of microbubble-based agents may improve renal tumor characterization on the basis of the contrast enhancement pattern, e.g., dotted or diffuse homogeneous enhancement in benign lesions, diffuse heterogeneous enhancement in malignant lesions, and absence of enhancement in renal metastases. Nevertheless, solid benign and malignant renal tumors may present an identical appearance after microbubble injection.

For this reason, renal tumor characterization still relies on contrast-enhanced helical CT or MR imaging (Zagoria 2000), which also allows staging assessment. Contrast-enhanced US has some advantages over baseline color and power Doppler US, such as the absence of motion and blooming artifacts and reduced dependence of the signal on the depth of the renal tumor.

Contrast-enhanced US may allow distinction between those renal tumors which should be characterized by cross-sectional imaging and those which can be exhaustively characterized by US, e.g., typical angiomyolipoma, hemorrhagic or hyperechoic cysts simulating a solid renal tumor, or simple or benign minimally complicated renal cysts. When diffuse homogeneous or heterogeneous contrast enhancement is identified in a solid renal tumor or peripheral

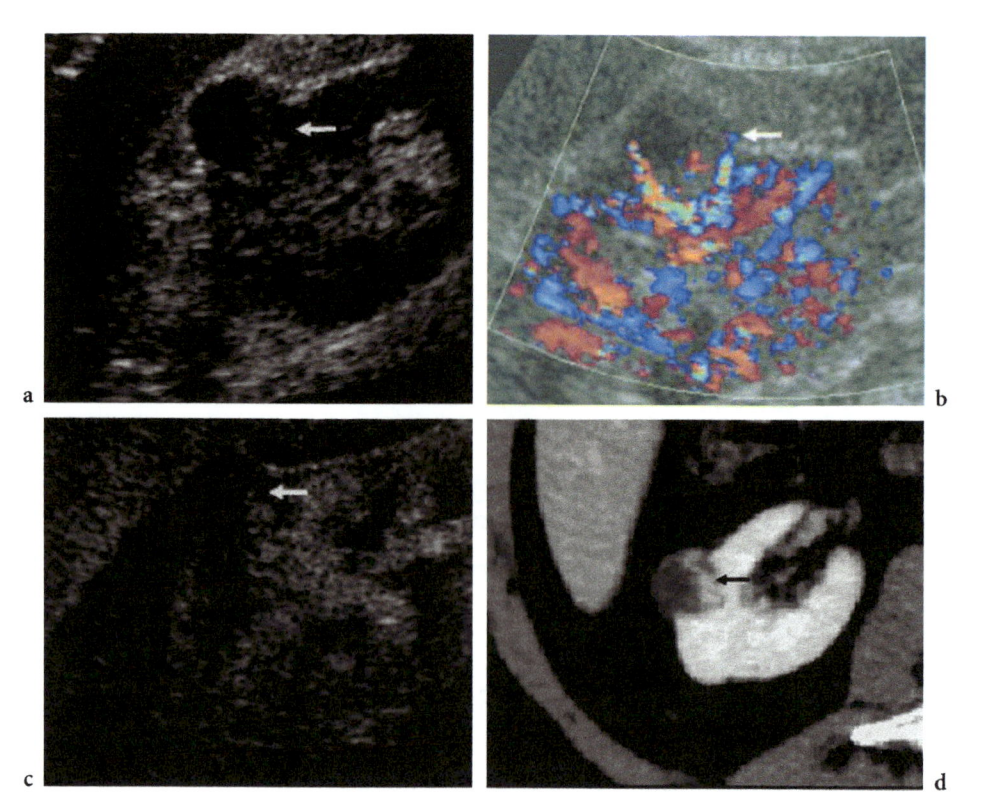

Fig. 15.17a–d. Cystic renal tumor with discontinuous rim-like peripheral enhancement. **a** Baseline US and **b** color Doppler US. A hypoechoic exophytic lesion (*arrow*) is identified at the right kidney with some vessels in the peripheral echogenic component. **c** Contrast-specific mode: Pulse Inversion Mode (Philips-ATL, WA, USA). Peripheral wall enhancement (*arrow*) is identified after the injection of air-filled microbubbles at intermittent high acoustic power insonation. **d** Contrast-enhanced CT. Peripheral contrast enhancement limited to the peripheral thickened wall (*arrow*) is identified after iodinated contrast agent injection. Cystic renal cell carcinoma of the clear cell type was diagnosed at histologic analysis of the surgical specimen.

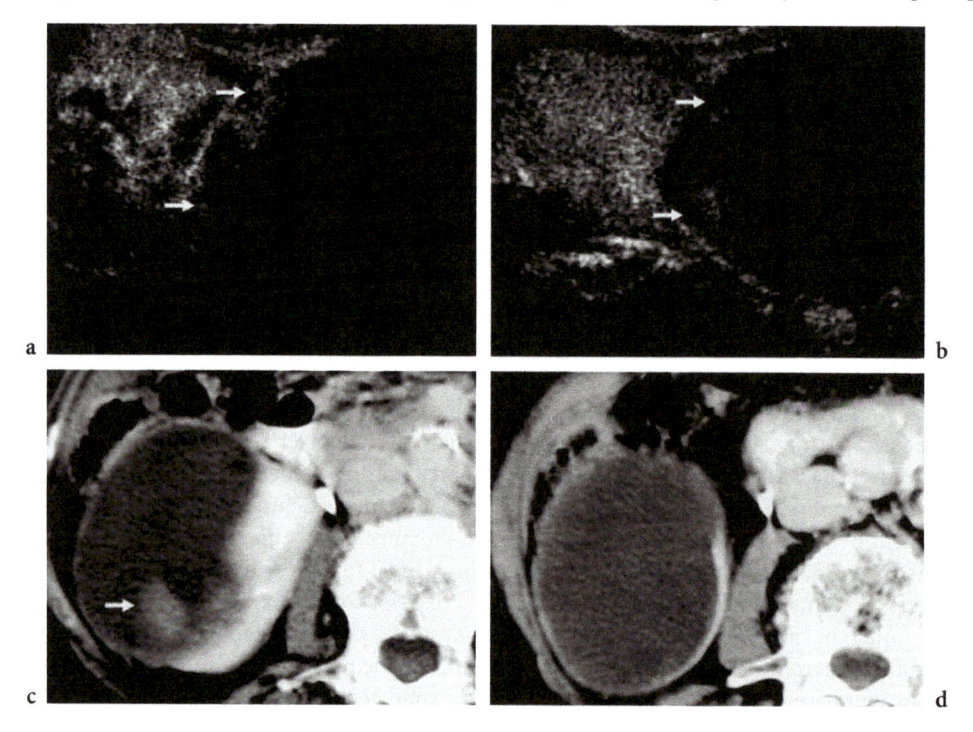

Fig. 15.18a–d. Cystic renal cell carcinoma with nodular peripheral enhancement. **a, b** Contrast-specific mode: Contrast Tuned Imaging (Esaote, Genoa, Italy) with low acoustic power insonation after the injection of sulfur hexafluoride-filled microbubbles. Contrast enhancement (*arrows*) is demonstrated in the solid peripheral nodular component of the tumor. **c, d** Contrast-enhanced CT. Peripheral contrast enhancement (*arrow*) is identified in the peripheral tumoral nodules, while the rest of the lesion presents a cystic appearance.

Characterization and Detection of Renal Tumors 241

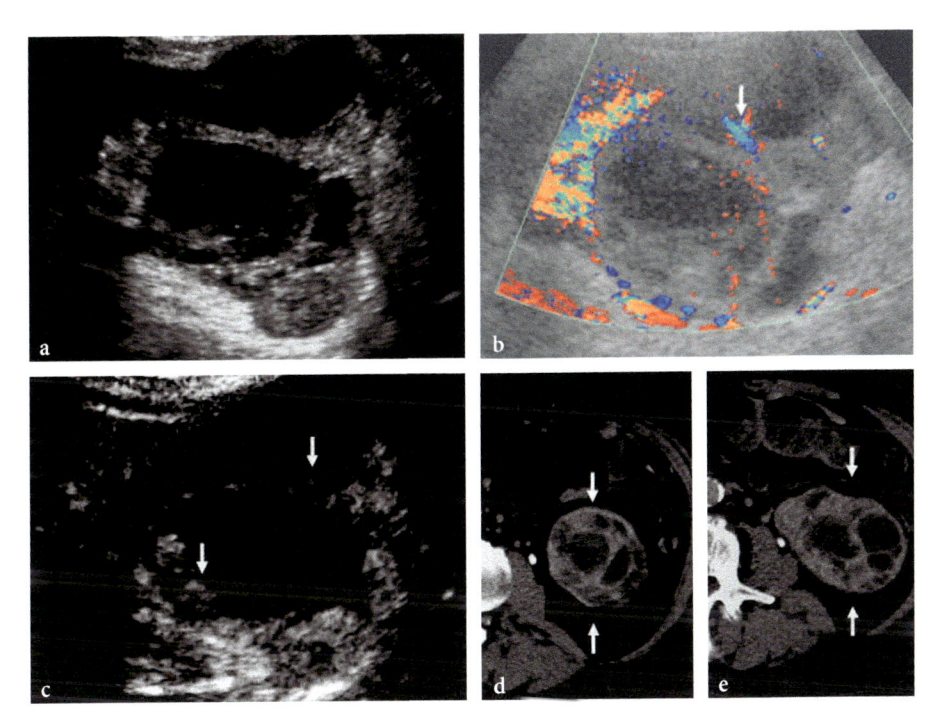

Fig. 15.19a–e. Cystic renal cell carcinoma. Diffuse nodular and septal enhancement. a Baseline US and b color Doppler US. A complex cystic renal mass shows a thickened peripheral wall and tumoral septa with evidence of vessels (*arrow*). c Contrast-specific mode: Contrast Tuned Imaging (Esaote, Genoa, Italy) with low acoustic power after the injection of sulfur hexafluoride-filled microbubbles. Diffuse septal and peripheral wall enhancement is demonstrated after microbubble injection. d, e Contrast-enhanced CT. Peripheral wall and septal enhancement (*arrows*) is identified after iodinated contrast agent injection.

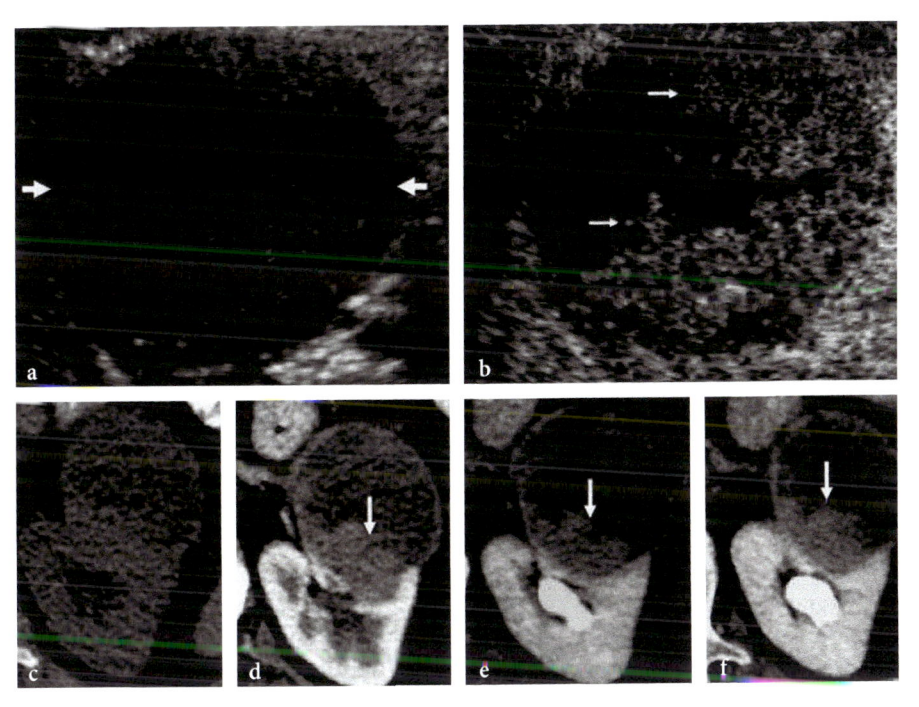

Fig. 15.20a–f. Cystic renal cell carcinoma with enhancement in the solid component. a Baseline US. A heterogeneous renal mass (*arrows*) displays a peripheral hyperechoic component and a central hypoechoic component. b Contrast-specific mode: Pulse Inversion Mode (Philips-ATL, WA, USA) with high acoustic power insonation after the injection of air-filled microbubbles. Peripheral contrast enhancement is revealed in the solid tumoral component (*arrows*), allowing better differentiation from the cystic tumoral component. c Non-enhanced CT and d-f contrast-enhanced CT. Peripheral contrast enhancement is identified in the peripheral solid component (*arrow*) of the cystic tumor, which appears progressively more evident from the corticomedullary (d) to the tubular (e) and excretory (f) phases.

or septal contrast enhancement is identified in a cystic renal tumor, the tumor has to be further examined by contrast-enhanced CT or MR imaging.

15.9
Detection of Renal Tumors

Baseline US. In addition to some technical and anatomical factors that may alter US performance, the detectability of renal tumors depends mainly on the size, location, and echogenicity of the lesion, with hyperechoic renal tumors being more easily visible. The main limitations of baseline US in the detection of renal tumors relate to small isoechoic intraparenchymal tumors and tumors of polar origin with extrarenal growth that may be obscured by bowel gas. Baseline US is less accurate than contrast-enhanced CT in demonstrating small renal masses, particularly when they are smaller than 3 cm (ZAGORIA 2000). Among small renal cell carcinomas (3 cm or less), 23–46% of solid tumors are iso- or hypoechoic compared with normal renal parenchyma (HÉLÉNON et al. 2001). Baseline color Doppler seems not to increase significantly the detection rate of small tumors (HÉLÉNON et al. 2001).

Contrast-enhanced CT and MR. Contrast-enhanced CT is considered a reliable technique for the detection of renal tumors (JAMIS-DOW et al. 1996; SZOLAR et al. 1997; ZAGORIA 2000). All renal masses can be detected by CT. Approximately 15% of renal masses detected on CT are benign, while the remaining 85% are malignant tumors (ZAGORIA 2000). For the accurate detection of renal masses, the nephrographic and excretory phases are optimal (SZOLAR et al. 1997; YUH and COHAN 1999; ZAGORIA 2000). The nephrographic and excretory phase images appear of similar value, but both are superior to corticomedullary phase images in terms of ability to detect and characterize renal masses. The corticomedullary phase should also be included for staging (KOPKA et al. 1997; ZAGORIA 2000).

Some diagnostic pitfalls have been described for contrast-enhanced CT (KOPKA et al. 1997; SZOLAR et al. 1997). The principal diagnostic difficulties are encountered in the presence of small hypervascular renal cell carcinomas with similar contrast enhancement to renal cortex, which may be mistaken for normal parenchyma in the corticomedullary phase, and centrally located tumors, which may be mistaken for normal hypoattenuating renal medulla (YUH and COHAN 1999).

Most studies indicate that MR imaging is comparable to CT for the detection of renal masses (SEMELKA et al. 1992; ZAGORIA 2000).

Contrast-enhanced US. The principal limitation of contrast-enhanced US in the detection of renal masses is that microbubble-based agents demonstrate only the corticomedullary phase without the possibility of a nephrographic phase. Since renal cell carcinomas present similar contrast enhancement to the adjacent renal parenchyma during the arterial corticomedullary phase, they become less evident after microbubble injection. Even though some studies seem to show an improvement in the detection of renal masses after microbubble injection (JENETT et al. 2000), malignant renal tumors are usually difficult to detect. The only exception may be renal hypovascular metastases, which present a persistent hypoechoic appearance after microbubble injection (QUAIA et al. 2003b) and appear as hypoechoic defects in the enhancing renal parenchyma.

15.10
When Should Microbubble-Based Agents Be Employed?

In typical angiomyolipoma, baseline US allows correct characterization (HÉLÉNON et al. 2001). Since the diagnostic performance of US in respect of malignancy has not been shown to improve significantly after microbubble injection (QUAIA et al. 2003b), microbubble-based agents should be employed only in selected other cases, e.g., to assess tumoral vascularity, to determine the extent of tumoral necrotic nonenhancing areas (Fig. 15.21), or to identify contrast enhancement in the tumoral thrombus. Every solid renal tumor which is indeterminate on both baseline US and contrast-enhanced CT or MR imaging has to be removed. Microbubble-based agents are also useful in differentiating renal tumors from pseudotumors such as hypertrophic column of Bertin. In pseudotumors, internal and peripheral vasculature exhibits smooth and homogeneous branching (CORREAS et al. 1999).

Simple (type 1) or minimally complicated (type 2) renal cysts are reliably assessed by baseline US. Microbubble-based agents should be employed to differentiate hemorrhagic and inflammatory renal cysts (Figs. 15.14, 15.15) from solid renal tumors. Indeterminate renal cysts (type 3) should always be assessed after microbubble injection to identify septal or mural

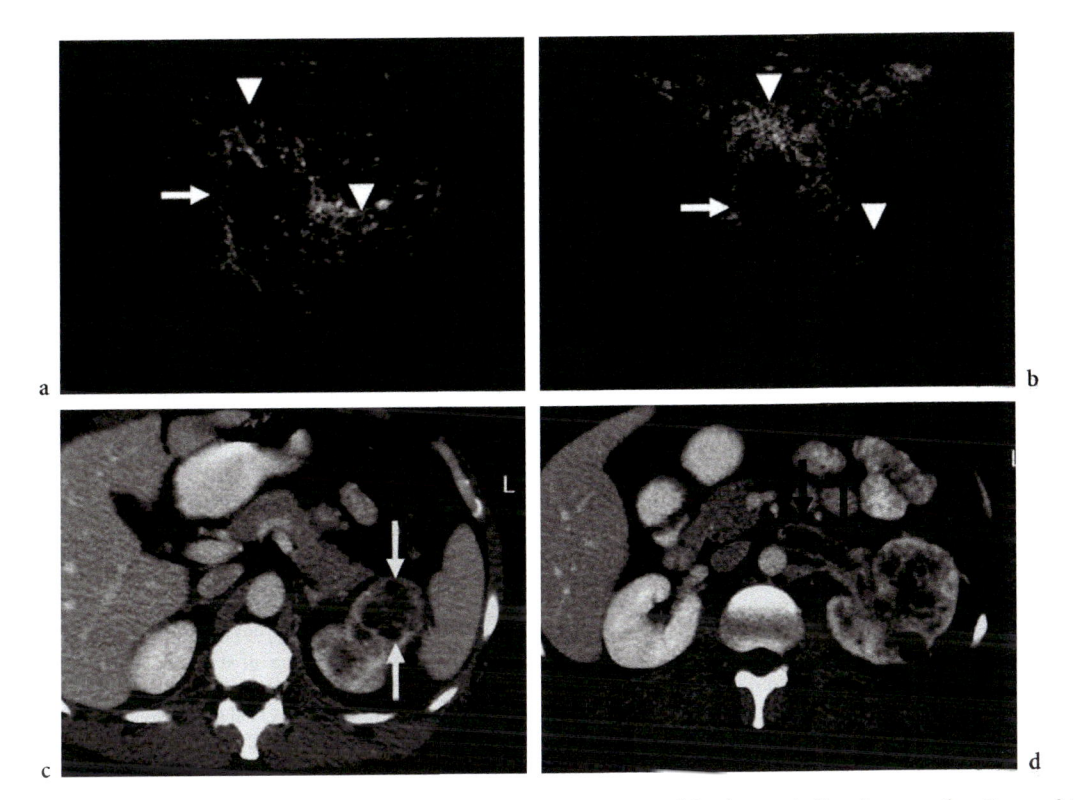

Fig. 15.21a–d. Large renal solid tumor that is extensively necrotic and displays an infiltrating growth pattern. **a, b** Heterogeneous diffuse contrast enhancement (*arrowheads*) is identified after microbubble injection, with central hypovascular necrotic regions (*arrow*). **c, d** Contrast-enhanced CT displays the tumor (*arrows*) in the upper left renal pole (**c**) with infiltrating growth towards the adjacent renal parenchyma (**d**) and complete thrombosis of the left renal vein (*arrows*).

nodule contrast enhancement, which is typical of malignant cysts. If these findings are identified, the renal cyst should be further examined by contrast-enhanced CT. In overt malignant renal cysts (type 4), microbubbles should be employed in selected cases, e.g., to distinguish solid from cystic, necrotic, nonenhancing components (Fig. 15.20).

In renal tumor detection, microbubbles should be employed only to detect renal metastases, which appear hypoechoic compared to the adjacent renal parenchyma on contrast-enhanced US.

References

Ambos MA, Bosniak MA, Valensi QJ (1978) Angiographic patterns in renal oncocytomas. Radiology 129:615-622

Amin MB, Crotty TB, Tickoo SK, Farrow GM (1997) Renal oncocytoma: a reappraisal of morphologic features with clinicopathologic findings in 80 cases. Am J Surg Pathol 21:1-12

Barr RG, Robbin ML, Peterson C (2001) Definity-enhanced ultrasound imaging of the kidney in patients with indeterminate masses: value of contrast harmonic imaging with bolus and infusion administration. Radiology [Suppl] 221:316

Bosniak MA (1986) The current radiological approach to renal cyst. Radiology 158:1-10

Bracken RB, Chica G, Johnson DE, Luna M (1979) Secondary renal neoplasms: an autopsy study. South Med J 72:806-807

Choyke PL, White EM, Zeman RK (1987) Renal metastases: clinicopathologic and radiologic correlation. Radiology 162:359-363

Choyke PL, Walther MM, Glenn GM et al (1997) Imaging features of hereditary papillary renal cancers. J Comput Assist Tomogr 21:737-741

Choyke PL, Glenn GM, Walther MM et al (2003) Hereditary renal cancers. Radiology 226:33-46

Claudon M, Tranquart F, Evans DH et al (2002) Advances in ultrasound. Eur Radiol 12:7-18

Correas JM, Hélénon O, Moreau JF (1999) Contrast-enhanced ultrasonography of native and transplanted kidney diseases. Eur Radiol 9 [Suppl 3]:S394-S400

Correas JM, Claudon M, Lesavre A et al (2001) Contrast-enhanced sonography of renal masses using FSO69: quantification of the enhancement with Pulse Inversion Imaging. Radiology [Suppl] 221:316

Correas JM, Claudon M, Tranquart F, Hélénon O (2003) Contrast-enhanced ultrasonography: renal applications. J Radiol 84:2041-2054

Dalla Palma L, Pozzi Mucelli F, Di Donna A, Pozzi Mucelli R (1990) Cystic renal tumors: US and CT findings. Urol Radiol 12:67-73

Davidson AJ, Hayes WS, Hartman DS (1993) Renal oncocytoma and carcinoma: failure of differentiation with CT. Radiology 186:693-696

De Carli P, Vidiri A, Lamanna L, Cantiani R (2000) Renal onco-

cytoma: image diagnostics and therapeutic aspects. J Exp Clin Cancer Res 19:287-290
Eilenberg SS, Lee JK, Brown J (1990) Renal masses: evaluation with gradient-echo Gd-DTPA-enhanced dynamic MR imaging. Radiology 176:333-338
Forman HP, Middleton WD, Melson GL, McLennan BL (1993) Hyperechoic renal cell carcinoma: increase in detection at US. Radiology 188:431-443
Hajri B, Ben Moualli S, Gelloub H et al (2001) Kidney oncocytoma. Report of 47 cases. Ann Urol 35:139-144
Hartman DS (1989) Renal cystic disease. AFIP atlas of radiologic-pathologic correlations. Saunders, Philadelphia, USA
Hartman DS (2001) Benign renal and adrenal tumors. Eur Radiol 11 [Suppl 2]:S195-S204
Hartman DS, Davidson AJ, Davis CJ, Goldman SM (1988) Infiltrative renal lesions: CT-sonographic-pathologic correlation. AJR Am J Roentgenol 150:1061-1064
Harvey CJ, Blomley MJ, Eckersley RJ et al (2000) Hepatic malignancies: improved detection with pulse inversion US in late phase of enhancement with SH U 508 A - early experience. Radiology 216:903-908
Hélénon O, Merran S, Paraf F et al (1997) Unusual fat-containing tumors of the kidney: a diagnostic dilemma. Radiographics 17:129-144
Hélénon O, Correas JM, Balleyguier C et al (2001) Ultrasound of renal tumors. Eur Radiol 11:1890-1901
Herts BR, Coll DM, Novick AC et al (2002) Enhancement characteristics of papillary renal neoplasms revealed on triphasic helical CT of the kidneys. AJR 178:367-372
Ho VB, Allen SF, Hood MN (2002) Renal masses: quantitative assessment of enhancement with dynamic MR imaging. Radiology 224:695-700
Israel G, Bosniak MA (2003a) Calcification in cystic renal masses: is it important in diagnosis? Radiology 226:47-52
Israel G, Bosniak MA (2003b) Renal imaging for diagnosis and staging of renal cell carcinoma. Urol Clin North Am 30:499-514
Jamis-Dow CA, Choyke PL, Jennings SB et al (1996) Small (<3-cm) renal masses: detection with CT versus US and pathologic correlation. Radiology 198:785-788
Jenett MA, Kessler C, Keberle MP et al (2000) Detection of renal lesions with contrast-enhanced wideband harmonic imaging. Radiology [Suppl] 217:559
Jinzaki M, Tanimoto A, Narimatsu Y et al (1997) Angiomyolipoma: imaging findings in lesions with minimal fat. Radiology 205:497-502
Jinzaki M, Ohkuma K, Tanimoto A et al (1998) Small solid renal lesions: usefulness of power Doppler US. Radiology 209:549-550
Kier R, Taylor KJ, Feyock AL, Ramos IM (1990) Renal masses: characterization with Doppler US. Radiology 176:703-707
Kim AY, Kim SH, Kim YJ, Lee IH (1999) Contrast-enhanced power Doppler sonography for the differentiation of cystic renal lesions: preliminary study. J Ultrasound Med 18:581-588
Kopka L, Fischer U, Zoeller G et al (1997) Dual-phase helical CT of the kidney: value of the corticomedullary and nephrographic phase for evaluation of renal lesions and preoperative staging of renal cell carcinoma. AJR Am J Roentgenol 169:1573-1578
Maki DD, Birnbaum BA, Chakraborty DP et al (1999) Renal cyst pseudoenhancement: beam-hardening effects on CT numbers. Radiology 213:468-472
Oyen R (1998) Renal parenchymal tumours. Halley Project 1998-2000, 2nd Refresher course series. Springer, Berlin Heidelberg New York
Oyen R, Verswijvel G, Van Poppel H, Roskams T (2001) Primary malignant renal parenchymal epithelial neoplasms. Eur Radiol 11 [Suppl 2]:S205-S217
Pickhardt PJ, Lonergan GJ, Davis CJ et al (2000) From the archives of AFIP. Infiltrative renal lesions: radiologic-pathologic correlation. Radiographics 20:215-243
Pozzi Mucelli R, Locatelli M (2002) Renal angiomyolipoma: typical and atypical features. Radiol Med 103:474-487
Pretorius ES, Wickstrom ML, Siegelman ES (2000) MR imaging of renal neoplasms. Magn Reson Imaging Clin North Am 8:813-836
Quaia E, Siracusano S, Bertolotto M et al (2003a) Characterization of renal tumours with pulse inversion harmonic imaging by intermittent high mechanical index technique. Preliminary results. Eur Radiol 13:1402-1412
Quaia E, Siracusano S, Bertolotto M et al (2003b) Characterization of renal masses scanned using low acoustic power US contrast specific mode after SonoVue injection (abstract). RSNA 2003. Scientific assembly and annual meeting program 666
Robert SC, Winick AB, Santi MR (1997) Papillary renal cell carcinoma: Diagnostic dilemma of a cystic renal mass. Radiographics 28:993-998
Semelka RC, Shoenut JP, Kroeker MA et al (1992) Renal lesions: controlled comparison between CT and 1.5-T MR imaging with nonenhanced and gadolinium-enhanced fat suppressed spin-echo and breath-hold FLASH techniques. Radiology 182:425-430
Sherman JL, Hartman DS, Friedman AC et al (1981) Angiomyolipomas: CT-pathologic correlations of 17 cases. AJR Am J Roentgenol 137:1221-1226
Sheth S, Scatarige JC, Horton KM (2001) Current concepts in the diagnosis and management of renal cell carcinoma: role of multidetector CT and three-dimensional CT. Radiographics 21:S237-S254
Silverman SG, Lee BY, Seltzer SE et al (1994) Small (<3-cm) renal masses: correlation of spiral CT features and pathologic findings. Am J Roentgenol 163:597-605
Soyer P, Dufresne AC, Klein I et al (1997) Renal cell carcinoma of clear cell type: correlation of CT features with tumor size, architectural patterns and pathologic staging. Eur Radiol 7:224-229
Storkel S, Eble JN, Adlakha K et al (1997) Classification of renal cell carcinoma: workgroup no 1. Union Internationale Contre le Cancer (UICC) and the American Joint Committee on Cancer (AJCC). Cancer 80:987-989
Szolar DH, Kammerhuber F, Altziebler S et al (1997) Multiphasic helical CT of the kidney: increased conspicuity for detection and characterization of small (<3-cm) renal masses. Radiology 202:211-217
Wagner BJ, Wong You Cheong JJ, Davis CJ (1997) From the archives of the AFIP. Adult renal hamartomas. Radiographics 17:155-169
Yamashita Y, Takahashi M, Watanabe O et al (1992) Small renal cell carcinoma: pathologic and radiologic correlation. Radiology 209:549-550
Yuh BI, Cohan RH (1999) Different phases of renal enhancement: role in detecting and characterizing renal masses during helical CT. AJR Am J Roentgenol 173:747-755
Zagoria RJ (2000) Imaging of small renal masses. A medical success story. Am J Roentgenol 175:945-955

16 Detection of Renal Perfusion Defects

Emilio Quaia and Salvatore Siracusano

CONTENTS

16.1 Introduction 245
16.2 Results in Animal Experimental Models 245
16.3 Results in Humans 246
16.3.1 Renal Perfusion Defects: Infarcts 246
16.3.2 Acute Renal Cortical Necrosis 249
16.3.3 Focal Acute Pyelonephritis and Renal Abscess 249
References 252

16.1 Introduction

Renal perfusion defects, often resulting in renal infarction, occur in a variety of clinical settings, such as thromboembolism, atherosclerosis, aneurysm of the aorta or renal artery, renal artery stenosis or occlusion, acute venous occlusion, subacute bacterial endocarditis (septic emboli), and vasculitis (Kawashima et al. 2000). Focal pyelonephritis manifests also as a perfusion defect. The most common cause is thromboembolism from cardiovascular disease which may determine also multifocal infarcts (Wong et al. 1984), while the most common clinical manifestation is sudden onset of flank or back pain with or without hematuria, proteinuria, fever, and leukocytosis.

Color and power Doppler US is a first-line imaging procedure to detect renal perfusion defect but presents clear limitations due to the relative insensitivity to low-velocity and low-amplitude flow states (Taylor et al. 1996). Coley et al. (1991) found a global accuracy of color Doppler US for detection of partial renal infarction of 20%. Contrast-enhanced color and power Doppler US are limited by blooming and flash artifacts, which may be attenuated by reducing the instrument gain settings and also diminishing the detection of focal abnormalities in renal blood flow (Taylor et al. 1996).

Contrast-material-enhanced CT represents a reference standard imaging technique to detect renal perfusion defects, which appear as focal wedge-shaped hypovascular lesions in normally perfused renal parenchyma.

Recent advances in microbubble-based contrast agents, and dedicated contrast-specific modes, have determined the achievement of increased image contrast in tissues. By transmitting at the fundamental frequency and receiving selectively harmonic frequencies, the background signal from stationary tissues is markedly suppressed resulting in a greater signal-to-noise ratio (Mattrey et al. 1998) and a better visibility of renal infarcts (Coley et al. 1991; Munzing et al. 1990; Girard et al. 2000). Blooming and flash artifacts are eliminated, shadowing artifacts are lessened, both spatial and temporal resolution are improved, and the brightness of gray-scale pixel does not depend on angle-dependent frequency shift estimates (Taylor et al. 1999). In contrast to iodinated contrast agent employed in CT, microbubbles are pure intravascular agents which are not excreted in renal tubules. Renal cortex rapidly enhances from 20 to 25 s after microbubble injection (Fig. 16.1a), while the vessels of renal medulla, which are less vascularized, are progressively filled from 30 to 35 s (Fig. 16.1b) and completely filled from 45 to 55 s (Fig. 16.1c) after microbubble injection.

16.2 Results in Animal Experimental Models

Animal models were firstly employed to assess the capabilities of contrast-enhanced US in detection of renal perfusion abnormalities (Taylor et al. 1998; Claudon et al. 1999; Quaia et al. 2004). We pro-

E. Quaia, MD
Assistant Professor of Radiology, Department of Radiology, Cattinara Hospital, University of Trieste, Strada di Fiume 447, 34149 Trieste, Italy
S. Siracusano, MD
Department of Urology, Cattinara Hospital, University of Trieste, Strada di Fiume 447, 34149 Trieste, Italy

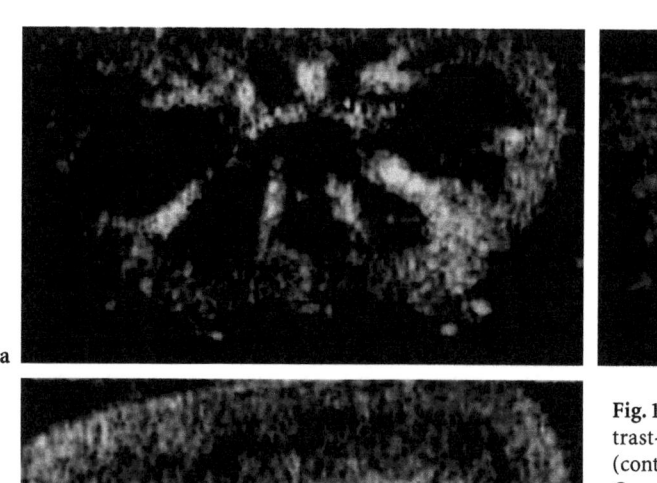

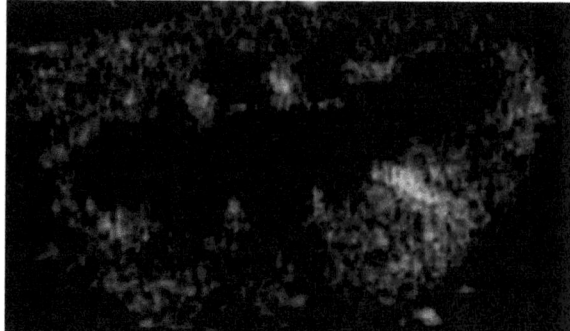

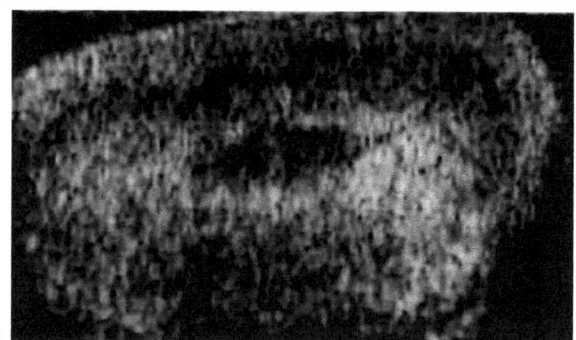

Fig. 16.1a–c. Animal model: New Zealand White rabbits. Contrast-enhanced US after microbubble-based agent injection (contrast-specific mode: contrast-tuned imaging; Esaote, Genoa, Italy). Cortico-medullary phase after microbubble-based agent injection. Normal renal perfusion at the early (**a**) arterial phase (15–20 s from injection) when only the cortical portion of the kidney is enhancing while the renal medulla is not yet filled by microbubbles. Normal renal perfusion at the late (**b**) arterial phase (25–40 s from injection) when both cortical and medullary portion of the kidney are enhancing. Normal renal perfusion at the late (**c**) phase (50–100 s from injection) when renal enhancement is homogeneous

posed an animal model) in which bilateral diffuse renal parenchymal embolization was performed in five adult New Zealand White rabbits (QUAIA et al. 2004). From 2 to 3 ml of polyvinyl alcohol particles (150–250 μm in diameter) were directly injected in the aorta 2 cm above the level of renal arteries. After embolization, both kidneys were surgically exposed at midline laparotomy. Each kidney was scanned at low acoustic power using a linear transducer before and after microbubble injection, 15 min after embolization, by placing the transducer on the surface of each kidney by interposing a gel pad to avoid reverberation artifacts. Digital subtraction angiography and macroscopic/histologic analysis of each kidney were considered as the reference standards.

After microbubble injection, renal perfusion defects appeared as single or multiple focal wedge-shaped areas of absent or diminished contrast enhancement in comparison with the adjacent renal parenchyma (Figs. 16.2, 16.3). Contrast-enhanced US revealed from 4 of 6 (66%) to 8 of 10 (80%) of renal perfusion defects confirmed by reference standards. The smallest renal perfusion defects identified by contrast-enhanced US revealed a diameter of 6 mm, while reference standards allowed detection of renal perfusion defects up to 3 mm in diameter. A significant increase in diagnostic confidence about presence or absence of renal perfusion defects was obtained by contrast-enhanced US in comparison with baseline US, even though it is limited in detection of renal perfusion defects smaller than 6 mm by volume average artifacts determined by the thickness of the US beam (about 5 mm).

16.3
Results in Humans

16.3.1
Renal Perfusion Defects: Infarcts

A) Baseline US and color Doppler US. Even though large renal perfusion defects or infarcts may be hypoechoic in comparison with the viable renal parenchyma, segmental renal infarcts are usually isoechoic or rarely hyperechoic if hemorrhagic component is present. Renal infarcts often reveal a wedge shape with capsular base. Even though baseline color Doppler US and power Doppler US present overt limitations to detect renal perfusion defects due to the low sensitivity to low-velocity and low-amplitude flow states, they may increase diagnostic capabilities of US in detecting renal infarcts, especially in elderly or obese patients and in patients with renal diseases. In renal infarct, color Doppler US and power Doppler US reveal absolute absence of renal cortical flows, even though it is very dif-

Detection of Renal Perfusion Defects

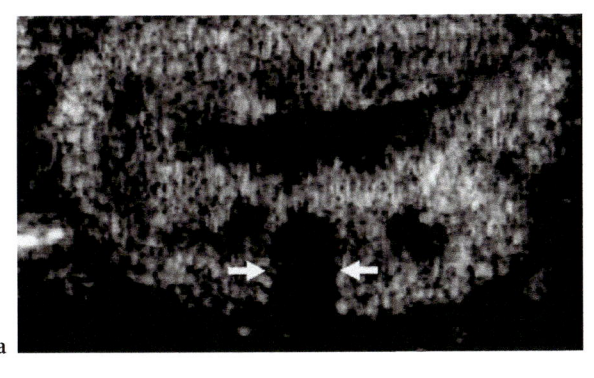

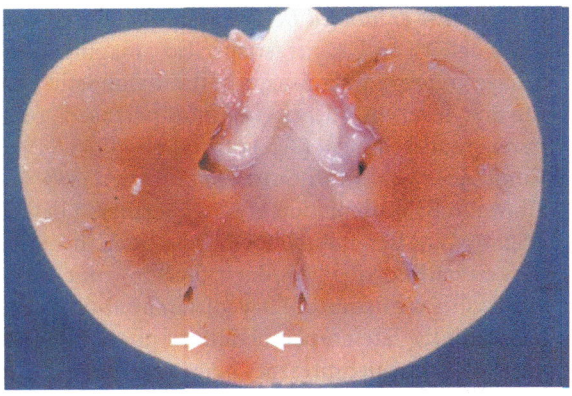

Fig. 16.2a,b Animal model: New Zealand White rabbits. Contrast-enhanced US after microbubble-based agent injection (contrast-specific mode: contrast-tuned imaging; Esaote, Genoa, Italy). Single focal renal perfusion defect (*arrows*) determined by random bilateral renal embolization by polyvinyl alcohol particles.

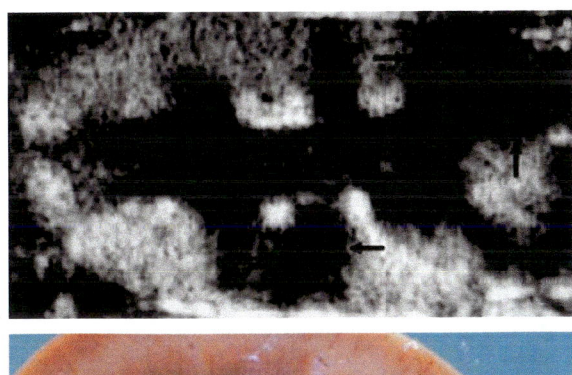

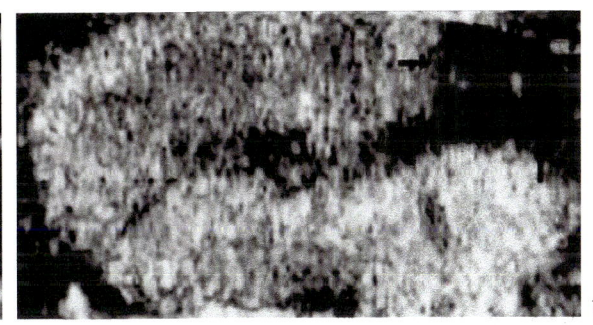

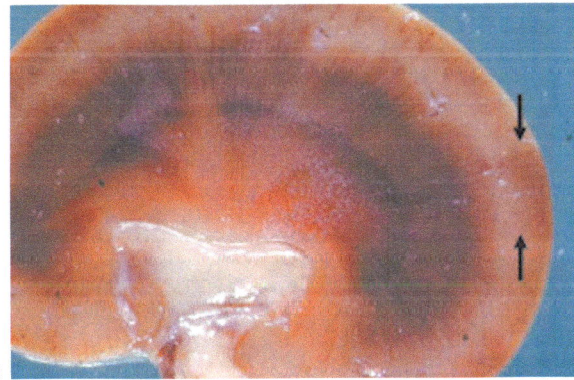

Fig. 16.3a–c. Animal model: New Zealand White rabbits. Contrast-enhanced US after microbubble-based agent injection (contrast-specific mode: contrast-tuned imaging; Esaote, Genoa, Italy). Different types for dimension and location of focal renal perfusion defects (*arrows*) determined by random bilateral renal embolization by polyvinyl alcohol particles. Contrast-enhanced US (a,b) allows a reliable depiction of renal perfusion defects which are confirmed at the gross specimen analysis (c).

ficult to differentiate renal segmental infarct from areas which appear poorly perfused due to underlying parenchymal disease, deep renal position, and artifacts. Moreover, color Doppler US presents a low accuracy in detection of small renal infarcts in the subcapsular region for limited spatial resolution and in the superior renal pole for the high Doppler angle and for the depth position (CORREAS et al. 2003).

B) Contrast-material-enhanced CT. Both CT and angiography are reference imaging techniques in renal infarct detection (KAWASHIMA et al. 2000). The parenchymal appearance of renal perfusion defects depends on the size of the embolus, the location of the arterial occlusion, and its age (KAWASHIMA et al. 2000). Contrast-material-enhanced CT shows the absence of enhancement in the affected renal tissue. Acute renal infarctions typically appear as wedge-shaped areas of decreased attenuation, while after the acute phase of renal infarction, atrophy begins and the infarcted tissue contracts, leaving a cortical scar.

C) Contrast-enhanced US. Microbubble-based contrast agents and contrast-specific imaging techniques improved significantly the diagnostic confidence level in identifying non-perfused renal parenchymal zones (TAYLOR et al. 1996, 1998; CORREAS et al. 1999; SCHMIEDL et al. 1999) and allow a reliable depiction of renal perfusion defects (Fig. 16.4). After microbubble injection, the early, or arterial, corticomedullary phase (from 20 to 40 s) with corticomedullary differentiation is followed by the late corticomedullary phase (from 45 up to 120 s), which presents homogeneous contrast enhancement of renal parenchyma sparing the renal collecting system. Both kidneys are scanned by low acoustic power in the longitudinal and axial plane during early and late corticomedullary phase. The renal poles are the most difficult regions to be assessed, since they are often hidden by interposing bowel gas. For this reason the position of the probe has to be dynamically modified during scanning to find the most effective acoustic window and to allow a complete visualization of each renal region. Renal perfusion defects appear as single or multiple focal wedge-shaped areas of absent, diminished, or delayed contrast enhancement in comparison with the adjacent renal parenchyma after microbubble injection (CORREAS et al. 2003).

The identification of small renal perfusion defects in the renal sub-capsular region is penalized by the limited spatial resolution of US which can not identify renal perfusion defects <5 mm. This is the case of cholesterinic renal embolization, since in this clinical situation the renal perfusion defects are often too small to be detected by contrast-enhanced US. If ≥5 mm, renal perfusions defects can be identified after microbubble injection (Fig. 16.5). Microbubble-based agents should be always employed to exclude renal infarcts in every old patient presenting with a renal colic-like pain in the flank region.

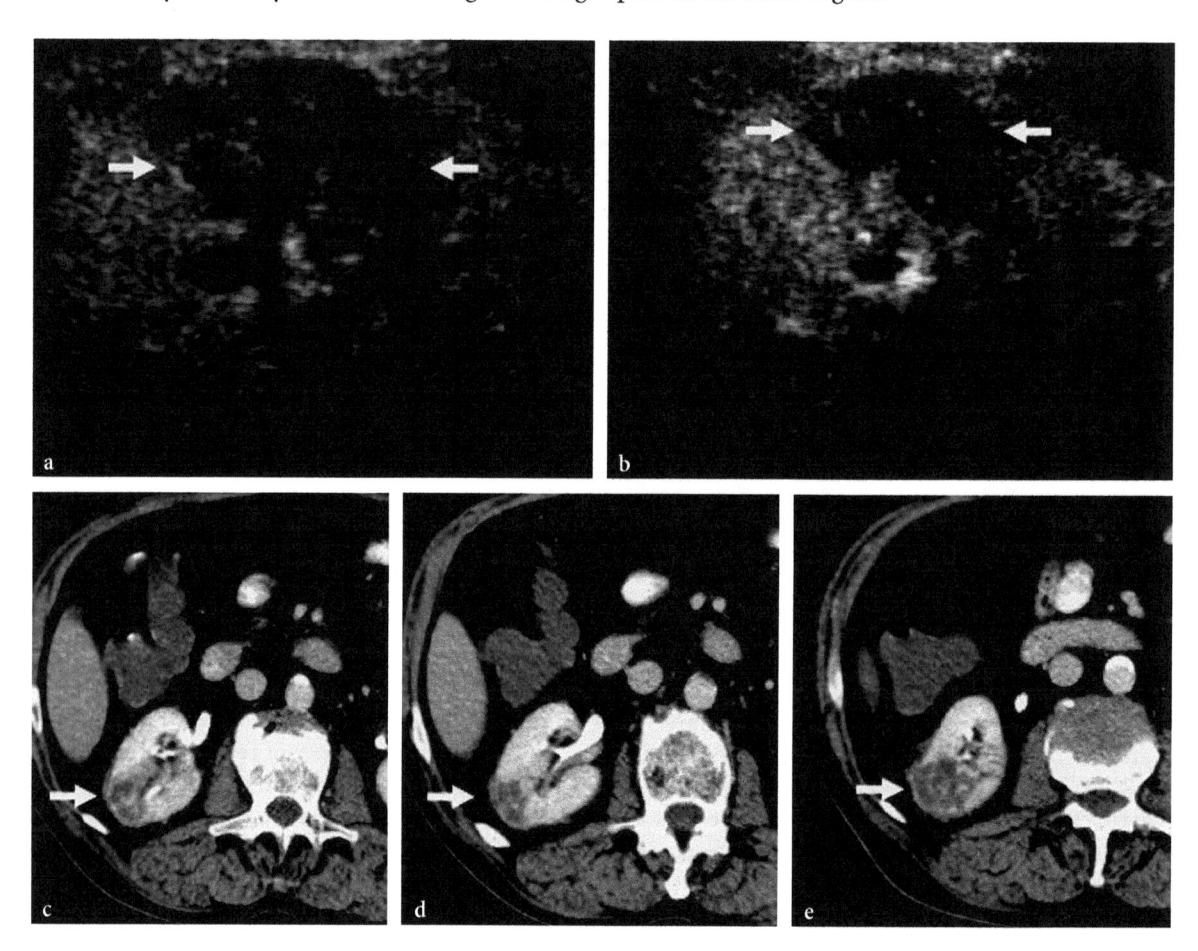

Fig. 16.4a–e. Human: focal renal perfusion defects. Contrast-enhanced US after microbubble-based agent injection (contrast-specific mode: pulse-inversion mode; Philips–ATL, Bothell, Wash.). Contrast-enhanced US (**a,b**) allows a reliable depiction of renal perfusion defect (*arrows*). The same renal perfusion defect (*arrow*) is confirmed at contrast-material-enhanced CT (**c–e**) after iodinated agent injection.

Detection of Renal Perfusion Defects

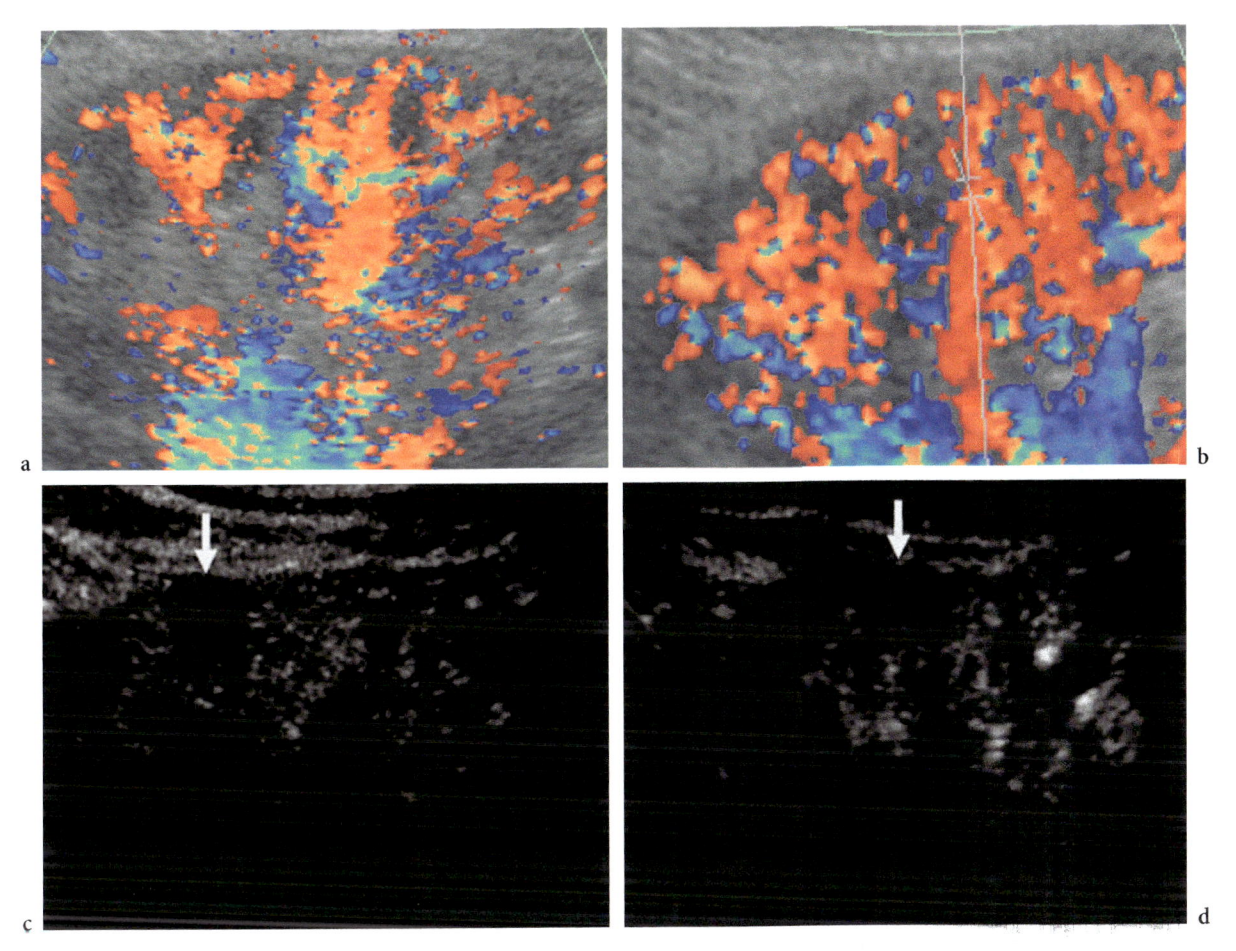

Fig. 16.5a–d. Human: cholesterinic renal embolization. Cholesterinic embolization proved by cutaneous biopsy. Contrast enhanced US after microbubble-based agent injection (contrast-specific mode: pulse-inversion mode; Philips–ATL, Bothell, Wash.). Baseline color Doppler US (**a,b**) does not allow identification of renal perfusion defects. Contrast-enhanced US (**c,d**) allows a reliable depiction of renal perfusion defect (*arrow*).

16.3.2
Acute Renal Cortical Necrosis

Acute renal cortical necrosis is a rare form of acute failure and results from ischemic necrosis of the renal cortex with sparing of the renal medulla. The process is either multifocal or diffuse; in most cases, it is bilateral. This condition is associated with complications of pregnancy, including abruptio placentae and septic abortion, sepsis, shock, or severe dehydration.

Contrast-material-enhanced CT scan shows enhancing interlobar and arcuate arteries adjacent to the nonenhancing cortex, enhancement of the medulla but no enhancement of the cortex, and/or a rim of subcapsular cortical enhancement (Kawashima et al. 2000; Jeong et al. 2002).

Acute renal cortical necrosis may be effectively represented by contrast-enhanced US (Fig. 16.6).

The necrotic cortex appears as a hypoechoic zone circumscribing the kidneys at contrast-enhanced US (Correas et al. 2003). Microbubble-based agents have to be always employed to exclude diffuse renal cortical necrosis, if it is clinically suspected.

16.3.3
Focal Acute Pyelonephritis and Renal Abscess

The visibility of focal pyelonephritis may be improved by color and power Doppler US in comparison with baseline gray-scale US (Quaia and Bertolotto 2002). Focal infective areas in acute pyelonephritis are prevalently less visible after microbubble injection in comparison with baseline gray-scale and color Doppler US (Fig. 16.7). This is because microbubbles remain entirely intravascular and renal vessels remain prevalently patent

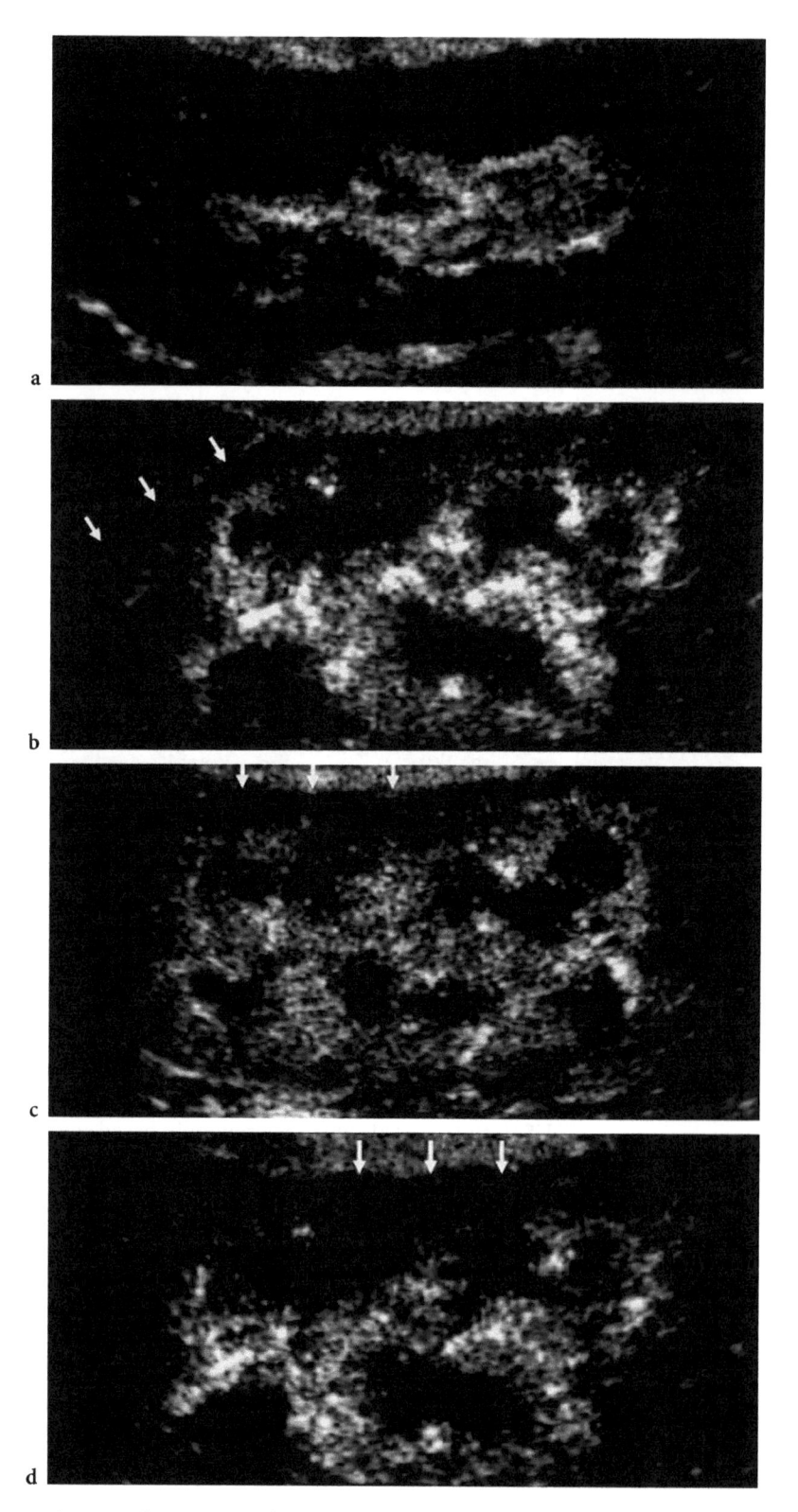

Fig. 16.6a–d. Human: renal acute cortical necrosis. An 80-year-old patient who was admitted to the emergency unit with acute renal failure. Baseline US (**a**) scan in the longitudinal plane did not demonstrate abnormalities as hydronephrosis. Absence of contrast enhancement in the superficial renal cortex identified after microbubbles injection (**b–d**; *arrows*). Acute cortical necrosis was confirmed at gross specimen and histologic analysis after patient death.

Detection of Renal Perfusion Defects

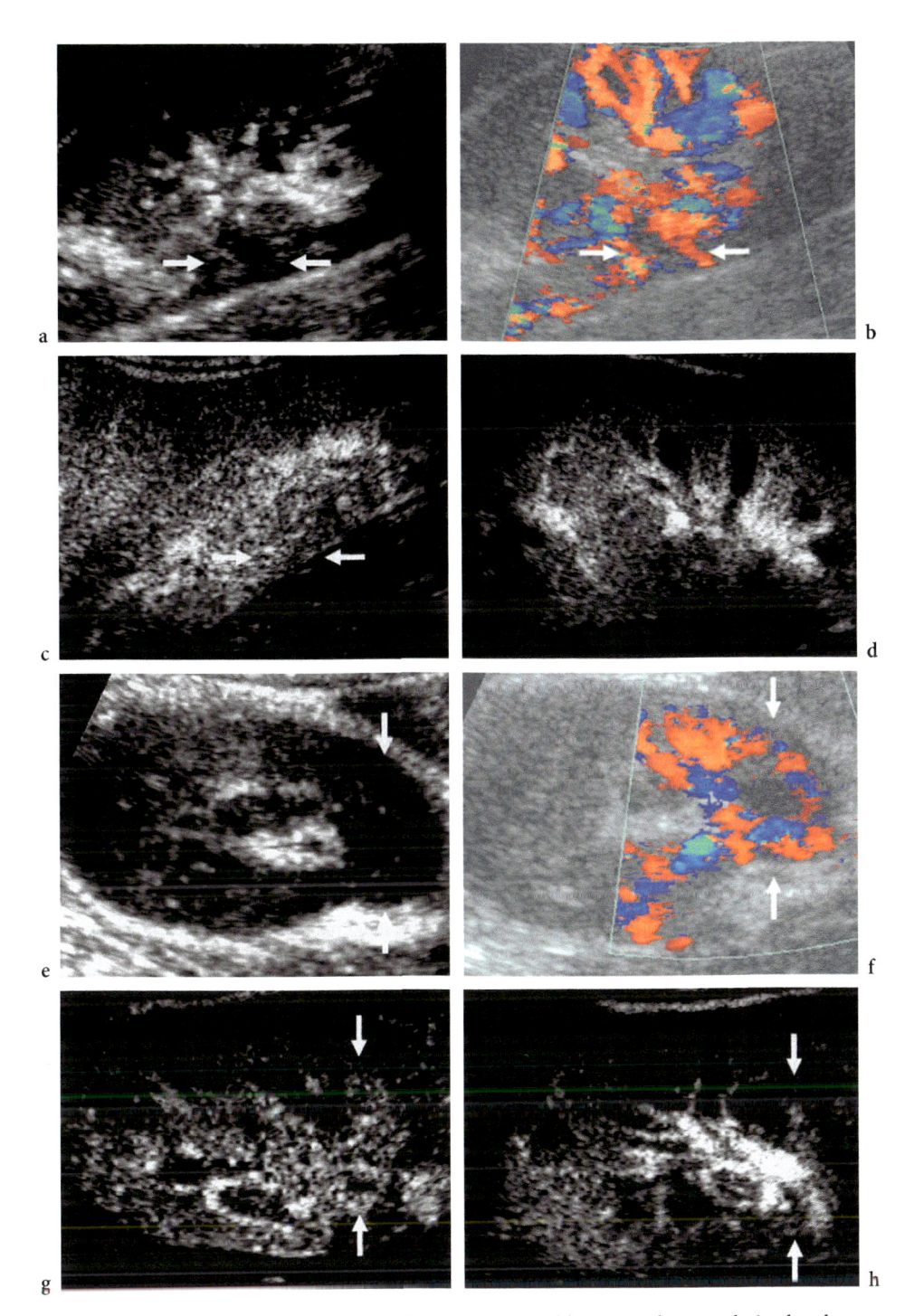

Fig. 16.7a–h. Human: acute focal pyelonephritis. A 32-year-old woman who was admitted to the emergency unit with fever and pain in the right flank. Two distinct areas of acute focal pyelonephritis in the right kidney are shown (*arrows*). The first area is located in the mesorenal region (**a–d**), while the second area is located in the lower renal pole (**e–h**). Baseline US (**a,c**) scan in the longitudinal plane shows a wedge-shaped hypoechoic area in the renal parenchyma which appears as an hypovascular region at color Doppler US (**b,f**). From 20 to 35 s after microbubble injection (**c,d,g,h**), renal parenchyma reveals homogeneous contrast enhancement (*arrows*) without evidence of renal perfusion defects.

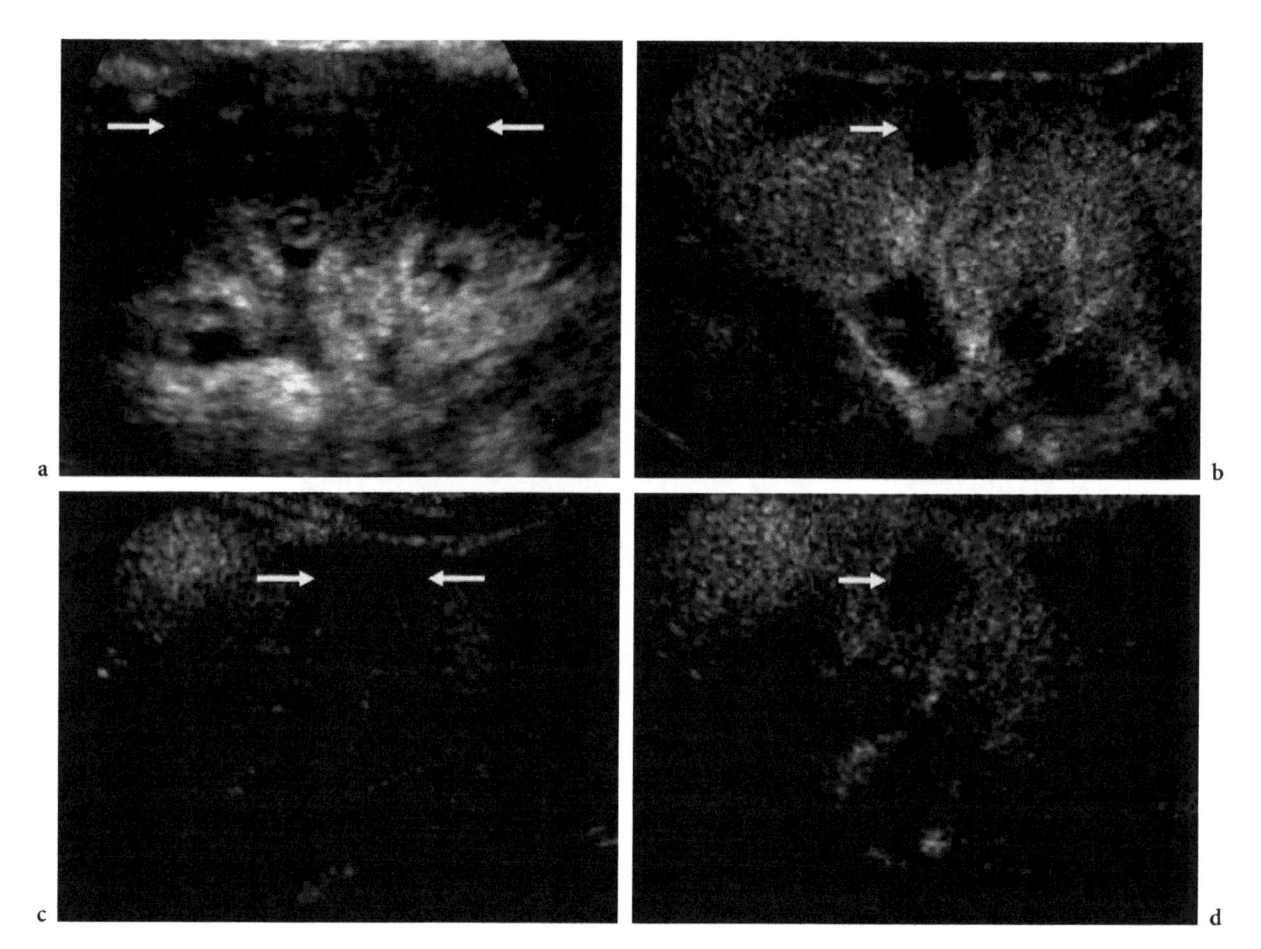

Fig. 16.8a–d. Human: renal abscess. A 38-year-old woman who was admitted to the emergency unit with fever, shivers, and pain in the left flank. Baseline US (**a**) scan in the longitudinal plane shows increased thickness and heterogeneous appearance (*arrows*) of the left renal parenchyma. After 25 s from microbubble injection (**b**), renal parenchyma revealed homogeneous contrast enhancement in the longitudinal plane except for a hypovascular lesion (*arrow*) corresponding to a small renal abscess. In the axial plane (**c**) a wedge-shaped renal perfusion defect (*arrows*) is identified corresponding to focal pyelonephritis, and the renal abscess (*arrow*) is confirmed (**d**).

in focal infective areas, while color Doppler US exclusively depicts large renal vessels which are prevalently displaced by inflammatory edema. Focal acute pyelonephritis may improve in conspicuity after microbubble injection if renal vessels are compressed by the adjacent edema revealing a triangular shape, similarly to the renal perfusion defects (Fig. 16.8). In fact, contrast-enhanced US was shown to improve the detection and conspicuity of renal parenchymal abnormalities in acute pyelonephritis in comparison with baseline US (KIM et al. 2001) and to improve the diagnosis of acute pyelonephritis (DUVAL et al. 2003).

Renal abscesses may be effectively represented after microbubble injection (Fig. 16.8), since they do not present intralesional vessels which are destroyed or displaced by the colliquative process (CORREAS et al. 2003).

References

Claudon M, Barnewolt C, Taylor GA et al (1999) Renal blood flow in pigs: changes depicted with contrast-enhanced harmonic US imaging during acute urinary obstruction. Radiology 212:725–731

Coley BD, Mattrey RF, Roberts A, Keane S (1991) Potential role of PFOB enhanced sonography of the kidney. II. Detection of partial infarction. Kidney Int 39:740–745

Correas JM, Helenon O, Moreau JF (1999) Contrast enhanced ultrasonography of native and transplant kidney diseases. Eur Radiol 9 (Suppl 3):394–400

Correas JM, Claudon M, Tranquart F, Hélenon O (2003) Contrast-enhanced ultrasonography: renal applications. J Radiol 84:2041–2054

Duval A, Correas JM, Morelon E (2003) The diagnosis of acute pyelonephritis in renal transplants using contrast-enhanced US (abstract). RSNA 2003

Girard MS, Mattrey RF, Baker KG et al (2000) Comparison of standard and second harmonic B-mode sonography in the detection of renal infarction with ultrasound contrast in a rabbit model. J Ultrasound Med 19:185–192

Jeong JY, Kim SH, Lee HJ (2002) Atypical low-signal-intensity renal parenchyma: causes and patterns. Radiographics 22:833–846

Kawashima A, Sandler CM, Ernst RD et al (2000) CT evaluation of renovascular disease. Radiographics 20:1321–1340

Kim B, Lim HK, Choi MH et al (2001) Detection of parenchymal abnormalities in acute pyelonephritis by pulse inversion harmonic imaging with or without microbubble ultrasonographic contrast agent. J Ultrasound Med 20:5–14

Mattrey RF, Steinbach G, Lee Y et al (1998) High-resolution harmonic gray-scale imaging of normal and abnormal vessels and tissues in animals. Acad Radiol 5 (Suppl): S63–S65

Munzing D, Mattrey RF, Reznik VM et al (1990) The potential role of PFOB enhanced sonography of the kidney, part I. Detection of renal function and acute tubular necrosis. Kidney Int 39:733–739

Quaia E, Bertolotto M (2002) Renal parenchymal diseases: Is characterization feasible with ultrasound? Eur Radiol 12:2006–2020

Quaia E, Siracusano S, Ciciliato S et al (2004) Detection of renal perfusion defects in rabbits using non-linear contrast specific modes with low transmit power imaging and SonoVue (abstract). ECR 2004

Schmiedl UP, Carter S, Martin RW et al (1999) Sonographic detection of acute parenchymal injury in an experimental porcine model of renal hemorrhage: gray-scale imaging using sonographic contrast agent. Am J Roentgenol 173:1289–1294

Taylor GA, Ecklund K, Dunning PS (1996) Renal cortical perfusion in rabbits: visualization with color amplitude imaging and an experimental mircobubble-based US contrast agent. Radiology 201:125–129

Taylor GA, Barnewolt CE, Adler BH, Dunning PS (1998) Renal cortical ischemia in rabbits revealed by contrast-enhanced power Doppler sonography. Am J Roentgenol 170:417–422

Taylor GA, Barnewolt CE, Claudon M, Dunning P (1999) Depiction of renal perfusion defects with contrast-enhanced harmonic sonography in a porcine model. Am J Roentgenol 173:757–760

Wong WS, Moss AA, Federle MP (1984) Renal infarction: CT diagnosis and correlation between CT findings and etiologies. Radiology 150:201–205

17 Quantitative Analysis of Renal Perfusion at Contrast-Enhanced US

Emilio Quaia

CONTENTS

17.1 Quantification of Perfusion by Doppler Techniques 255
17.1.1 Spectral Doppler 256
17.1.2 Power Doppler 256
17.2 Speckle Decorrelation 256
17.3 Quantitation of Renal Perfusion by Microbubble-Based Agents 256
17.3.1 Intermittent High-Transmit-Power Technique 257
17.3.2 Continuous Low-Transmit-Power Technique 257
17.4 Microbubble Injection 257
17.5 Objective Analysis of Echo Signal Intensity 257
17.6 Approximation by Mathematical Functions 259
17.6.1 Wash-in/Wash-out Curves (Gamma Variate) 259
17.6.2 Negative Exponential 260
17.6.3 Sigmoid 260
17.6.4 Other Mathematical Functions and Drawbacks in Mathematical Approximation 261
17.7 Clinical Applications of Renal Perfusion Quantitation 262
References 263

17.1 Quantification of Perfusion by Doppler Techniques

Tissue viability and function may be maintained only in the presence of adequate perfusion, which is tightly regulated to maintain factors such as nutrient delivery, gas exchange, and fluid balance. The ability to accurately quantify blood flow in solid organs is essential for a variety of reasons, including confirmation of organ or tissue viability, assessment of tumor ablation procedures, postoperative imaging where rejection or vascular complications may occur, and determination of the response to angiogenesis-modulating drugs.

Different parameters have to be considered in blood-flow quantitation. Firstly, the blood velocity which corresponds to the speed of red blood cells (in centimeters per second) in the analyzed region. Secondly, the blood flow which is volume of blood passing in a section of tissue per unit of time (cubic centimeters per second), corresponding to the blood velocity x section of perfused parenchymal tissue (expressed in square centimeters per second). The parenchymal perfusion corresponds to the parenchymal blood flow equalized for the volume or weight of the perfused parenchyma – or the amount of flow in a volume of tissue per unit of time – and it is expressed in cm^3/seconds/cm^3 or grams. Thirdly, the fractional vascular volume is an index of the physiological vascularity of a region and is the proportion of tissue occupied by blood.

Many imaging techniques, including radionuclide single-photon emission computed tomography (SPECT), ultrafast computed tomography (CT), magnetic resonance (MR) imaging, and positron emission tomography (PET), have been used to evaluate tissue blood flow; however, those techniques are not portable and expensive and present some inherent limitations such as the low availability and the patient exposition to irradiation or nuclear tracers.

The progressive improvement of microbubble and ultrasound (US) contrast-specific modes has determined the advent of a new non-invasive, portable, and relatively inexpensive modality for the assessment of tissue blood flow. Ultrasound provides excellent spatial resolution (<1 mm axially) and temporal resolution (240 Hz), which is even better than many other imaging modalities.

Microbubble-based contrast agents consist of stabilized microbubbles, filled by air or perfluorocarbon gas and covered by a peripheral shell of various composition and rigidity. Microbubbles remain entirely intravascular, mix uniformly with blood in the circulation, and possess the same intravascular rheology as red blood cells when injected intravenously. Perfluorocarbon or sulfur hexafluoride-filled agents (SCHNEIDER et al. 1995) present a strong harmonic behavior at low transmit power and are made by stabilized microbubbles of gases of high

E. QUAIA, MD
Assistant Professor of Radiology, Department of Radiology, Cattinara Hospital, University of Trieste, Strada di Fiume 447, 34149 Trieste, Italy

molecular weight and low solubility in water which provides a longer persistence in the bloodstream than air-filled agents. Doppler, speckle decorrelation, and contrast-specific modes may be employed to assess flow (amount of blood passing per unit time, in milliliters per minute), perfusion (amount of flow in a volume of tissue per unit of time, in milliliters per minute per milligram), and fractional blood or vascular volume (tissue occupied by blood, in milliliters per milligram).

17.1.1
Spectral Doppler

Spectral Doppler may be employed to estimate the mean velocity of blood in a vessel, and if the cross-sectional area of the vessel is also measured, the product gives the mean flow rate. Due to difficulty of accurately measuring the vessel area and the time-averaged mean velocity, this estimation remains subject to serious errors and is operator dependent. Microbubble-based US contrast agents increase the intensity of spectral Doppler signal, which may be quantified via a sound card or a dedicated A-to-D audio converter to obtain time–intensity curves.

The mean transit time (MTT) may be derived from time–intensity curves (COSGROVE et al. 2001), through deconvolution mathematical procedures, and corresponds to the average persistence of a microbubble in the circulation of a region of tissue as it travels from an inflow to an outflow vessel. The MTT is also related to the renal blood flow (RBF) and fractional renal blood volume (RBV) by the central volume principle:

$$RBF = \frac{RBV}{MTT}.$$

17.1.2
Power Doppler

Power Doppler signals are log-compressed and proportional to the number of moving reflectors. After quantification and appropriate transformation (antilogging and correction for color post-processing), a power Doppler image should give a map of regional red-cell concentration and of fractional blood volume. After microbubble injection, a time–intensity curve can be obtained by analyzing the increase of signal intensity in a region of interest (ROI). Fractional blood volume could be calculated by dividing the area under the time–intensity curve obtained from a parenchymal region by that obtained from a vascular region of interest, while perfusion may be quantified by measuring the concentration of microbubbles in vivo.

17.2
Speckle Decorrelation

Because US is a coherent imaging method, the amplitude of the received US signal fluctuates as a result of the relative spatial arrangement of sub-resolution scatterers, which generate speckle (RUBIN et al. 1999). The phenomenon manifests in B-mode images as fluctuations in time of the amplitude of speckle and is also observed in Doppler US as fluctuations of the signal amplitude. Decorrelation is caused by a change in the speckle pattern in a given sample volume determined by the dimensions of the US beam and the pulse length. Ideally, this speckle pattern change would be caused completely by fluid movement through the sample volume. Ultrasound gray-scale speckle decorrelation with bubble contrast agents may be useful for measuring blood flow in vivo (RUBIN et al. 1999).

17.3
Quantitation of Renal Perfusion by Microbubble-Based Agents

The accurate quantitation of parenchymal perfusion in solid organs is essential for confirmation of organ or tissue viability and determination of response to angiogenesis-modulating drugs. Presently, quantitation of organ perfusion can be performed non-invasively using dedicated US contrast-specific modes and microbubble-based contrast agents. A linear relation exists between microbubble concentration and the video signal intensity (CORREAS et al. 2000), which may be quantified by dedicated software to produce time–intensity curves.

With expanded use and development of microbubble-based contrast agents, a variety of innovative applications have been developed. The intravenous injection of microbubble-based contrast agents allows estimation of relative blood flow and fractional blood volume of the microvasculature in an ROI (WEI et al. 1998a). The first phenomenon which has to be elicited is microbubble destruction in the insonated tissue by applying a high-transmit power train. The major factors influencing microbubble destruction are the transmit frequency and the transmit power which actually constitute the mechanical index (MI), inversely related to transducer frequency and directly to the transmit power and representing the amount of US energy being transmitted (WEI et al. 1997; CORREAS et al. 2002). After initial microbubble destruction, other trains of destructive high transmit power may be transmitted at increasing pulsing intervals or a continuous low transmit power may be employed to image tissue replenishment in real time. For both technique the fundamental assumption is that the relation between microbubble concentration and video intensity is linear up to the achievement of a plateau phase (CORREAS et al. 2000).

17.3.1
Intermittent High-Transmit-Power Technique

By setting up an infusion of microbubbles to produce a steady blood concentration, the bubbles in a imaged slice may be destroyed by applying a train of high-transmit power frames. After microbubbles have been destroyed, the speed of tissue replenishment by microbubbles will depend on time interval between destructive pulses and the flow velocity of microbubbles. When the next destructive beam is applied, the intensity of the echoes depends on the number of bubbles that have flowed into the slice and so increased with longer intervals (WEI et al. 1998). If the process is repeated at a series of intervals, a time–intensity curve may be created and its slope is related to the speed of blood moving into the slice and the maximum level reached (the asymptote or plateau phase) relates to the vascular blood volume. This method is sensitive to relative movements between probe and the tissue because such movements expose a new slice of tissue that contains bubbles that have not been removed by the previous frame thus introducing errors.

17.3.2
Continuous Low-Transmit-Power Technique

Because US can destroy microbubbles, the change in echogenicity after tissue has been cleared of microbubbles can be imaged and quantified to obtain destruction–replenishment curve. This technique is also known as negative bolus since a void of microbubbles is created in the insonated tissue which is refilled progressively by incoming bubbles (Fig. 17.1). With the recent introduction of bubble-specific imaging methods that operate at very low MI (0.08–0.21), such as power pulse inversion or pulse inversion mode, continuous interrogation can be performed without destroying bubbles in the slice so that the refill can be observed in real time and with much less likelihood of probe movements.

17.4
Microbubble Injection

In order for the concentration of microbubbles to be quantifiable, microbubbles have to be carefully administered to maintain concentrations in the circulation below the level of signal saturation. When a dilute solution of microbubbles is administered as a constant infusion, the concentration of microbubbles in circulation will reach a steady state (WEI et al. 1998). At steady state the number of microbubbles entering or leaving any microcirculatory unit is constant and depends on the flow rate. The bolus injection in a peripheral vein may be employed only to assess the mean organ transit time, while it must be avoided in contrast-specific modes since bolus dispersion in peripheral circulation do not allow assumption of a steady state in microcirculation. If microbubbles are injected directly as a discrete bolus in an artery supplying the organ, their mean transit rate through the parenchyma reflects the flow per unit volume (parenchymal blood flow/total artery blood flow), while the same relation does not apply if microbubbles are injected in a peripheral vein. Consequently to dispersion of microbubbles into the organ parenchyma, the parenchyma output function is wider that the input function. This problem can be partially solved by complex deconvolution mathematical procedures which are difficult and not always applicable.

17.5
Objective Analysis of Echo Signal Intensity

Determination of the degree of tissue contrast enhancement relies on accurate distinction between backscatterer signals originating from microbubbles and the intrinsic signal emanating from tissues which varies widely within the US sector for inhomogeneities of acoustic power and differences in

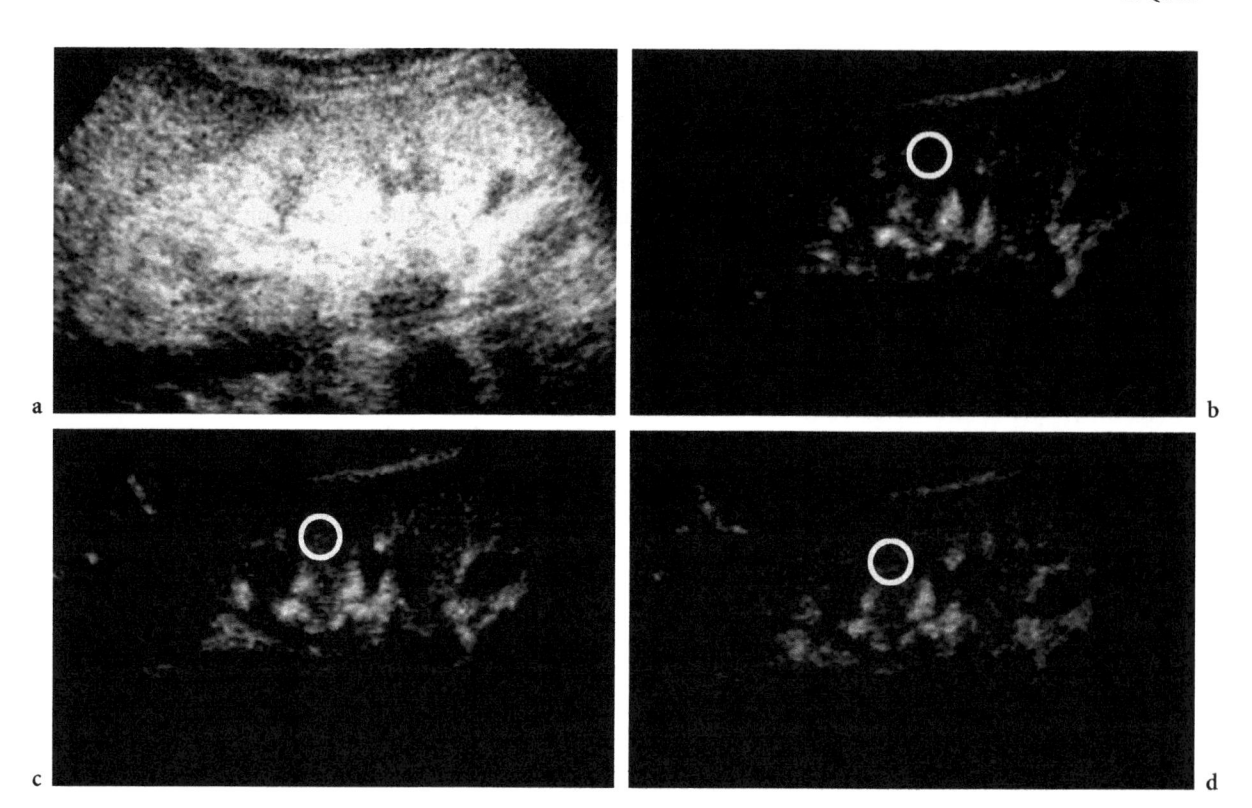

Fig. 17.1a-d. Progressive refilling of renal parenchyma at low acoustic power insonation after microbubble destruction. After image alignment and background subtraction, the echo signal intensity may be quantified by manually defined regions of interest (ROI) positioned in a region of renal parenchyma. A preliminary high acoustic power train of US pulses (**a**) destroy all the microbubbles comprised in the imaged slice of renal parenchyma. The progressive refilling of renal parenchyma by microbubbles is monitored at low acoustic power (**b-d**). The progressive higher echo signal intensity of renal parenchyma is determined by the progressive microbubble accumulation in the imaged slice.

attenuation and absorption of US energy by tissue. Direct visual assessment of the degree of contrast enhancement is the less accurate method.

Accurate quantitation of the degree of contrast enhancement requires assessment of the change in echo-signal intensity between the baseline and contrast-enhanced images. Digital image-processing techniques, such as image alignment, averaging, video densitometry, and background subtraction, are essential and may be performed by calculation software packages produced by the scanner manufacturers which have access to the raw data before applications of non-linear modifications (HDIlab from Philips/ATL, Bothell, Wash.). These dedicated softwares allow to anti-log the gray-scale signals which are log-compressed for video presentation. Log-compressed video-intensity can be considered as:

$$10 * \log_{10}\left(\frac{I}{I_{ref}}\right),$$

where I is the acoustic intensity and I_{ref} is an intensity level determined through equipment gain.

The other possibility is to quantify directly the log-compressed video intensity of a digital cine clip. The log-compressed video-intensity does not provide a reliable quantification of microbubble signal, since several stages of post-processing in an ultrasound equipment for image video presentation, including log-compression, modify the original features of the signal. Moreover, the log-compressed video-intensity signal does provide quantification of what is displayed and used for qualitative clinical assessment (PHILLIPS and GARDNER 2004).

The echo signal intensity, linearized or log-compressed, may be quantified by positioning manually defined circular or rectangular ROIs in a region of renal parenchyma (Fig. 17.2), and by correlating time with the measured echo-signal video intensity in linear or logarithmic scale. Since the renal medulla presents a much lower perfusion (190 ml/min per 100 g) than the renal cortex (400 ml/min per 100 g; Fig. 17.2), it is preferable to encompass with a single manually defined ROI (Fig. 17.3) all the renal cortex excluding renal medulla.

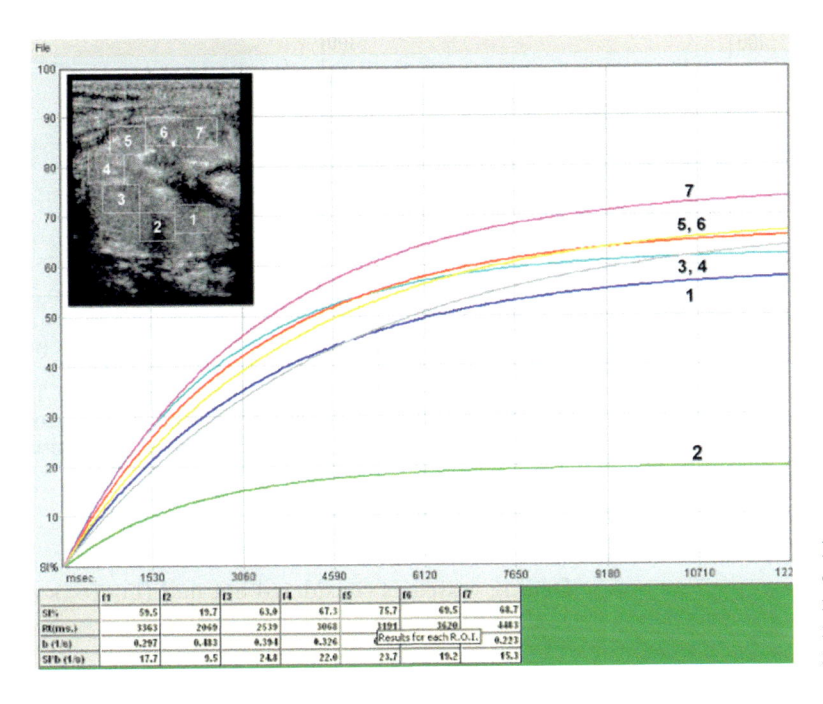

Fig. 17.2 Different refilling profile between different regions of interest positioned in renal cortex (regions 1 and 3–7) and one region of interest positioned in the renal medulla (region 2)

17.6
Approximation by Mathematical Functions

Different mathematical functions (Fig. 17.4) have been proposed to fit echo-signal intensity raw data vs time (Li and Yang 2003). The most employed is exponential negative ($A(1-e^{-\alpha t})$) based on a single-compartment model (Wei et al. 1998). The slope of the first ascending tract is related to microbubble velocity, while the plateau phase is related to fractional blood volume. This model, however, is based on continuous microbubble infusion into a single open compartment and is valid only if we assume that a constant number of microbubbles enters the region of interest per unit time. Recently, the exponential negative function was shown (Lucidarme et al. 2003a) to present distortion toward a sigmoid curve if the percentage of bubbles destruction in the feeding vessels is not null. Even though both these functions could represent a reliable model, a wide variability between subjects exists: the first ascending tract of the curve presents a large interpolating error determined by the few available points, and both ascending and plateau phase tracts present large points dispersion.

17.6.1
Wash-in/Wash-out Curves (Gamma Variate)

The gamma variate (Fig. 17.4a) has the form $y=At\,e^{-\alpha t}+C$, where A=the amplitude of the curve above

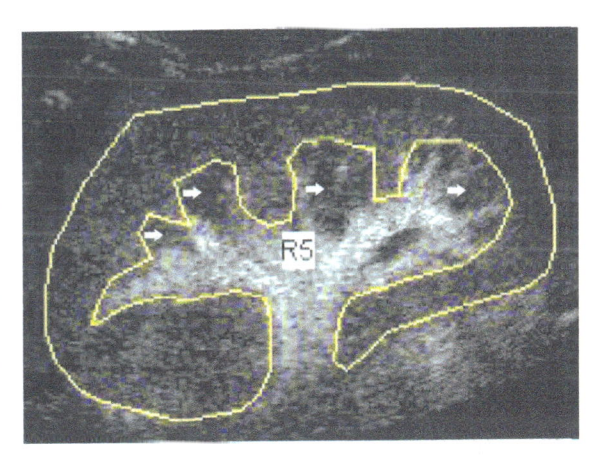

Fig. 17.3 It is possible to encompass with a single manually defined ROI all the renal parenchyma, excluding renal medulla (*arrows*), which presents a much lower perfusion value (190 ml/min per 100 g) if compared with renal cortex (400 ml/min per 100 g).

baseline, α=the initial slope of the curve, and C=the intensity at baseline (the zero crossing point of the y-axis). Wash in/out curves is generally described by a two-compartment filling and outflow model, which is mathematically represented by the gamma-variate function. Data from bolus injections of contrast, which have a distinct wash-in and wash-out phase, can be fit using this function. This protocol of injection is suitable for calculation of the MTT in an organ.

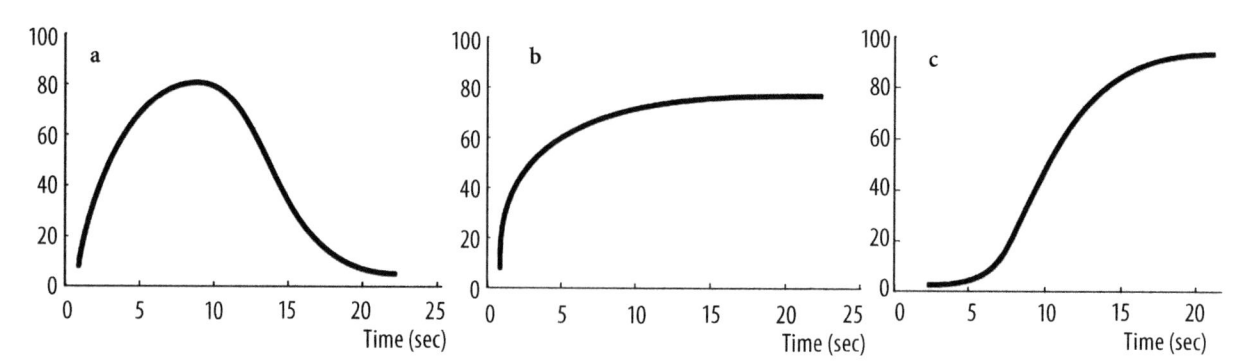

Fig. 17.4a–c. The most important mathematical models employed to fit echo-signal intensity vs time in renal parenchyma. The gamma variate (**a**) is suitable for intravenous bolus injection. When intravenous contrast infusion is employed the negative exponential (**b**) and the sigmoid (**c**) function are proposed to represent the refilling kinetic from microbubbles after destructive insonation.

17.6.2
Negative Exponential

The negative exponential function (Fig. 17.4b) has the form y=A(1-e$^{-\alpha t}$)+C, where A=the amplitude of the curve above baseline, α=the? initial slope of the curve, and C=the intensity at baseline (the zero crossing point of the y-axis). It is based on a single-compartment model (WEI et al. 1998, 2001) which has generally been proposed to fit time/intensity curves. According to this equation, the mean microbubble velocity in the microcirculation is related directly to α, the slope of the increasing function, and the plateau echo enhancement A correlates with the fractional blood volume (Fig. 17.5), provided that the microbubble destruction rate induced by the US field was considered null. Moreover, this exponential model is valid only if the concentration of microbubbles entering the ROI, immediately after the train of destructive pulses, is constant.

17.6.3
Sigmoid

SCHLOSSER et al. (2001) showed that different forms of function are observed for the replenishment curves from renal hilum vessels up to the renal cortex. The hilum replenishment exhibited an exponential that asymptotically approached a maximum, but the cortical replenishment showed a sigmoid curve. Recently, the exponential negative function was confirmed to present distortion toward a sigmoid curve (Fig. 17.4c), with a low initial slope that increases secondarily up to an inflexion point, if the percentage of bubble destruction in the ROI

feeding vessels is considered not null (LUCIDARME et al. 2003a).

The equation is $C_n(t) = \dfrac{C_0}{(1+\tau\lambda)^n} \times \left[1 - \left(1 + \sum\limits_{i=1}^{n-1} \dfrac{\beta^i t^i}{i!} \right) e^{-\beta t} \right]$

and describes a curve with a low initial slope that increases secondarily to an inflexion point and is derived from the classic indicator dilution theory, by considering a series of subvolumes in the US field placed serially with respect to flow direction.

$C_n(t)$ is the refilling evolution of the microbubble concentration in the subvolume n, C_0 is the concentration of microbubbles in blood vessels that enter the ROI (number of microbubbles per liter), which is assumed to be constant with time, t is time, λ represents the fraction of microbubbles destroyed by the US beam per second, which is assumed to be constant,

$\dfrac{1}{\tau} = \dfrac{F}{V_b}$, where F is the rate of the inflow (equals to the rate of outflow) and Vb is the volume of flow in the ROI,

and β is $\dfrac{(1+\tau\lambda)}{\tau}$.

In a sigmoid curve, the initial slope is theoretically equal to zero, and the slope measured at the inflexion point, even with a constant flow rate and a constant microbubble concentration in the circulation, decreases when the length of the path followed by the microbubbles in the US field increases before they reach the ROI. Consequently, microbubble velocity in the ROI estimated from the initial slope (α) of the refill curve, in the classic model described by an exponential function that approaches a maxi-

Quantitative Analysis of Renal Perfusion at Contrast-Enhanced US

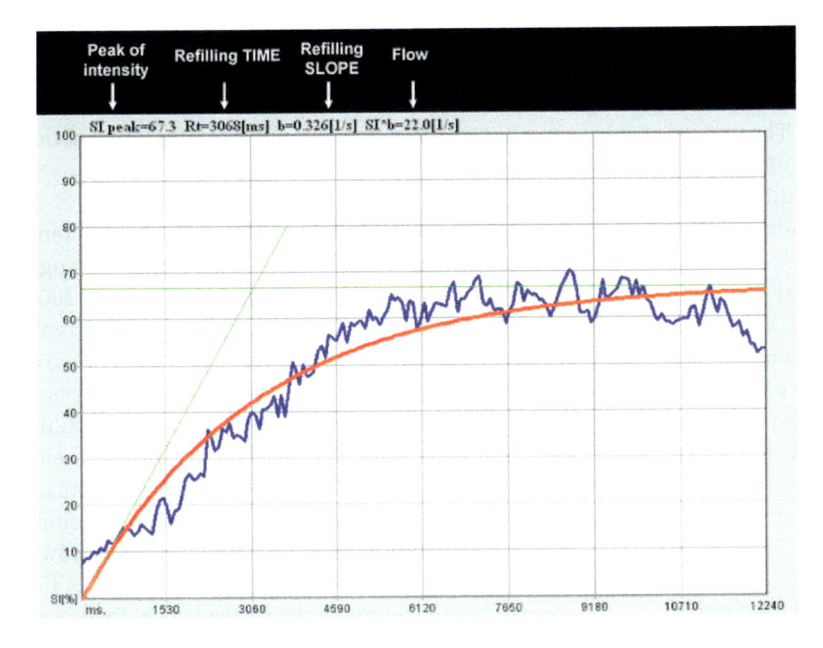

Fig. 17.5 Different mathematical parameters are calculated from negative exponential approximation of renal parenchyma refilling. The refilling time and the slope of the first ascending tract of the curve (b value) are related to the speed of the blood entering in the imaging slice. The peak of intensity in the plateau phase is related to the fractional blood volume in renal parenchyma. The flow is estimated by the product of the slope of the first ascending tract of the curve for the peak intensity value in the plateau phase.

mum, is not correct if microbubble destruction occurs in the feeding vessels.

17.6.4
Other Mathematical Functions and Drawbacks in Mathematical Approximation

Even though both negative exponential and sigmoid functions represent a reliable model to represent refilling kinetic in renal parenchyma, the first ascending tract of the curve is difficult to be fitted for the low availability of points which produces a large error of approximation (Fig. 17.6). As a further problem, the time-intensity curves present a large points dispersion both during the first ascending tract and the second plateau-phase tract of the curve (Fig. 17.6). A wide variability exists and further mathematical functions have been proposed to represent the refilling kinetic from microbubbles, such as the inverse negative exponential (LUCIDARME et al. 2003b) and the hyperbolic (KRIX et al. 2003).

Recently, a further mathematical model (QUAIA and TORELLI 2005) has been proposed which was derived from the biological models theory about progressive volume filling. The system was represented by a three-compartmental model, in which the large afferent vessels (segmentary, interlobar, and arciform arteries) represent the first compartment, the small cortical vessels (interlobular arteries and glomeruli) the second compartment ($K_{1,2}$=transfer constant from the first to the second compartment), and the small medullary vessels (the vasa recta capillaries) the third compartment ($K_{2,3}$=transfer constant from the second to the third compartment).

Different variables are present in this model: (a) The direction of the vessels compared with the US beam. The refilling is almost instantaneous in the renal vessels which present a perpendicular direction to the US beam, while the refilling follows a complex kinetic in vessels parallel to the US beam; (b) Velocity of the blood in the vessels. Microbubble velocity entering the volume was considered as a multi-directional variable of control since the microbubbles refill the imaging volume from all the directions. The refilling is rapid in arterial vessels (segmentary, interlobar, and arciform), while it is

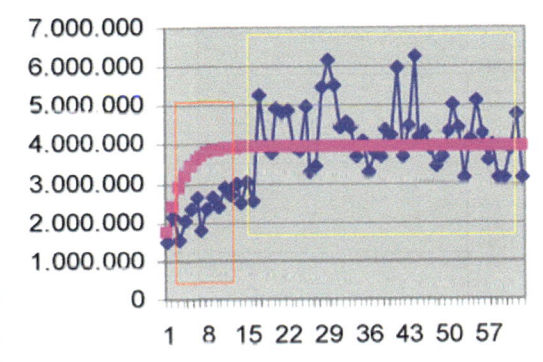

Fig. 17.6 The principal drawbacks in mathematical approximation of refilling kinetic in renal parenchyma. *Red square*=few points are available to approximate the first ascending tract of the curve; *yellow square*=the plateau phase presents a wide dispersion of data due to the variability of US signal.

more slow in the small cortical (interlobular, afferent, and efferent artery) and medullary (vasa recta) arteries and in the venous vessels; (c) Percentage of volume filled by the microbubbles. The imaged renal volume (thickness of the US beam ≈5 mm) was considered as a not conservative variable of state since the volume replenishment is dependent on the grade of filling.

A system of partial differential equations was derived including the velocity of volume replenishment, time, the volume percentage occupied by microbubbles, the percentage of microbubbles destroyed in the volume, and the percentage of microbubbles leaving the volume and not replaced.

17.7
Clinical Applications of Renal Perfusion Quantitation

Renal perfusion quantitation may be employed in different clinical situations with the aim of revealing a reduced perfusion of renal parenchyma.

Renal artery stenosis. One of the most important fields of application is the assessment of renal parenchyma perfusion in tight renal artery stenosis. The normally perfused kidney presents a higher slope of the first ascending tract of the curve and an higher value of gray-scale intensity at the plateau phase in comparison with the kidney presenting a tight renal artery stenosis (Fig. 17.7), revealing, respectively, a higher velocity in the blood entering the scanning plane and a higher fractional blood volume. These results seem encouraging, even though renal stenosis has to be tight (>80%) for renal perfusion differences to become manifest at quantitative contrast-enhanced US.

Urinary obstruction. Contrast-enhanced US may depict changes in renal blood flow during acute obstruction, by revealing a lower area under the time–intensity curve during ureteral obstruction (CLAUDON et al. 1999).

Renal perfusion differences related to age. The renal perfusion is dependent on age, reflecting the changes in vessel structure. We analyzed (QUAIA et al. 2003) 50 normal volunteers (25 men and 25 women), 25 with age range between 27 and 48 years, and 25 between 61 and 80 years, with well-functioning native kidneys all without clinical and laboratory signs of renal failure after SonoVue peripheral intravenous slow infusion (4.8 ml at a flow rate of 4.0 ml/min) by automatic injector. After the blood concentration of microbubbles reached equilibrium, four high-transmit power (MI: 1.2–1.4) pulses were sent to destroy bubbles filling renal parenchyma in the imaged slice. By using a low-transmit power (MI: 0.06–0.08), the progressive replenishment of renal cortex was imaged in real time during apnea to avoid breathing-related movements for at least 6 s. Both kidneys were scanned.

The progressive refilling of renal cortex was quantified in linear scale after anti-log gray-scale transformation. Slope of the first ascending tract of the curve (α, 1/s) was related to the speed of blood (in centimeters per second) moving into the selected slice. To reduce variability between subjects due to the different signal gain, focal position, and anatomical features, the plateau values of renal cortex were equalized with those measured in the interlobar artery and the Ar/Ai (plateau intensity ratios in renal cortex, r; and interlobar renal artery, i) and AUCr/AUCi (area-under-curve ratio in renal cortex, r; and interlobar renal artery, i) were related to the fractional blood volume. Since the fractional blood volume is related to the area of the capillary bed, the

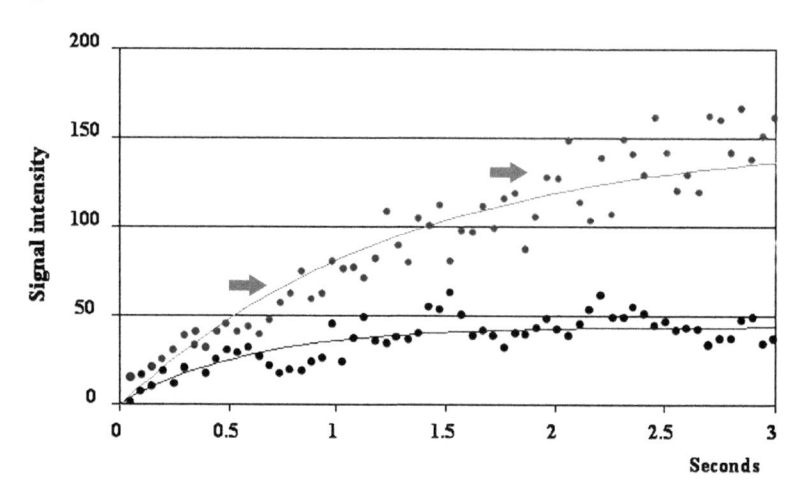

Fig. 17.7 Quantitation of renal perfusion through contrast-enhanced US, after sulfur hexafluoride-filled microbubble injection and at low acoustic power insonation. Difference in the refilling kinetics of renal parenchyma due to renal artery stenosis. The normally perfused kidney (*arrows*) presents a higher slope of the first ascending tract of the curve and a higher value of echo signal intensity at the plateau phase in comparison with the kidney which presents a tight renal artery stenosis (*black points*)

renal flow was related to the products α× Ar/Ai and α× AUCr/AUCi (Fig. 17.5).

No significant difference in cortical perfusion was found between the right and left kidneys in each volunteer, and between the cortical refilling time of group 1 to group 2 (4.4±1.6 s vs 4.9±1.3 s; $p=0.23$, Mann-Whitney U test). Despite that group 1 revealed an α value higher than group 2 (0.78±0.16 vs 0.70±0.43), the difference was not significant ($p=0.21$). Statistically significant difference was found between the Ar/Ai (0.048±0.025 vs 0.016±0.004; $p<0.05$), AUCr/AUCi (0.15±0.19 vs 0.12±0.14; $p<0.05$), β×Ar/As (0.037±0.017 vs 0.01±0.006; $p<0.05$) and α×AUCr/AUCi (0.12±0.20 vs 0.008±0.09; $p<0.05$) of group 1 vs group 2. These results showed that the principal differences in renal perfusion in different age groups can be quantitatively analyzed by contrast-enhanced US (Fig. 17.8).

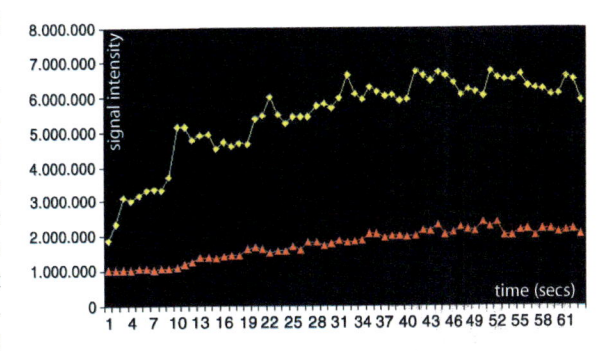

Fig. 17.8 Quantitation of renal perfusion through contrast-enhanced US, after sulfur hexafluoride-filled microbubble injection and at low acoustic power insonation. Difference in the refilling kinetics of renal parenchyma due to age. The kidney of a young volunteer (25 years of age) presents a higher slope of the first ascending tract of the curve (*yellow*) and a higher value of intensity at the plateau phase in comparison with the curve (*red*) obtained from a 65-year-old volunteer.

References

Claudon M, Barnewolt CE, Taylor GA et al (1999) Renal blood flow in pigs: changes depicted with contrast-enhanced harmonic US imaging during acute urinary obstruction. Radiology 212:725–731

Correas JM, Burns PN, Lai X, Qi X (2000) Infusion versus bolus of an ultrasound contrast agent: in vivo dose-response measurements of BR1. Invest Radiol 35:72–79

Correas JM, Kurtisovski E, Bridal SF et al (2002) Optimizing an ultrasound contrast agent's stability using an in vitro measurement. Invest Radiol 37:672–679

Cosgrove DO, Eckersley R, Blomley M, Harvey C (2001) Quantification of blood flow. Eur Radiol 11:1338–1344

Krix M, Kiessling F, Farhan N et al (2003) A multivessel model describing replenishment kinetics of ultrasound contrast agent for quantification of tissue perfusion. US Med Biol 29:1421–1430

Li PC, Ynag MJ (2003) Transfer function analysis of ultrasonic time–intensity measurements. US Med Biol 29:1493–1500

Lucidarme O, Franchi-Abella S, Correas JM et al (2003a) Blood flow quantification with contrast-enhanced US: entrance in the section phenomenon – phantom and rabbit study. Radiology 228:473–479

Lucidarme O, Kono Y, Corbeil J, Choi SH, Mattrey RF (2003b) Validation of ultrasound contrast destruction imaging for flow quantification. Ultrasound Med Biol 29:1697–1704

Phillips P, Gardner E (2004) Contrast-agent detection and quantification. Eur Radiol 14 (Suppl 8):P4–P10

Quaia E, Torelli L (2005) Proposal of an appropriate mathematical model representing replenishment kinetic of renal parenchyma after microbubbles destruction to assess numerical parameters related to perfusion [abstract]. European Congress of Radiology 2005

Quaia E, Bertolotto M, Lubin E et al (2003) Evaluation of renal cortical perfusion by pulse inversion harmonic imaging with SonoVue: preliminary experience. European Congress Radiology 2003. Eur Radiol 13 [Suppl 1]

Rubin JM, Fowlkes JB, Tuthill TA et al (1999) Speckle decorrelation flow measurement with B-mode US of contrast agent flow in a phantom and in rabbit kidney. Radiology 213:429–437

Schlosser T, Pohl C, Veltmann C et al (2001) Feasibility of the FLASH-replenishment concept in renal tissue: Which parameters affect the assessment of the contrast replenishment? Ultrasound Med Biol 27:937–944

Schneider M, Arditi M, Barrau MB et al (1995) BR1: a new ultrasonographic contrast agent based on sulfur hexafluoride-filled microbubbles. Invest Radiol 30:451–457

Wei K, Skyba DM, Firschke C et al (1997) Interactions between microbubbles and ultrasound: in vitro and in vivo observations. J Am Coll Cardiol 29:1081–1088

Wei K, Ananda R, Jayaweera AR et al (1998a) Quantification of myocardial blood flow with ultrasound-induced destruction of microbubbles administered as a constant venous infusion. Circulation 97:473–483

Wei K, Jayaweera AR, Firoozan S et al (1998b) Basis for detection of stenosis using venous administration of microbubbles during myocardial contrast echocardiography: bolus or continuous infusion? J Am Coll Cardiol 32:252–260

Wei K, Le E, Bin JP et al (2001) Quantification of renal blood flow with contrast-enhanced ultrasound. J Am Coll Cardiol 37:1135–1140

Cardiac Applications

18 Assessment of Regional Myocardial Blood Flow

Saul Kalvaitis and Kevin Wei

CONTENTS

18.1 Introduction 267
18.2 Microbubbles as Perfusion Agents in the Myocardium 267
18.3 Image Processing for Quantification of Myocardial Perfusion 268
18.4 Quantification of Myocardial Blood Flow 271
18.5 High vs Low Acoustic Power for Quantification of Myocardial Blood Velocity 272
18.6 Clinical Applications for Quantitative Parameters Derived Using Contrast-enhanced US 274
18.7 Conclusion 274
References 276

18.1 Introduction

Contrast echocardiography is a technology that has evolved greatly over the past 4 decades. From its initial description in the late 1960s, contrast echocardiography has been used to identify cardiac structures, detect intracardiac shunts, visualize blood flow on M-mode echocardiography, detect valvular regurgitation, and quantify cardiac output using indicator–dilution curve theory. During the past decade, tremendous advances have been made to both ultrasound (US) technology and microbubble-based contrast agents, which have expanded applications of contrast echocardiography to the systemic circulation, including enhanced detection of left ventricular endocardial borders and left sided Doppler signals. Most recently, contrast echocardiography now allows assessment of myocardial perfusion with US and microbubble-based contrast agents. Myocardial contrast echocardiography has been incorporated into the detection of coronary artery disease, assessment of acute myocardial infarction, and evaluation of myocardial viability. All of these accomplishments are bringing us closer to the era when myocardial perfusion imaging with contrast echocardiography will be used not only as a research tool, but as a clinical technique for the management of a wide range of cardiovascular and other diseases.

Contrast echocardiography is a technique that can non-invasively evaluate both the temporal and spatial aspects of myocardial perfusion. This chapter discusses basic principles behind assessment of myocardial perfusion imaging by contrast echocardiography and reviews important interactions between US and microbubbles that form the basis of those imaging techniques.

The ability of US to destroy microbubbles is also an important component of the method that allows contrast echocardiography to quantify myocardial blood flow, and therefore allows the assessment of the temporal aspect of myocardial perfusion. Furthermore, evaluating the replenishment of microbubbles into the coronary microcirculation has become the de facto method for myocardial perfusion imaging.

18.2 Microbubbles as Perfusion Agents in the Myocardium

Although larger microbubbles produce much greater acoustic signals, their maximum size is limited by the diameter of the capillary so that intravenously administered agents may cross the pulmonary microcirculation, which is approximately 5 µm. The limitations of a small microbubble became evident with the first commercial air-filled microbubble agent that was made by sonication of a solution of 5% human albumin. The mean microbubble size of 4.3 µm allowed it to clear the pulmonary circulation following an intravenous injection, but the air rapidly diffused out along the concentration gra

---

S. Kalvaitis, MD; K. Wei, MD
Cardiac Imaging Center, Cardiovascular Division, University of Virginia School of Medicine, Charlottesville, VA 22908-0158, USA

dient into the surrounding blood, with a resultant decrease in bubble size and backscatter signal. This inevitably meant that by the time the microbubbles had cleared the pulmonary circulation, their ability to opacify the myocardium was already substantially diminished; therefore, the majority of studies using this agent for myocardial perfusion relied on direct intra-coronary injections.

The need to improve microbubble persistence in the circulation was eventually overcome by the incorporation of high molecular weight gases with low diffusibility and solubility, or by the use of gas-impermeable polymer shells into new generation microbubbles. The gas proved to diffuse out of the microbubbles at a much slower rate, which meant that microbubbles had the ability to maintain their size and significantly increase their half-life within the circulation. The new-generation microbubbles currently approved for clinical use in the United States (Optison, Amersham Health Inc., Princeton, NJ; Definity, Bristol-Myers Squibb Medical Imaging, North Billerica, Mass.; and Imagent, Imcor Pharmaceuticals, San Diego, Calif.) share a number of similarities in that they are composed of a thin shell that encloses a core of perfluorocarbon gas. A number of other microbubbles are in various phases of development and approval.

Apart from their stability, microbubble-based contrast agents possess a number of unique properties that distinguish them from tracers used with other non-invasive imaging technologies. The microbubbles remain entirely intravascular, unlike nuclear tracers such as thallium or ^{99m}Tc-sestamibi which are extracted by myocytes, or radiologic contrast agents for CT or gadolinium tracers for MR imaging that diffuse into the interstitial space. The microbubbles are also hemodynamically inert, so they do not affect local or systemic blood flow (KELLER et al. 1988). By comparing the transit of microbubbles with Tc-labeled red blood cells, or by direct visualization of fluorescently labeled microbubbles and red blood cells, the in vivo myocardial kinetics and rheology of microbubbles have been shown to be very close to that of red blood cells (KELLER et al. 1989; JAYAWEERA et al. 1994; SKYBA et al. 1996).

The behavior of microbubbles in the normal circulation depends on more than just their size and deformability. Microbubble interactions with the endothelium and its glycocalyx may also affect their transit (MOORE et al. 1986; VILLANUEVA et al. 1997; FISHER et al. 2002). For the most part, microbubble shells minimize their interaction with cellular elements. For example, most lipid shells are essentially neutral in charge, and some contain polyethyleneglycol, which prevents interactions with serum proteins and cells (KLIBANOV et al. 1990; TORCHLIN et al. 1994). These measures extend the intravascular life span of microbubbles by reducing cellular uptake in reticuloendothelial organs. Lipid microbubbles with a highly negative charge that lack polyethylene glycol can be retained within capillaries of normal tissue due to interactions with the vascular endothelium (KLIBANOV et al. 1990).

At very high acoustic pressures, exaggerated microbubble oscillation leads to microbubble destruction by one of several mechanisms (WEI et al. 1997; DAYTON et al. 1999; DE JONG et al. 2000a; CHOMAS et al. 2001) Microbubble compression can increase surface tension and cause outward diffusion of the microbubble gas during each high-pressure US cycle, resulting in a gradual reduction in microbubble volume. Exaggerated radial oscillations can result in permanent defects in the microbubble shell, which results in rapid loss of gas from the microbubbles. Finally, abrupt fragmentation of microbubbles have been visualized with only a single high-energy US pulse (Fig. 18.1; PELBERG et al. 1999). Harmonic power Doppler is one of the most sensitive high-acoustic-power techniques for perfusion imaging (Fig. 18.2) and offers the best signal-to-noise ratio (BURNS et al. 1996; DE JONG et al. 2000b).

18.3
Image Processing for Quantification of Myocardial Perfusion

Backscatter signals from microbubbles are processed into pixels of brightness, or video intensity in the US system. In order to quantitate the microbubble backscatter signal, the relationship between microbubble concentration and video intensity must be known. Figure 18.3 shows that at low concentration of microbubbles, the relationship between video intensity and microbubble concentration is linear (SKYBA et al. 1994), but the relation reaches a plateau as microbubble concentration increases. At even higher concentrations, the video intensity actually decreases due to attenuation of US by the microbubbles themselves. It is essential to ensure that the microbubble concentration is maintained within the linear range so that video intensity remains directly proportional to microbubble con-

Assessment of Regional Myocardial Blood Flow

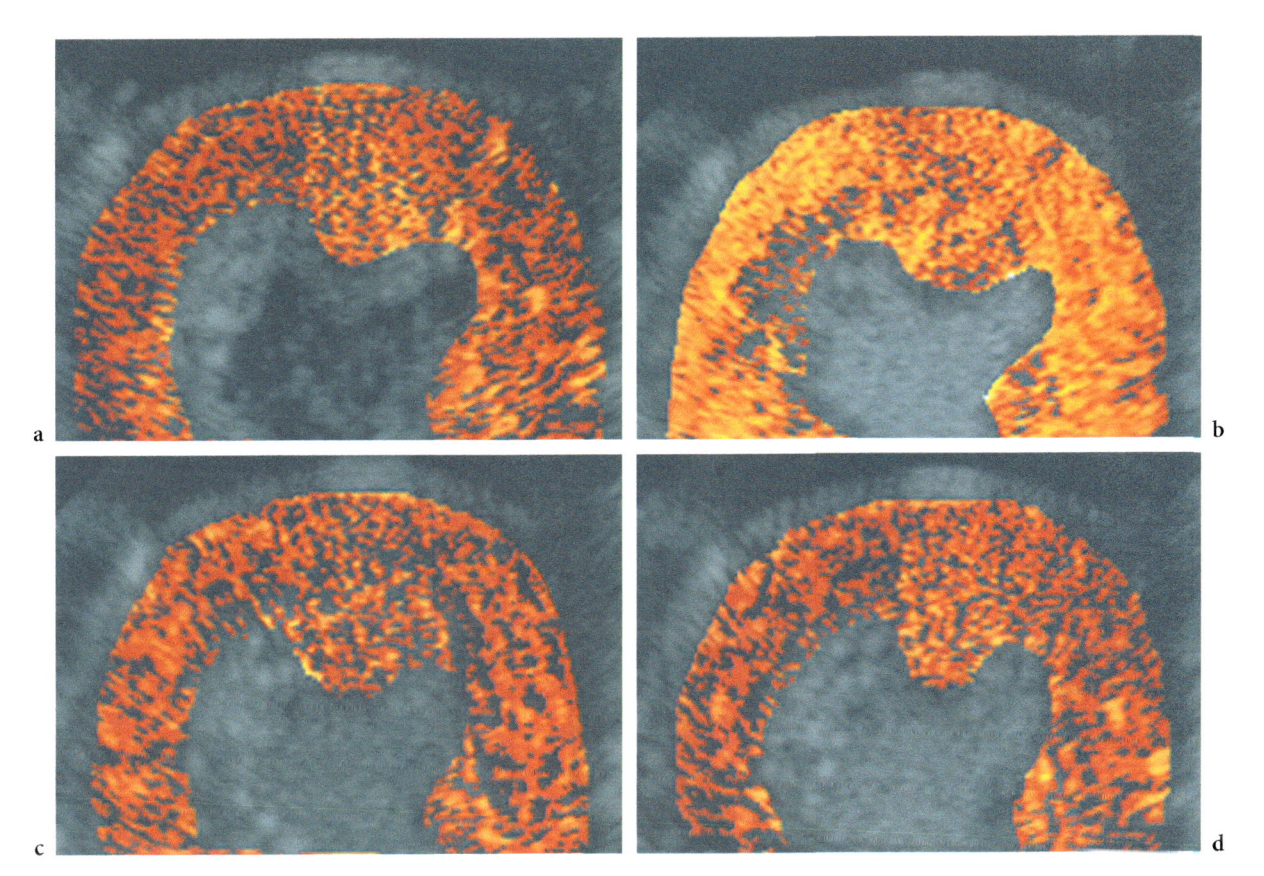

Fig. 18.1a–d. Animal model. **a** Background-subtracted color-coded images obtained at baseline pre-contrast which is predominantly red due to the lack of myocardial contrast enhancement. **b** Steady state during continuous infusion of microbubbles, which shows confluent myocardial opacification, is seen with the first US high-acoustic-power pulse. **c,d** Images obtained from the first three US pulses after microbubbles in the circulation had reached steady-state levels and the first two images obtained at 30 and 50 ms after the achievement of a steady state (**c,d**). Absent confluent myocardial opacification in the image produced by the second US pulse transmitted only 30 ms later (**c**). The rapid decrease in myocardial contrast enhancement is secondary to microbubble destruction induced by the first US pulse. No further decreases in myocardial video intensity is seen with subsequent US pulses (**d**), since the concentration of microbubbles in tissue is already below the detection threshold of the US system. (From Pelberg et al. 1999)

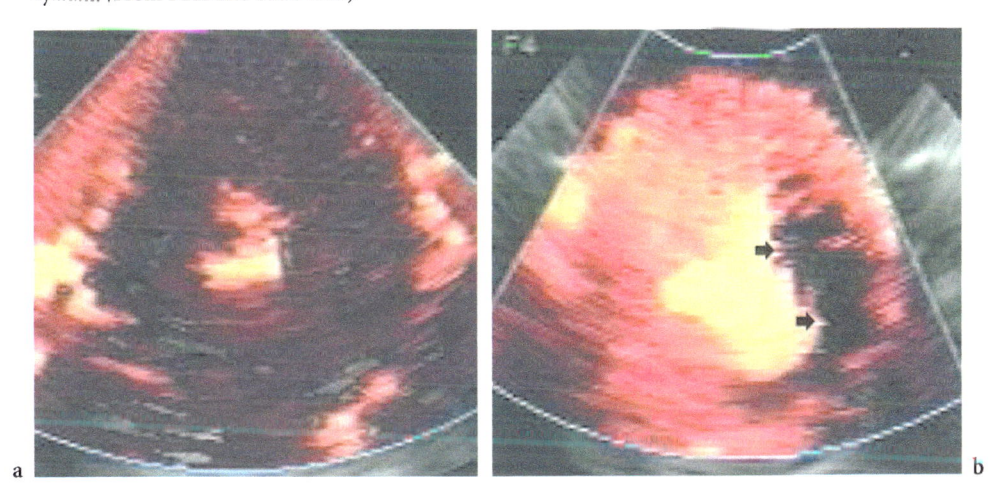

Fig. 18.2a,b. Baseline (**a**) and contrast-enhanced (**b**) harmonic power Doppler images. Prior to administration of microbubbles, tissue signal is almost completely absent (**a**). Strong homogeneous contrast enhancement is noted throughout the myocardium after microbubble injection (**b**), except in the lateral wall (*arrows*) where microbubbles were excluded by occlusion of the left circumflex coronary artery – and displays a near transmural perfusion defect.

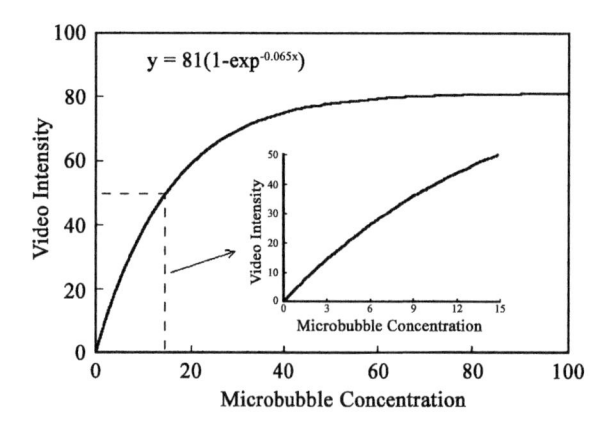

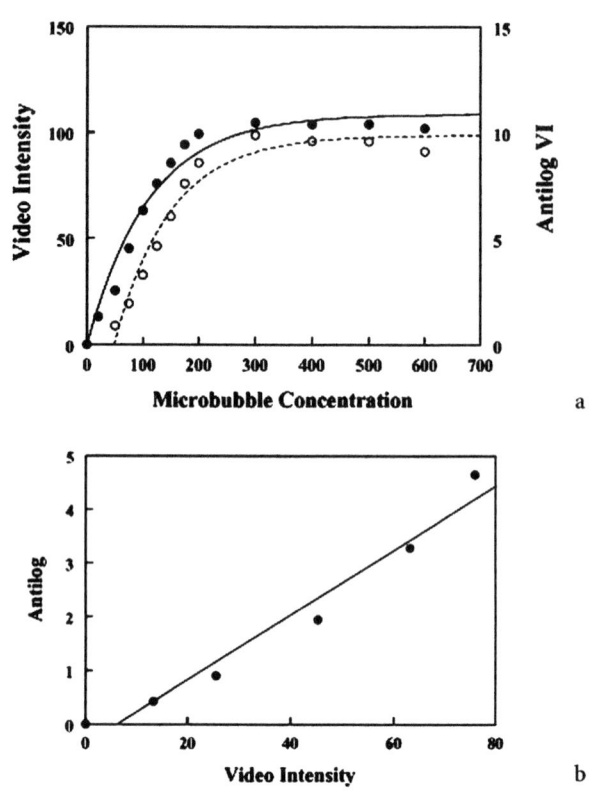

Fig. 18.3 Relation between microbubble concentration (microbubbles per microliter) and video intensity determined in an in vitro system. The relationship is exponential, with linear range occurring at lower concentrations (*inset*). (Reproduced with permission from SKYBA et al. 1994)

centration. A simple way of ensuring that saturation has not been reached within the myocardium is to keep myocardial enhancement visually lower than that of the left ventricular cavity.

Although many of the contrast-specific imaging modalities have improved the microbubble signal-to-tissue noise ratio, there are still situations when tissue harmonic signals are not well suppressed. The process of quantification requires a determination of the change in video intensity between baseline and contrast-enhanced images. Visual determination of these changes may be extremely difficult, as the background tissue signal varies widely within the US sector, due to inhomogeneities of acoustic power (WEYMAN 1994), and to regional differences in attenuation and absorption of US energy by tissue. Non-uniform tissue characteristics, such as fibrosis after myocardial infarction, also produces high harmonic signals and bright tissue. In this situation, after normal myocardial beds become enhanced with microbubbles, the entire myocardium appears bright, and it is not possible to visually appreciate a "perfusion defect" in the infarcted segment. To remove the tissue noise, digital-image processing techniques, such as image alignment, background-subtraction, averaging, and video densitometry, become essential.

To perform background subtraction, baseline (pre-contrast) and contrast-enhanced images are aligned and all video-intensity values within a region of interest from the baseline image are digitally subtracted from the contrast-enhanced image. It is important, however, to understand that video-intensity data are logarithmic, and that log A-log B=log A/B (A=microbubbles; B=background or baseline). Consequently, subtraction of baseline video-intensity values is actually a calculation of the logarithm of a ratio between echo intensities. Background subtraction should therefore ideally be performed after logarithmic video-intensity data have been converted to linear data using an antilog function. From a practical standpoint, application of an antilog function within the linear range of the microbubble concentration vs video-intensity relation does not extend the linear range or significantly alter the near linearity of the relation between these two variables (Fig. 18.4).

When microbubbles are administered as a constant infusion, steady state is achieved after 2–3 min, where their concentration in any blood pool (left

Fig. 18.4. a Relation between microbubble concentration (microbubbles per microliter) and video intensity (VI; left y-axis) as well as antilog video intensity (right y-axis). The plateau in both cases starts at a microbubble concentration of approximately 200 microbubbles/ml. Since the antilog function does not extend the linear range, the myocardial blood volume must be small enough so that system saturation never occurs, even with the use of high concentrations of microbubbles. **b** At low microbubble concentrations the relation between video intensity and its corresponding antilog values is linear. For practical purposes, tissue background video intensity signal can be subtracted from contrast-enhanced myocardial video intensity signal without requiring antilog conversion.

ventricular cavity, myocardium, etc.) is constant and proportional to the blood volume fraction of that pool. For example, during normal conditions, for every 100 microbubbles within a sample volume in the left ventricular cavity, there will be 8 microbubbles within a similar-sized sample volume in the myocardium. The video intensity measured from the myocardium normalized to that from the left ventricular cavity provides a measure of mean blood volume fraction (since the left ventricular cavity is 100% blood; Kassab et al. 1994a). In order to normalize myocardial video intensity to that of the left ventricular cavity, the microbubble concentration vs video-intensity relation must be linear within both compartments (Fig. 18.5).

18.4
Quantification of Myocardial Blood Flow

As mentioned above, microbubble contrast agents are hemodynamically inert, remain entirely intravascular, and also have the same rheology as red blood cells. They are therefore ideal tracers of red blood cell kinetics. Because the microbubbles used during contrast echocardiography are pure intravascular tracers, an understanding of the anatomy of the coronary microcirculation is required to appreciate the physiologic information represented by myocardial contrast echocardiography images. Although the coronary microcirculation is reviewed in greater detail in the next chapter, which deals with myocardial blood volume, aspects that are required in order to understand quantification of myocardial blood flow (velocity = myocardial blood × myocardial blood volume) with contrast echocardiography are reviewed here.

The 45 ml of blood in the adult human coronary circulation is divided nearly equally between the arterial, venous, and microcirculatory networks (Kassab et al. 1994a). Most of the blood in the arterial and venous compartments are situated on the epicardial surface of the heart. Within the myocardium itself, approximately 8% of the left ventricular mass is constituted by blood present in the microcirculation (Kassab et al. 1994b). There are approximately 8 million capillaries in the human heart which contain 90% of the myocardial blood volume (Kaul and Jayaweera 1997). The velocity of blood in the coronary vessels is related to their size. At the capillary level (mean length and diameter of 0.5 mm × 7 μm), the mean red cell velocity at rest is very low and averages about 1 mm s-1 (Kaul and Jayaweera 1997).

At steady state during a continuous infusion of microbubbles, the inflow and outflow of microbubbles in any microcirculatory unit is constant and is dependent only on the flow rate of microbubbles. Since microbubbles within the myocardium can be destroyed with high-acoustic-power insonation, they can be rapidly eliminated from the myocardium. By measuring the rate of microbubble reappearance, red blood cell velocity can be determined (Wei et al. 1998). High-acoustic-power insonation can effectively destroy microbubbles within the entire elevation (thickness) of the beam, which measures approximately 5 mm in thickness; thus, in order for microbubbles to completely replenish the capillary bed within the US elevation (thickness), the frame rate of US must be reduced to <0.2 Hz (1 frame every 5 s).

Because flow constitutes a volume of blood moving at a certain mean velocity, the product of myocardial blood volume fraction and velocity of myocardial blood flow reflects myocardial microvascular flow. This value can also be represented per gram of tissue by knowing the sample volume size and specific gravity of the myocardium, although for most clinical applications it is not necessary to do so.

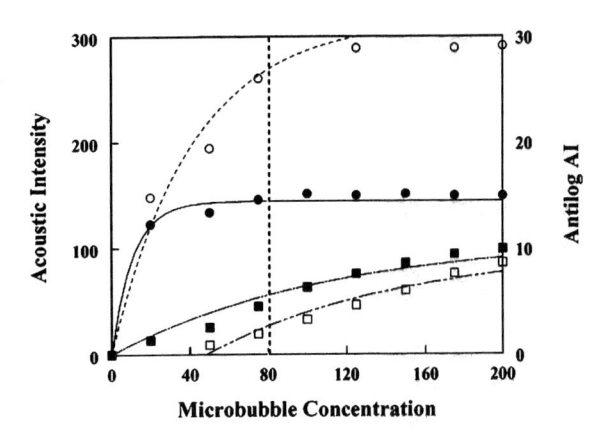

Fig. 18.5 Relation between microbubble concentration (microbubbles per microliter) and video intensity (VI; *solid circles*, left y-axis) as well as antilog video intensity (*open circles*, right y-axis) derived from the left ventricular cavity, and myocardial video intensity (*solid squares*, left y-axis) and the corresponding myocardial antilog data (*open squares*, right y-axis). The left ventricular cavity video intensity reaches a plateau at microbubble concentrations <40 that are inadequate to produce significant myocardial contrast enhancement. Unlike the myocardium, the linear range of the left ventricular cavity is extended after antilog conversion of video-intensity data, and allows normalization of signals between the myocardium and left ventricular cavity even at concentrations that result in myocardial contrast enhancement (*vertical dotted line*).

To understand this concept mathematically, assume that all microbubbles within a US field are destroyed by a single US pulse, and that the elevation (thickness) of the US beam E is uniform (Fig. 18.6a). If new microbubbles enter this field with a flat profile at a velocity v, then the distance (d) they will travel within the beam elevation as the pulsing interval is prolonged (t_1 to t_4; Fig. 18.6b–e) will be given by the equation: $E=vt$; thus, as the time interval between consecutive destructive US pulses is increased, more time is allowed for microbubble replenishment, which is dependent on the velocity of the microbubbles. As pulsing interval lengthens, the rise in microbubble concentration is displayed as a corresponding rise in myocardial video intensity, provided that the relationship between video intensity and microbubble concentration remains linear. As shown in Fig. 18.6f, when the pulsing interval exceeds T, video intensity remains constant. This plateau phase reflects the effective microbubble concentration within the myocardial microcirculation. At any given concentration of microbubbles, the video intensity at the plateau phase will be proportional to the sum of the cross-sectional area of microvessels (a) within the beam elevation (thickness).

The model predicts a sharp demarcation between the upslope and plateau phases of the pulsing interval–video intensity relation. In reality, however, neither the beam elevation (thickness) nor the degree of microbubble destruction are expected to be entirely uniform. The profile of the microbubbles is also not expected to be entirely flat. The actual relation between video intensity and pulsing interval is therefore more likely to be curvilinear and can be described by the exponential function: $y=A(1-e^{\beta t})$, where y is video intensity at a pulsing interval of t, A is the plateau video intensity, and β is the rate constant that determines the rate of rise of video intensity.

Because the slope of the tangent to the curve is given by $dv/dt=A\beta E^{-\beta t}$, the slope at the origin ($t=0$) is $A\beta$.

As shown in Fig. 18.6f, this slope is also equal to A/T; therefore, $T=1/\beta$. Eliminating T between equations results in: $v=E\beta$; thus, for a given beam elevation (thickness at a given distance from the transducer), the mean velocity of microbubbles is proportional to β. If flow, f, occurs through an area, a, then: $f=av$.

If E is constant, then a will be proportional to A; therefore, with rearrangement substitution for v we get: $f \propto A\beta E$. When E is constant, f is proportional to $A\beta$.

If E is known, then v can be expressed in centimeters per second. Similarly, if the microvascular cross-sectional area is known, then A can be expressed in square centimeters. The product of A and v will then represent f in milliliters per second (WEI et al. 1998).

In experimental studies, an excellent linear relationship between absolute myocardial blood flow measured with radiolabeled microspheres and myocardial contrast echocardiography-derived microbubble velocity or myocardial blood flow were found (WEI et al. 1998). In humans, significant correlations have also been found between positron emission tomography and contrast echocardiography-derived myocardial blood flow (AY et al. 2001); thus, contrast echocardiography allows quantification of myocardial blood flow velocity (β), mean blood volume (A), and myocardial blood flow ($A\beta$) in both experimental and clinical settings.

18.5
High vs Low Acoustic Power for Quantification of Myocardial Blood Velocity

The method for quantification of myocardial blood flow with contrast echocardiography is based on an assessment of microbubble transit through the

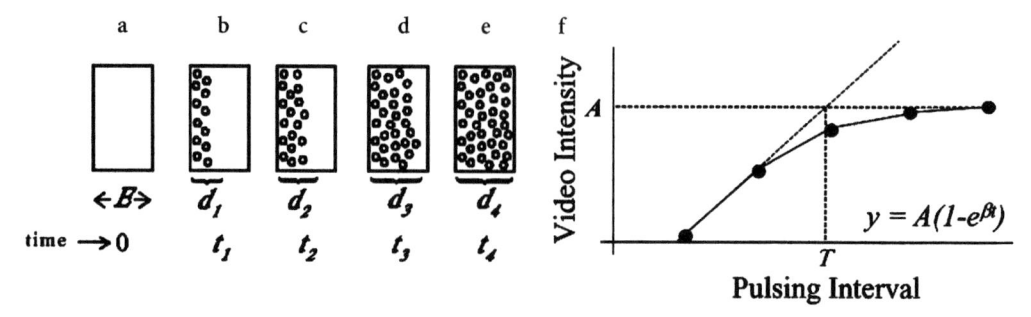

Fig. 18.6 a–f. Progressive replenishment of microbubbles into the US beam elevation (E) at increasing pulsing intervals (t_1–t_4). Pulsing interval vs myocardial acoustic intensity relation fitted to an exponential function is also shown (f).

myocardial capillary bed. Myocardial vessels fill with blood when myocardial elasticity is low in diastole. In systole, the high elasticity compresses intramyocardial arterioles which empty out retrogradely (CHILIAN and MARCUS 1982). Likewise, intramyocardial veins are compressed during systole, which propels blood forward into the coronary sinus (KAJIYA et al. 1985). Because arterioles and venules are larger than capillaries, their compression would occur earlier in systole, causing an increase in their resistance that would result in the functional isolation of capillaries (WEI et al. 2002). Capillary pressure would thus increase concurrently with intramyocardial pressure during systole, preventing appreciable changes in capillary dimensions (TOYOTA et al. 2002; WEI et al. 2002). Since large intramyocardial vessels do not fill anterogradely during systole, the progressive replenishment of microbubbles in the capillary bed alone is determined using intermittent high-acoustic-power imaging triggered in systole.

With low acoustic power imaging, a "flash" impulse consisting of several high-power US frames can be used to destroy the microbubbles within the beam elevation, and microbubble replenishment into the microcirculation can then be followed while imaging is continued at a relatively high frame rate (>15 Hz; PORTER et al. 2001; SHIMONI et al. 2001). Apart from the ability to visualize both perfusion and myocardial function simultaneously, the main advantage of these techniques for evaluation of myocardial blood flow is the rapidity with which the entire microbubble replenishment curve can be acquired (15 s compared with >5 min for intermittent imaging techniques).

With real-time imaging, frames throughout the cardiac cycle are acquired after each flash impulse. In diastole, however, large intra-myocardial vessels rapidly replenish with microbubbles due to their high flow velocity (LEONG-POI et al. 2001); therefore, capillary replenishment is not being evaluated during diastole, and fitting a replenishment curve to sequential end-diastolic frames results in overestimation of the velocity of myocardial blood flow by 41% (LEONG-POI et al. 2001). Fitting the exponential function to all frames (including diastolic and systolic) within the cardiac cycle overestimates the velocity of myocardial blood flow by 24% (LEONG-POI et al. 2001). Myocardial blood flow derived from end-diastolic frames also correlates poorly with relative flows derived from radiolabeled microspheres ($r=0.53$, $p=0.04$; LEONG-POI et al. 2001). Accurate quantification of the velocity of myocardial blood flow and of myocardial blood flow is achieved by using only end-systolic frames. The use of systolic frames also allows quantification of stenosis severity ($r=0.94$, $p<0.001$).

Despite assessment of only end-systolic frames with both high- and low-acoustic-power imaging techniques, differences in the quantitative parameters are still obtained using the two modalities. The ability of the two modalities to assess the physiologic significance of coronary stenoses were recently compared with ^{99m}Tc-sestamibi single photon emission tomography (SPECT) in patients (DAWSON et al. 2003).

Intermittent ultra-harmonic imaging and power modulation were performed during continuous infusions of microbubbles at rest and after dipyridamole stress in 39 patients. The ^{99m}Tc-sestamibi SPECT was performed simultaneously. Myocardial blood flow velocity and myocardial blood flow velocity reserve (hyperemic/resting myocardial blood flow velocity) were quantified from pulsing interval vs video-intensity curves. Myocardial blood flow velocity derived from both myocardial contrast echocardiography methods increased significantly after dipyridamole in normal patients, compared with those with either reversible or fixed defects on SPECT. Consequently, myocardial blood flow velocity reserve was significantly greater in patients with normal perfusion using both techniques. Receiver-operator-characteristics curves obtained for myocardial blood flow velocity reserve provided a sensitivity 82 vs 64% for low mechanical index imaging for detection of defects compared with SPECT. The absolute value of β was also significantly lower during low- compared with high-mechanical-index imaging.

There are several potential reasons for the difference in absolute β between the techniques, as well as for the lower sensitivity of quantitative parameters derived from the low-acoustic-power technique. Excessive destruction of microbubbles in the left ventricular cavity from multiple flash frames could result in distortion of the myocardial input function and prolongation of the output function. Microbubble destruction may also occur due to high frame rates despite the low acoustic power. More importantly, however, the error probably occurs from differences in dynamic range, incorrect curve fitting, and noise (DAWSON et al. 2003). Despite these differences, quantitative parameters derived using low-acoustic-power techniques that are relative (either between myocardial beds, or between resting and hyperemic stages) are equivalent to those derived from high-acoustic techniques.

18.6
Clinical Applications for Quantitative Parameters Derived Using Contrast-enhanced US

During hyperemia (Fig. 18.7), the normal myocardium replenishes rapidly after microbubble destruction (1–1.5 s), while in regions subserved by stenoses the rate of filling is slower depending on the severity of stenosis (Fig. 18.8). The filling abnormalities are frequently seen to be more marked in the endocardium and, in the case of milder stenoses, may be localized only within the endocardium (LINKA et al. 1998). It is for this reason that contrast echocardiography has been shown to be more sensitive than SPECT in the detection of coronary stenoses in patients with normal regional function and only moderate coronary artery disease (SOMAN et al. 2001).

Because of its poorer spatial resolution (centimeters vs millimeters) compared with contrast echocardiography, SPECT cannot detect defects located only in the endocardium. Contrast echocardiography is also superior in identifying multi-vessel coronary artery disease, because each myocardial segment at stress is compared with itself at rest, while on SPECT the comparison is across segments, so that left main or "balanced" multi-vessel coronary artery disease can be missed.

The contrast echocardiography methods to quantify regional myocardial blood flow can also be used to detect coronary stenoses in the clinical setting, and can non-invasively determine the physiologic significance of stenoses in patients (WEI et al. 2001b). The use of relative differences in myocardial blood volume from contrast echocardiography is discussed in the following chapter.

These experiments were performed in the cardiac catheterization laboratory where coronary blood flow velocity was measured using a Doppler flow wire simultaneously with contrast echocardiography measurements (Fig. 18.8). Since hyperemic myocardial blood flow is lower in the presence of a physiologically significant stenosis, microbubble replenishment into a bed subtended by a stenosis is slower than a normal bed and results in a relative perfusion defect at short pulsing interval. In a case of milder stenosis, only abnormalities in velocity of myocardial blood flow may be detected, while changes in myocardial blood flow may be difficult to detect, since replenishment at longer pulsing intervals may be normal due to collateral-supplied myocardial blood flow.

Stenosis severity can be quantified from contrast echocardiography. By dividing hyperemic velocity of myocardial blood flow by that at rest, myocardial blood flow velocity reserve can be calculated. In Figure 18.9 the relation between percent luminal diameter narrowing derived using quantitative coronary angiography vs contrast echocardiography-derived reserve in velocity of myocardial blood flow is shown. The relation closely resembles that described by GOULD and LIPSCOMB (1974). Myocardial blood flow velocity reserve <1.5 indicates the presence of >70% epicardial stenosis (WEI et al. 2001). These results demonstrate the ability of contrast echocardiography to noninvasively determine the presence, and quantify the severity, of coronary artery disease in patients.

18.7
Conclusion

Noninvasive perfusion imaging with contrast echocardiography is now a feasible clinical tool. In this chapter we review the wide array of perfusion imaging methods that are currently used during

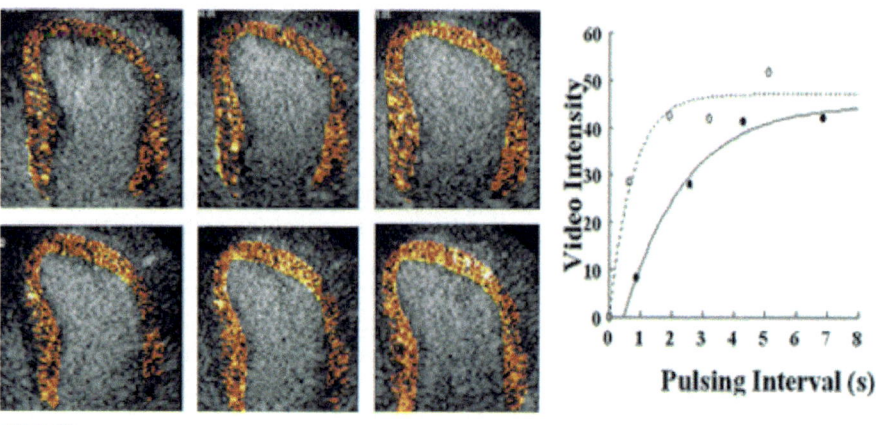

Fig. 18.7. During hyperemia, the normal myocardium replenishes rapidly after microbubble destruction. Difference in the first ascending tract of the war at rest (•) and after dopartine (ΔP) stress (o).

Assessment of Regional Myocardial Blood Flow

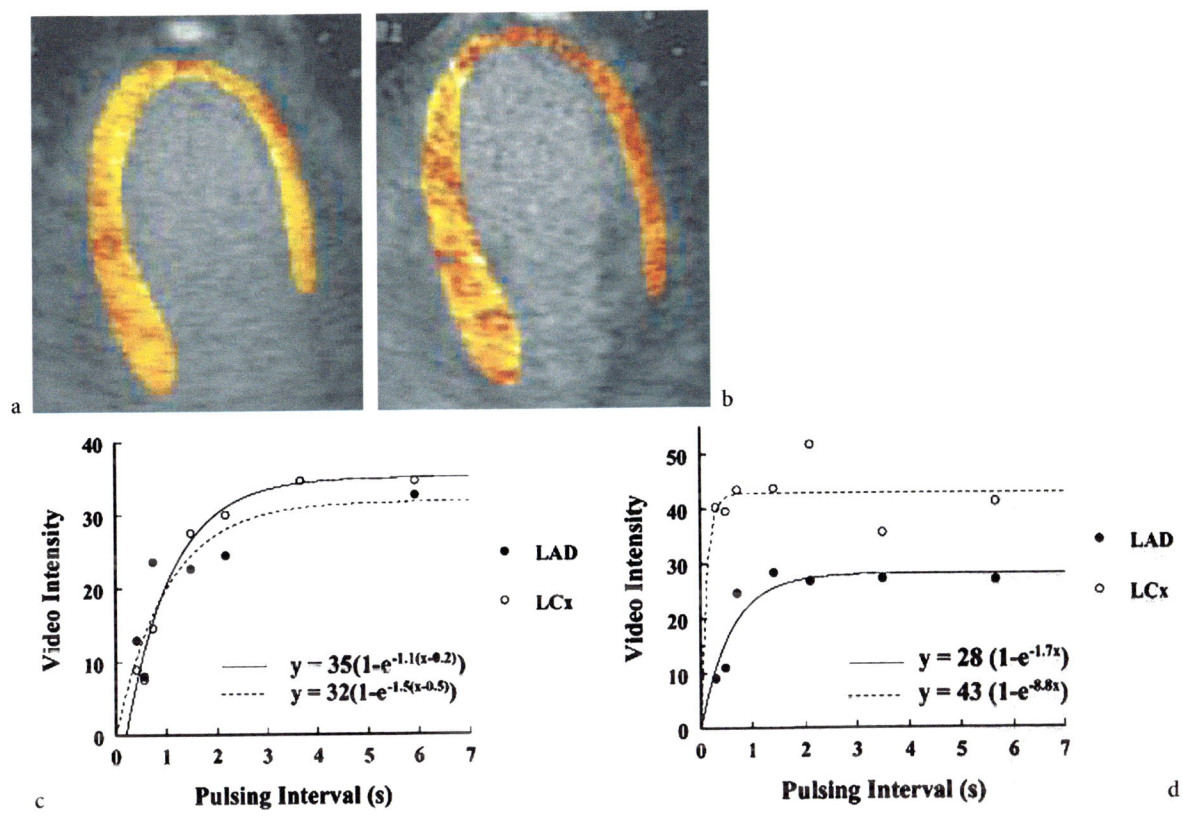

Fig. 18.8a–d. Data from a patient with a 60% left anterior descending (*LAD*) coronary artery stenosis measured using quantitative coronary angiography. **a,b** Pulsing intervals of 2 s. Background-subtracted color-coded apical myocardial contrast echocardiography images from the apical two-chamber view obtained at rest (**a**), and during hyperemia induced with 140 µg kg^{-1} min^{-1} of adenosine (**b**). All pixels with a gray-scale value >10 were assigned a color based on the degree of contrast enhancement. Shades of *red*, progressing to hues of *orange, yellow,* and *white* represent incremental contrast opacification. Equal and homogeneous opacification in both myocardial beds is showed at rest (**a**). **c,d** Corresponding pulsing interval vs video-intensity curves are shown. At rest (**c**), both left circumflex coronary artery (*LCx*) and left anterior descending (*LAD*) coronary artery beds show similar myocardial blood volume and velocity of myocardial blood flow. During hyperemia (**d**), the two pulsing interval vs video-intensity curves show rapid replenishment of microbubbles into the normal myocardium (left circumflex coronary artery bed) at 1 s, while the left anterior descending coronary artery bed shows a slower replenishment due to the presence of increased vascular resistance in that bed (**d**). (From WEI et al. 2001b)

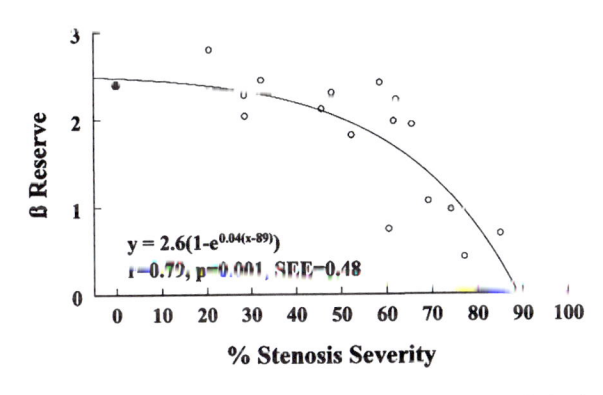

Fig. 18.9. Relation between percentage of stenosis severity derived from quantitative coronary angiography and myocardial contrast echocardiography-derived myocardial blood flow velocity (β) reserve. See text for details. (From WEI et al. 2001b)

myocardial contrast echocardiography. Instead of being considered confusing, the choices available in contrast echocardiography provide a great deal of flexibility that allows almost any patient to have a successful perfusion study.

We also discuss the ability of contrast echocardiography to quantify regional velocity of myocardial blood flow at rest and during hyperemia. We used detection and quantification of coronary stenosis severity to highlight one application of this technology.

Given the flexibility, portability, and wide availability of US, we expect contrast echocardiography to play an increasingly important role in patient management and noninvasive imaging in the future. Furthermore, not only can the principles outlined herein be used for cardiac imaging, they can also be applied to any organ that is accessible to US (WEI et al. 2001a; MEAIRS et al. 2000; BURNS et al. 2000).

References

Ay T, London V, d'Hondt AM et al (2001) Quantification of coronary flow reserve with myocardial contrast echocardiography in humans: comparison with positron emission tomography (abstract). Circulation 104 (Suppl II):589

Burns P, Powers JE, Simpson DH et al (1996) Harmonic imaging principles and preliminary results. Clin Radiol 51(Suppl):50–55

Burns PN, Wilson SR, Simpson DH (2000) Pulse inversion imaging of liver blood flow. Improved method for characterizing focal masses with microbubble contrast. Invest Radiol 35:58–71

Chilian WM, Marcus ML (1982) Phasic coronary blood flow velocity in intramural and epicardial coronary arteries. Circ Res 50:772–781

Chomas JE, Dayton P, Allen J et al (2001) Mechanisms of contrast agent destruction. IEEE Trans Ultrason Ferr Freq Control 48:232–248

Dawson D, Rinkevich D, Belcik T (2003) Measurement of myocardial blood flow velocity reserve with myocardial contrast echocardiography in patients with suspected coronary artery disease: comparison with quantitative gated ^{99m}Tc sestamibi SPECT. J Am Soc Echocardiogr 16:1171–1177

Dayton PA, Morgan KE, Klibanov AL et al (1999) Optical and acoustical observations of the effects of ultrasound on contrast agents. IEEE Trans Ultrason Ferr Freq Contr 46:220–232

De Jong N, Frinking PJ, Bouakaz A (2000a) Optical imaging of contrast agent microbubbles in an ultrasound field with a 100-MHx camera. Ultrasound Med Biol 26:487–492

De Jong N, Frinking PJA, Bouakaz A, Ten Cate FT (2000b) Detection procedures of ultrasound contrast agents. Ultrasonics 38:87–92

Fisher NG, Christiansen JP, Klibanov AL et al (2002) Influence of surface charge on capillary transit and myocardial contrast enhancement. J Am Coll Cardiol 40:811–819

Gould KL, Lipscomb K (1974) Effects of coronary stenoses on coronary flow reserve and resistance. Am J Cardiol 34:48–55

Jayaweera AR, Edwards N, Glasheen WP et al (1994) In vivo myocardial kinetics of air-filled albumin microbubbles during myocardial contrast echocardiography. Comparison with radiolabeled red blood cells. Circ Res 74:1157–1165

Kajiya F, Tsujioka K, Goto M et al (1985) Evaluation of phasic blood flow velocity in the great cardiac vein by a laser Doppler method. Heart Vessels 1:16–23

Kassab GS, Lin DH, Fung YB (1994a) Topology and dimensions of pig coronary capillary network. Am J Physiol 267:H319–H325

Kassab GS, Lin DH, Fung YB (1994b) Morphometry of pig coronary venous system. Am J Physiol 267:H2100–H2113

Kaul S, Jayaweera AR (1997) Coronary and myocardial blood volumes: Noninvasive tools to assess the coronary microcirculation? Circulation 96:719–724

Keller MW, Glasheen WP, Teja K et al (1988) Myocardial contrast echocardiography without significant hemodynamic effects or reactive hyperemia: a major advantage in the imaging of myocardial perfusion. J Am Coll Cardiol 12:1039–1047

Keller MW, Segal SS, Kaul S, Duling BR (1989) The behavior of sonicated albumin microbubbles within the microcirculation: a basis for their use during myocardial contrast echocardiography. Circ Res 65:458–467

Klibanov AL, Maruyama K, Torchilin VP, Huang L (1990) Amphipathic polyethyleneglycols effectively prolong the circulation time of liposomes. FEBS Lett 268:235–237

Leong-Poi H, Le E, Rim SJ et al (2001) Quantification of myocardial perfusion and determination of coronary stenosis severity during hyperemia using real-time myocardial contrast echocardiography. J Am Soc Echocardiogr 14:1173–1182

Linka AZ, Sklenar J, Wei K et al (1998) Spatial distribution of microbubble velocity and concentration within the myocardium: insights into the transmural distribution of myocardial blood flow and volume. Circulation 98:1912–1920

Meairs S, Daffertshofer M, Neff W et al (2000) Pulse-inversion contrast harmonic imaging: ultrasonographic assessment of cerebral perfusion. Lancet 355:550–551

Moore CA, Smucker ML, Kaul S (1986) Myocardial contrast echocardiography in humans. I. Safety: A comparison with routine coronary arteriography. J Am Coll Cardiol 8:1066–1072

Pelberg RA, Wei K, Kamiyama N et al (1999) Advantages of "Flash Echocardiography": a new technique for assessing myocardial perfusion. J Am Soc Echocardiogr 12:85–93

Porter TR, Xie F, Silver M et al (2001) Real-time perfusion imaging with low mechanical index pulse inversion Doppler imaging. J Am Coll Cardiol 37:748–753

Shimoni S, Zoghbi WA, Xie F et al (2001) Real-time assessment of myocardial perfusion and wall motion during bicycle and treadmill exercise echocardiography: comparison with single photon emission computed tomography. J Am Coll Cardiol 37:741–747

Skyba DM, Jayaweera AR, Goodman NC et al (1994) Quantification of myocardial perfusion with myocardial contrast echocardiography during left atrial injection of contrast: implications for venous injection. Circulation 90:1513–1521

Skyba DM, Camarano G, Goodman NC et al (1996) Hemodynamic characteristics, myocardial kinetics and microvascular rheology of FS-069, a second-generation echocardiographic contrast agent capable of producing myocardial opacification from a venous injection. J Am Coll Cardiol 28:1292–1300

Soman P, Taillefer R, DePuey EG et al (2001) Enhanced detection of reversible perfusion defects by Tc-99m sestamibi compared to Tc-99m tetrofosmin during vasodilator stress SPECT imaging in mild-to-moderate coronary artery disease. J Am Coll Cardiol 37:458–462

Torchilin VP, Omelyanenko VG, Papisov MI et al (1994) Poly(ethylene glycol) on the liposome surface: on the mechanism of polymer-coated liposome longevity. Biochim Biophys Acta 1195:11–20

Toyota E, Fujimoto K, Ogasawara Y et al (2002) Dynamic changes in three-dimensional architecture and vascular volume of transmural coronary microvasculature between diastolic- and systolic-arrested rat hearts. Circulation 105:621–626

Villanueva FS, Jankowski RJ, Manaugh C, Wagner WR (1997) Albumin microbubble adherence to human coronary endothelium: implications for assessment of endothelial function using myocardial contrast echocardiography. J Am Coll Cardiol 30:689–693

Wei K, Skyba DM, Firschke C et al (1997) Interaction between microbubbles and ultrasound: in vitro and in vivo observations. J Am Coll Cardiol 29:1081–1088

Wei K, Jayaweera AR, Firoozan S et al (1998) Quantification of myocardial blood flow with ultrasound-induced destruction of microbubbles administered as a constant infusion. Circulation 97:473–483

Wei K, Le E, Bin J-P et al (2001a) Quantification of total and regional renal blood flow using contrast-enhanced ultrasonography. J Am Coll Cardiol 37:1135–1140

Wei K, Ragosta M, Thorpe J et al (2001b) Non-invasive quantification of coronary blood flow reserve in humans using myocardial contrast echocardiography. Circulation 103:2560–2565

Wei K (2002) Assessment of myocardial blood flow and volume using myocardial contrast echocardiography. Echocardiography 19(5):409–416

Weyman AE (1994) Physical principles of ultrasound. In: Weyman AE (ed) Principles and practice of echocardiography. Lea and Febiger, Philadelphia

19 Assessment of Myocardial Blood Volume

Kevin Wei

CONTENTS

19.1 Introduction 277
19.2 Coronary Microcirculation 277
19.3 Myocardial Contrast Enhancement and Capillary Blood Volume 278
19.3.1 Fixed Perfusion Defects 279
19.3.2 Reversible Perfusion Defects 284
19.4 Coupling Between Capillary Derecruitment and Hyperemic Flow 288
19.5 Conclusion 289
References 289

19.1
Introduction

Myocardial contrast echocardiography uses microbubbles as a perfusion tracer. The microbubbles approximate the size of red blood cells (2–5 μm), and they remain entirely intravascular; thus, detection of these microbubbles can provide important insights into the integrity of the myocardial microvasculature. Ultrasound has excellent spatial resolution (<1 mm axially), which allows assessment of even transmural differences in myocardial perfusion (Linka et al. 1998; Villanueva et al. 1993). Myocardial contrast echocardiography is therefore ideally suited to evaluate the location, size, and transmural extent of myocardial perfusion defects.

This chapter reviews important aspects of the coronary microcirculation that are pertinent for understanding normal and abnormal myocardial perfusion on contrast echocardiography. The ability of contrast echocardiography to assess spatial aspects of myocardial perfusion (i.e., fixed and reversible perfusion defects), and the pathophysiologic changes that occur in the coronary microcirculation to produce such defects, are discussed. The discussion on perfusion defects focus on applications of contrast echocardiography in the setting of acute myocardial infarction, and on the development of reversible perfusion defects during stress in the setting of coronary artery disease.

19.2
Coronary Microcirculation

Coronary microcirculation is directly or indirectly involved in a wide array of pathologic states. Its behavior in different diseases and situations can therefore provide important insights into coronary pathophysiology in humans. Having an understanding of microvascular anatomy and characteristics is therefore important for interpreting myocardial contrast echocardiography images.

Detailed descriptions of the coronary systems of many species are now available (Bassingthwaighte et al. 1974; Marcus 1983; Tschabitscher 1984; Anderson et al. 1988; Kassab et al. 1993; Kassab et al. 1994a,b). In particular, studies of the pig heart have provided an understanding of the distribution of blood within the coronary system (Kassab et al. 1993, 1994a,b) and allowed us to appreciate what a myocardial contrast echocardiography image represents.

The arterial and venous systems have branching vessels that can be mathematically characterized as fractals. The venous system has arcading veins in the epicardial and endocardial surfaces in pigs. Arcading arteries are present on the epicardial surface in pigs (Kassab et al. 1993), but they exist on the endocardial surface in humans. The majority of venules drain into the coronary sinus, but some (Thebesian veins) drain directly into the ventricular cavities (Kassab et al. 1994a). For each order of branching, veins in the myocardium are larger than arteries of the same order.

K. Wei, MD
Cardiac Imaging Center, Cardiovascular Division, University of Virginia School of Medicine, P.O. Box 800158, Charlottesville, VA 22908-0158, USA

Additionally, myocardial veins are more irregularly shaped than arteries. The myocardial veins are also interconnected, and more than one vein may drain a myocardial region served by a single artery (Kassab et al. 1994a).

Unlike the arterial and venous systems, most capillaries traverse the length of a myocyte, and their orientation is parallel to that of myocardial muscle fibers. The arterioles feeding the capillaries are approximately 10 µm in diameter (the smallest order of branches). Capillaries can also branch directly from up to third-order vessels (the main trunk being eleventh order; Kassab et al. 1994a). Approximately 50% of feeding arterioles run parallel to the capillary bed, and each can give rise to several capillaries.

About 25% of the feeding arterioles course transversely toward the myocyte and give off two capillaries at right angles. The remaining arterioles are a mixture of these two patterns (Kassab et al. 1994a). The draining venules run in the same direction as capillaries before turning obliquely to join higher-order veins. Even though most capillaries drain into first-order venules, they may drain into up to seventh-order venules (the coronary sinus being the thirteenth order) (Kassab et al. 1994b).

Capillaries have been characterized as Y, H, or T depending on their shape. The mean capillary diameter is approximately 6 µm, and the mean length is 0.5–1 mm, depending on the species. The mean intercapillary distance is 15–20 µm (Kassab et al. 1994b; Bassingthwaighte et al. 1974). To provide efficient oxygen delivery, capillaries traverse the length of myocytes, and each capillary has a domain and is responsible for its nutrition. The rate of oxygen diffusion across tissue, and the rate of oxygen consumption by tissue, determine the size of the domain (Gayeski and Honig 1991). The number of capillaries and the intercapillary distance within a tissue depend on the oxygen needs of the specific tissue (Kassab et al. 1994b; Bassingthwaighte et al. 1974). Under resting conditions, not all capillaries allow red blood cell flow. Red blood cell flux is seen in only about half of the capillaries in cardiac muscle (Tillmans et al. 1987). Because myocardial oxygen extraction is already near maximal at rest, adequate oxygen delivery can be met only through increases in myocardial blood flow when myocardial oxygen consumption increases (Le et al. 2002). A mild increase in myocyte oxygen requirements results in a mild increase in red blood cell velocity through capillaries. Further increases in demand, however, require additional mechanisms to increase nutrient delivery. One mechanism for the increase in myocardial O_2 delivery during stress is functional recruitment of capillaries, allowing more red blood cells to pass through more capillaries (Friedman et al. 1995; Le et al. 2002).

The volume of blood within the entire coronary circulation at rest in diastole is approximately 12 ml/100 g of left ventricular myocardium (Kassab et al. 1994a). This volume is distributed almost equally between the arterial (epicardial coronary artery to 200-µm arterioles), microcirculatory (200-µm arterioles to 200-µm venules), and venous compartments (200-µm venules to coronary sinus) – with 3.5, 3.8, and 4.9 ml/100 g in each compartment, respectively. Most of the arterial and venous blood volumes, however, are located on the epicardial surface of the heart. Within the myocardium itself, the capillaries numerically outnumber all other vessels (with a density of 3000–4000/mm^2), and contain almost all the myocardial blood volume. Only 5–10% of myocardial blood volume is contained within intramyocardial arterioles and venules (Kassab et al. 1994a).

19.3
Myocardial Contrast Enhancement and Capillary Blood Volume

The microbubble agents used to evaluate myocardial perfusion during contrast echocardiography are efficient scatterers of US energy. A linear relation exists between low microbubble concentrations and the corresponding backscatter signal displayed on contrast echocardiography, so their relative concentrations in tissue can be quantified (Skyba et al. 1994). The microbubbles are unlike the tracers used with other non-invasive cardiac imaging techniques (such as PET, SPECT, MRI, or CT), because they are hemodynamically inert, and also remain entirely intravascular (Keller et al. 1989).

Relative concentration (or regional video intensity on myocardial contrast echocardiography) of microbubbles in different areas of the myocardium therefore reflect the blood volume in those regions (Linka et al. 1998; Wei et al. 1998a).

Since the largest proportion of myocardial blood volume is contained within capillaries, regional video intensity reflects capillary blood volume; thus, provided that the relation between signal amplitude and tracer concentration is linear, changes in myocardial blood volume are reflected by proportional changes in video intensity on contrast echocardiography (Fig. 19.1) expressing as perfusion defects.

Assessment of Myocardial Blood Volume

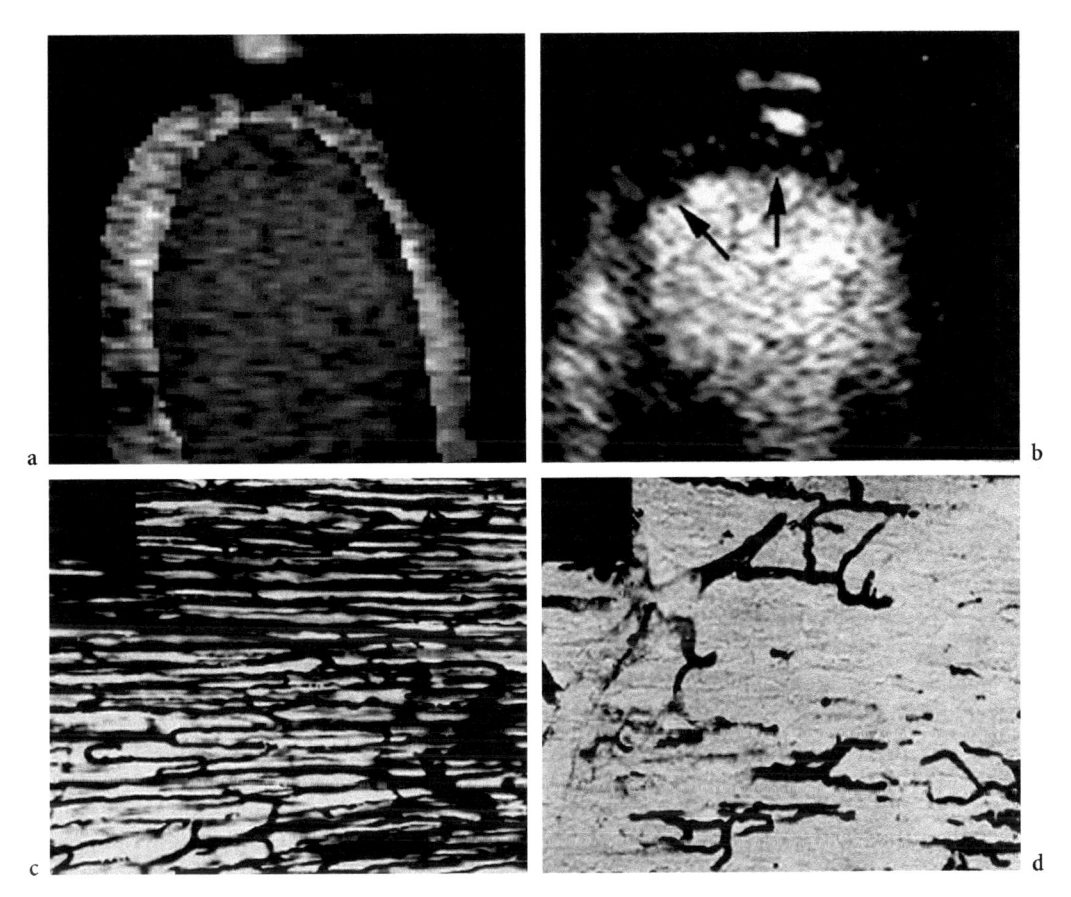

Fig. 19.1a–d. Contrast-enhanced apical three-chamber view shows homogeneous myocardial opacification in all perfusion territories (a) representing normal capillary integrity (c). A focal subendocardial perfusion defect in patient with prior apical infarction (b) is seen (*arrows*) in the presence of capillary damage (d).

19.3.1
Fixed Perfusion Defects

The fixed myocardial perfusion defects are those which are evident both during resting and during physical or pharmacologic stress.

a) Application of contrast echocardiography in acute myocardial infarction. Experimental studies in dogs have shown that the time course of cell death begins approximately 30–40 min after acute coronary occlusion (REIMER and JENNINGS 1979). Necrosis extends from the subendocardium where ischemia is the most severe, towards the subepicardium, and becomes transmural after 6 h. Reperfusion within 2 h can result in functional recovery of the ischemic tissue; thus, early reperfusion of the infarct-related artery has been shown to salvage viable myocardium within the infarct bed. Zones of severe myocellular injury or death are associated with microvascular damage or plugging. Microbubbles will therefore be excluded from these areas, which will manifest as perfusion defects on myocardial contrast echocardiography.

Apart from the duration of occlusion, determinants of infarct size include the size of the risk area, as well as the adequacy of collateral flow (KAUL et al. 1987; LEVIN 1974; PIEK and BECKER 1988).

With the advent of contrast echocardiography, there is now a non-invasive method that can assess both of these latter parameters rapidly at the patient's bedside. Furthermore, contrast echocardiography can be used to determine the success of reperfusion. Since the microbubbles have only a short half-life in the circulation, contrast echocardiography can also be used serially to study the effects of interventions in patients with acute myocardial infarction. With its portability and excellent spatial resolution (<1 mm axially), contrast echocardiography may be very useful if incorporated into the assessment of patients with acute myocardial infarction.

b) Detection of Risk Area.

The region of myocardium subtended by an occluded coronary artery that may eventually develop necrosis is termed the risk area (KAUL et al. 1984). On myocardial contrast echocardiography, the risk area is a well demarcated zone of hypoperfusion adjacent to neighboring areas of normal myocardial blood flow. After a direct intracoronary injection of microbubbles, the risk area appears as a non-enhanced region of myocardium with a distinct border. In animal models, direct intracoronary (KAUL et al. 1985, 1986), aortic root (FIRSCHKE et al. 1997a), right or left atrial (VILLANUEVA et al. 1993; FIRSCHKE et al. 1997a), and most recently intravenous (GRAYBURN et al. 1995; FIRSCHKE et al. 1997b; LINDNER et al. 1998) injections of microbubbles have all been shown to successfully define the risk area with excellent concordance (LINDNER et al. 1998) to intracoronary injections of color dyes or technetium autoradiography (Fig. 19.2).

In acute animal models, it has been shown that the size of the risk area matches closely with the extent of abnormal wall motion on echocardiography (KAUL et al. 1984, 1986). In patients, however, preexisting wall motion abnormalities may be present from prior infarction, acute or chronic ischemia, or cardiomyopathic causes. Evaluation of wall motion alone may not be adequate for the assessment of risk area in many patients, and an assessment of perfusion may provide useful adjunctive information.

Defining the spatial extent of the area at risk may help to guide therapy in the future. For example, patients with a small risk area who have relative contraindications to thrombolytic therapy may have an unacceptable risk of bleeding compared with the benefit of modest myocardial salvage from reperfusion. On the other hand, a large perfusion defect may help to define patients who would derive the greatest benefit from urgent primary angioplasty. It is also possible that the evaluation of perfusion defect size and severity with contrast echocardiography may help identify patients with non-ST ECG trace elevation myocardial infarction who have greater clot burden and may benefit from early institution of potent antiplatelet agents, thrombolytics, or angioplasty. These issues await further clinical studies to demonstrate clinical efficacy.

c) Assessment of the Success of Reperfusion and Determination of Infarct Size.

Both morbidity and mortality from myocardial infarction are significantly affected by infarct size, which can be characterized by the endocardial length and/or the transmural extent of the perfusion defect on contrast echocardiography.

Early reperfusion remains the mainstay of therapy for patients presenting with acute myocardial infarction. Clinical markers, including resolution of ST, segment of ECG elevation, alleviation of angina, and ventricular arrhythmias, such as an accelerated idioventricular rhythm, are indicative of tissue reperfusion, but are neither sensitive nor specific (CALIFF et al. 1988). Wall thickening on echocardiography cannot reliably determine the success of reperfusion either, due to the development of stunning from prolonged ischemia.

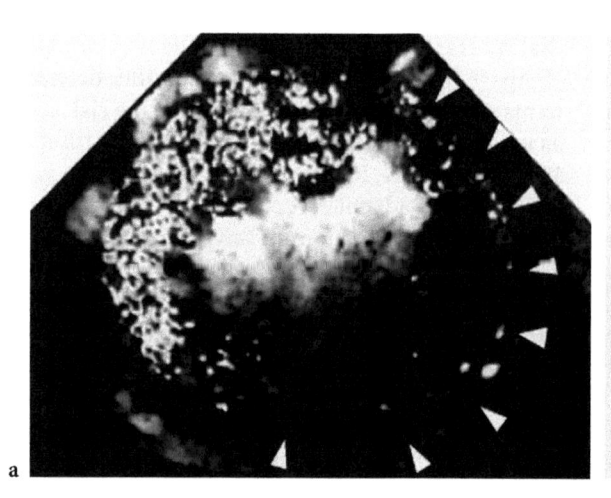

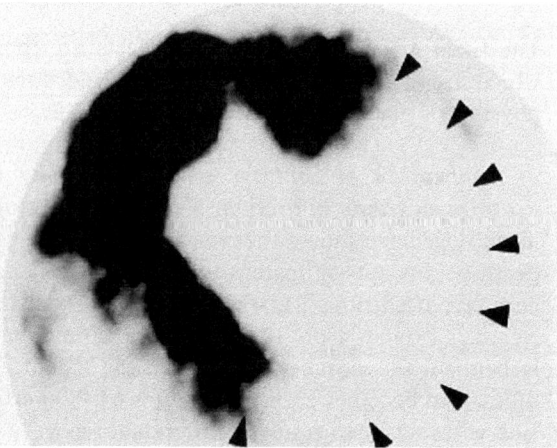

Fig. 19.2a,b. A color-coded short-axis image of the left ventricle after a peripheral intravenous injection of microbubbles in a dog with an occlusion of the left circumflex coronary artery (a). A technetium autoradiograph obtained from the same short-axis level is also shown (b). The lateral wall (*arrows*) has a well-defined area without contrast enhancement which is clearly separated from the normal bed. The spatial location and extent of the risk area on myocardial contrast echocardiography closely approximates the "cold spot" on the technetium autoradiograph.

A non-invasive perfusion method that can easily and rapidly define the re-establishment of tissue flow would therefore be useful. Apart from assessing the success of therapy, determining those patients with unsuccessful thrombolysis may be beneficial, as they may require further interventions such as rescue angioplasty (BELENKIE et al. 1992; ELLIS et al. 1994). Myocardial contrast echocardiography therefore has the potential to provide important adjunctive information that may impact the management of patients presenting with acute myocardial infarction.

Even in patients who undergo primary angioplasty, it is now recognized that simple recanalization of the infarct-related artery is inadequate to ensure a good outcome. Perfusion must also be restored at a microvascular level; thus, after blood flow is restored to an occluded bed, myocardial opacification should be seen within regions with successful reperfusion on myocardial contrast echocardiography. Despite patency of the infarct-related artery, myocardial contrast echocardiography can define regions with significant myocellular injury (necrosis) and microvascular disruption, since they show no opacification – or no reflow. This phenomenon may be due to reduced microvascular flow from small vessel spasm or microvessels could be plugged by thrombi, inflammatory cells, or debris.

Due to the excellent spatial resolution of US, the spatial extent and location of even subendocardial infarction can be defined on myocardial contrast echocardiography (Fig. 19.1), and has been shown in animal studies to correlate well with 2,3,5-triphenyltetrazolium chloride assessments of infarct size (FIRSCHKE et al. 1997b; LINDNER et al. 1998).

Clinical studies have evaluated the relationship between antegrade epicardial flow using the Thrombolysis in Myocardial Infarction study group grading system, and the adequacy of microvascular perfusion on contrast echocardiography. A number of landmark studies have shown that patients with Thrombolysis in Myocardial Infarction grades 1 and 2 flow have a higher incidence of no-reflow on contrast echocardiography compared with those with Thrombolysis in Myocardial Infarction grade 3 flow (ITO et al. 1996a; IWAKURA et al. 1996). Even in patients with Thrombolysis in Myocardial Infarction grade 3 flow, however, 16% had microvascular no-reflow on contrast echocardiography (ITO et al. 1996a), and other studies have found even higher incidences (PORTER et al. 1998).

The extent of no-reflow on contrast echocardiography has been shown to have significant consequences. Patients with low- or no-reflow had poor recovery of left ventricular function, greater infarct expansion, remodeling, and left ventricular dilation (ITO et al. 1996b; PORTER et al. 1998). Moreover, patients with poor microvascular reperfusion have a significantly higher incidence of cardiac events including cardiac death, non-fatal myocardial infarction, and congestive heart failure over a 1-year follow-up period (SAKUMA et al. 1998).

More recent studies done with intravenously administered contrast agents show good concordance between contrast echocardiography and SPECT for detection of viability (Fig. 19.2). Dysfunctional segments that demonstrated contrast enhancement had better recovery of wall motion than segments with no-reflow (ROCCHI et al. 2001). The presence of reflow defined by myocardial contrast echocardiography 24 h after reperfusion has been found to be associated with higher coronary flow reserve than patients with no-reflow, and these authors also found that these segments had better improvement in regional and global ventricular function at follow-up (LEPPER et al. 2000).

d) Evaluation of Collateral Flow in Acute Myocardial Infarction with Contrast Echocardiography.

Defining infarct size by assessment of the no-reflow zone is performed only after reperfusion (DITTRICH et al. 1995). As mentioned above, the adequacy of collateral flow to the occluded bed influences the extent of necrosis and ultimate infarct size (MARUOKA et al. 1986; SABIA et al. 1992); thus, for any given size of risk area and duration of coronary occlusion, the magnitude and extent of collateral flow into the risk area will determine the degree of necrosis and ultimate infarct size.

Prior to the development of new-generation microbubble agents, the ability of direct intracoronary injections of microbubbles to define the presence of collateral flow in patients with recent acute myocardial infarction was shown (MARUOKA et al. 1986; SABIA et al. 1992). Even though collaterals may not be present de novo in normal subjects, patients with chronic coronary artery disease have been shown to develop abundant collaterals to ischemic territories (SABIA et al. 1992). Even with persistent coronary occlusion and prolonged absence of antegrade flow, adequate levels of collateral-derived blood flow can allow maintenance of myocardial viability and spares tissue from necrosis (SABIA et al. 1992).

More recently, COGGINS et al. (2001) demonstrated that collateral flow can be assessed using intravenously administered microbubbles. The method is based on providing enough time for microbubble replenishment into the risk area after their destruction, so that slow collateral-derived flow (COGGINS et al. 2001) can be imaged (Fig. 19.3). Not only does the presence of contrast enhancement within the risk area define the presence of collateral flow, but myocardial opacification is only seen when myocardial blood flow exceeds approximately 20% of normal resting levels. Since myocytes may remain viable at levels of 25% of normal resting myocardial blood flow (MARUOKA et al. 1986; COGGINS et al. 2001), the spatial distribution of perfusion within the risk area identifies tissue that may be spared from necrosis despite persistent coronary occlusion; thus, despite a prolonged 6-h occlusion in the animal shown in Fig. 19.3, no infarction developed. Figure 19.3 illustrates how collateral flow can prevent myocellular necrosis and can modulate infarct size despite prolonged occlusion of the epicardial coronary artery. In the same study, the circumferential extent of abnormal wall thickening was found to correlate well with the size of the initial risk area on myocardial contrast echocardiography, but overestimated the eventual infarct size (COGGINS et al. 2001). This finding confirmed those of previous studies (VILLANUEVA et al. 1993).

Thus, despite adequate collateral flow to maintain viability, it is insufficient to preserve normal wall

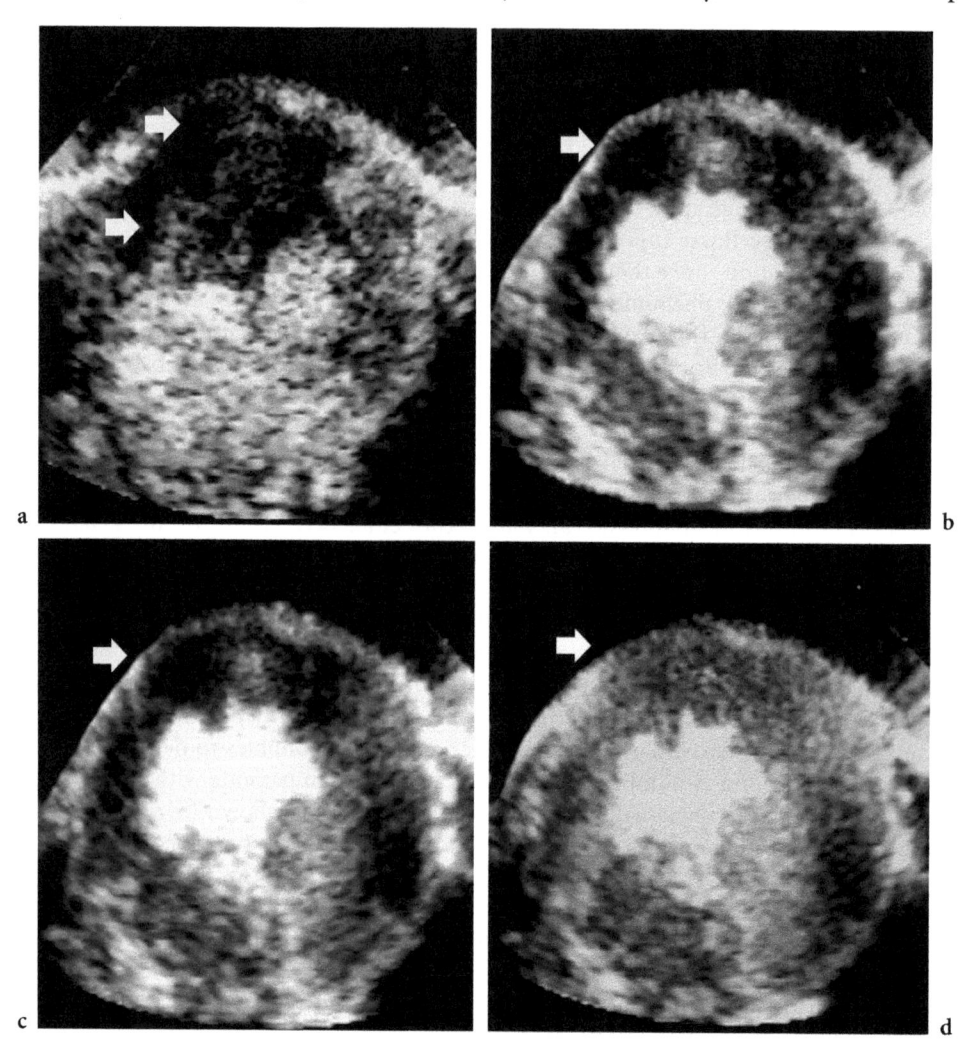

Fig. 19.3a–d. Short-axis images obtained in the presence of an occlusion of the left anterior descending coronary artery, during a continuous intravenous infusion of microbubbles. At the shortest pulsing interval (a), a clear demarcation is noted between the inferoposterior wall which has normal myocardial perfusion and the occluded anterior bed, which shows no contrast enhancement (*arrows*). The hypoperfused zone at this pulsing interval represents the risk area. At a longer pulsing intervals of 1.5 and 2.5 s, border zones of the anterior myocardium supplied by collateral flow has started to replenish with microbubbles (b,c). At an interval of 10 s, the entire risk area has become homogeneously opacified from collateral-derived myocardial blood flow (d). (From COGGINS et al. 2001)

thickening. Again, assessments of wall thickening alone therefore provide only limited information in patients presenting with acute myocardial infarction. It cannot be used to predict eventual infarct size, as wall thickening remains severely abnormal even in the presence of adequate collateral flow.

Because the spatial distribution of regions with adequate collateral flow to maintain viability despite persistent coronary occlusion can be defined with myocardial contrast echocardiography, this method can potentially predict infarct size even prior to reperfusion, by defining areas that will be destined to necrose unless reperfusion is achieved (COGGINS et al. 2001). As a corollary to the example shown in Fig. 19.3, the short-axis images displayed in Fig. 19.4 demonstrate an animal with a left circumflex coronary occlusion with minimal collateral flow.

Myocardial contrast echocardiography can therefore provide significant information in patients presenting with acute myocardial infarction. It can be used to define the location and spatial extent of the risk area, to evaluate the degree of collateral flow within the risk area, and therefore it can be used to predict eventual infarct size by determining which areas within the risk area will be protected from necrosis by adequate levels of collateral-derived nutrient perfusion. Myocardial contrast echocardiography can also be used serially to evaluate the success of reperfusion therapy, and the assessment of eventual infarct size can provide prognostic infor-

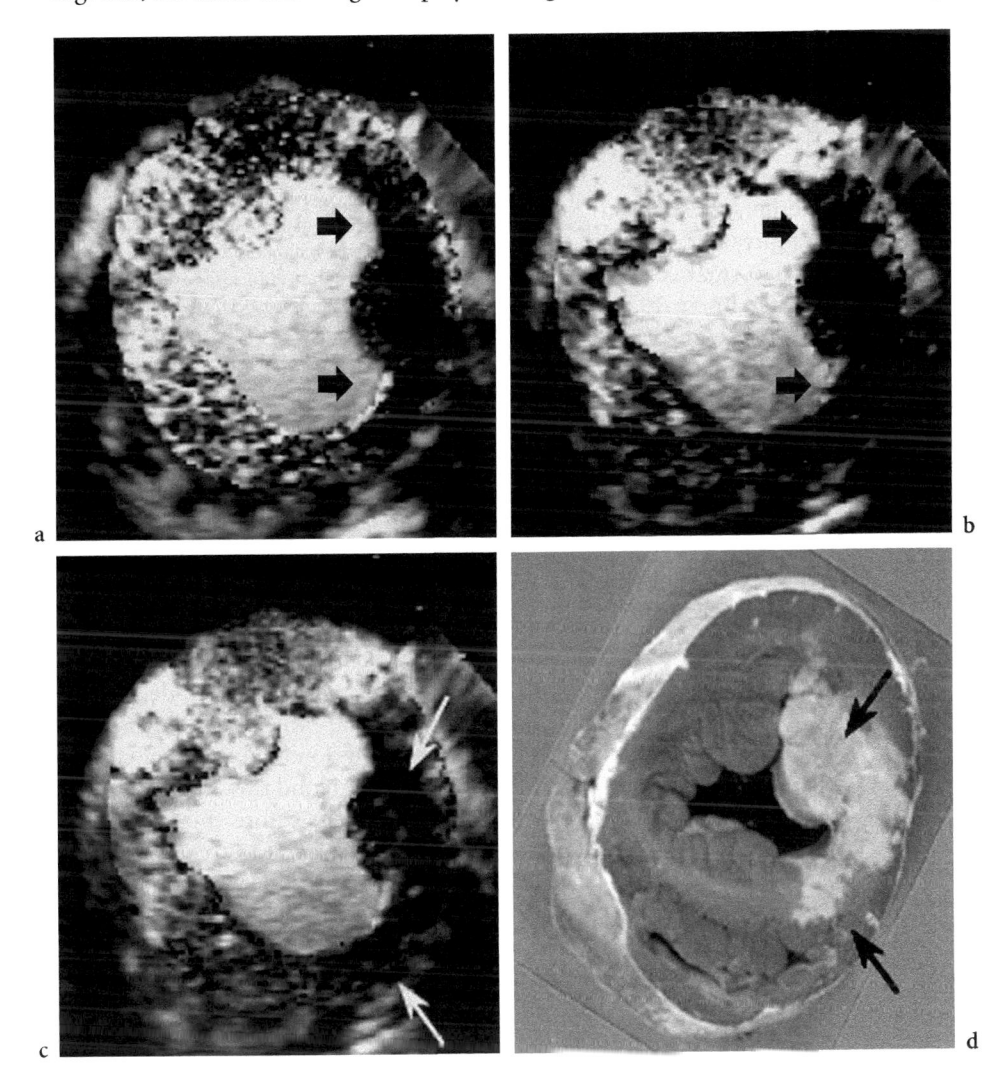

Fig. 19.4a-d. Absence of collateral flow in the risk area during left circumflex occlusion (a-c) and subsequent transmural lateral wall infarction (d). The risk area in the lateral wall is again seen as a distinct zone of hypoperfusion (*arrows*) at the shortest pulsing interval (a). Despite progressive prolongation of the pulsing interval up to 9 s, however, no significant replenishment of microbubbles (*arrows*) is noted within the risk area (b-c). After 6 h of occlusion, this animal developed a transmural infarct in the lateral wall demonstrated by the absence of triphenyl tetrazolium chloride staining (*arrows*; d). (From COGGINS et al. 2001)

mation; however, the exact role of contrast echocardiography in acute myocardial infarction remains to be determined in clinical trials.

19.3.2
Reversible Perfusion Defects

The reversible myocardial perfusion defects are those which become evident during physical or pharmacologic stress and disappear during resting. In the absence of prior myocardial injury, both resting coronary blood flow (Table 19.1) and left ventricular function remain normal even in the presence of an epicardial coronary stenosis up to 85–90% in severity (Fig. 19.5; GOULD and LIPSCOMB 1974). This ability of the myocardium to maintain normal resting myocardial blood flow (Table 19.1) is due to autoregulation, a mechanism by which increases in resistance in one part of the circulation (stenosis in the epicardial coronary artery) are counterbalanced by decreases in another (resistance arterioles; Table 19.1). A histogram representing the distribution of resistances across the normal coronary circulation at baseline is illustrated in Fig. 19.6 (CHILIAN et al. 1986; JOHNSON 1986; JAYAWEERA et al. 1999). This process of autoregulation is operative until a stenosis exceeds approximately 85% in severity, when arteriolar vasodilatory reserve is

Table 19.1 Fundamental formulas of myocardial perfusion.

MBF = Velocity of MBF × MBV
P = CBF × R (= autoregulation formula)

MBF myocardial blood flow, *MBV* myocardial blood volume, *CBF* coronary blood flow, *P* coronary driving pressure, *R* resistance of coronary circulation

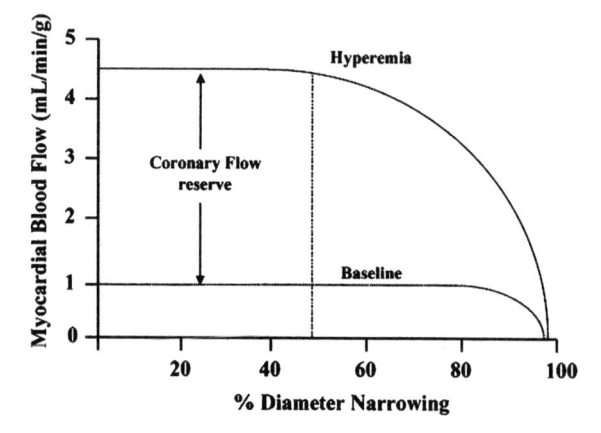

Fig. 19.5 Relation between percentage of stenosis severity and myocardial blood flow at rest and during hyperemia. See text for details. (Redrawn from GOULD and LIPSCOMB 1974)

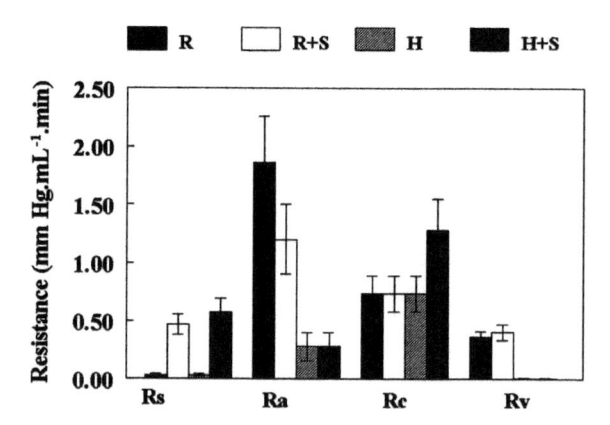

Fig. 19.6 Resistances across the stenosis (Rs), arterioles (Ra), capillaries (Rc), and venules (Rv) are shown at rest (R), during non-critical stenosis ($R+S$), and during hyperemia in the absence (H) and presence of non-critical stenosis ($H+S$). At rest in the absence of stenosis (R), the mean aortic pressure of approximately 90 mmHg is reduced to a pre-capillary pressure of 45 mmHg because of arteriolar resistance (R_a), which is the site of greatest resistance to coronary blood flow at rest. There is a further 30 mmHg drop of pressure across the capillary bed. The capillaries are very small in size and offer high resistance, but since they are arranged in parallel, the total capillary resistance decreases with increasing numbers of capillaries (R_c). The drop across the venous bed is only 15 mmHg since these are high-capacitance vessels, which nevertheless have some smooth muscle. Thus, at rest approximately 60% of total myocardial vascular resistance is offered by the arterioles, 25% by the capillaries, and 15% by the venules (R_v). In the presence of a non-critical coronary stenosis ($R+S$), trans-stenotic resistance (R_s) increases, which results in a decrease in the distal coronary pressure as well as the coronary driving pressure. In this situation, arteriolar vasodilation occurs to decrease arteriolar tone and resistance (R_a). The decrease in arteriolar resistance balances the increase in trans-stenotic resistance, allowing blood flow, pre-capillary arteriolar pressure, and capillary hydrostatic pressure to be maintained at normal resting levels.

exhausted. After this point, further decreases in coronary driving pressure will result in decreases in resting coronary blood flow. Since neither coronary blood flow, myocardial blood flow, nor wall motion abnormalities are evident before this, non-critical stenoses cannot be detected at rest using non-invasive perfusion imaging techniques or assessments of resting left ventricular function.

In order to meet increases in myocardial oxygen demand induced by exercise or other forms of stress, coronary blood flow can usually increase four to five times that of resting levels. Coronary arteries with stenoses that encroach more than 50% of the luminal diameter, however, show an attenuated hyperemic response (Fig. 19.5). To detect non-flow limiting stenoses with echocardiography, therefore, adequate exercise or pharmacologic stress is used to produce supply/demand mismatch and ischemia, which results in the development of a regional wall motion abnormality.

With the advent of perfusion imaging during contrast echocardiography, regional differences in myocardial video intensity between beds with and without stenosis during hyperemia have also been found using intra-arterial, right and left atrial, as well as intravenous bolus injections of microbubbles (ISMAIL et al. 1995; FIRSCHKE et al. 1997b; WEI et al. 1998b). It has been shown in animal models that the severity of reversible perfusion defects that develop on contrast echocardiography correlate with myocardial blood flow mismatch between the normal and stenosed beds determined using radiolabeled microspheres, and that the spatial extent of myocardial contrast echocardiography perfusion defects corresponds to the region showing hypoperfusion by radiolabeled microspheres.

Background-subtracted color-coded images from an animal experiment obtained during hyperemia at baseline and in the presence of left anterior descending coronary artery stenoses of varying severity are shown in Fig. 19.7 which shows the difference between reversible (low-grade coronary stenosis) and fixed (high-grade coronary stenosis) perfusion defects. A good correlation was found between the myocardial video-intensity ratio between the stenosed and normal beds and the degree of myocardial blood flow mismatch between those beds (WEI et al. 1998b).

Similarly, clinical studies performed using bolus injections of microbubbles have shown that abnormal perfusion at rest and during dipyridamole stress can be defined using contrast echocardiography (KAUL et al. 1997; PORTER et al. 1997; HEINLE et al. 2000). The location of the perfusion defects, and their physiologic relevance (fixed or reversible) are similar to those obtained with ^{99m}Tc-sestamibi SPECT (KAUL et al. 1997; HEINLE et al. 2000). Excellent concordance was found when analyses were performed on a segment-by-segment (92%, κ=0.99), territory-by-territory (90%, κ=0.77), or patient-by-patient basis (86%, κ=0.71; KAUL et al. 1997).

a) Mechanism Underlying the Development of Reversible Perfusion Defects on Myocardial Contrast Echocardiography. As with all perfusion defects on myocardial contrast echocardiography, the presence of a reversible perfusion defect denotes the development of relative differences in myocardial blood volume between the stenosed and normal beds after stress that reverses at rest. With bolus injections of microbubbles, however, it was not possible to determine whether the defect was due to an absolute decrease in myocardial blood volume in the stenosed bed, or to an increase in myocardial blood volume in the normal bed during stress (WEI et al. 1998b).

We now know using continuous infusions of microbubbles that capillary derecruitment (or an absolute decrease in myocardial blood volume)

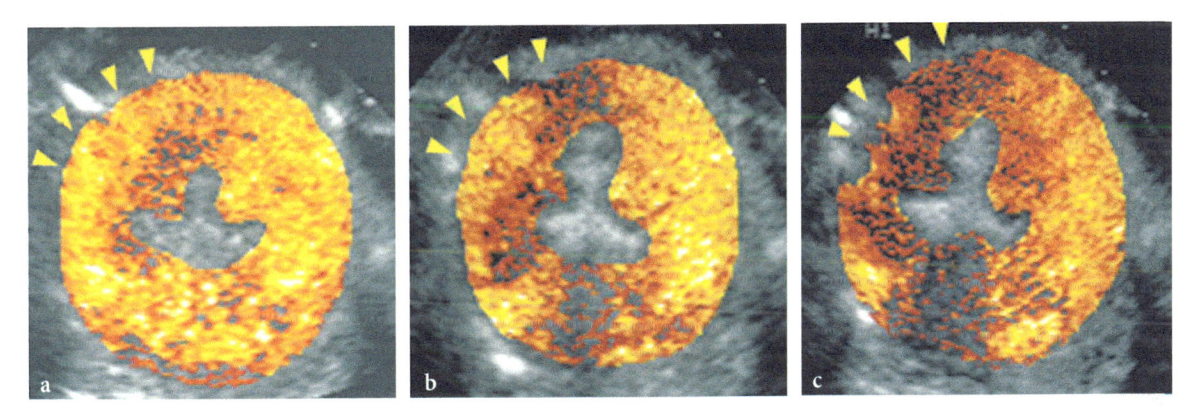

Fig. 19.7a–c. Contrast-enhanced images during hyperemia before (**a**) and in the presence of a mild (**b**) and moderate (**c**) left anterior descending coronary artery stenosis. High concentrations of microbubbles in the left ventricular cavity due to bolus injections produces some attenuation of far-field structures in all the images. Before stenosis placement (**a**), myocardial video intensity is similar between the left anterior descending (*arrows*; 8 to 10 o'clock) and circumflex coronary artery (1 to 5 o'clock) beds. After placement (**b**) of a mild stenosis (trans-stenotic pressure gradient of 14 mmHg), the color in the left anterior descending coronary artery bed takes on more hues of orange and red, denoting a lower myocardial blood volume in the left anterior descending coronary artery (*arrows*) compared with the left circumflex coronary artery bed. Further capillary derecruitment (**c**) develops in the presence of a moderate stenosis (trans-stenotic pressure gradient of 22 mmHg) during hyperemia, causing myocardial video intensity in the left anterior descending coronary artery (*arrows*) bed to also decrease further.

develops in the stenosed bed during stress. We have confirmed that myocardial blood volume decreases in the presence of a stenosis during hyperemia by measuring the myocardial vascular resistance (Fig. 19.8; WEI 2001). We believe that capillaries derecruit distal to a stenosis during hyperemia in order to maintain capillary hydrostatic pressure.

This hypothesis was tested in a model of the coronary circulation consisting of a series of resistances representing the arterial, capillary, and venous beds (JAYAWEERA et al. 1999). The model assumes that the regulation of coronary blood flow is secondary to changes in resistance of these various compartments, and that the main reason for autoregulation is maintenance of homeostasis and capillary hydrostatic pressure. Using hemodynamic data acquired from animal experiments at four different stages (baseline, maximal hyperemia, epicardial coronary stenosis, and stenosis+hyperemia), resistances from the three circulatory components were derived from the model.

The resistance across the stenosis and the model-derived resistances from the three compartments during the four different experimental settings are shown in Fig. 19.6. When hyperemia was induced in the absence of a stenosis (H), equivalent proportional decreases (approximately 90%) in R_a and R_v developed. The increase in pressure gradient across the capillary bed produces a proportional increase in hyperemic flow, and allows R_c to remain unchanged. During hyperemia (H), however, it is apparent that the compartment with the highest resistance to flow has shifted from the arterioles to the capillaries (Fig. 19.6). When hyperemia was induced in the presence of a non-critical stenosis (H+S), capillary resistance increased further secondary to capillary derecruitment.

Since the length of a capillary does not change, capillary resistance can only increase by reductions of capillary cross-sectional area, or by capillary derecruitment (JAYAWEERA et al. 1999). The mechanism underlying the derecruitment of capillaries is unclear but occurs in an attempt to maintain capillary hydrostatic pressure (JAYAWEERA et al. 1999). This mechanism likely prevents unacceptable shifts in fluid distribution between the intra- and extravascular spaces.

JARHULT and MELLANDER (1973) have previously shown that net transcapillary fluid movement (a measure of capillary hydrostatic pressure) remained essentially constant as skeletal muscle perfusion pressure was varied from 20 to 180 mmHg. Below the lower limit of the autoregulatory range, however, capillary hydrostatic pressure was maintained by increases in postcapillary resistance. It was hypothesized that the increase in venular resistance possibly resulted from passive venular collapse, rheological factors such as increased viscosity at low shear rates, or postcapillary aggregation of red or white blood cells (JARHULT and MELLANDER 1973). Increases in resistance at the distal end of the capillaries may essentially close the capillary to blood flow.

Investigators have also shown that a severe decrease in perfusion pressure in poststenotic arterioles resulted in capillary derecruitment as determined by an increase in the intercapillary distance visualized by fluorescein-tagged high-molecular dextran (TILLMANS and KUEBLER 1984). Using

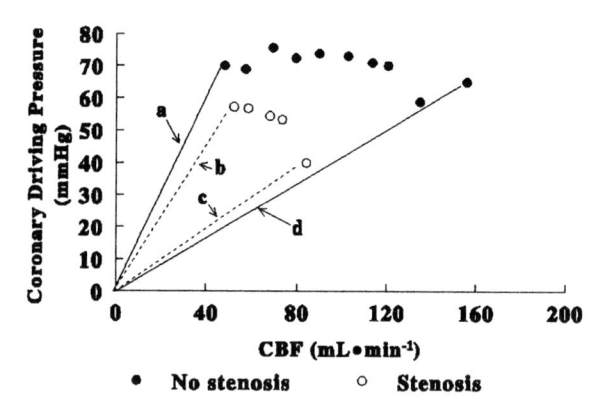

Fig. 19.8 Relation between epicardial coronary blood flow (CBF) and coronary driving pressure (coronary artery pressure–right atrial pressure) derived from an animal in the presence (*open circle*) and absence (*closed circle*) of a non-critical coronary stenosis at rest, and during infusion of adenosine. Myocardial vascular resistance at any level of coronary blood flow and coronary driving pressure is represented by the slope from the origin to that data point. In the absence of a stenosis at rest, coronary driving pressure measured approximately 80 mmHg, with a baseline myocardial blood flow of about 45 ml min^{-1}, and a myocardial vascular resistance denoted by the line a. During peak hyperemia, a significant decrease in myocardial vascular resistance (line d compared with line a) due to arteriolar vasodilation resulted in an almost fourfold increase in coronary blood flow. With placement of a non-flow limiting coronary stenosis, coronary blood flow remains unchanged at 45 ml min^{-1}, but the pressure gradient across the stenosis decreases distal coronary pressure, resulting in a decrease in coronary driving pressure. Resting coronary blood flow remains constant due to a decrease in myocardial vascular resistance (line b compared with line a), which results from arteriolar vasodilation secondary to autoregulation. When maximal hyperemia is induced in the presence of a stenosis, however, myocardial vascular resistance is higher than expected (line c compared with line d). Maximal arteriolar vasodilation would have been expected to reduce the myocardial vascular resistance again to line d, but instead, capillary derecruitment that occurs distal to the stenosis during hyperemia increases the myocardial vascular resistance. (From WEI 2001-)

direct intravital microscopy, TILLMANS et al. (1991) also showed that in the setting of critical arterial stenosis, capillary and venular diameters did not change significantly, but the ratio of capillaries containing red cells to those containing plasma alone was significantly reduced, producing a functional derecruitment of capillaries.

The decrease in myocardial blood volume that occurs distal to a stenosis during hyperemia underlies the development of reversible perfusion defects not only on contrast echocardiography, but also with other tracers, such as ^{99m}Tc sestamibi. It is currently believed that flow mismatch which develops between the stenosed and normal myocardial beds during hyperemia is the cause of reversible perfusion defects on ^{99m}Tc sestamibi images (BELLER and WATSON 1991). For flow mismatch to produce a reversible perfusion defect, the uptake of a tracer must be proportional to flow. Relative Tc sestamibi uptake between the hyperemic and control beds, however, remains fairly constant over a wide range of hyperemic flows (GLOVER and OKADA 1990; GLOVER et al. 1995).

We have recently evaluated the relation between Tc-uptake, regional myocardial blood flow, and myocardial blood volume (WEI et al. 2001). In the first group of dogs, myocardial blood flow was selectively increased in the left anterior descending coronary artery bed with intracoronary infusions of adenosine. During adenosine infusion, mean myocardial blood flow (from all animals) in the left anterior descending coronary artery bed was increased almost three times, while myocardial blood flow in the left circumflex coronary artery bed remained unchanged. Myocardial blood volume between the hyperemic and control beds remained unchanged despite the large regional disparity in myocardial blood flow. Figure 19.9 shows an example of a color-coded parametric image representing myocardial blood volume from a dog where the myocardial blood flow of the left anterior descending coronary artery bed was selectively increased approximately four times that of the control left circumflex coronary artery bed during intracoronary infusion of adenosine; thus, in the absence of changes in capillary blood volume, Tc uptake remains equal despite the presence of significant flow disparity between myocardial beds (WEI et al. 2001). In a second group of dogs, hyperemic flow was induced in both the left anterior descending and the left circumflex coronary artery beds with left main infusions of adenosine. While myocardial blood flow was increased, myocardial blood volume was decreased to different degrees with non-flow-limiting stenoses of different severities in only the left anterior descending coronary artery bed (Fig. 19.10).

These studies indicate that uptake of Tc sestamibi is not dependent on changes in myocardial blood flow, but rather on changes in myocardial blood volume. In the presence of a coronary stenosis during hyperemia, there is capillary derecruitment in the bed distal to a stenosis, which results in a lower capillary surface area for uptake of Tc sestamibi. Decreases in myocardial blood volume, therefore, form the basis for reversible perfusion defects seen on both myocardial contrast echocardiography and Tc sestamibi radionuclide imaging (WEI et al. 2001).

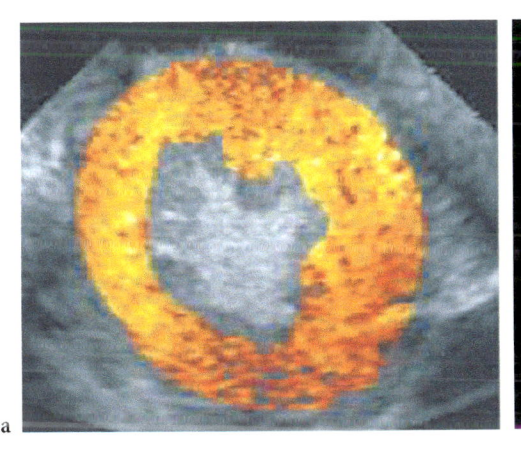

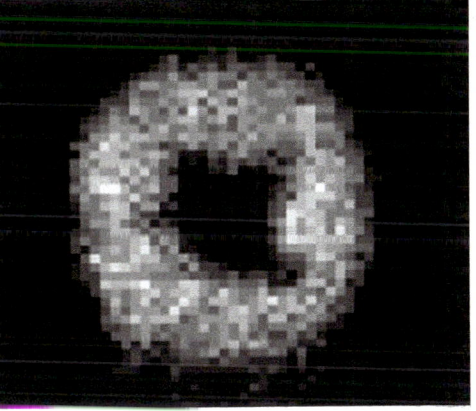

Fig. 19.9a,b. Background-subtracted color-coded contrast echocardiography image (a) and corresponding ex vivo Tc-sestamibi image (b) obtained during selective left anterior descending hyperemia (10 to 1 o'clock). Despite the large disparity in regional flow between myocardial beds, the entire myocardium shows homogeneous contrast enhancement indicating a similar capillary blood volume in both beds. The corresponding ex vivo Tc-sestamibi image of the same short-axis heart slice also shows equal uptake of sestamibi in the entire myocardium. (From WEI et al. 2001)

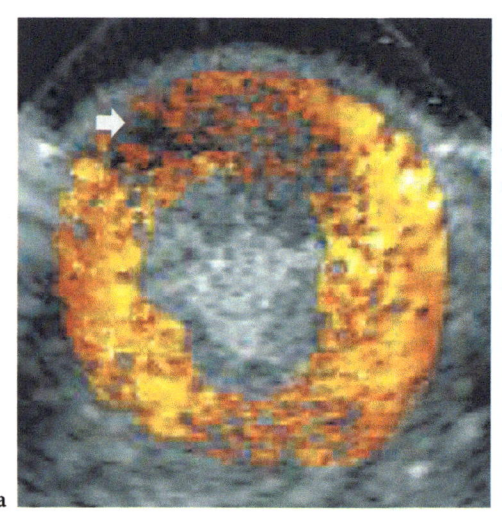

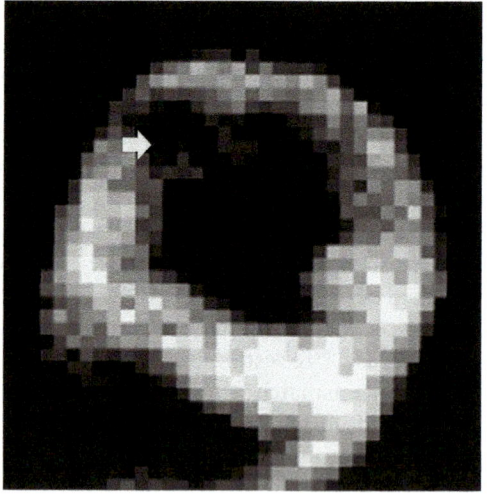

Fig. 19.10a,b. Animal with a moderate left anterior descending coronary artery stenosis. Background-subtracted color-coded contrast echocardiography image (a) and corresponding ex vivo Tc-sestamibi image (b) obtained during left main infusions of adenosine in the presence of a non-critical left anterior descending stenosis (10 to 1 o'clock). During left main adenosine, myocardial blood flow in the left anterior descending coronary artery bed increased from 1.0 to 2.0 ml min^{-1} g^{-1}. A perfusion defect (*arrow*), indicating a decrease in capillary blood volume, is seen in the left anterior descending coronary artery bed despite the increase in absolute left anterior descending coronary artery flow during hyperemia. The corresponding ex vivo Tc image (B) also shows a perfusion defect (*arrow*) that corresponds both in location and spatial extent to the region with decreased capillary blood volume on the myocardial contrast echocardiography image. (From WEI et al. 2001)

b) Summary. A fixed perfusion defect (which means rest and stress perfusion defects) coupled with akinetic wall motion is indicative of myocardial necrosis, while a reversible perfusion defect (stress defect with a normal resting perfusion) coupled with inducible wall motion abnormalities is indicative of myocardial ischemia (MILLER and NANDA 2004). In this chapter the myocardial stunning and myocardial hibernation were not mentioned for brevity. Myocardial stunning is defined as a wall motion abnormality in a myocardial territory with a normal perfusion after a recent ischemic insult. Myocardial hibernation is a chronic state of impaired myocardial function at rest, represented by hypokinetic and hypoperfused myocardium, which results from reduced coronary blood flow caused by a critical coronary stenosis and which may be reversed by improving blood flow to the affected myocardium.

19.4
Coupling Between Capillary Derecruitment and Hyperemic Flow

Irrespective of the mechanism producing capillary derecruitment in the presence of a stenosis during hyperemia, the increase in capillary resistance affects hyperemic myocardial blood flow. As discussed, capillaries offer the greatest resistance to hyperemic flow. Increases in capillary resistance therefore reduce hyperemic flow, resulting in a coupling between decreases in capillary blood volume and hyperemic myocardial blood flow and producing reversible perfusion defects. The more severe the stenosis, the greater the degree of capillary derecruitment, the greater the increase in capillary resistance during hyperemia, and the greater the limitation of hyperemic flow.

As shown in the previous and current chapters, myocardial contrast echocardiography has the ability to separately assess both components of myocardial blood flow, namely, velocity of myocardial blood flow as well as myocardial blood volume (Table 19.1). With ^{99m}Tc-sestamibi SPECT, however, only regional decreases in myocardial blood volume are assessed. In the presence of mild or moderate stenoses, subtle differences in myocardial blood volume may not be detectable due to insufficient disparity in counts (<25%) between beds (GLOVER et al. 1995). On the other hand, contrast echocardiography has far superior spatial resolution (<1 vs 15 mm) and can detect mild subendocardial defects more readily. Furthermore, even if subtle decreases in myocardial blood volume are not detectable on myocardial contrast echocardiography, regional differences in myocardial blood flow velocity reserve during hyperemia may allow detection of coronary artery disease.

Myocardial contrast echocardiography therefore has features that may allow greater sensitivity for detection of coronary artery disease, and preliminary evidence shows that the combined assessment of myocardial blood flow velocity reserve and myocardial blood volume with myocardial contrast echocardiography may improve detection of mild to moderate coronary artery disease compared with SPECT (WEI et al. 2003).

19.5 Conclusion

Myocardial contrast echocardiogarphy is a versatile technique with excellent spatial and temporal resolution. Perfusion defects on contrast echocardiogarphy, irrespective of whether they are fixed or reversible, are related to relative differences in myocardial blood volume. More importantly, the presence of contrast enhancement on myocardial contrast echocardiogarphy provides an assessment of microvascular integrity, and thus, myocardial viability. Combined with the ability to evaluate red blood cell kinetics, myocardial contrast echocardiogarphy can be used to define the risk area, the adequacy of collateral flow, success of reperfusion, and eventual infarct size in the setting of acute myocardial infarction. These insights may provide new management paradigms for these patients.

Myocardial contrast echocardiogarphy has also provided new insights into the pathophysiologic behavior of the capillary bed in the presence of coronary artery disease during hyperemia, and has allowed us to demonstrate the important role of capillaries in regulating hyperemic flow. Contrast echocardiogarphy has also provided a cohesive relation between changes in myocardial blood volume and myocardial blood flow reserve, and the assessment of either variable can be used to detect and quantify coronary stenosis severity. Because myocardial contrast echocardiogarphy can non-invasively evaluate both specific components of myocardial blood flow, it is a powerful tool that can be used in a broad range of patients with coronary artery disease, extending from the diagnosis of occult stenosis to acute myocardial infarction.

References

Anderson WD, Anderson WB, Seguin RJ (1988) Microvasculature of the bear heart demonstrated by scanning electron microscopy. Acta Anat 131:305-313

Bassingthwaighte JB, Yipintsoi T, Harvey RB (1974) Microvasculature of the dog left ventricular myocardium. Microvasc Res 7:229-249

Belenkie I, Trabousi M, Hall C et al (1992) Rescue angioplasty during myocardial infarction has a beneficial effect on mortality: a tenable hypothesis. Can J Cardiol 8:357-362

Beller GA, Watson DD (1991) Physiological basis of myocardial perfusion imaging with the technetium-99m agents. Semin Nucl Med 21:173-181

Califf RM, O'Neill W, Stacks RS et al (1988) Failure of simple clinical measurements to predict perfusion status after intravenous thrombolysis. Ann Intern Med 108:658-662

Chilian WM, Harrison DG, Haws CW et al (1986) Adrenergic coronary tone during submaximal exercise in the dog is produced by circulating catecolatives. Evidence for adrenergic denervation supersensitivity in the myocardium but not in coronary vessels. Circ Res 58(1)68-82

Coggins MP, Sklenar J, Le E et al (2001) Noninvasive prediction of ultimate infarct size at the time of acute coronary occlusion based on the extent and magnitude of collateral-derived myocardial blood flow. Circulation 104:2471-2477

Dittrich HC, Bales GL, Kuvelas T et al (1995) Myocardial contrast echocardiography in experimental coronary artery occlusion with a new intravenously administered contrast agent. J Am Soc Echocardogr 8:465-474

Ellis SG, da Silva ER, Heyndrickx G et al (1994) Randomized comparison of rescue angioplasty with conservative management of patients with early failure of thrombolysis for acute anterior myocardial infarction. Circulation 90:2280-2284

Firschke C, Lindner JR, Goodman NC et al (1997a) Myocardial contrast echocardiography in acute myocardial infarction using aortic root injections of microbubbles in conjunction with harmonic imaging: potential application in the cardiac catheterization laboratory. J Am Coll Cardiol 29:207-216

Firschke C, Lindner JR, Wei K et al (1997b) Myocardial perfusion imaging in the setting of coronary artery stenosis and acute myocardial infarction using venous injection of a second-generation echocardiographic contrast agent. Circulation 96:959-967

Friedman BJ, Grinberg OY, Isaacs KA et al (1995) Myocardial oxygen tension and relative capillary density in isolated perfused rat hearts. J Mol Cell Cardiol 27:2551-2558

Gayeski TE, Honig CR (1991) Intracellular PO2 in individual cardiomyocytes in dogs, cats, rabbits, ferrets, and rats. Am J Physiol 260:H552-H531

Glover DK, Okada RD (1990) Myocardial kinetics of Tc-MIBI in canine myocardium after dipyridamole. Circulation 81:628-637

Glover DK, Ruiz M, Edwards NC et al (1995) Comparison between ^{201}Tl and [99m]Tc Sestamibi uptake during adenosine induced vasodilation as a function of coronary stenosis severity. Circulation 91:813-820

Gould KL, Lipscomb K (1974) Effects of coronary stenoses

on coronary flow reserve and resistance. Am J Cardiol 34:48–55
Grayburn PA, Erickson JM, Escobar J et al (1995) Peripheral intravenous myocardial contrast echocardiography using a 2% dodecafluoropentane emulsion: identification of myocardial risk area and infarct size in the canine model of ischemia. J Am Coll Cardiol 26:1340–1347
Heinle SK, Noblin J, Goree-Best P et al (2000) Assessment of myocardial perfusion by harmonic power Doppler imaging at rest and during adenosine stress. Comparison with ^{99m}Tc-sestamibi SPECT imaging. Circulation 102:55–60
Ismail S, Jayaweera AR, Goodman NC et al (1995) Detection of coronary stenosesand quantification of the degree and spatial extent of blood flow mismatch during coronary hyperemia with myocardial contrast echocardiography. Circulation 91:821–830
Ito H, Okamura A, Iwakura K et al (1996a) Myocardial perfusion patterns related to thrombolysis in myocardial infarction perfusion grades after coronary angioplasty in patinets with acute anterior wall myocardial infarction. Circulation 93:1993–1999
Ito H, Maruyama A, Iwakura K (1996b) Clinical implications of the "no reflow" phenomenon. A predictor of complications and left ventricular remodeling in reperfused anterior wall myocardial infarction. Circulation 93:223–228
Iwakura K, Ito H, Takiuchi S et al (1996) Alternation in the coronary blood flow velocity pattern in patients with no reflow and reperfused acute myocardial infarction. Circulation 94:1269–1275
Jarhult J, Mellander S (1973) Autoregulation of capilalry hydrostatic pressure in skeletal muscle during regional arterial hypo- and hypertension. Acta Physiol Scand 91:32–41
Jayaweera AR, Jayaweera AR, Wei K et al (1999) Fate of capillaries distal to a stenosis. Their role in determining coronary blood flow reserve. Am J Physiol 46:H2363–H2372
Johnson Paul C (1986) Autoregulation of blood flow. Circ Res 59:483–495
Kassab GS, Lin DH, Fung YB (1993) Morphometry of pig coronary arterial trees. Am J Physiol 265:H350–H365
Kassab GS, Lin DH, Fung YB (1994a) Morphometry of the pig coronary venous system. Am J Physiol 267:H2100–2113
Kassab GS, Lin DH, Fung YB (1994b) Topology and dimensions of pig coronary capillary network. Am J Physiol 267:H319–H325
Kaul S, Pandian NG, Okada RD et al (1984) Contrast echocardiography in acute myocardial ischemia. I. In vivo determination of total left ventricular "area at risk". J Am Coll Cardiol 4:1272–1282
Kaul S, Gillam L, Weyman AE (1985) Contrast echocardiography in acute myocardial ischemia. II. The effect of site of injection of contrast agent on the estimation of area at risk for necrosis after coronary occlusion. J Am Coll Cardiol 6:825–830
Kaul S, Pandian NG, Gillam LD et al (1986) Contrast echocardiography in acute myocardial ischemia. III. An in-vivo comparison of the extent of abnormal wall motion with the "area at risk" for necrosis. J Am Coll Cardiol 7:383–392
Kaul S, Pandian NG, Guerrero L et al (1987) Effects of selectively altering collateral driving pressure on regional perfusion and function in occluded coronary bed in the dog. Circ Res 61:77–85
Kaul S, Senior R, Dittrich H et al (1997) Detection of coronary artery disease using myocardial contrast echocardiography: comparison with 99mTc sestamibi single photon emission computed tomography. Circulation 96:785–792
Keller MW, Segal SS, Kaul S, Duling B (1989) The behaviour of sonicated albumin microbubbles within the microcirculation: a basis for their use during myocardial contrast echocardiography. Circ Res 65:458–467
Le DE, Bin JP, Coggins MP et al (2002) Relation between myocardial oxygen consumption and myocardial blood volume: a study using myocardial contrast echocardiography. J Am Soc Echocardiogr 15:857–863
Lepper W, Hoffmann R, Kamp O et al (2000) Assessment of myocardial reperfusion by intravenous myocardial contrast echocardiography and coronary flow reserve after primary percutaneous transluminal coronary angiography in patients with acute myocardial infarction. Circulation 101:2368–2374
Levin DC (1974) Pathways and functional significance of the coronary collateral circulation. Circulation 50:831–837
Lindner JR, Firschke C, Wei K et al (1998) Myocardial perfusion characteristics and hemodynamic profile of MRX-115, a venous echocardiographic contrast agent, during acute myocardial infarction. J Am Soc Echocardiogr 11:36–46
Linka AZ, Sklenar J, Wei K et al (1998) Spatial distribution of microbubble velocity and concentration within the myocardium: insights into the transmural distribution of myocardial blood flow and volume. Circulation 98:1912–1920
Marcus ML (1983) Anatomy of the coronary vasculature. In: Marcus ML (ed) The coronary circulation in health and disease. McGraw-ill, New York, pp 3–21
Maruoka Y, Tomoike H, Kawachi Y et al (1986) Relations between collateral flow and tissue salvage in the risk area after acute coronary occlusion in dogs: a topographical analysis. Br J Exp Pathol 67:33–42
Miller AP, Nanda NC (2004) Contrast echocardiography: new agents. Ultrasound Med Biol 30:425–434
Piek J, Becker AE (1988) Collateral blood supply to the myocardium at risk in human myocardial infarction: a quantitative postmortem assessment. J Am Coll Cardiol 11:1290–1296
Porter TR, Li S, Kilzer K, Deligonul U (1997) Effect of significant two-vessel versus one-vessel coronary artery stenosis on myocardial contrast defects observed with intermittent harmonic imaging after intravenous contrast injection during dobutamine stress echocardiography. J Am Coll Cardiol 30:1399–1406
Porter TR, Li S, Oster R, Deligonul U (1998) The clinical implications of no reflow demonstrated with intravenous perfluorocarbon containing microbubbles following restoration of thrombolysis in myocardial infarction (TIMI) 3 flow in patients with acute myocardial infarction. Am J Cardiol 82:1173–1177
Reimer KA, Jennings RB (1979) The "wavefront phenomenon" of myocardial ischemic cell death. II. Transmural progression of necrosis within the framework of ischemic bed size (myocardium at risk) and collateral flow. Lab Invest 40:633–644
Rocchi G, Kasprzak JD, Galema TW et al (2001) Usefulness of power Doppler contrast echocardiography to identify reperfusion after acute myocardial infarction. Am J Cardiol 87:278–282

Sabia PJ, Powers ER, Jayaweera AR et al (1992) Functional significance of collateral blood flow in patients with recent acute myocardial infarction: a study using myocardial contrast echocardiography. Circulation 85:2080–2089

Sakuma T, Hayashi Y, Sumii K et al (1998) Prediction of short- and intermediate-term prognoses of patients with acute myocardial infarction using myocardial contrast echocardiography one day after recanalization. J Am Coll Cardiol 32:890–897

Skyba DM, Jayaweera AR, Goodman NC et al (1994) Quantification of myocardial perfusion with myocardial contrast echocardiography from left atrial injection of contrast: implications for venous injection. Circulation 90:1513–1521

Tillmanns H, Kuebler W (1984) What happens in the microcirculation? In: Hearse DJ, Yellon DM (eds) Approaches to myocardial infarct size limitation. Raven, New York

Tillmans H, Leinberger H, Neumann FJ et al (1987) Myocardial microcirculation in the beating heart: in vivo microscopic studies. In: Spaan JAE, Bruschke AVG, Gittenberger-de Groot AC (eds) Coronary virculation. Nijhoff, Dordrecht, pp 88–94

Tillmanns H, Steinhausen M, Leinberger H et al (1991) Hemodynamics of the coronary microcirculation during myocardial ischemia. Circulation (Suppl) IV:40

Tschabitscher M (1984) Anatomy of coronary veins. In: Mohl W, Wolner E, Glogar D (eds) The coronary sinus: proceedings of the first international symposium on myocardial protection via the coronary sinus. Steinkopff, Darmstadt, pp 8–25

Villanueva FS, Glasheen WP, Sklenar J, Kaul S (1993) Assessment of risk area during coronary occlusion and infarct size after reperfusion with myocardial contrast echocardiography using left and right atrial injections of contrast. Circulation 88:596–604

Wei K, Jayaweera AR, Firoozan S et al (1998a) Quantification of myocardial blood flow using ultrasound-induced destruction of microbubbles administered as a constant venous infusion. Circulation 97:473–483

Wei K, Jayaweera AR, Firoozan S et al (1998b) Basis for detection of stenosis using venous administration of microbubbles during myocardial contrast echocardiography: Bolus or continuous infusion? J Am Coll Cardiol 32:252–260

Wei K (2001) Detection and quantification of coronary stenosis severity with myocardial contrast echocardiography. Prog Cardiovasc Dis 44:81–100

Wei K, Le E, Bin JP, Coggins M et al (2001) Mechanism of reversible ^{99m}Tc-sestamibi perfusion defects during pharmacologically induced coronary vasodilation. Am J Physiol 280:H1896–H1904

Wei K, Crouse L, Weiss J et al (2003) PB127 phase 2 trial results: detection of coronary disease with rest and dipyridamole stress myocardial contrast echocardiography compared to ^{99m}Tc-sestamibi single photon emission computed tomography. Am J Cardiol 91:1293–1298

Special Topics

20 Abdominal Traumas

Emilio Quaia

CONTENTS

20.1 Introduction 295
20.2 Baseline US 295
20.3 Contrast-Enhanced US 296
20.4 When Microbubble-Based Agents Should Be Employed 299
References 299

20.1
Introduction

Abdominal ultrasound (US) is useful in screening for injury in patients with blunt abdominal trauma, and it presents high (82–96%) sensitivity (Poletti et al. 2003) and high (94–100%) specificity (Kimura and Otsuka 1991; McKenney 1999; Dondelinger et al. 2004) to detect free fluid in blunt abdominal trauma. On the other hand, the sensitivity of US is very low (40–55%) for directly demonstrating organ injury (Poletti et al. 2003).

The detection of free intraperitoneal fluid by US is considered very useful in hemodynamically unstable patients, while the value of US in hemodynamically stable patients is not clear for the large percentage of organ injuries that are not associated with free fluid (Shanmuganathan et al. 1999; Poletti et al. 2004); however, the combination of negative US findings and negative clinical observation virtually excludes abdominal injury in patients who are admitted and observed for at least 12–24 h (Sirlin et al. 2004).

Contrast-enhanced computed tomography (CT) is the reference imaging procedure for diagnosing traumatic abdominal injuries (Poletti et al. 2002; Huppert 2004). Contrast-enhanced CT is used when screening US findings are positive or when injury is clinically suspected despite negative US findings (Brown et al. 2001), and it is generally performed only in hemodynamically stable patients. Anyway, contrast-enhanced CT presents a lower sensitivity compared with US in detecting abdominal free fluid (Poletti et al. 2003) and presents higher costs and radiation exposure.

Diagnostic peritoneal lavage to clarify free fluid has been replaced in Europe by US and CT. If a large amount of free fluid is found and the patient is hemodynamically unstable, an emergency laparotomy is performed (Zügel et al. 2004).

20.2
Baseline US

The first post-traumatic lesion in abdominal organs is parenchymal contusion, which is defined as an area of abnormal vascularization and edema, but with only little collected hemorrhage (Dondelinger et al. 2004). Parenchymal contusion appears as a hypoechoic area which does not show any signal of perfusion at color or power Doppler US (Dondelinger et al. 2004).

Acute hematoma appears as a hyperechoic rounded lesion with sharp margins at baseline US. When the location is subcapsular, the shape of hematoma is lenticular and the normal hepatic parenchyma is displaced centrally (Dondelinger et al. 2004). When clot organization is completed, the hematoma presents an anechoic pattern if the clot lysis is prevalent or a calcific pattern with posterior acoustic shadowing if the solid component persists.

Parenchymal tear or laceration is defined as a parenchymal interruption without connection to the opposite margins. Parenchymal fracture is defined as a complete parenchymal interruption with opposite-margins connection. Abdominal free fluid is always present in parenchymal laceration or fracture. Both parenchymal tears and fractures appear as hyperechoic bands, lines, or stellate strands (Dondelinger et al. 2004).

E. Quaia, MD
Department of Radiology, Cattinara Hospital, University of Trieste, Strada di Fiume 447, 34149 Trieste, Italy

20.3
Contrast-Enhanced US

In comparison with baseline US, contrast-enhanced US improves the visibility of injuries in all abdominal parenchymas, the spleen (Figs. 20.1, 20.2), the liver (Fig. 20.3), and the kidneys (Fig. 20.4; POLETTI et al. 2004). Microbubbles injection improves the visibility of parenchymal hematoma, lacerations, and fractures (Fig. 20.2), by increasing the contrast resolution in comparison with the adjacent normal parenchyma. In fact, after microbubble-based agent injection, hematoma appears as a hypovascular intraparenchymal lesion, while parenchymal fracture and lacerations (Figs. 20.1, 20.3) appear as wedge-shaped avascular zones. Post-traumatic lesion of the hilar branches of the main renal artery may determine focal perfusion defects in the renal parenchyma appearing as hypovascular wedge-shaped lesions (Figs. 20.4).

Even though the improvement in visibility of abdominal organs injuries is improved after microbubble injection, if compared with baseline US, some recent clinical studies showed clear limitations of contrast-enhanced US in detecting parenchymal injuries in hemodynamically stable patients (POLETTI et al. 2004). The only exception was the intraparenchymal pseudoaneurysms from vascular injuries which appear as focal pooling of microbubbles (Fig. 20.5) in the injured parenchyma correlating with contrast extravasation in CT (CATALANO et al. 2003; POLETTI et al. 2004). Contrast-enhanced US was found effective also in revealing the active bleeding in the injured spleen, liver and kidney parenchyma, and in abdominal aortic aneurysm rupture. Active contrast medium extravasation is a known angiography and CT sign of ongoing bleeding. Owing to the current possibilities of real-time, contrast-specific US systems, it is now possible to detect contrast leakage by using contrast-enhanced US, frequently the first image option in screening patients with abdominal emergencies (CUSATI et al. 2004). At contrast-enhanced US, the active bleeding appears as a subcontinuous hyperechoic jet which tends to pool dependently. It should be differentiated from calcifications, opacified normal vessels, small pseudoaneurysm, and still-vascularized areas within injuries parenchyma (CUSATI et al. 2004).

Some studies have reported the high accuracy of contrast-enhanced US in the visibility of parenchymal lesions in children (OLDENBURG et al. 2004), in whom the splenic injury is the most common complication in blunt abdominal traumas. Even though contrast-enhanced CT is the most accurate imaging procedure to identify splenic injuries (KRUPNICK et al. 1997), US has several advantages over CT in children, such as the absence of radiation (particularly important in children), lower costs, no sedation, and the possibility of imaging at the bedside (OLDENBURG et al. 2004).

Fig. 20.2a–d. Splenic fracture in a 20-year-old man after car accident. At baseline US (a) the spleen appears homogeneous. At contrast-enhanced US, both as longitudinal (b) and axial (c) plane, splenic fracture (*arrows*) connecting opposite organ margins is evident. Contrast-enhanced CT (d) confirms splenic fracture (*arrows*).

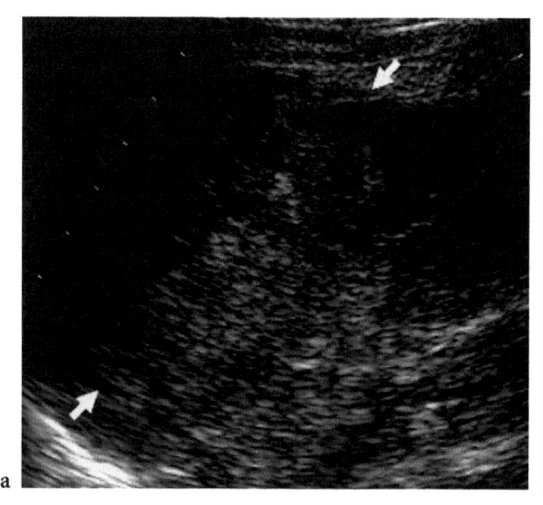

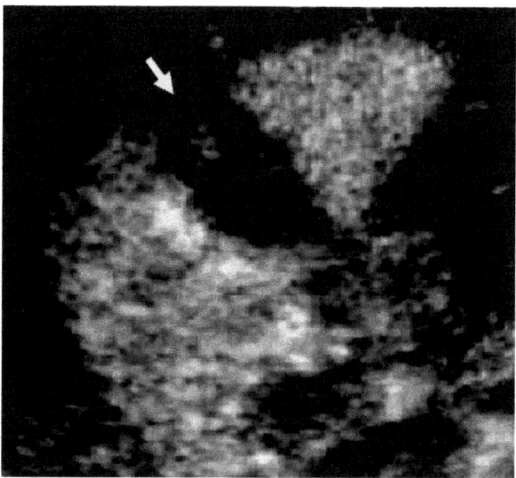

Fig. 20.1a,b. Splenic laceration. At baseline US (a) the spleen (*arrows*) appears diffusely heterogeneous. At contrast-enhanced US (b) an avascular wedge-shaped parenchymal zone becomes evident.

Abdominal Traumas

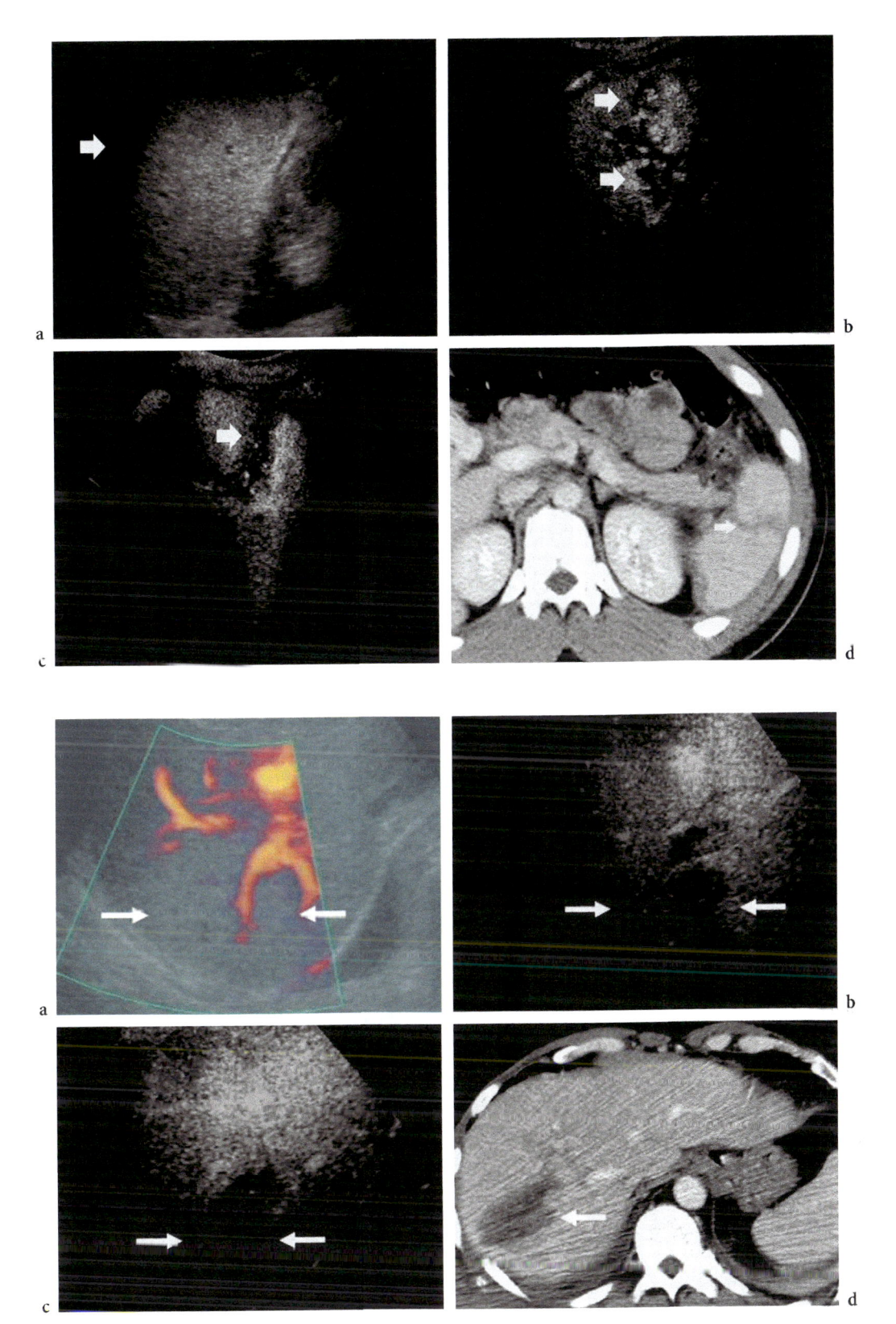

Fig. 20.3a–d Liver laceration in a 33 year-old man after a motorbike accident. At baseline power Doppler US (a) a heterogeneous area (*arrows*) is identified in the liver parenchyma. At contrast-enhanced US a liver parenchyma laceration becomes evident (*arrows*) in different scan planes (b,c). Contrast-enhanced CT (d) confirms liver laceration (*arrow*).

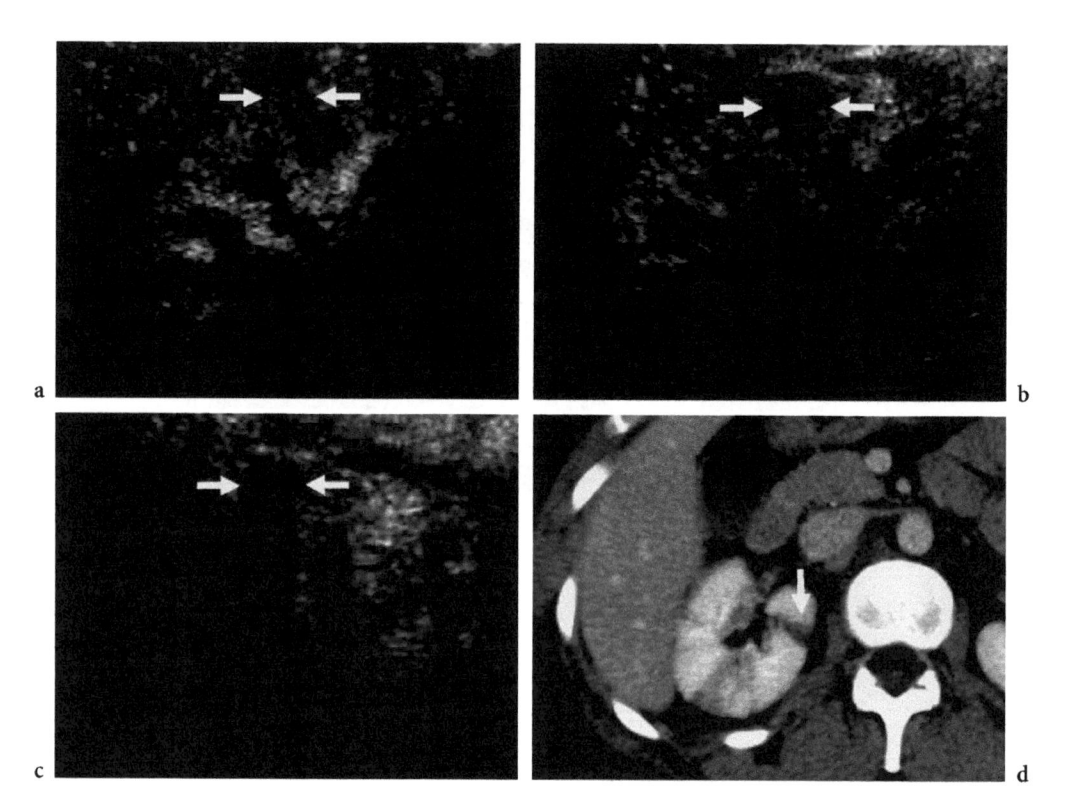

Fig. 20.4a–d. Post-traumatic renal perfusion defects in a 32-year-old woman after a car accident. Immediately after the accident, the patient revealed hematuria. a–c At contrast-enhanced US a wedge-shaped renal perfusion defects (*arrows*) is evident in renal parenchyma after microbubble injection. Contrast-enhanced CT (d) reveals a similar finding (*arrow*) also with evidence of renal parenchyma interruption. A small and covered renal parenchyma laceration was found at surgical laparoscopy.

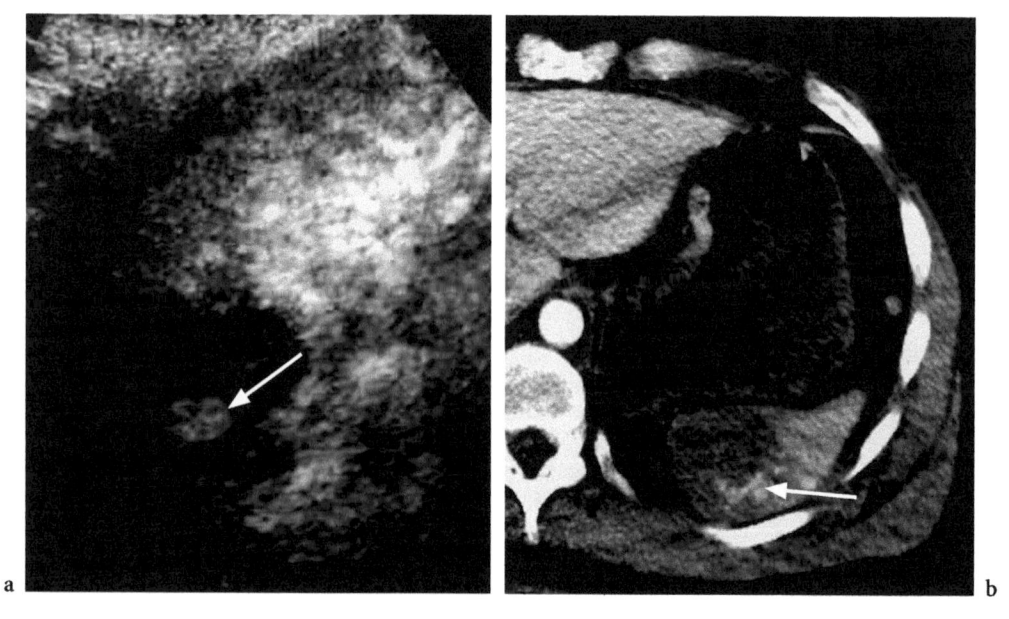

Fig. 20.5a,b. a Intraparenchymal focal pooling of microbubbles from vascular injuries in splenic trauma. b Contrast-enhanced CT revealed contrast extravasation at arterial phase 30 s after iodinated agent injection. (Courtesy of O. Catalano)

20.4
When Microbubble-Based Agents Should Be Employed

The employment of microbubble-based agents in the abdominal traumas is not still defined. Microbubbles should be employed in hemodynamically stable patients, without or with evidence of free fluid at baseline US, to improve the accuracy of US in detection of parenchymal injuries. Contrast-enhanced US has been showed to be particularly useful to detect splenic injuries in children, principally for the absence of radiation and sedation (OLDENBURG et al. 2004). Moreover, some recent studies have shown the low accuracy of contrast-enhanced US in detecting organ injuries (POLETTI et al. 2004), except for the depiction of delayed splenic pseudoaneurysm from trauma. According to these studies, contrast-enhanced US cannot be recommended to replace CT in the triage of hemodynamically stable patients with negative findings on abdominal US at admission (POLETTI et al. 2004).

In conclusion, contrast-enhanced CT still has to be performed if free fluid or pathological findings are shown by US. In hemodynamically unstable patients surgical laparoscopy remains the unique procedure.

References

Brown MA, Casola G, Sirlin CB et al (2001) Blunt abdominal trauma: screening US in 2683 patients. Radiology 218:352-358

Catalano O, Lobianco R, Sandomenico F, Siani A (2003) Splenic trauma: evaluation with contrast-specific sonography and a second generation contrast medium: preliminary experience. J Ultrasound Med 22:467-477

Cusati B, Catalano O, Nunziata A (2004) Contrast medium extravasation as an indicator of active bleeding: demonstration with contrast-enhanced sonography (abstract). RSNA 2004

Dondelinger RF, Cornet O, Boverie JH (2004) Injuries of the liver. In: Dondelinger RF (ed) Imaging and intervention in abdominal trauma. Springer, Berlin Heidelberg New York, pp 67-112

Huppert P (2004) CT examinations protocols in abdominal trauma. In: Dondelinger RF (ed) Imaging and intervention in abdominal trauma. Springer, Berlin Heidelberg New York, pp 17-23

Kimura A, Otsuka T (1991) Emergency center ultrasonography in the evaluation of hemoperitoneum: a prospective study. J Trauma 31:20-23

Krupnick AS, Teitelbaum DH, Geiger JD et al (1997) Use of abdominal ultrasonography to assess pediatric splenic trauma: potential pitfall in the diagnosis. Ann Surg 225:408-414

McKenney KL (1999) Ultrasound of blunt abdominal trauma. Radiol Clin North Am 37:879-893

Oldenburg A, Hohmann J, Skrok J, Albrecht T (2004) Imaging of paediatric splenic injury with contrast-enhanced ultrasonograpgy. Pediatr Radiol 34:351-354

Poletti PA, Wintermark M, Schnyder P et al (2002) Traumatic injuries: role of imaging in the management of the polytrauma victim (conservative expectation). Eur Radiol 12:969-978

Poletti PA, Kinkel K, Vermeulen B et al (2003) Blunt abdominal trauma: Should US be used to detect both free fluid and organ injuries? Radiology 227:95-103

Poletti PA, Platon A, Becker CD et al (2004) Blunt abdominal trauma: Does the use of a second generation sonographic contrast agent help to detect solid organs injuries? Am J Roentgenol 183:1293-1301

Shanmuganathan K, Mirvis SE, Sherbourne CD et al (1999) Hemoperitoneum as the sole indicator of abdominal visceral injuries: a potential limitation of screening abdominal US for trauma. Radiology 212:423-430

Sirlin CB, Brown MA, Andrade-Barreto OA et al (2004) Blunt abdominal trauma: clinical value of negative screening US scans. Radiology 230:661-668

Zügel N, Breitschaft K, Mayr E, Häuser H (2004) Relevance of imaging to surgical management of abdominal injuries. In: Dondelinger RF (ed) Imaging and intervention in abdominal trauma. Springer, Berlin Heidelberg New York, pp 635-647

21 Breast

GIORGIO RIZZATTO, ROBERTA CHERSEVANI, and GITA RALLEIGH

CONTENTS

21.1 Introduction 301
21.2 Conventional Vascular US 301
21.3 Early Experience in Contrast-Enhanced Vascular Assessment 303
21.4 Ultrasonography of the Breast with New-Generation Contrast Agents 304
21.4.1 Lesion Characterization 305
21.4.2 Evaluation of Lesions Preliminarily Identified with MR Imaging 307
21.4.3 Detection of Lymph Node Metastases as an Alternative to the Sentinel Lymph Node Procedure 309
21.4.4 Monitoring the Response of Advanced Breast Cancers to Neoadjuvant Therapy 311
21.4.5 Evaluation of Microcalcification in Ductal Carcinoma In Situ 312
21.5 Future Developments 312
References 313

21.1 Introduction

Although the use of contrast-enhanced ultrasonography for breast imaging is less established than other applications, it is an exciting technique with great potential. The principles of contrast-enhanced ultrasonography of breast cancers are similar to those for all tumors, and are based on the detection of tumor-associated neoangiogenesis. In the breast, neoangiogenesis is characteristic of both invasive disease and in situ cancer including high-grade ductal carcinoma in situ. Breast tumors present with increased vascular density, irregular and often chaotic branching and penetrating vessels, and sometimes incomplete vascular walls that permit leakage of contrast agent into the surrounding tissue; this diagnostic clue for malignancy is currently used with magnetic resonance imaging (MR) imaging. Since angiogenesis correlates with tumor grade (and presence of metastatic disease), a patient's prognosis can be partly determined from the degree of angiogenesis observed at diagnostic imaging.

21.2 Conventional Vascular US

Continuous progression in ultrasound (US) technology and related software has greatly refined the diagnostic capability of this technique in breast pathology.

Vascular assessment has progressed enough to depict vessels in almost all the tumors and in most fibroadenomas (RIZZATTO 2001). Modern US scanners have sufficient sensitivity to detect blood flow through small blood vessels of 1 mm or less in diameter and with blood flow on the order of 1 cm/s. This allows visualization of arterioles and venules, but does not reveal flow through smaller blood vessels at capillary level.

Fibroadenomas are the most common benign tumor in the breast. Clinically, these tumors tend to be soft and mobile, and are seen mostly in younger women. On color and power Doppler US, fibroadenomas generally have poor vascularity; vessels are peripheral, with a nest arrangement, regular and small.

In contrast, malignant tumors have numerous central and penetrating, branching vessels with irregular caliper and velocities. These patterns reflect the abnormalities that are peculiar for rapidly growing tumors: irregular and variable vessel caliber, elongated and coiled vessels, arteriovenous shunts, disturbed dichotomous branching and decreasing of caliber, and incomplete vascular wall (LESS et al. 1991). The correlation between the vascular disorganization and the grade of tumoral anaplasia is very close.

G. RIZZATTO, MD; R. CHERSEVANI, MD
Department of Diagnostic Imaging, General Hospital, via Vittorio Veneto 171, Gorizia, 34170, Italy
G. RALLEIGH, MD
Department of Radiology, King's College Hospital, Denmark Hill, London, SE5 9RS, UK

Benign tumors may have one vascular pole while malignant tumors can have more than one.

The best results are obtained when Doppler frequency is higher than 5 MHz, pulse repetition frequency is between 600 and 800 Hz, and the area of interest is scanned with minimal compression. The relative risk for malignancy is higher when the vessels exhibit irregular morphology and irregular velocities (Table 21.1); these two characteristics contribute to define the "mosaic" pattern (Figure 21.1).

Information obtained with conventional color Doppler is very helpful for detecting small lesions and axillary nodes with large fatty infiltration of the hilum. In most cases vascularity enables correct diagnosis of intramammary nodes and acts as major alert for inflammation and malignancies. OZDEMIR et al. (2001) prospectively examined 112 lesions with Doppler (70 malignant and 42 benign) detected with mammography and sonography; Doppler studies increased the specificity of mammography and gray scale sonography for lesions 10 mm and smaller (from 88.9% to 100%) and for those larger than 10 mm (from 70% to 96.6%).

There is some overlap, however, in the vascular properties of breast lesions. At conventional ultrasonography, false-positive results are mostly given by hypervascularized inflammatory lesions, proliferating and juvenile fibroadenomas and phylloid tumors. There are also false negatives, particularly small tubular or ductal lesions with intense fibrosis

Table 21.1. Malignant characteristics of the vascularity in solid breast nodules

Characteristic	Relative risk Masses <15 mm	Relative risk Masses >15 mm
Irregular morphology	5.8	4.7
Irregular velocities	3.2	4.3
Multiple poles	2.1	2.0
Central vessels only	2.6	3.4
Peripheral vessels only	1.2	1.4

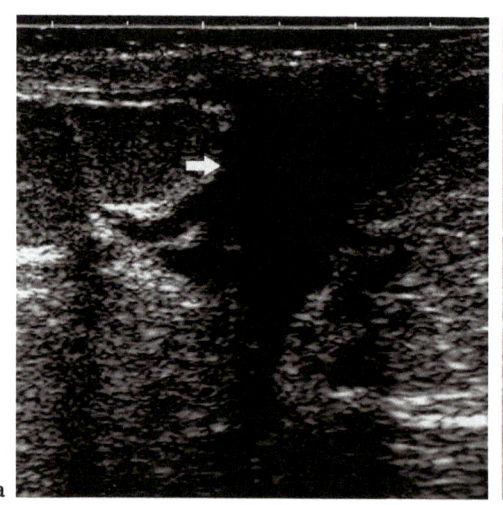

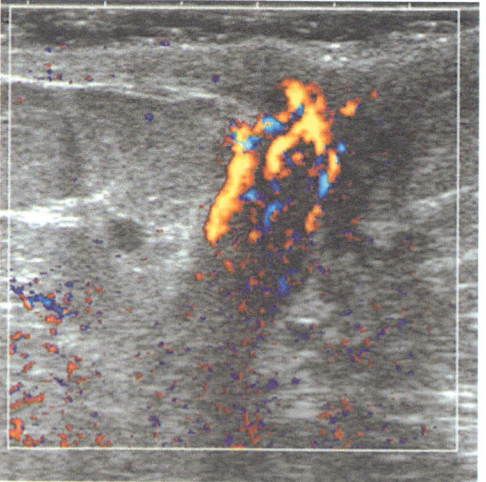

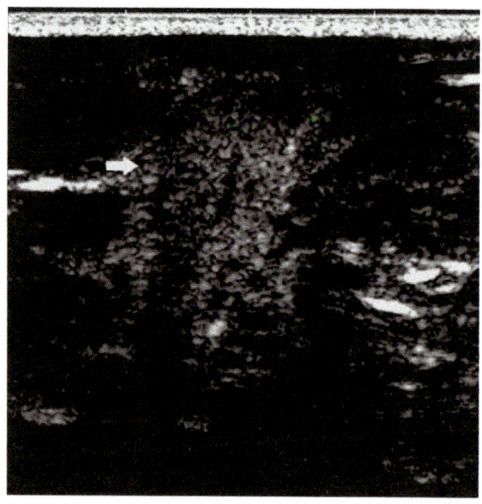

Fig. 21.1a–c. a Small superficial ductal invasive carcinoma (*arrow*). b Conventional Doppler imaging demonstrates a typical "mosaic" pattern, with different flow velocities and directions represented by multiple pseudo-color maps. c Perfusion imaging, 22 s after the end of microbubble injection, shows a homogeneous enhancement of all the tumor (*arrow*)

giving an avascular appearance. Intraductal carcinoma is covered by the original basement membrane and is supplied by perfusion only from capillary vessels out of the ducts; the only exception is a papillary form with fibrovascular cores (WU et al. 2002). In invasive carcinoma tumoral cells are accompanied by the surrounding angiogenesis, and are supplied from capillary vessels in the circumference.

21.3
Early Experience in Contrast-Enhanced Vascular Assessment

Initially, contrast-enhanced US was used in breast imaging to increase the sensitivity and specificity of color Doppler US (RIZZATTO and CHERSEVANI 1998). The use of contrast agents markedly improved visualization of the intratumoral vascular architecture (today similar images are obtained with conventional Doppler and accurate technique).

Using the presence of vascularity as a criterion for malignancy, MOON et al. (2000) found an increase in sensitivity (36%–95%), positive and negative predictive values, but a reduction in specificity (86%–79%) due to the hypervascularity of some benign lesions. WEIND et al. (1988) had already demonstrated an overlapping in the microvessel distribution between carcinomas and fibroadenomas. ELLIS (1999), re-evaluating their results, pointed out that the higher was the grade of tumor in their series the higher the distribution ratio and that fibroadenomas and grade I tumors had no substantial difference in vascular distribution. These results confirm that frequently there is little functional difference between low-grade invasive tumors and benign tumors.

SCHROEDER et al. (2003) have compared the different published studies with unenhanced and enhanced color Doppler and found that the diagnostic accuracy has improved by contrast enhancement. This was mainly caused by better assessment of the vascular architecture and better depiction of the hypervascularity of malignancies.

STUHRMANN et al. (1998) tested the possibility of improving the evaluation of benign breast lesions at Doppler sonography in patients scheduled for surgical resection. They measured the degree of enhancement provided by Levovist (Schering, Berlin, Germany), scored on a 5-points scale, the number of tumor vessels, the time to maximal enhancement, and vascular morphology and course (classified as: avascular lesions; lesions with monomorphic or peripheral vessels; and lesions with irregular penetrating vessels). They observed more vessels and faster, stronger enhancement in malignant tumors compared to benign lesions, but the best distinction was afforded by vascular morphology and course, with 90% sensitivity. However, the 81% specificity limited the clinical utility of this approach. Later reports confirmed that irregularities in the morphology and course of tumoral vessels may be highly suggestive of malignancies leading to a sensitivity of 95% and specificity of 83% or higher (SCHROEDER et al. 1999; SEHGAL et al. 2000). As reported by ZDEMIR et al. (2004), really only in the category BI-RADS 4 may the combination of mammography–gray scale sonography and contrast-enhanced Doppler achieve a higher specificity (71%) and positive predictive value (70%) than mammography–gray scale US (39% and 53%, respectively).

Contrast-enhanced Doppler was also tested in the difficult distinction between postoperative scar and tumor recurrence. Many studies have confirmed that contrast-enhanced hypervascularity may suggest recurrence (SCHROEDER et al. 2003). Contrast-enhanced US was found to substantially reduce biopsy rates (WINEHOUSE et al. 1999) and was suggested as an alternative to MR imaging, particularly in the first 18 postoperative months, when nodular scars or granulomas may also be vascularized with decreasing tendency parallel to the increasing age of the scar (STUHRMANN et al. 2000).

Unfortunately most of the results originating from all the published series on breast masses did not correlate well with the microvessel density determined histopathologically, and so far this imaging modality has not translated into increased diagnostic accuracy. Since the breast is a relatively superficial organ, diagnostic biopsy is considered safe and is performed as a gold standard. Thus, there is less demand for an imaging technique to differentiate between malignant and benign lesions.

Doppler US, even with contrast agents, enables visualization of blood vessels at the level of arterioles and venules, but does not reveal flow through the capillary bed. The relatively poor correlation between Doppler flow parameters and histopathological analysis of microvessel density confirms that Doppler US visualizes mainly tumoral macrovasculature. Therefore, there is need for an imaging modality that provides information about a lesion's microvasculature, because of the correlation with markers such as HER2 positivity, lymphovascular invasion, metastatic disease and poorer prognosis.

The specificity and sensitivity of evaluating breast lesions with MR imaging is improved by performing quantitative imaging with the aid of contrast agents: malignant tumors show early enhancement followed by washout or plateau, whereas benign lesions exhibit a gradual increase in enhancement from early to late phases. To determine if this phenomenon is also observed during dynamic contrast-enhanced US, Huber et al. (1998) studied 47 patients with breast lesions and measured color pixel density on Doppler US for 3 min after injection of Levovist. They reported a shorter time to peak enhancement for carcinoma than for benign tumors. Different time–intensity curves have been found for carcinomas, fibroadenomas and scars (Rizzatto et al. 2001). Focal inflammations, due to their markedly increased vascularity, showed the same curves of malignancies. But the wash-out behavior, although different, was adversely influenced by the continuous bubble destruction induced by the high US mechanical pressure.

21.4
Ultrasonography of the Breast with New-Generation Contrast Agents

New contrast agents are less fragile and allow the use of specific softwares that reveal the perfusional flow even in the smallest vessels (Rizzatto 2003). Actual experience is based on the use of a blood-pool echo contrast agent. SonoVue (Bracco, Milan, Italy) consists of microbubbles containing sulfur hexafluoride and encapsulated by a flexible phospholipid shell. These microbubbles have a mean diameter of 2.5 µm, with 99% smaller than 11 µm, allowing a free passage of capillaries but keeping the agent within the vascular lumen (intravascular tracer). The microbubble suspension contains 8 µl/ml SF6 gas. The best results in the breast are obtained with bolus injections of 4.8 ml administered intravenously through a three-way connector, followed by an injection of 5 ml saline solution for flushing.

Due to the flexibility of the microbubble phospholipid shell the reflectivity of SonoVue is very high. This results in a strong echo enhancement. Due to the poor solubility and diffusivity of sulfur hexafluoride gas this agent is also highly resistant to pressure.

Depending on the frequency and amplitude (mechanical index, MI) of the ultrasound wave, SonoVue microbubbles may reflect the incident wave repeatedly without being altered (low MI continuous imaging). The reflected wave contains harmonic frequency components caused by the non-linear bubble oscillations. Because the microbubbles are very flexible, significant harmonic response is obtained even at very low MI.

Although harmonics are also generated during propagation of ultrasound waves in tissues, SonoVue microbubbles generate echoes that are considerably larger than tissue echoes at harmonic frequencies. Contrast-specific imaging modes have been developed in order to accurately discriminate between the harmonic response from microbubbles and the response from tissue.

This results in perfusional images of the tumoral microcirculation based only on microbubble response. Microvascular blood velocities in the order of 0.1–10 mm/s, that cannot be detected with conventional Doppler methods, can be demonstrated with this technique.

Actual experience is based on the use of contrast tuned imaging that is a low MI technique proposed by Esaote (Genoa, Italy) in which the fundamental echo is filtered out and only the second harmonic echo is detected by the US probe. The best perfusional imaging in the breast is obtained with MI values between 0.1 and 0.08, without reducing the field of view to much to avoid superficial artifacts and with the focal zone positioned just behind the deeper lesion margin.

Perfusion is seen as an area of enhancement on the background of a nearly absent tissue signal and with minimal microbubble destruction. The resolution is rather poor in harmonic mode, and may be problematic for detecting small lesions (Fig. 21.2).

Linear hyperechoic structures, like ligaments, often act as reference structures to keep the right scanning position. Contrast tuned imaging mode has the capability to render the time–intensity curves. The signal perfusion intensity is monitored over time in selected tumor regions of interest (ROIs) and plotted on a final graph. Curves can be filtered and normalized according to the baseline signal intensity in the selected ROIs.

A group of European physicians (G. Rizzatto, R. Chersevani, E. Cassano, and A. Gambaro, Italy; J. Camps Herrero, Spain; S. Paebke, Germany; and G. Ralleigh, United Kingdom) is participating in the multicenter project PUMEB 04–05 (Perfusion Ultrasound Multicenter European Breast study) to determine appropriate uses of low MI contrast tuned imaging in the evaluation of breast cancers. The clinical applications of contrast-enhanced US that are being evaluated in PUMEB 04–05 are described in the following sections.

21.4.1
Lesion Characterization

There is a major difference in the behavior of the contrast agents that are used in MR imaging and US; therefore, both the size of the enhanced area and the time–intensity curves may differ, especially in the later phases.

Tumor angiogenesis is a sequential process. During the organization of tumor-associated capillary networks neovessels progressively acquire their distinctive structural and functional characteristics (SCOAZEC 2000). Their lining is formed by fenestrated endothelial cells limited by a discontinuous basement membrane; as a result the neoangiogenetic vessels are more permeable than the normal ones.

Vascular endothelial growth factor is the cytokine that directly stimulates endothelial cell division and migration; it strongly increases permeability allowing the extravasation of plasma proteins and resulting in the formation of an extravascular gel conducive to neovascular growth (ROSEN 2002).

In contrast-enhanced MR imaging the actual tracers cross the tumor microvessels and extravasate in the extravascular tumoral space; this capability is responsible for the major capability of MR imaging to differentiate between varying angiogenetic properties and to assess changes in angiogenesis during neoadjuvant therapy (KNOPP et al. 1999).

In contrast, the diameter of SonoVue microbubbles keeps the agent within the vascular lumen (intravascular tracer). Therefore the area of perfusion and the correlated time–intensity

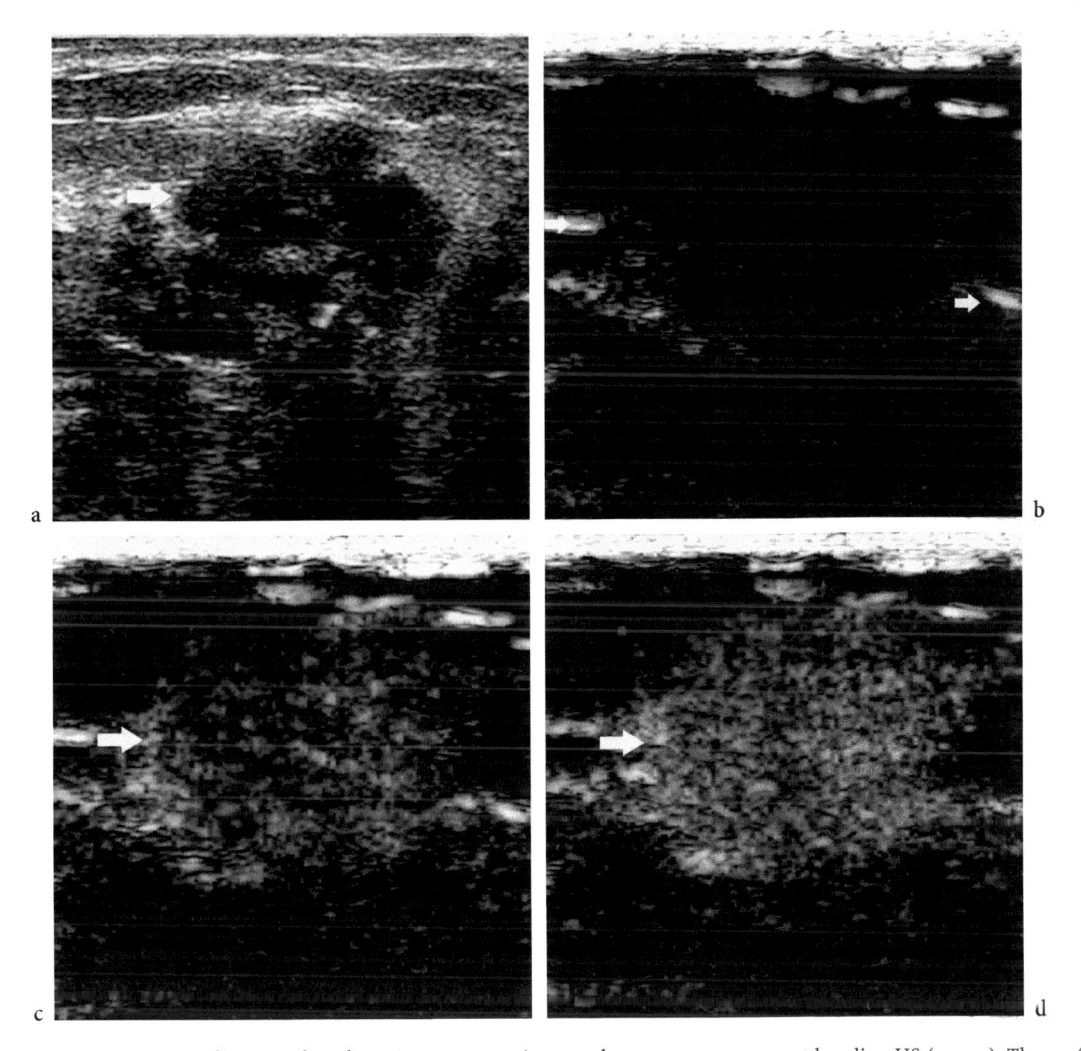

Fig. 21.2a–d. a Infiltrating ductal carcinoma appearing as a heterogeneous mass at baseline US (*arrow*). The perfusion image, before microbubble injection (b), is very poor and only the hyperechoic ligaments (*small arrows*) assure that the scanning plane is correct. c,d Perfusion imaging (18 and 23 s from microbubble injection) demonstrates a progressive homogeneous enhancement (*arrow*)

curves strictly correspond to the neoangiogenetic vascular bed, and not to the extravascular tumor space.

Some new characteristics have been identified through clinical use of contrast tuned imaging mode:
- Avascular lesions (adenosis, fibrotic changes, scars) do not exhibit internal perfusion
- Fibroadenomas usually have only a peripheral rim of perfusion (Fig. 21.3).
- Some fibroadenomas (Fig. 21.4) have diffuse perfusion and a peripheral rim during the latest phases (75 s and more).
- The perfused area in malignancies is always larger than the vascular area seen with contrast-enhanced Doppler. Conspicuity differs mainly in infiltrating tumors with acoustic shadowing and in lobular carcinomas growing without mass (Fig. 21.5).
- Tumoral perfusion may be inhomogeneous, mainly in larger or treated tumors (Fig. 21.6).
- Tumoral perfusion slightly differs in the same patient with different injections; this might be related to the differences induced by the manual injection and/or the correlation with the cardiac cycle.
- Tumoral perfusion is lower in older patients (60 years and above).
- Time-to-peak is usually shorter for malignancies (20–25 s) than for benign lesions (30 s and more) (Figs. 21.4 and 21.7).

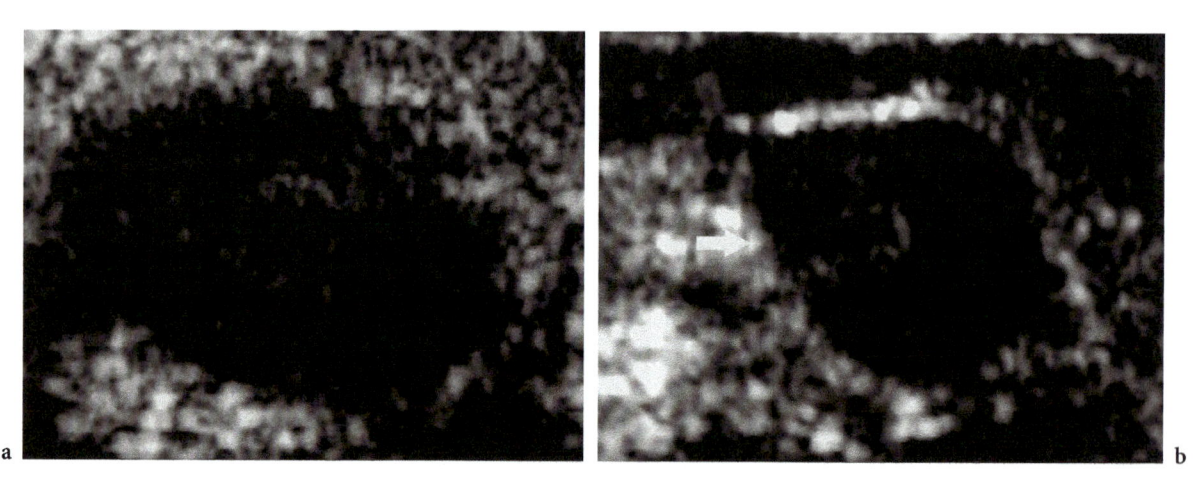

Fig. 21.3a,b. Fibroadenomas. After microbubble injection, fibroadenomas reveal a very low perfusion, also with a peripheral hyperechoic, slowly enhancing, rim (*arrow*)

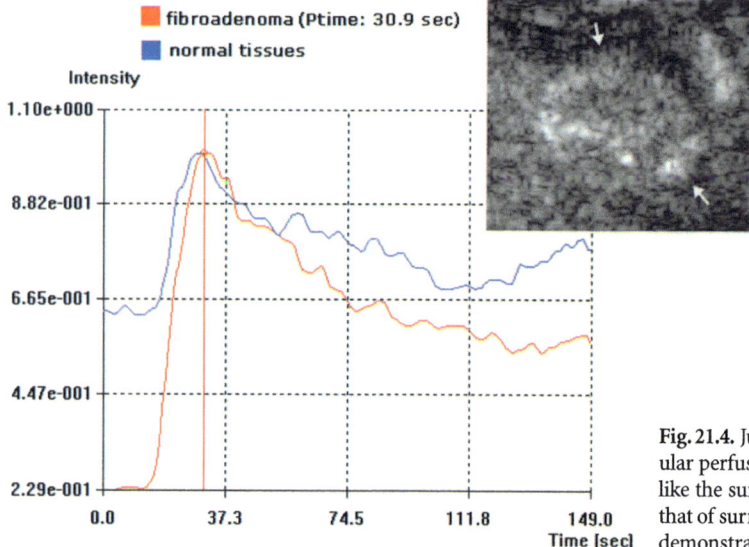

Fig. 21.4. Juvenile fibroadenoma showing also intranodular perfusion. Enhancement reaches the peak after 30 s like the surrounding gland. Wash-out plateau is close to that of surrounding tissues. After 90 s perfusion imaging demonstrates a hyperechoic rim (*arrows*)

- Time-to-peak is slightly increased for in situ and low grade invasive carcinomas.
- Time–intensity curves in invasive tumors, probably due to the presence of important arteriovenous shunts, exhibit a very rapid wash-out (Fig. 21.7).
- Time-intensity curves in benign lesions or in situ carcinomas have a longer plateau and/or a less steep gradient during the wash-out phase (Fig. 21.8).

Many of these characteristics seem to correlate very well to the different vascular arrangements of breast pathologies. This is only a preliminary experience and must be supported by larger series of cases; but it gives an idea of the potential of US perfusion imaging. There is no doubt that biopsies offer more reassuring information, but we must foresee whether these possibilities will have an impact on some breast clinical and imaging problems, and the new therapies.

21.4.2
Evaluation of Lesions Preliminarily Identified with MR Imaging

Currently, MR imaging is the most sensitive technique for detecting breast cancer; although specificity is high, biopsy is still required for non-palpable lesions evident only on MR images. Expertise to perform MR-guided biopsy or localization presently exists only in few centers; moreover, MR-guided procedures are time consuming and have a technical failure rate of 20%.

MR-detected lesions may be localized with "second-look" US to obtain additional information or to guide real time biopsy. LaTrenta et al. (2003) identified 23% of 93 suspicious, non-palpable and mammographically occult lesions with a median size of 0.9 mm. The likelihood of carcinoma was higher among lesions with a US correlate (43% carcinoma) than lesions without a US correlate (14% carcinoma). Conventional US, however, may be inef-

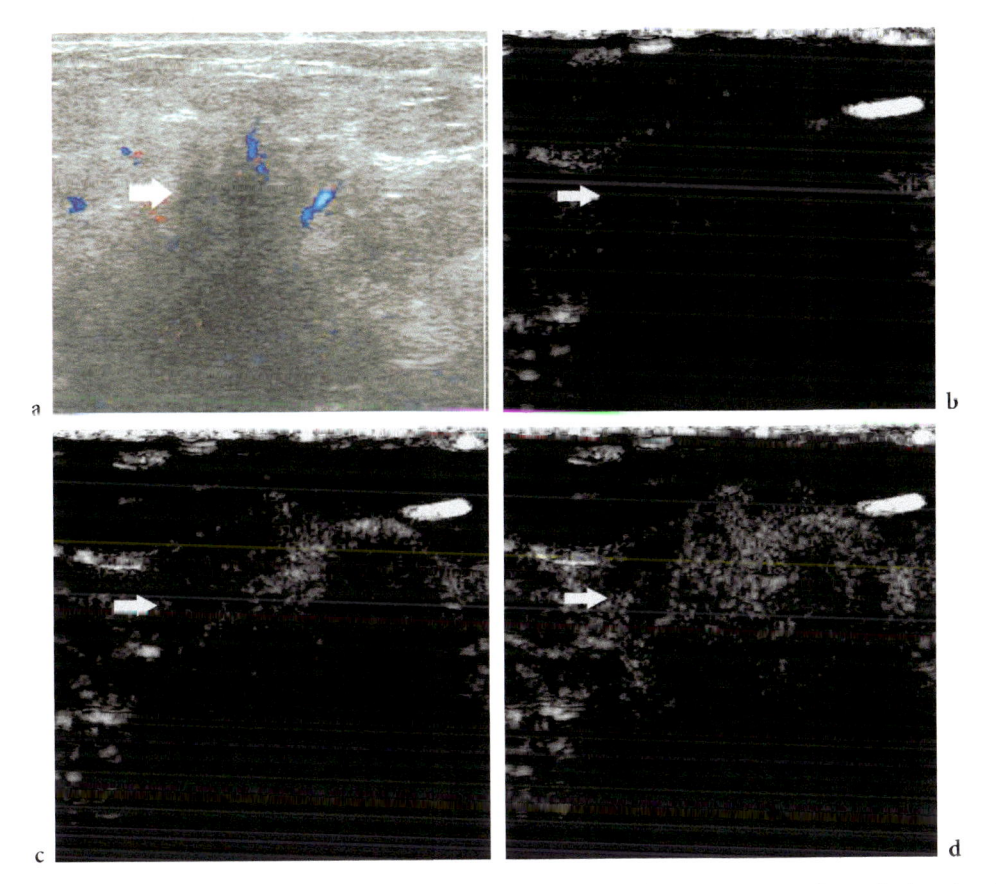

Fig. 21.5a–d. Infiltrating ductal carcinoma with acoustic shadowing. a Conventional Doppler imaging shows only penetrating vessels at the periphery of the tumor (arrow). b–d Perfusion imaging (baseline, 15 and 23 s from microbubble injection) demonstrates significant intratumoral vascularity (arrow)

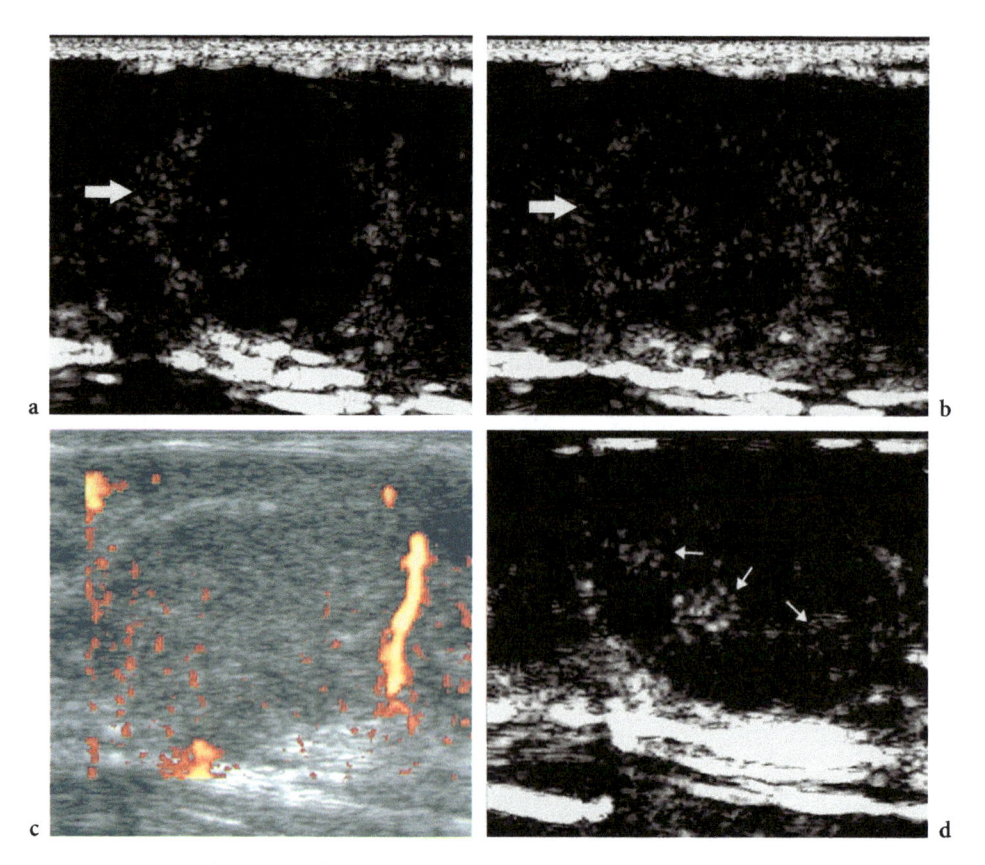

Fig. 21.6a–d. Locally advanced breast cancer treated with neoadjuvant chemotherapy. **a,b** Before treatment contrast-enhanced US (18 and 28 s) shows heterogeneous perfusion pattern (*arrow*). **c** After four cycles of a combination of cytotoxics contrast-enhanced power Doppler US demonstrates only peripheral vessels. **d** Contrast-specific mode clearly depicts some residual areas of intratumoral vascularity (*arrows*)

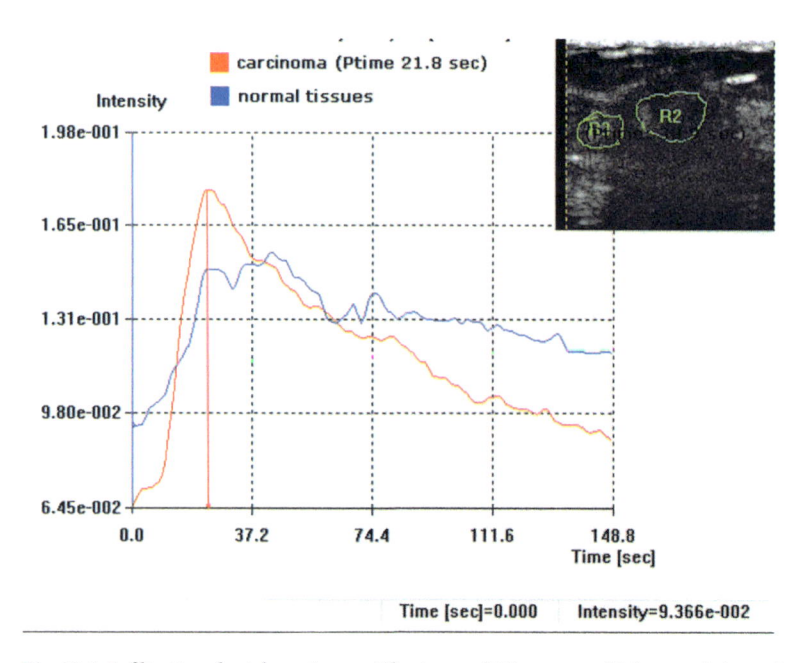

Fig. 21.7. Infiltrating ductal carcinoma. The tumor (*R2*) presents higher peak intensity value than surrounding tissues (*R3*). In the tumor, the perfusion time-to-peak is very short and the wash-out curve is very steep, probably due to the arteriovenous shunts

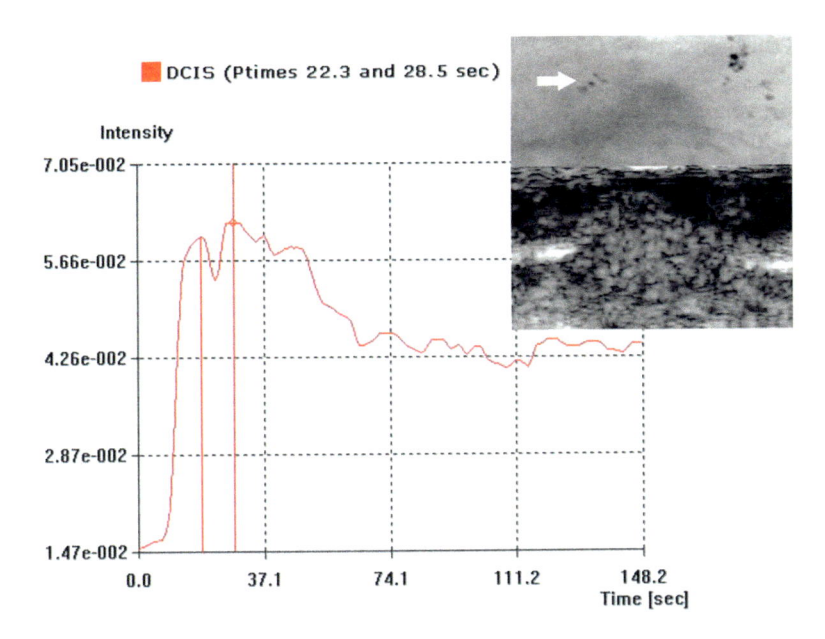

Fig. 21.8. Comedo-type ductal carcinoma in situ. Perfusion imaging demonstrates an area of enhancement corresponding to the location of multiple suspicious calcifications (*arrow*) depicted by digital mammography. The intensity curve shows two major peaks and, instead of the steep wash-out typical of infiltrating carcinomas, the curve reveals a late plateau

fective in locating the malignant lesion in patients who have multiple benign cysts or fibroadenomas.

With dynamic contrast-enhanced US, it may be easier to locate the malignant lesion on the basis of an enhancement time course similar to that observed at MR. This application is important because it may permit accurate guidance for biopsy.

21.4.3
Detection of Lymph Node Metastases as an Alternative to the Sentinel Lymph Node Procedure

Today, most patients with breast cancer undergo local resection or mastectomy, as well as axillary lymph node dissection if a sentinel lymph node procedure has provided evidence of malignancy. This procedure involves biopsy and histopathological analysis of the first draining (sentinel) lymph node, identified by following the clearance through the lymphatic system of a radioactive or colored dye injected into the breast near the tumor.

Use of the sentinel lymph node procedure is justified by the knowledge that when the sentinel node is negative for malignancy, there is very low likelihood that the tumor has metastasized to the axillary nodes; in this case many surgical groups now avoid axillary dissection. In general, sentinel lymph node is an accurate procedure, but pitfalls exist. Studies correlating the results of sentinel lymph node biopsy with axillary dissection in more than 3000 patients have shown that sentinel lymph node biopsy has a technical success rate of 88%, sensitivity of 93%, and accuracy of 97% (LIBERMAN 2003). VERONESI et al. (2003) have found 32% of positive sentinel lymph nodes in 516 patients with primary breast cancer in whom the tumor was less than or equal to 2 cm in diameter; in 34% the sentinel lymph nodes were seeded only by micrometastases (foci ≤2 mm in diameter).

US can usually identify enlarged reactive or metastatic nodes. In vitro studies demonstrate that metastatic disease is often indicated by an enlarged and round shaped node, the absence of an echogenic hilum, a marginal bulging or a small hypoechoic area within the echogenic cortex (FEU et al. 1997; TATEISHI et al. 1999). Doppler studies show a reduced vascularity inside the metastatic deposits; in the case of massive metastatic infiltration the remaining vessels are displaced at the periphery of the node (YANG et al. 2000). Conventional US has great potential; both specificity and positive predictive value are high (RIZZATTO 2001). US-guided biopsy can confirm a positive diagnosis (DE KANTER et al. 1999) and these patients can be immediately scheduled for nodal dissection.

US actual resolution is within the range of macrometastases (3 mm or more); this situation is expected in around 20%–25% of all the breast cancer patients.

Some new characteristics have been identified through clinical use of contrast tuned imaging:
- Normal or reactive cortex always has intense, homogeneous perfusion.
- Marginal bulgings without lack of perfusion may reflect normal morphologic variability.
- In the early phase of metastatic seeding the node is highly reactive, with diffuse and homogeneous enhancement.
- Contrast tuned imaging has insufficient resolution to depict micrometastases (≤2 mm in diameter) but small deposits larger than 3 mm are clearly seen as non-perfused "black" areas not always predictable on the basis of conventional imaging and Doppler (Fig. 21.9).
- In the case of massive infiltration the perfused non-involved area is always larger than shown with conventional imaging and Doppler (Fig. 21.10).
- In the case of enlarged nodes with Doppler massive vascularity the behavior of perfusion progression may suggest different pathologies.

Many imaging groups dealing with a large number of breast cancers have already appreciated the accuracy and advantages offered by sonography in assessing nodal status (Rizzatto 2001). Nodes can be assessed in a very early phase and US can guide a needle very precisely in the suspicious areas.

Perfusion imaging offers a unique capability in picking up the metastatic areas in all the different nodal locations that may be involved by breast carcinoma. Small deposits, 3 mm and more, located in the normal cortex are easily discovered and are precisely assessed with biopsy. False positives may be related to small fibrotic changes or granulomas. In the case of enlarged nodes that exhibit poor vascularity on conventional Doppler the needle is guided in the metastatic areas that are usually smaller than with conventional imaging. In other cases the intense but inhomogeneous speckled enhancement in the early arterial phase, that seems to be mostly related to lymphomas (Rubaltelli et al. 2004), is accurate enough to readdress the patient.

Perfusion imaging actually increases the already high positive predictive value of US in nodal assess-

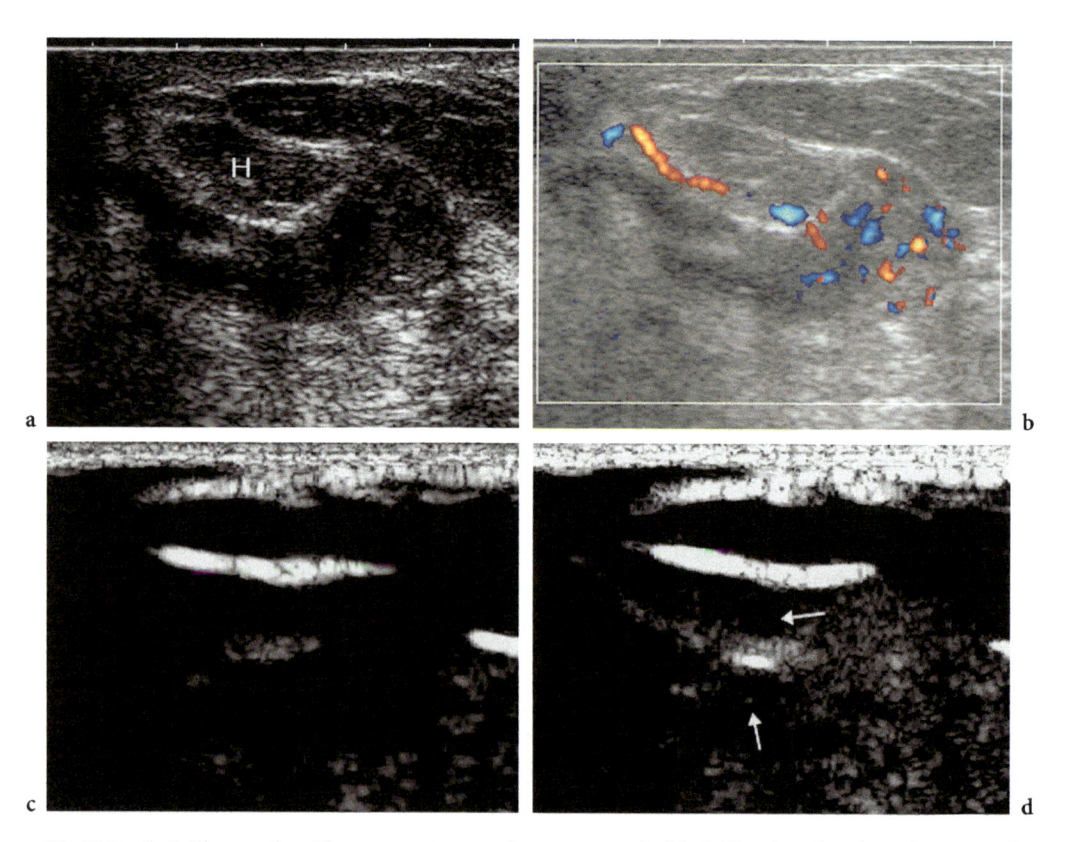

Fig. 21.9a–d. Axillary node with macrometastases from a non-palpable infiltrating ductal carcinoma. **a** The node (*arrow*) is mainly enlarged due to fatty infiltration of the hilum (*H*). **b** Conventional Doppler shows a slightly reduced cortical vascularity. **c,d** Perfusion imaging, 20 s after microbubble injection, clearly depicts macrometastases of 3.5 mm in diameter (*arrows*) and enabled guidance for accurate fine-needle aspiration

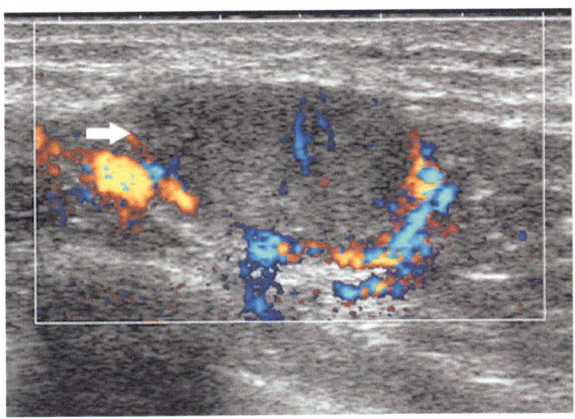

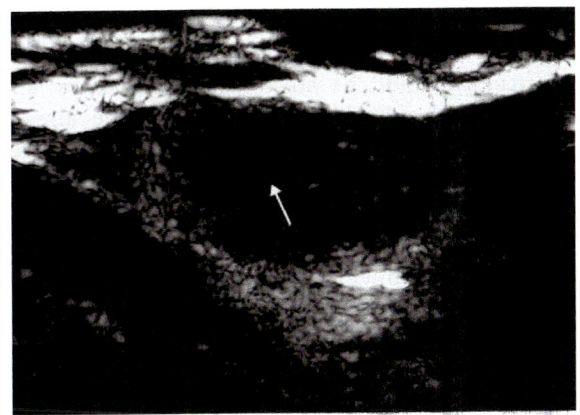

Fig. 21.10a,b. Enlarged metastatic axillary node from locally advanced breast cancer. a The node (*arrow*) keeps its normal oval shape but conventional Doppler shows a suspicious peripheral displacement of the vessels and the echo pattern seems homogeneous. b After microbubble injection, perfusion imaging presents a heterogeneous pattern also with a 9-mm non-enhancing area (*arrow*). Biopsy was US-guided in this area for more accurate sampling

ment. When a node is positive on US and biopsy the patient is scheduled for axillary dissection and a sentinel lymph node procedure is avoided. This happens in around 20% of patients with breast cancer. Imaging impact is very high because of the reduced cost of the diagnostic procedure and the better scheduling of the operating room.

21.4.4
Monitoring the Response of Advanced Breast Cancers to Neoadjuvant Therapy

Advanced breast cancers include local recurrence, disseminated disease or locally advanced breast cancer. In this last stage the tumor in the breast is usually more than 5 cm across or it has destroyed the superficial fascia and invaded the subcutaneous lymphatic network, or it has spread to the axillary nodes or to other nodes or tissues near the breast.

Neoadjuvant therapy includes standard cytotoxic and/or hormonal manipulation. About 75% of these locally advanced breast cancer regress with cytotoxic treatment allowing surgery with disease free margins. In more than 50% of these patients there is no tumor left or only microscopic tumor (HUNKOOP et al. 1997). In the responsive area cancer tissue is transformed to a xanthogranulomatous lesion with the infiltration of macrophages and lymphocytes (WU et al. 2002). It is replaced by myxomatous fibrous tissue and then by cicatricial tissue. The cases with a high proportion of intraductal component have lower response (WU et al. 2002); the larger number of residual cancer cells are found within the ducts and preserve their proliferative activity. In all the tumors there is a consistent reduction in mitotic activity and in global microvessel density. Complete response to neoadjuvant chemotherapy is also documented for axillary nodal metastases. KUERER et al. (1999) reported complete axillary conversion in 23% of patients. ARIMAPPAMAGAN et al. (2004) found a complete response in 22% of patients; in 10% conversion was complete for both axilla and primary tumor.

The management of advanced breast cancer is really an expanding field. Many trials are now going on to evaluate also the potentials of novel combinations or new cytotoxics like anthracyclines and taxanes, or the effects of monoclonal antibodies. Future developments will include host response modifiers like agents which suppress angiogenesis.

The challenges for breast imaging lie in the ability to incorporate technologies to ensure both accurate staging and effective monitoring of tumor response.

Mammography and conventional US have limited efficiency; they usually measure the tumor response evaluating the changes of its diameter, morphology and echo pattern. MR imaging seems to be the most accurate imaging modality (DELILLE et al. 2003; WASSER et al. 2003). The correlation between tumor diameter measured by histopathology and MRI is very high; a clear reduction in size is usually seen only after the third cycle. Size reduction is usually associated with a decrease of the contrast enhancement parameters.

MR imaging is not universally available. Optimization of a US protocol to monitor treatment outcomes would be advantageous clinically and economically. Huber et al. (2000) have already documented an increased US efficiency when color Doppler flow imaging is added to conventional US. Good efficiency has also been proven for very short interval monitoring of the neoangiogenetic vascularity of inflammatory lesions undergoing antibiotic therapy (Rizzatto and Chersevani 1998).

More recently Pollard et al. (2003) documented the potentials of a destruction-replenishment US technique in monitoring the antineoangiogenetic effects of therapy in rat models. Preliminary experience with contrast tuned imaging demonstrates that contrast-enhanced Doppler may give false negative vascular patterns while perfusion imaging still registers important residual intratumoral vascularity (Fig. 21.6).

Actually perfusion US must be considered the only alternative to MR imaging; moreover, it offers the possibility of guiding further biopsies in the residual areas. In the future, with the clinical introduction of new therapies, it will be very important to understand if monitoring should be restricted to the tumoral vessels or also include the extravascular bed. This decision will determine the choice in favor of perfusion US or MR imaging.

21.4.5
Evaluation of Microcalcification in Ductal Carcinoma In Situ

Patients with ductal carcinoma in situ usually present with clinically occult screen-detected microcalcification, which is biopsied using stereotactic guidance. Stereotactic biopsy can significantly underestimate (by approximately 8%–20%) the presence of invasive disease necessitating delayed axillary node sampling and multiple operations (Hoorntje et al. 2003; Leifland et al. 2003).

Investigators have previously demonstrated that large clusters (>10 mm) of microcalcifications are visible with high frequency US (Yang and Tse 2004). In addition ductal carcinoma in situ may manifest as a hypoechoic mass, acoustic shadowing and/or intraductal abnormality. Abnormal vascularity has previously been demonstrated using power Doppler in areas of ductal carcinoma in situ (Teh et al. 2000).

Currently, areas of microcalcification are biopsied during lengthy stereotactic procedures. The ability to guide biopsy by contrast-enhanced US would render the procedure more comfortable for the patient and would permit clinicians to excise the most intensely vascularized lesions; this may translate into an improved detection of invasive foci within areas of ductal carcinoma in situ. High-grade ductal carcinoma in situ is associated with increased microvessel density next to the arm, negative ER and positive HER2 status, and poor prognosis. Contrast-enhanced ultrasonography may contribute in the evaluation of these patients by stratifying lesions, describing tumor biology, and providing information regarding prognosis and the likelihood of success with systemic therapies. The use of SonoVue during contrast tuned imaging may be a useful adjunct to mammography and percutaneous biopsy in the assessment of these lesions (Fig. 21.8).

21.5
Future Developments

Future developments are needed both in terms of technology and contrast agents. Probably large matrix transducers will help in acquiring larger 3D volumes and computer-aided diagnosis will increase the recognition of small enhancing lesions, thereby facilitating screening procedures. Tracers, however, must change in terms of their properties, with both longer recirculating time and higher resolution without movement artifacts.

Two major interests are linked to US perfusion imaging. First the capability to store drugs or other components within the microbubble. They will be targeted and linked to specific tissues; or they will be monitored up to the peak perfusion within the tumor, or even benign pathologies like inflammations. Fusion with molecular imaging and optical probes might be part of this future. The same transducer will use higher energies to destroy the microbubbles or to partially fragment their shells and to release the drug in the proper time. The same perfusion US imaging will monitor the effects of therapy.

The second improvement will be the capability of new contrast agents to enter the lymphatic stream and to fully replace radiotracers in the sentinel lymph node procedure. Some of these future applications are already working within ongoing projects on animal models (Allen et al. 2002; Dayton and Ferrara 2002; May et al. 2002; Mattrey et al. 2002; Wisner et al. 2003; Choi et al. 2004; Goldberg et al. 2004).

References

Allen JS, May DJ, Ferrara KW (2002) Dynamics of therapeutic ultrasound contrast agents. Ultrasound Med Biol 28:805-816

Arimappamagan A, Kadambari D, Srinivasan K et al (2004) Complete axillary conversion after neoadjuvant chemotherapy in locally advanced breast cancer: a step towards conserving axilla? Indian J Cancer 41:13-17

Choi SH, Kono Y, Corbeil J et al (2004) Model to quantify lymph node enhancement on indirect sonographic lymphography. AJR Am J Roentgenol 183:513-517

Dayton PA, Ferrara KW (2002) Targeted imaging using ultrasound. J Magn Reson Imaging 16:362-377

De Kanter AY, van Eijck CH, van Geel AN et al (1999) Multicentre study of ultrasonographically guided axillary node biopsy in patients with breast cancer. Br J Surg 86:1459-1462

Delille JP, Slanetz PJ, Yeh ED et al (2003) Invasive ductal breast carcinoma response to neoadjuvant chemotherapy: noninvasive monitoring with functional MR imaging pilot study. Radiology 228:63-69

Ellis RL (1999) Differentiation of benign versus malignant breast disease. Radiology 210:878-880

Feu J, Tresserra F, Fabregas R et al (1997) Metastatic breast carcinoma in axillary lymph nodes: in vitro US detection. Radiology 205:831-835

Goldberg BB, Merton DA, Liu JB et al (2004) Sentinel lymph nodes in a swine model with melanoma: contrast-enhanced lymphatic US. Radiology 230:727-734

Honkoop AH, Pinedo HM, de Jong JS et al (1997) Effects of chemotherapy on pathologic and biologic characteristics of locally advanced breast cancer. Am J Clin Pathol 107:211-218

Hoorntje LE, Schipper ME, Peeters PH et al (2003) The finding of invasive cancer after a preoperative diagnosis of ductal carcinoma-in-situ: causes of ductal carcinoma-in-situ underestimates with stereotactic 14-gauge needle biopsy. Ann Surg Oncol 10:748-753

Huber S, Helbich T, Kettenbach J et al (1988) Effects of a microbubble contrast agent on breast tumors: computer-assisted quantitative assessment with color Doppler US-early experience. Radiology 208:485-489

Huber S, Medl M, Helbich T et al (2000) Locally advanced breast carcinoma: computer assisted semiquantitative analysis of color Doppler ultrasonography in the evaluation of tumor response to neoadjuvant chemotherapy (work in progress). J Ultrasound Med 19:601-607

Knopp MV, Weiss E, Sinn HP et al (1999) Pathophysiologic basis of contrast enhancement in breast tumors. J Magn Reson Imaging 10:260-266

Kuerer HM, Sahin AA, Hunt KK et al (1999) Incidence and impact of documented eradication of breast cancer axillary lymph node metastases before surgery in patients treated with neoadjuvant chemotherapy. Ann Surg 230:72-78

LaTrenta LR, Menell JH, Morris EA et al (2003) Breast lesions detected with MR imaging: utility and importance of identification with US. Radiology 227:856-861

Leifland K, Lundquist H, Lagerstedt U et al (2003) Comparison of preoperative simultaneous stereotactic fine needle aspiration biopsy and stereotactic core needle biopsy in ductal carcinoma in situ of the breast. Acta Radiol 44:213-217

Less JR, Skalak TC, Sevick EM et al (1991) Microvascular architecture in a mammary carcinoma: branching patterns and vessel dimensions. Cancer Res 51:265-273

Liberman L (2003) Lymphoscintigraphy for lymphatic mapping in breast carcinoma. Radiology 228:313-315

Mattrey RF, Kono Y, Baker K et al (2002) Sentinel lymph node imaging with microbubble ultrasound contrast material. Acad Radiol 9 [Suppl 1]:S231-S235

May DJ, Allen JS, Ferrara KW (2002) Dynamics and fragmentation of thick-shelled microbubbles. IEEE Trans Ultrason Ferroelectr Freq Control 49:1400-1410

Moon WK, Im JG, Noh DY et al (2000) Nonpalpable breast lesions: evaluation with power Doppler US and a microbubble contrast agent-initial experience. Radiology 217:240-246

Ozdemir A, Ozdemir H, Maral I et al (2001) Differential diagnosis of solid breast lesions. Contribution of Doppler studies to mammography and gray scale imaging. J Ultrasound Med 20:1091-1101

Pollard RE, Sadlowski AR, Bloch SH et al (2003) Contrast-assisted destruction-replenishment ultrasound for the assessment of tumor microvasculature in a rat model. Technol Cancer Res Treat 1:459-470

Rizzatto G (2001) Towards a more sophisticated use of breast ultrasound. Eur Radiol 11:2425-2435

Rizzatto G (2003) Contrast-enhanced ultrasound examination of breast lesions. Eur Radiol 13:D63-D65

Rizzatto G, Chersevani R (1998) Breast ultrasound and new technologies. Eur J Radiol 27:S242-S249

Rizzatto G, Martegani A, Chersevani R et al (2001) Importance of staging of breast cancer and role of contrast ultrasound. Eur Radiol 11[Suppl 3]:E47-E52

Rosen LS (2002) Clinical experience with angiogenesis signaling inhibitors: focus on vascular endothelial growth factor (VEGF) blockers. Cancer Control 9:36-44

Rubaltelli L, Khadivi Y, Tregnaghi A et al (2004) Evaluation of lymph node perfusion using continuous mode harmonic ultrasonography with a second-generation contrast agent. J Ultrasound Med 23:829-836

Schroeder RJ, Maeurer J, Vogl TJ et al (1999) D-galactose based signal-enhanced color Doppler sonography of breast tumors and tumorlike lesions. Invest Radiol 34:109-115

Schroeder RJ, Bostanjoglo M, Rademaker J et al (2003) Role of power Doppler techniques and ultrasound contrast enhancement in the differential diagnosis of focal breast lesions. Eur Radiol 13:68-79

Scoazec J (2000) Tumor angiogenesis. Ann Pathol 20:25-37

Sehgal CM, Arger PH, Rowling SE et al (2000) Quantitative vascularity of breast masses by Doppler imaging: regional variations and diagnostic implications. J Ultrasound Med 19:427-440

Stuhrmann M, Aronius R, Roefke C et al (1998) Vascularization of breast tumors: use of ultrasound contrast medium in evaluating tumor entity. Preliminary results. Röfo Fortschr Geb Röntgenstr Neuen Bildgeb Verfahr 169:360-364

Stuhrmann M, Aronius R, Schietzel M (2000) Tumor vascularity of breast lesions: potentials and limits of contrast-enhanced Doppler sonography. AJR Am J Roentgenol 175:1585-1589

Tateishi T, Machi J, Feleppa EJ et al (1999) In vitro B-mode ultrasonographic criteria for diagnosing axillary lymph node metastasis of breast cancer. J Ultrasound Med 18:349-356

Teh WL, Wilson AR, Evans AJ et al (2000) Ultrasound guided core biopsy of suspicious mammographic calcifications using high frequency and power Doppler ultrasound. Clin Radiol 55:390-394

Veronesi U, Paganelli G, Viale G et al (2003) A randomized comparison of sentinel-node biopsy with routine axillary dissection in breast cancer. N Engl J Med 349:546-553

Wasser K, Klein SK, Fink C et al (2003) Evaluation of neoadjuvant chemotherapeutic response of breast cancer using dynamic MRI with high temporal resolution. Eur Radiol 13:80-87

Weind KL, Maier CF, Rutt BK et al (1998) Invasive carcinomas and fibroadenomas of the breast: comparison of microvessel distributions. Implications for imaging modalities. Radiology 208:477-483

Winehouse J, Douek M, Holz K et al (1999) Contrast-enhanced color Doppler ultrasonography in suspected breast cancer recurrence. Br J Surg 86:1198-1201

Wisner ER, Ferrara KW, Short RE et al (2003) Sentinel node detection using contrast-enhanced power Doppler ultrasound lymphography. Invest Radiol 38:358-365

Wu W, Kamma H, Ueno E et al (2002) The intraductal component of breast cancer is poorly responsive to neo-adjuvant chemotherapy. Oncol Rep 9:1027-1031

Yang WT, Tse GM (2004) Sonographic, mammographic, and histopathologic correlation of symptomatic ductal carcinoma in situ. AJR Am J Roentgenol 182:101-110

Yang WT, Chang J, Metreweli C (2000) Patients with breast cancer: differences in color Doppler flow and gray-scale US features of benign and malignant axillary lymph nodes. Radiology 215:568-573

Zdemir A, Kilic K, Ozdemir H et al (2004) Contrast-enhanced power Doppler sonography in breast lesions: effect on differential diagnosis after mammography and gray scale sonography. J Ultrasound Med 23:183-195

22 Lymph Nodes

Leopoldo Rubaltelli, Alberto Tregnaghi, and Roberto Stramare

CONTENTS

22.1 Introduction 315
22.2 Conventional Baseline US 315
22.3 Color and Power Doppler US 316
22.4 Computed Tomography and Magnetic Resonance Imaging 316
22.5 Contrast-Enhanced Color Doppler 317
22.6 Evaluation of Lymph Node Perfusion 317
22.6.1 Qualitative Study 317
22.6.2 Quantitative Study 321
22.7 Sentinel Lymph Node – Lymphosonography 321
22.8 Conclusions 321
References 322

22.1
Introduction

The role of imaging to evaluate lymphadenopathies is of fundamental importance. The presence or absence of lymph node metastases directly influences not only the prognosis of oncologic patients, but also the appropriate therapeutic approach. Similarly, the characterization of enlarged lymph nodes in patients without a previous history of neoplastic disease is of primary importance.

Baseline ultrasound (US) is commonly employed to assess lymph nodes in the superficial anatomical regions (cervical, axillary, and inguinal) and the role of high-resolution US is well established (Marchal et al. 1985; Rubaltelli et al. 1990; Vassallo et al. 1992, 1993; Adibelli et al. 1998; Ahuja and Ying 2002, 2003). Besides the information supplied by gray-scale US, nowadays additional data on lymph node vascularity may be provided by color and power Doppler US, which is even more sensitive (Ahuja et al. 2001; Giovagnorio et al. 1997, 2002; Yang and Metreweli 1998; Ying et al. 2000, 2001).

The latest acquisition in this field consists in the capability of studying lymph node perfusion in real time by means of microbubble-based contrast agents in combination with gray-scale tissue harmonic imaging techniques. Consequently, it is possible to assess lymph node vascularity in greater detail than Doppler US techniques and with a degree of definition that is comparable with high-resolution US probes.

22.2
Conventional Baseline US

High frequency (10–13 MHz) and high-resolution transducers still represent the fundamental basis for the evaluation of the superficial lymph nodes. Normal, or reactive, lymph nodes appear as oval or fusiform shapes with a hyperechoic central part, defined as the hilus, surrounded by the hypoechoic and homogeneous cortex. The echogenic hilus is, in reality, the representation of the lymph node medulla where numerous interfaces produced by the blood vessels, lymphatic sinuses and fatty tissue are present (Marchal et al. 1985; Perin et al. 1987; Rubaltelli et al. 1990; Vassallo et al. 1993; Ahuja and Ying 2002, 2003; Ying and Ahuja 2003).

The morphological and structural parameters useful for distinguishing between benign and malignant lymph nodes are: the dimensions, the shape, the presence or absence of the echogenic hilus, the thickness and structure of cortex (Vassallo et al. 1992). The absence of the echogenic hilus and the round shape (longitudinal to transverse ratio <2) are the most characteristic signs of metastatic lymph nodes (Vassallo et al. 1992; Ahuja and Ying 2003), and they were found in, respectively, 88.1% and 87.1% of the metastatic lymph nodes investigated during a recent study on cervical lymph nodes (Ahuja and Ying 2002).

These parameters are employed only in superficial lymph nodes, whereas the study of abdominal lymph

L. Rubaltelli, MD; A. Tregnaghi, MD; R. Stramare, MD
Department of Medical Diagnostic Sciences and Special Therapies, University of Padua, Via Giustiniani 2, 35128 Padua, Italy

nodes requires US transducers with both lower frequency and resolution. Moreover, the obesity and meteorism represent still further limitations, and when the visualization of abdominal lymph nodes is possible, baseline US is generally limited to the dimensional evaluation without any possibility to assess lymph node structural parameters.

22.3
Color and Power Doppler US

At color or power Doppler US, normal lymph nodes reveal hilar vascularization since the principal vessels are found in the hilus while no peripheral vessels are identified at the boundary of the capsule (STEINKAMP et al. 1998; TSCHAMMLER et al. 1998; AHUJA et al. 2001; AHUJA and YING 2002). The smallest lymph nodes, with a maximum transverse diameter of less than 5 mm, can be apparently avascular at color or power Doppler US (YING et al. 2001). This aspect is more frequently identified in cervical rather than in axillary or inguinal lymph nodes, especially in the posterior triangle (YING et al. 2000), and the avascular appearance is highly frequent in the elderly. Among cervical lymph nodes the greatest extent of vascularization is found in the sub-mandibular region (YING et al. 2000, 2001), and it may be related to inflammation of the upper respiratory tract which, although asymptomatic, is nevertheless able to activate regional lymph nodes.

Metastatic lymph nodes tend to have either peripheral vascularization along the boundary of the capsule with the presence of numerous vascular poles, or a mixed, peripheral, and hilar vascularization (GIOVAGNORIO et al. 1997; NA et al. 1997; STEINKAMP et al. 1998; TSCHAMMLER et al. 1998). This framework of peripheral vascularization is determined by the fact that the neoplastic cells arrive at the lymph node from the lymphatic afferents, perforate the capsule on its convexity, and colonize the outer part to invade the inner part of the lymph node reaching the medulla and hilus.

The presence of hypertrophic vessels, branching away from the hilus and associated to peripheral vessels, is frequently observed in lymphomas (GIOVAGNORIO et al. 1997). However, peripheral vessels are less frequently observed then in metastases, since lymphoma originate in the context of lymph node cortex and later invade the central part, while the lymph node periphery may remain normal (GIOVAGNORIO et al. 2002).

The vascular pattern at color Doppler US of lymph nodes in lymphomas may appear similar to inflammatory lymph nodes (ADIBELLI et al. 1998), especially in low-grade lymphomas.

However, the most significant finding to differentiate benign from malignant lymph nodes is the evidence of peripheral vascularization, which should always induce one to perform some further diagnostic investigations. Lastly, it should be underlined that lymph nodes which appear avascular at color Doppler US, but are morphologically altered at grayscale US, can be metastatic with extensive areas of necrosis and obliteration of the newly-formed vessels.

The complete absence of visible vessels at color Doppler US has also been reported in tubercular lymphadenopathies in relation to necrosis and fibrosis. The dislocation of intranodal vessels, reported both in metastases (STEINKAMP et al. 1998) and in tuberculosis (AHUJA and YING 2003), is not considered a frequent aspect.

The resistivity (RI) and pulsatility indices (PI), calculated from the Doppler interrogation of lymph node arterial vessels, are lower in reactive lymph nodes than in metastatic lymph nodes (CHOI et al. 1995; NA et al. 1997; HO et al. 2000), although there is no consensus on the optimal cut-off to obtain an accurate differentiation (ADIBELLI et al. 1998). Furthermore, if one considers the differential diagnosis between benign and malignant lymph nodes (metastases and lymphomas), the role of RI and PI becomes even less significant since lymphomas tend to have lower RI and PI than metastases (FERRARI et al. 1997; ADIBELLI et al. 1998).

22.4
Computed Tomography and Magnetic Resonance Imaging

The panoramic aspect and high spatial resolution of computed tomography (CT) and magnetic resonance (MR) imaging guarantee notable sensitivity in the recognition of even small and deep lymph nodes. However, such sensitivity is not accompanied by an equally high specificity since CT and MR imaging of lymph node pathology are substantially related to dimensional parameters, with variable limits of measurement in the various anatomical districts, and to recognition of areas of necrosis.

The aim of intravenously administered contrast agents, iodinated for CT and paramagnetic for MR imaging, is to differentiate lymph nodes from other structures (vessels, intestinal loops) and to identify intranodal areas of altered vascularity. Notable improvement is expected from the employment of superparamagnetic contrast agents, composed by extremely minute corpuscular elements, capable of passing through the pulmonary circle and eventually phagocytized by the lymph node cells of the reticuloendothelial system (BELLIN et al. 2000; WEIMANN et al. 2003).

To date, the performed studies indicate the utility of these contrast agents for MR imaging (MACK et al. 2002; SIGAL et al. 2002), but precise evaluation of their diagnostic efficacy will only be possible in the future.

22.5
Contrast-Enhanced Color Doppler

Intravenously administered air-filled microbubble based contrast agents were initially utilized to increase intranodal vascular signals at Doppler US and some studies have reported that this technique has improved diagnostic accuracy in the evaluation of cervical lymph nodes (MAURER et al. 1997; WILLAM et al. 1998; MORITZ et al. 2000). After microbubble-based agent injection, cervical lymph nodes in patients with metastatic squamous carcinoma revealed nodal vessels not identified before microbubble injection, with improvement in the assessment of vascular pattern both in benign and malignant lymph nodes (MAURER et al. 1997). The improved visualization of Doppler signals in lymph nodes after microbubble injection, was particularly significant in reactive lymph nodes. This is because baseline color Doppler US represents as avascular those lymph nodes which reveal hilar vascularization at contrast-enhanced US, which is considered a benignancy finding (MAURER et al. 1997; WILLAM et al. 1998).

In a more recent study, including 94 cervical lymph nodes in 39 patients with oral cavity carcinoma assessed by color Doppler US after air-filled microbubble injection, high sensitivity (100%) and specificity (98%) in differentiating benign from malignant lymph nodes were observed (MORITZ et al. 2000). Such results, although brilliant, are somehow difficult to reproduce due to limitations of contrast enhanced color Doppler US, particularly evident in lymph nodes close to pulsating structures such as the arterial vessels. Moreover, the resolution of contrast-enhanced color Doppler US is too low to identify small intranodal lesions, even though some vascular signals are found in approximately 90% of lymph nodes having a maximum transverse diameter >5 mm (YANG and METREWELI 1998).

At the current state of the art, the employment of microbubble-based contrast agents to amplify Doppler signals has to be considered obsolete since microbubble-based agents are not able to improve the intrinsic limits of color and power Doppler and only information regarding lymph nodes macrovascularization is provided. Dedicated US contrast-specific techniques are necessary to assess lymph node perfusion after microbubble injection.

22.6
Evaluation of Lymph Node Perfusion

22.6.1
Qualitative Study

The most recent contribution to advancement in US imaging lies in the possibility of evaluating lymph node perfusion by means of gray-scale harmonic imaging after intravenous administration of perfluorocarbon or sulfur hexafluoride-filled microbubbles. The application of contrast-enhanced US in structures of small dimensions, and with relatively low rates of flow such as lymph nodes, is recent. Actually, nowadays only some US equipment provides good results in this field, due to the low sensitivity of the high frequency linear-array transducers to microbubble harmonic signals.

22.6.1.1
Methodology of scanning

After perfluorocarbon or sulfur hexafluoride-filled contrast agent injection (SOLBIATI et al. 2002), dedicated contrast-specific modes selectively register the signal emitted by the microbubbles and thereby eliminate all the redundant signals. Initially, clinical applications utilized a 7.5-MHz linear transducer equipped with continuous harmonic imaging advanced technology.

The low acoustic power (mechanical index: 0.05–0.2) insonation produces microbubble oscillation at maximum intensity, but without the risk of being destroyed. A 4.8-ml dose of the contrast agent is bolus-injected into a peripheral vein, followed by a 10-ml injection of physiological saline solution. This technique makes it possible to achieve high resolution both in the arterial (15–30 s after injection) and late-parenchymal phase (40–90 s after injection), and to identify diffuse or partial alterations of the lymph node perfusion, also in the case of lymph nodes having a maximum diameter <1 cm.

22.6.1.2
Enhancement Patterns

The experience gained in our department with this technique has led to interesting, although still preliminary, results. Different contrast enhancement patterns (Fig. 22.1) were identified in lymph nodes.

Reactive lymph nodes give rise to diffuse intense and homogeneous contrast enhancement (Figs. 22.2 and 22.3) due to the intense vascularization with a rich cortical capillary circulation (GADRE et al. 1994).

Nodal metastases are generally less vascularized than the adjacent normal lymph node parenchyma, and they appear as perfusion defects inside the lymph nodes after microbubble injection (Figs. 22.1 and 22.4). In metastatic lymph nodes, the presence of completely avascular areas of necrosis (CASTELIJNS and VAN DEN BREKEL 2002) is frequently observed, and contrast enhancement may be very low or totally absent due to the confluence of wide areas of necrosis extending also to the entire node. It should be underlined that the presence of necrosis, which is considered a specific sign of metastasis under investigation with CT and MR imaging (CASTELIJNS and VAN DEN BREKEL 2002), may be the result of a phlogistic process, such as in tubercular nodes and lymphadenitis.

Contrast-enhancement patterns after microbubble-based agent injection in lymphomas present a more variable appearance (Fig. 22.1), which is partially similar to the patterns of reactive and metastatic lymph nodes. Lymphomas often present diffuse and heterogeneous contrast enhancement with a dotted appearance at arterial phase (Fig. 22.5). However, lymphomas may reveal a diffuse contrast enhancement pattern after microbubble injection, especially in low-grade malignity lymphomas, similarly to reactive or inflammatory lymph nodes. Dotted contrast enhancement at arterial phase was observed only in lymphomas, and it is probably related to the presence of hypertrophic arterial vessels larger than those present in the other forms of lymphadenopathies which appear punctiform throughout the parenchyma (RUBALTELLI et al. 2004).

22.6.1.3
Personal Experience

The study of lymph node perfusion after microbubble-based agent injection was performed in 56 histologically analyzed lymph nodes. The assessment of lymph node appearance after microbubble injection,

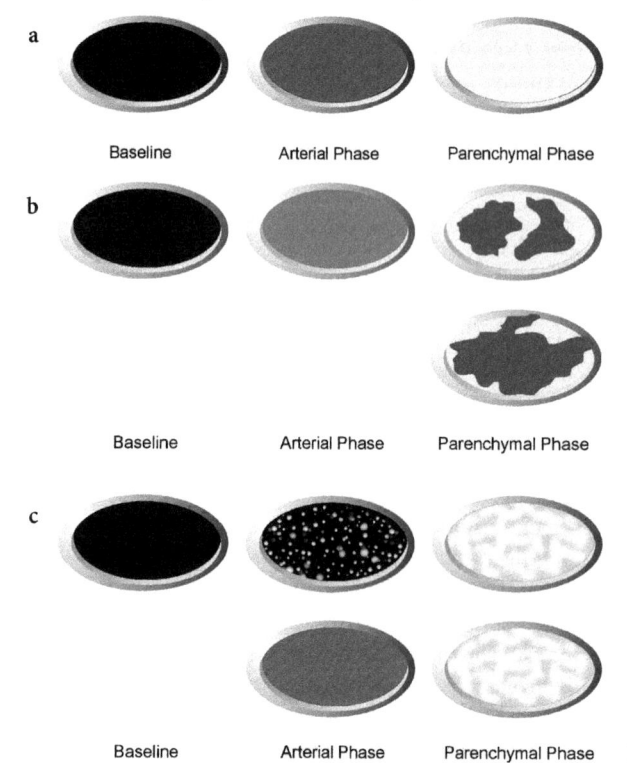

Fig. 22.1a–c. The different contrast enhancement patterns in lymph nodes after microbubble injection. **a** Normal or reactive lymph nodes. In normal or reactive lymph nodes contrast enhancement appears low at arterial phase and diffusely homogeneous at late (parenchymal) phase. **b** Metastases. At arterial phase contrast enhancement appears low. At late (parenchymal) phase metastases are characterized by heterogeneous contrast enhancement due to perfusion defects from tumoral infiltration and necrosis. **c** Lymphomas. In lymphomas different contrast enhancement patterns may be observed. At arterial phase contrast enhancement may appear dotted, related to the presence of tumoral vessels arising from neoangiogenesis, or diffuse as in reactive lymph nodes. At late (parenchymal) phase contrast enhancement appear diffusely heterogeneous

Lymph Nodes

Fig. 22.2a-c. Reactive lymph node. **a** Baseline US of reactive lymph node (*arrows*) of the neck with oval shape, regular margins and homogeneous hypoechoic structure. **b** Contrast specific mode (Contrast Tuned Imaging; Esaote, Genoa, Italy) before injection of contrast agent. **c** After injection of sulfur hexafluoride-filled microbubbles, the node, in the late (parenchymal) phase, shows diffuse contrast enhancement

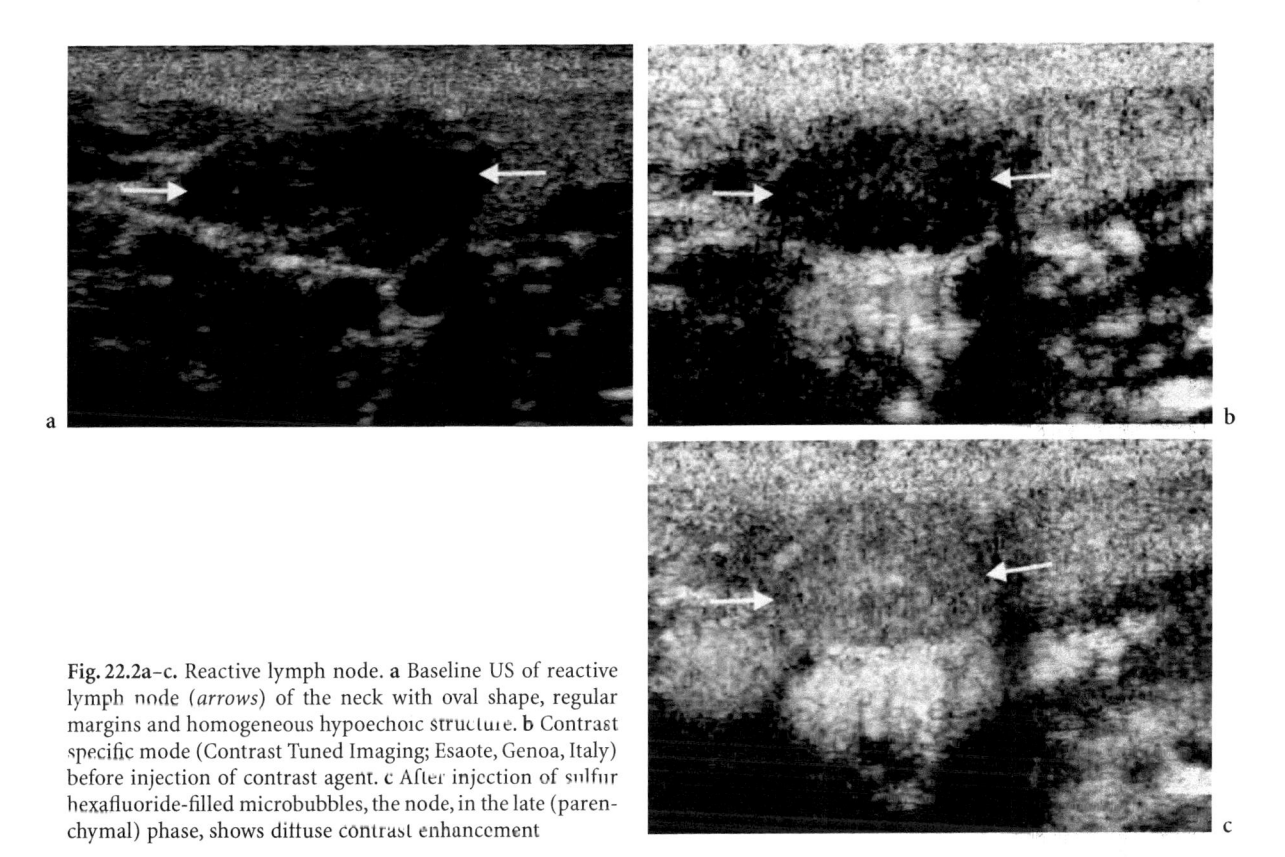

Fig. 22.3a,b. Reactive lymph node. **a** Baseline US shows round lymph node (*arrows*) without echogenic hilus. **b** Contrast-enhanced US shows diffuse and homogeneous contrast enhancement in the late (parenchymal) phase

correctly modified nine (16%) diagnoses firstly proposed on baseline US and power Doppler US, whereas in three lymph nodes the diagnostic conclusion was incorrect. Only one lymph node, correctly assessed as neoplastic (non-HD lymphoma) after baseline US, was incorrectly classified as benign following microbubble injection (RUBALTELLI et al. 2004).

In conclusion, these results show that contrast-enhanced US provides highly accurate differentiation between benign and malignant lymph nodes. Furthermore, after detection of a perfusion defect also in lymph nodes of smaller than 1 cm, contrast-enhanced US may be considered a means to indicate the most opportune site for fine-needle sampling.

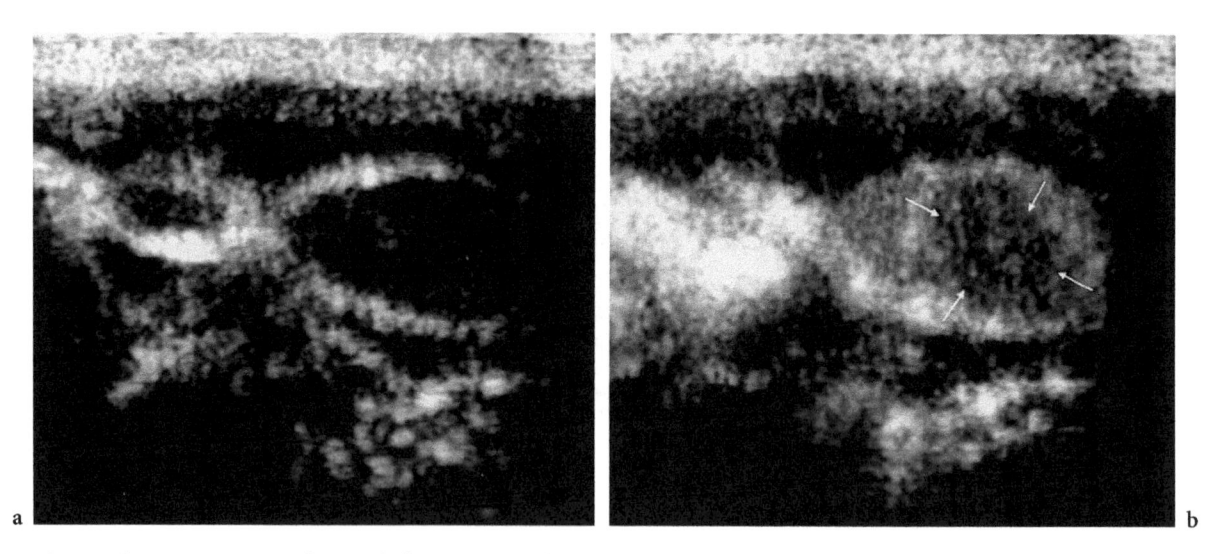

Fig. 22.4a,b. Metastasis. **a** Baseline US before injection of contrast agent shows oval-shaped lymph node with regular margins and homogeneous structure. **b** Contrast-enhanced US shows diffuse contrast enhancement in the normal parenchyma and a central hypoechoic perfusion defect (*arrows*) due to intranodal metastasis in late (parenchymal) phase. [Reproduced with permission from RUBALTELLI et al. (2004)

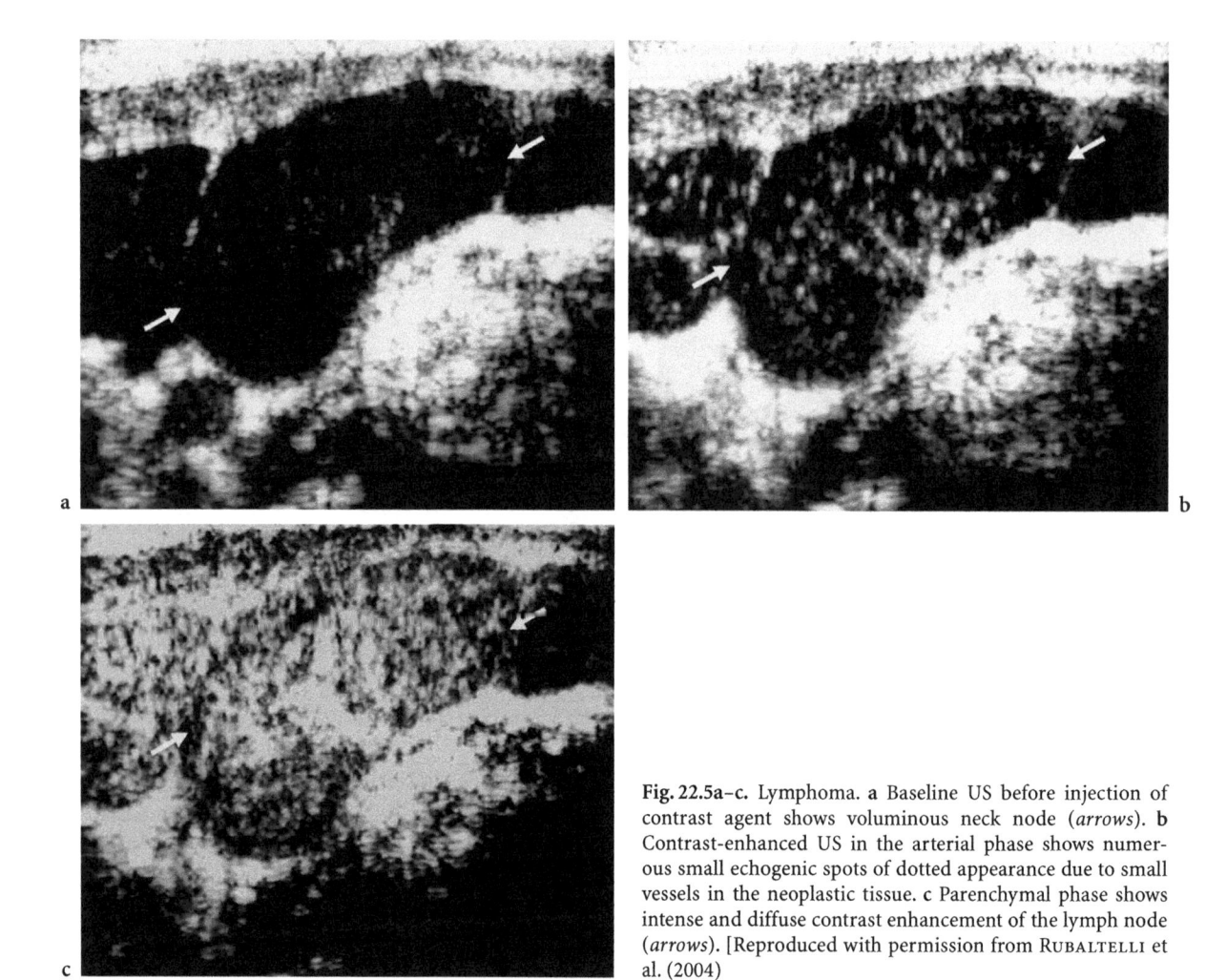

Fig. 22.5a–c. Lymphoma. **a** Baseline US before injection of contrast agent shows voluminous neck node (*arrows*). **b** Contrast-enhanced US in the arterial phase shows numerous small echogenic spots of dotted appearance due to small vessels in the neoplastic tissue. **c** Parenchymal phase shows intense and diffuse contrast enhancement of the lymph node (*arrows*). [Reproduced with permission from RUBALTELLI et al. (2004)

22.6.2
Quantitative Study

The video sequences obtained after microbubble-based contrast agent injection and stored in digital format can be analyzed off-site by means of proprietary softwares, enabling objective evaluation of the quantitative parameters of perfusion. Images are processed automatically, and the video intensity of the signal is analyzed in every pixel to generate chromatic parametric maps of the various perfusion parameters such as the highest echo-signal intensity value reached in each pixel, the time to reach 50% of the highest echo-signal intensity value, the difference between the maximum and minimum value of echo-signal intensity and the slope of signal intensity increase. Such parametric maps permit immediate evaluation of the perfusion properties of the entire lymph node, according to the shape or size of the region of interest selected by the operator. The same procedure may be employed to compare the perfusion characteristics of the area of the lymph node to the other reference areas, such as the surrounding tissues or the large vessels.

Dedicated equipment and softwares may graphically represent the relation between the echo-signal video-intensity with time. These qualitative studies are still experimental in the case of lymph nodes, even though it is also possible to obtain quantitative objective data to differentiate areas of normal tissue from perfusion defects (Fig. 22.6).

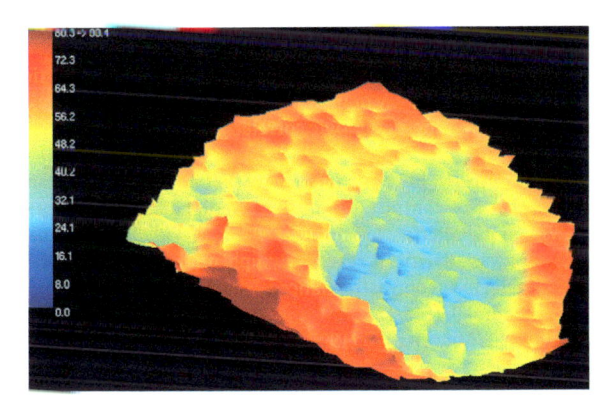

Fig. 22.6. Quantitative evaluation of perfusion in a metastatic lymph node. The maximum intensity of the signal in each pixel after microbubble-based contrast agent injection is represented by the map with a color scale from *dark red* (maximum contrast enhancement) to *dark blue* (absence of contrast enhancement). In this case, the map reveals the presence of a widespread perfusion defect

22.7
Sentinel Lymph Node – Lymphosonography

The identification and intraoperative biopsy of the sentinel lymph node is utilized in surgery for mammary carcinoma and cutaneous melanoma. Location is commonly achieved by lymphoscintigraphy, by means of an interstitial perilesional injection of 99-m Tc human albumin nanocolloids.

Recently, the use of contrast-enhanced US has been proposed after interstitial (subcutaneous or submucosal) injection of microbubble-based contrast agents to identify the sentinel lymph node (Tornes et al. 2002; Goldberg et al. 2004), and this technique is named lymphosonography. It is possible to trace the lymphatic channels from the injection site up to the draining sentinel lymph node(s) by lymphosonography. These studies have provided encouraging results, but such techniques are still experimental and currently only applied on animals. The advantage of lymphosonography over lymphoscintigraphy is the possibility to identify intranodal metastases (Goldberg et al. 2004).

Similar methodology has been proposed to obtain indirect US lymphography, which showed homogeneous contrast enhancement in normal lymph nodes after microbubble-based agent injection and the presence of perfusion defects or heterogeneous enhancement in metastatic lymph nodes (Kono et al. 2002).

22.8
Conclusions

High-resolution US and color/power Doppler US are commonly utilized for the study of superficial lymph nodes. The evaluation of morphology, echo structure, and vascularity of lymph nodes, together with the clinical and laboratory data, enables the selection of those cases to be examined either by US-guided fine-needle aspiration or by surgical biopsy.

The most recent harmonic imaging techniques combined with intravenous administration of a microbubble-based contrast agent can supply further useful information in cases where doubt has arisen with conventional techniques. The possibility to obtain data in relation to lymph node microvascularity represents a further step, even though the results are still preliminary and necessitate further confirmation over a wider range of cases.

Contrast-enhanced US was showed to differentiate benign from neoplastic lymph nodes to a high degree of accuracy in comparison to baseline US, and revealed capabilities to identify perfusion defects also in lymph nodes <1 cm. In addition to the diagnostic significance, contrast-enhanced US may guide US-guided fine-needle aspiration to the most suitable lymph node portion for cytology.

References

Adibelli ZH, Unal G, Gul E et al (1998) Differentiation of benign and malignant cervical lymph nodes: value of B.mode and color Doppler sonography. Eur J Radiol 28:230-234

Ahuja A, Ying M (2002) An overview of neck node sonography. Invest Radiol 37:333-342

Ahuja A, Ying M (2003) Sonography of neck lymph nodes, part II. Abnormal lymph nodes. Clin Radiol 58:359-366

Ahuja A, Ying M, Ho SSY, Metreweli C (2001) Distribution of intranodal vessels in differentiating benign from metastatic neck nodes. Clin Radiol 56:197-201

Bellin MF, Beigelman C, Precetti-Morel S (2000) Iron oxide-enhanced MR lymphography: initial experience. Eur J Radiol 34:257-264

Castelijns JA, van den Brekel MW (2002) Imaging of lymphadenopathy in the neck. Eur Radiol 12:727-738

Choi MY, Lee JW, Jang KJ (1995) Distinction between benign and malignant causes of cervical, axillary and inguinal lymphadenopathy: value of Doppler spectral waveform analysis. AJR 165:981-984

Ferrari FS, Cozza S, Guazzi G et al (1997) Ruolo del Color Doppler nella diagnosi differenziale delle adenopatie benigne e maligne. Radiol Med 93:242-245

Gadre A, Briner W, O'Leary M (1994) A scanning electron microscope study of the human cervical lymph node. Acta Otolaryngol 114:87-90

Giovagnorio F, Caiazzo R, Avitto A (1997) Evaluation of vascular patterns of cervical lymph nodes with power doppler sonography. J Clin Ultrasound 25:71-76

Giovagnorio F, Galluzzo M, Andreoli C et al (2002) Color Doppler sonography in the evaluation of superficial lymphomatous lymph nodes. J Ultrasound Med 21:403-408

Goldberg BB, Merton DA, Liu JB et al (2004) Sentinel lymph nodes in a swine model with melanoma: contrast-enhanced lymphatic US. Radiology 230:727-734

Ho SS, Ahuja AT, Kew J, Metreweli C (2000) Differentiation of lymphadenopathy in different forms of carcinoma with Doppler sonography. Clin Radiol 55:627-631

Kono Y, Choi S, Corbeil J et al (2002) Indirect US lymphography to distinguish normal from metastatic lymph nodes (abstract) Radiology 225:586

Mack MG, Balzer JO, Straub R et al (2002) Superparamagnetic iron oxide-enhanced MR imaging of head and neck lymph nodes. Radiology 222:239-244

Marchal G, Oyen R, Verschakelen J et al (1985) Sonographic appearance of normal lymph nodes. J Ultrasound Med 4:417-419

Maurer J, William C, Schroeder R et al (1997) Evaluation of metastases and reactive lymoh nodes in Doppler sonography using an ultrasound contrast enhancer. Invest Radiol 32:441-446

Moritz JD, Ludwig A, Oestmann JW (2000) Contrast-enhanced color Doppler sonography for evaluation of enlarged cervical lymph nodes in head and neck tumors. AJR 174:1279-1284

Na DG, Lim HK, Byun HS et al (1997) Differential diagnosis of cervical lymphadenopathy: usefulness of color Doppler sonography. AJR 168:1311-1316

Perin B, Gardellin G, Nisi E et al (1987) Ultrasonic diagnosis of the central hyperechogenic area in lymph nodes. A sign of benign lymphadenopathy. Radiol Med 74:535-538

Rubaltelli L, Proto E, Salmaso R et al (1990) Sonography of abnormal lymph nodes in vitro: correlation of sonographic and histologic findings. AJR Am J Roentgenol 155:1241-1244

Rubaltelli L, Khadivi Y, Tregnaghi A et al (2004) Evaluation of lymph node perfusion using continuous mode harmonic ultrasound with a second generation contrast agent. J Ultrasound Med 23:829-836

Sigal R, Vogl T, Casselman J et al (2002) Lymph node metastases from head and neck squamous cell carcinoma: MR imaging with ultrasmall superparamagnetic oxide particles (Sinerem MR) - results of phase-III multicentric clinical trial. Eur Radiol 12:1104-1113

Solbiati L, Cova L, Tonolini M et al (2002) Improved characterization of reactive and malignant superficial lymph nodes using harmonic ultrasound with second generation contrast agent (abstract). Radiology 225:586

Steinkamp HJ, Mueffelmann M, Bock JC et al (1998) Differential diagnosis of lymph node lesions: a semiquantitative approach with colour Doppler ultrasound. Br J Radiol 71:828-833

Tornes A, Rasmussen H, Goldberg BB et al (2002) Sentinel lymph node identification with an ultrasound contrast agent. Experimental study in pigs (abstract). Radiology 225:586-587

Tschammler A, Ott G, Schang T et al (1998) Lymphadenopathy: differentiation of benign from malignant disease – color Doppler US assessment of intranodal angioarchitecture. Radiology 208:117-123

Vassallo P, Wernecke K, Roos N, Peters PE (1992) Differentiation of benign from malignant superficial lymphadenopathy: the role of high-resolution US. Radiology 183:215-220

Vassallo P, Edel G, Roos N et al (1993) In-vitro high-resolution ultrasonography of benign and malignant lymph nodes: a sonographic-pathologic correlation. Invest Radiol 28:698-705

Weinmann HJ, Ebert W, Misselwitz B et al (2003) Tissue-specific MR contrast agents. Eur J Radiol 46:33-44

Willam C, Maurer J, Schroeder R et al (1998) Assessment of vascularity in reactive lymph nodes by means of D-galactose contrast-enhanced Doppler sonography. Invest Radiol 33:146-152

Yang WT, Metreweli C (1998) Colour Doppler flow in normal axillary lymph nodes. Br J Radiol 71:381-383

Ying M, Ahuja A (2003) Sonography of neck lymph nodes, part I. Normal lymph nodes. Clin Radiol 58:351-358

Ying M, Ahuja A, Brook F, Metreweli C (2000) Power Doppler sonography of normal cervical lymph nodes. J Ultrasound Med 19:511-517

Ying M, Ahuja A, Brook F, Metreweli C (2001) Vascularity and grey-scale sonographic features of normal cervical lymph nodes: variations with nodal size. Clin Radiol 56:416-419

23 Female Pelvis

ANTONIA CARLA TESTA, ERIKA FRUSCELLA, GABRIELLA FERRANDINA,
MARINELLA MALAGGESE, GIOVANNI SCAMBIA, CATERINA EXACOUSTOS,
and EMILIO QUAIA

CONTENTS

23.1 Introduction 323
23.2 Ovarian Tumors 323
23.3 Uterine Fibroids 325
23.4 Evaluation of Fallopian Tube Patency 327
References 328

23.1
Introduction

Ultrasound (US) is considered the preferred imaging procedure in the study of female pelvis because it is widely available, non-invasive and able to provide definitive diagnostic information in many pathologies (DERCHI et al. 2001). As a first step, the female pelvis has to be examined by transabdominal US to provide global delineation of all organs and to allow a panoramic and complete evaluation of large lesions. Transvaginal US should be employed after transabdominal US and is the best examination technique to evaluate the female pelvis (DERCHI et al. 2001). Sonohysterography is an examination technique which provides a better analysis of the endometrial surface through distension of the endometrial lumen with 30 ml of sterile saline.

Microbubble-based contrast agents have been used in gynecological and obstetric US (ORDÉN et al. 1999a,b). The principal application is the assessment of vascularization of ovarian tumors. Other applications include the assessment of vascularization of uterine fibromas and the assessment of tubal patency.

23.2
Ovarian Tumors

Even though ovarian tumors are less frequent than uterine tumors, these lesions are the principal cause of death from gynecological malignancy (DERCHI et al. 2001). Since ovarian tumors determine non-specific symptoms in early stages, they are commonly discovered at advanced stages. Most ovarian tumors are benign, while 15% are malignant and 5% are secondary tumors (DERCHI et al. 2001). Epithelial tumors are the most common (70%–75% of all cases), and can be serous, mucinous, and endometrioid (DERCHI et al. 2001). Although the final diagnosis of an adnexal mass is based on findings at histologic examination, it is desirable to differentiate preoperatively between benign and malignant tumors to select the time, place, and type of surgery.

US is a well-established imaging modality for the assessment of pelvic masses and a subjective evaluation of the gray-scale US image by an expert sonographer can reach an accuracy of more than 90% in discriminating between benign and malignant adnexal masses (VALENTIN 1997). The absence of solid components and the absence of irregularities in an adnexal mass at US suggest benignity, whereas any irregularity – be it in the outline, the cyst wall or in the echogenicity of a tumor – suggests malignancy (VALENTIN 2004).

Malignant tumors are generally well-vascularized, with flow signals both at the periphery and in the central regions of the mass, while benign ovarian tumors appear relatively poorly vascularized (DERCHI et al. 2001). Malignant ovarian tumors have certain specific characteristics, such as neovessels with irregular course and arteriovenous shunts with high blood flow velocities. Muscularization of the

---

A. C. TESTA, MD; E. FRUSCELLA, MD; G. FERRANDINA, MD;
M. MALAGGESE, MD
Gynecologic Oncology Unit, Catholic University of Sacred Heart, L.go A. Gemelli 8, 00168 Rome, Italy
G. SCAMBIA, MD
Oncology Department, Catholic University of Sacred Heart, Centro di Ricerca e Formazione ad Alta Tecnologia nelle Scienze Biomediche, Campobasso, Italy
C. EXACOUSTOS, MD
Department of Surgery, Obstetrics and Gynecology Unit, University of Rome "Tor Vergata", Rome, Italy
E. QUAIA, MD
Department of Radiology, Cattinara Hospital, University of Trieste, Strada di Fiume 447, 34149 Trieste, Italy

vessel walls is incomplete and results in formation of tumoral lakes, low resistance to flow, and little systolic-diastolic variation in blood flow velocity. Color Doppler and power Doppler US can be used to detect neovascularization characteristic of malignant lesions (TEKAY and JOUPPILA 1992). However, the combination of gray-scale US morphology and Doppler flow imaging information does not seem to yield much improvement in diagnostic accuracy (STEIN et al. 1995), even though it may increase the diagnostic confidence to make a correct diagnosis of benignity or malignancy (VALENTIN 2004).

Recently, a multicenter study (International Ovarian Tumor Analysis, IOTA) based on artificial intelligence models has been conducted in >1000 patients. The preliminary results of this study demonstrate that the parameter (presence of solid vascularized parts in an adnexal lesion) is highly predictive of malignancy (TIMMERMAN et al. 2004). However, some pelvic masses with solid parts and some multilocular cysts with a high number of locules remain difficult to be classified as benign or malignant.

Microbubble-based contrast agents have been used to enhance Doppler signal in tumoral vessels (SUREN et al. 1994; ORDÉN et al. 1999a,b, 2000). Recently, dedicated contrast-enhanced US technologies, such as contrast tuned imaging, have been developed to optimize the use of microbubble-based contrast agents and to produce microbubble insonation at low acoustic power for several minutes. Dedicated contrast specific techniques at low acoustic power insonation with perfluorocarbon or sulfur hexafluoride microbubbles allow visualization of a dramatically higher number of intralesional vessels in comparison to color Doppler US.

In our preliminary experience in the evaluation of uncertain pelvic masses the application of contrast tuned imaging with sulfur hexafluoride-filled microbubbles (SonoVue, Bracco, Italy) provided an improvement in the diagnostic confidence of the operator to distinguish benign from malignant adnexal lesions. In particular, the absence of perfusion in uncertain pelvic masses, with no detectable vessels in the solid intracystic tissue, improved the

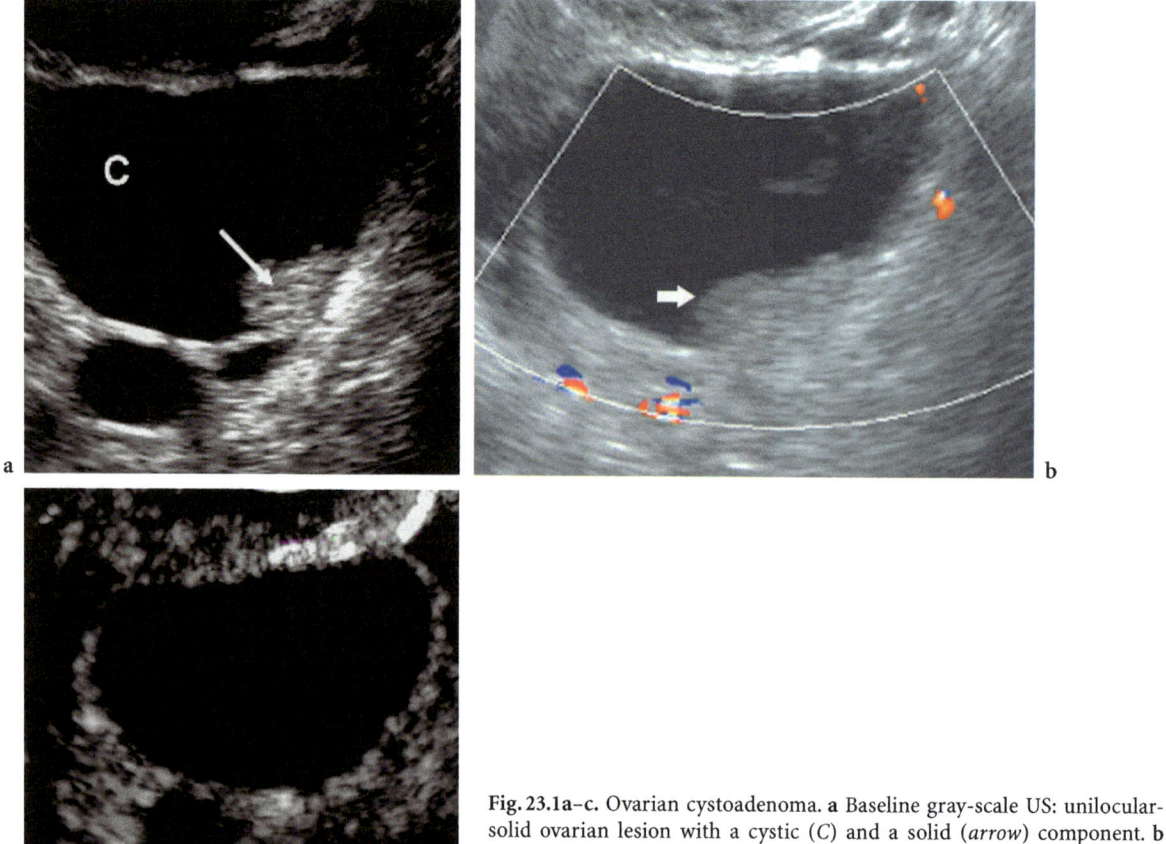

Fig. 23.1a–c. Ovarian cystoadenoma. **a** Baseline gray-scale US: unilocular-solid ovarian lesion with a cystic (*C*) and a solid (*arrow*) component. **b** Color Doppler US revealing no flow signals in the solid component (*arrow*) of the tumor. **c** Contrast-enhanced US reveals absence of contrast enhancement in the solid component

diagnostic confidence of the operator in making a benignity diagnosis confirmed by histology (Figs. 23.1 and Fig. 23.2), while the presence of perfusion in uncertain pelvic masses, with detectable vessels in the solid intracystic tissue, could play an important role to confirm the diagnosis of malignancy (Fig. 23.3) (Testa et al. 2003b).

An objective digital analysis of kinetics of an air-filled microbubble-based contrast agent in imaging benign and malignant adnexal tumors, with a special focus on the timing of the transit of the microbubble bolus, was shown in a recent study (Ordén et al. 2003). After a quick rise in intensity, the washout phase was biphasic, firstly with a fast linear decrease (distribution phase) and, secondly, with a slow linear decrease (elimination phase). Both the baseline and maximum power Doppler intensities, as the rise in intensity compared to time, were significantly higher in malignant than in benign ovarian tumors. The microbubbles arrival time was significantly shorter in malignant than it was in benign tumors. This could be caused by the high-velocity flow through the arteriovenous shunts that are typically found in malignant neovascularization.

Besides changes in echo-signal intensity, the duration of contrast enhancement and the value of the area under the time-intensity curve appeared to be the best discriminating factors between benign and malignant tumors. Ordén et al. (2003) found that the mean duration of microbubble contrast effect was 190.4 s in malignant tumors, and 103.6 s in benign tumors. The longer persistence of enhancement in malignant lesions could be explained by microbubbles pooling of the contrast agent in dilated and blind-ending vessels. The bypass of capillary beds through arteriovenous shunts will reduce the rate of bubble destruction and will result in an higher microbubble concentration in malignant tumors vasculature.

New softwares performing qualitative and quantitative analysis of the time intensity curves are under evaluation. Qontrast (Contrast Quantification Tool, AMID and R&D, Bracco, Milan, Italy) software analyzes the time sequences of digitally stored perfusion images and enables objective evaluation of quantitative perfusion parameters of any portion of an organ during each set of frames. The resulting parametric maps allow the visual assessment of perfusion features over the entire selected region (Fig. 23.4). The aim of this representation is to maximize accuracy and reproducibility of results in contrast enhancement analysis and to minimize the inter- and intra-operator variability.

23.3
Uterine Fibroids

Uterine fibroids (fibroleiomyomas) are the most common tumors of the uterus and the most common cause of uterine enlargement. They are benign tumors made of smooth muscle fibers intermixed

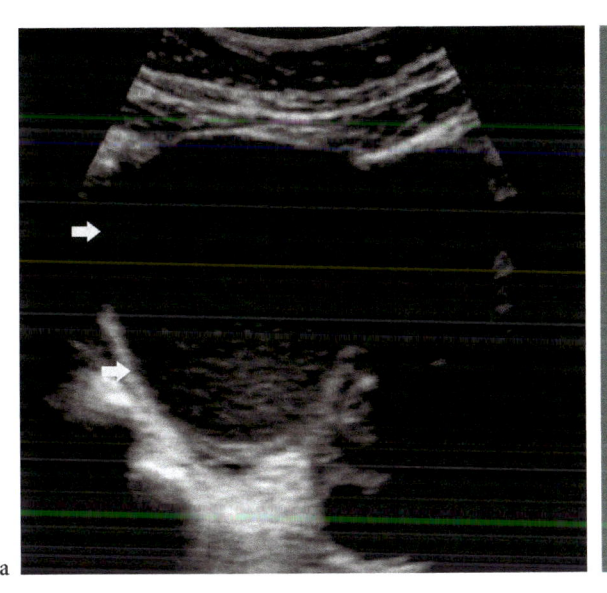

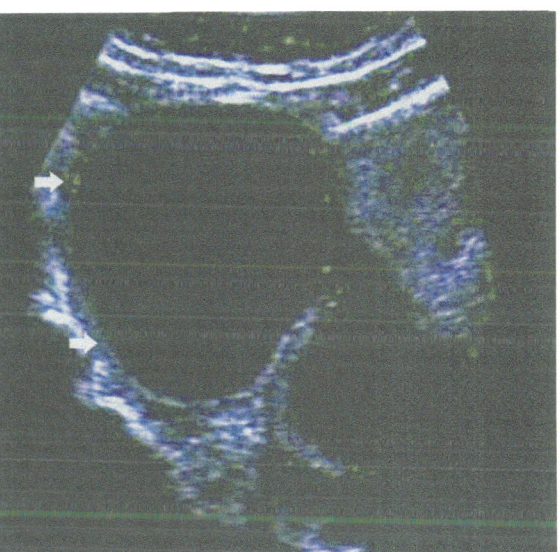

Fig. 23.2a,b. Cystic endometriosis in the right ovary. a Baseline US reveals a round lesion with corpuscular content (*arrows*). b Contrast-enhanced US reveals absence of contrast enhancement in the context of the lesion (*arrows*) which reveals only a slight peripheral enhancement in the cystic wall. [Images courtesy of Dr. Roberta Padovan, Aloka, Tokyo, Japan]

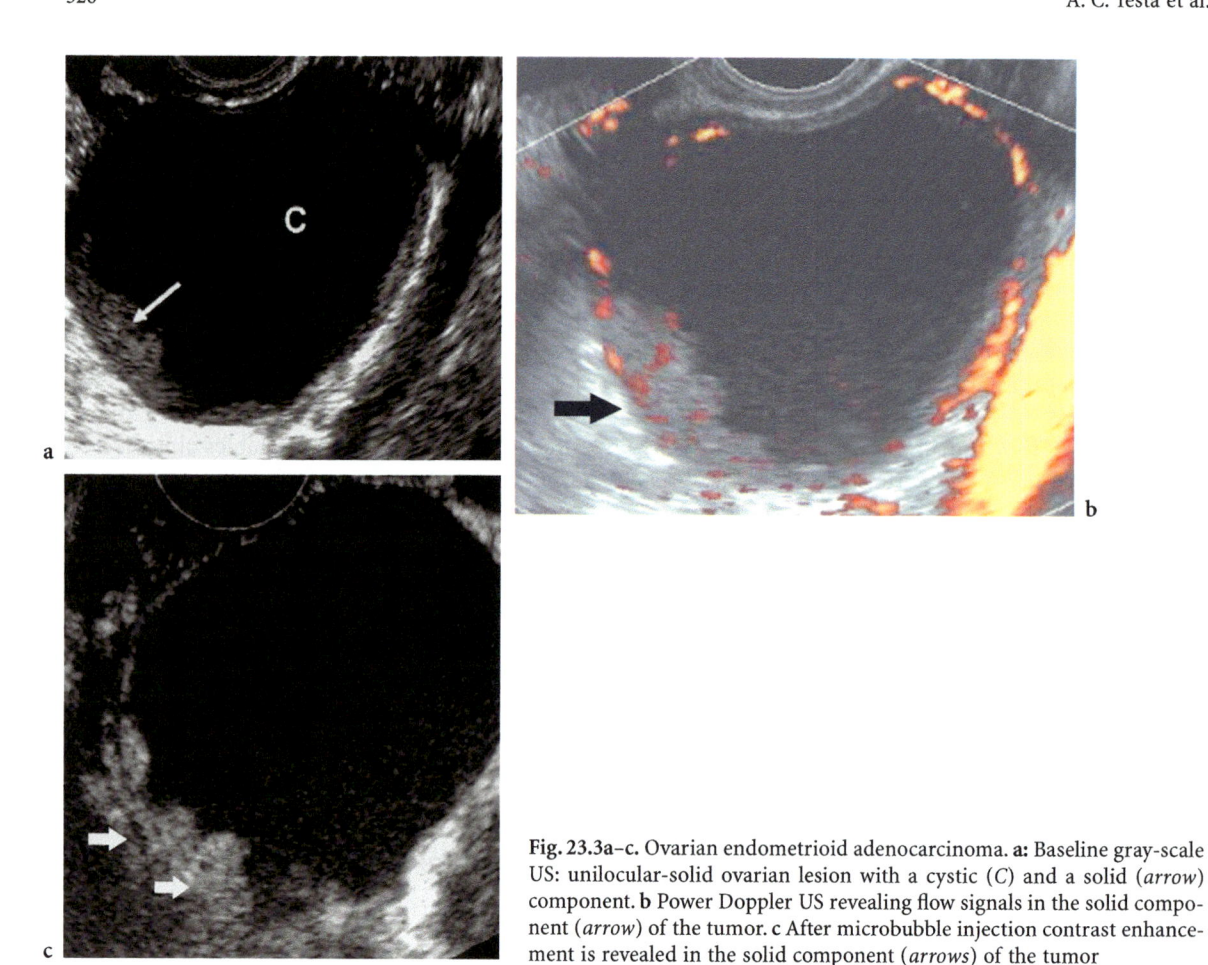

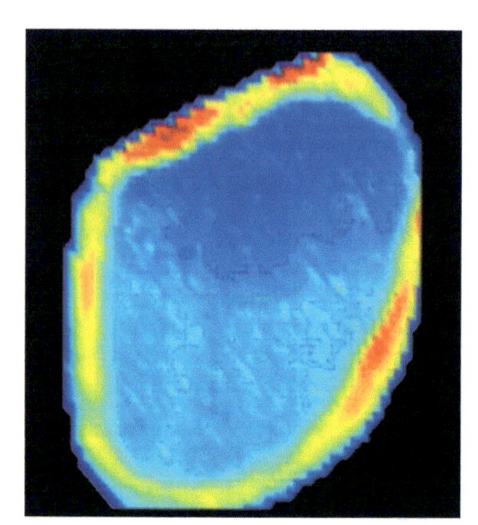

Fig. 23.3a–c. Ovarian endometrioid adenocarcinoma. a: Baseline gray-scale US: unilocular-solid ovarian lesion with a cystic (*C*) and a solid (*arrow*) component. b Power Doppler US revealing flow signals in the solid component (*arrow*) of the tumor. c After microbubble injection contrast enhancement is revealed in the solid component (*arrows*) of the tumor

Fig. 23.4. The "QONTRAST" software application to contrast-enhanced US examination of a unilocular ovarian lesion. The resulting parametric map, in which different colors express a different microbubble uptake, allows a visual assessment of perfusion properties over the entire selected region at once

with a variable amount of fibrous connective tissue (DERCHI et al. 2001). Fibroids are usually multiple and grow under estrogen influence. They are most commonly located in the intramural myometrium, while submucosal and subserosal fibroids may determine respectively abnormal uterine bleeding or simulate an adnexal mass. At baseline US, uterine fibroids appear as well-defined masses with a hypoechoic, or less frequently hyper- or isoechoic, echostructure if compared to myometrium.

Baseline color and power Doppler US are effective to reveal the vascularization in uterine fibroids. In our experience (TESTA et al. 2003a) the preoperative Doppler evaluation of uterine fibroids did not provide predictive information about the proliferative status of the tumor. A significant correlation was found between the size of the fibroid and the resistive index, as well as between the volume of the fibroid and resistive index. The injection of sulfur hexafluoride-filled microbubbles did not add any further useful information to baseline US (Fig. 23.5).

Female Pelvis

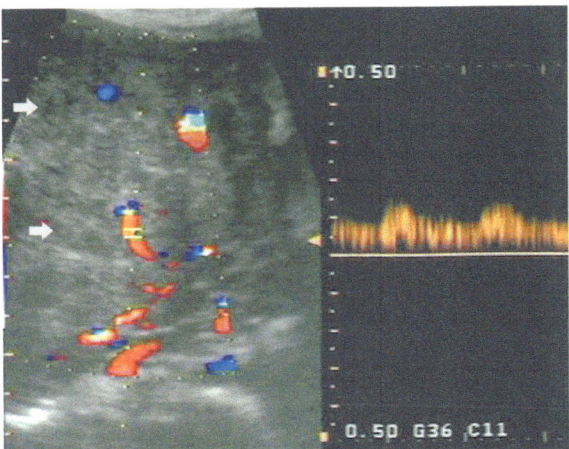

Fig. 23.5a–c. Uterine fibroid. Baseline color Doppler US (a) reveals only some peripheral vessels with arterial flow at Doppler interrogation. Contrast-enhanced US reveals diffuse contrast enhancement in the uterine fibroid during arterial phase (b), also with evidence of tumoral vessels, and microbubble washout at late phase (c)

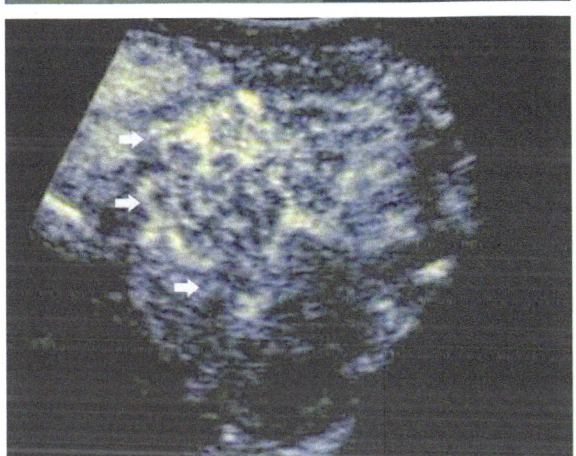

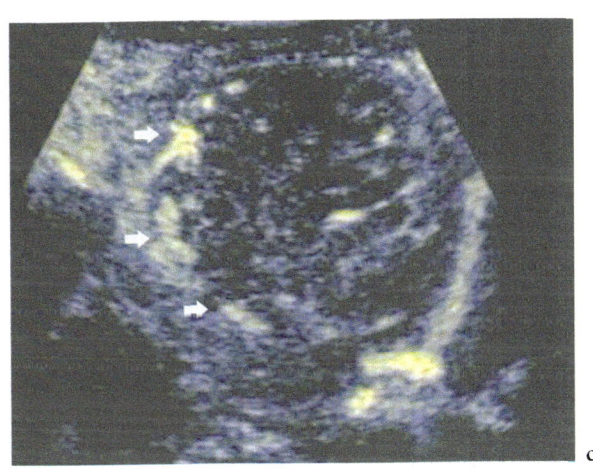

23.4
Evaluation of Fallopian Tube Patency

Infertility is a common problem in the developing world, affecting 10%–15% of the couples (CHENIA et al. 1997). An important part of any protocol for investigation of the infertile couple is the assessment of fallopian tube patency in the woman, as this can influence the future course of treatment. Several authors have suggested saline solution as the first-choice agent to assess the endometrial cavity (PARSONS and LENSE 1993; GOLDSTEIN 1996). X-ray hysterosalpingography and laparoscopic dye-test are currently the main procedures for investigating tubal patency.

The recent development of hysterosalpingo contrast sonography may offer some benefits over these two methods. Hysterosalpingo contrast sonography involves a transvaginal US investigation of the fallopian tubes both before and after the injection of a microbubble-based contrast agent into the tubes via the uterine cavity. After initial precontrast transvaginal US, the cervix and vagina are cleansed with sterile sodium chloride solution. A 5-F intrauterine balloon catheter is then introduced transcervically without the use of a tenaculum, unless catheterization is hindered by marked anteversion, retroversion, or flexion of the uterine corpus. The intrauterine balloon catheter is employed to avoid reflux of contrast through the cervical os (CAMPBELL et al. 1994; DIETRICH et al. 1996; DERCHI et al. 2001). The uterine cavity is then analyzed using sterile saline solution and, finally, after Echovist (SHU 454, Schering, Berlin, Germany) or SonoVue (Bracco, Milan, Italy) injection. Microbubbles are slowly injected through the catheter in 1- to 2-ml boluses under US control (HAMILTON et al. 1998). Microbubbles firstly fill the isthmic portion of each fallopian tube, while later they fill the whole tube up to the distal portion (Fig. 23.6). Both the passage of microbubbles through the tubes and spillage into the peritoneal cavity can be assessed by color Doppler or dedicated contrast specific modes (DERCHI et al. 2001).

Hysterosalpingo contrast sonography is considered a first-line screening method to select infertile women

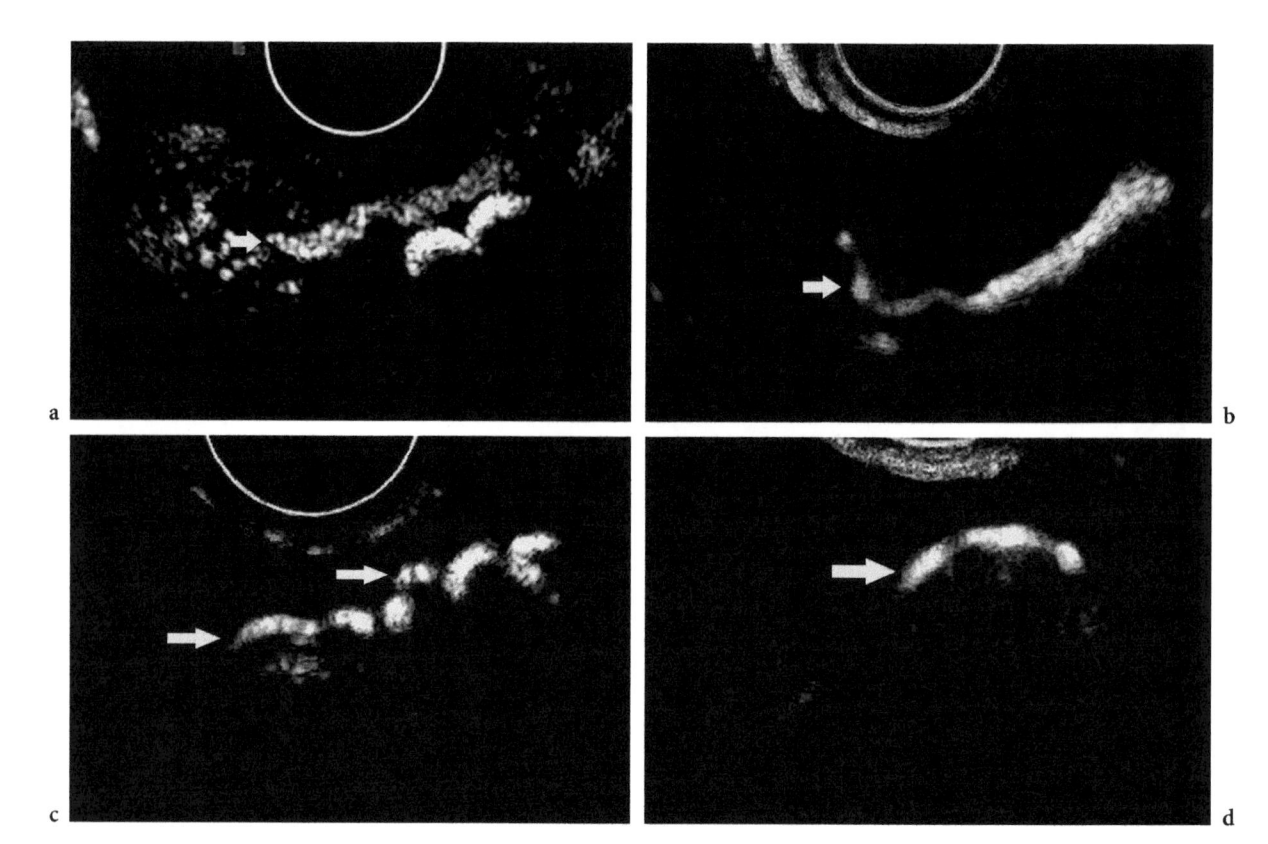

Fig. 23.6a-d. Hysterosalpingo contrast-sonography. a,b Transverse section through the uterine fundus following SonoVue injection. The isthmic portion of the left fallopian tube is visualized (*arrow*). c Normal left fallopian tube which is depicted from the isthmic uterine tract up to the distal tract (*arrows*), where it spills adjacent to the ovary. d Distal portion of the normal fallopian tube with spill from fimbrial end (*arrow*)

in whom more invasive investigations are likely to reveal pathology (HAMILTON et al. 1998; EXACOUSTOS et al. 2003). Hysterosalpingography with saline solution is limited in demonstrating fallopian tube patency, especially in the corneal region (CHENIA et al. 1997; HAMILTON et al. 1998), while hysterosalpingo contrast sonography provides a complete tubal assessment limiting the number of visits that infertile women must undergo (HAMILTON et al. 1998).

References

Campbell S, Bourne TH, Tan SL, Collins WP (1994) Hysterosalpingo contrast sonography (HyCoSy) and its future role within the investigation of infertility in Europe. Ultrasound Obstet Gynecol 1:245-253

Chenia F, Hofmeyer GJ, Moolla S, Oratis P (1997) Sonographic hydrotubation using agitated saline: a new technique for improving fallopian tube visualization. Br J Radiol 70:833-836

Derchi L, Serafini G, Gandolfo N et al (2001) Ultrasound in gynecology. Eur Radiol 11:2137-2155

Dietrich M, Suren A, Hinney B (1996) Evaluation of tubal patency by hysterocontrast sonography (HyCoSy, Echovist) and its correlation with laparoscopic findings. J Clin Ultrasound 24:523-527

Exacoustos C, Zupi E, Carusotti C et al (2003) Hysterosalpingo-contrast sonography compared with hysterosalpingography and laparoscopic dye perturbation to evaluate tubal patency. J Am Assoc Gynecol Lapar 10:29-32

Goldstein SR (1996) Saline infusion sonohysterography. Clin Obstet Gynecol 39:248-258

Hamilton JA, Larson AJ, Lower AM et al (1998) Evaluation of the performance of hysterosalpingo contrast sonography in 500 consecutive, unselected, infertile women. Hum Reprod 13:1519-1526

Ordén MR, Gudmundsson S, Kirkinen P (1999a) Intravascular ultrasound contrast agent: an aid in imaging intervillous blood flow? Placenta 20:235-240

Ordén MR, Gudmundsson S, Helin HL, Kirkinen P (1999b) Intravascular contrast agent in the ultrasonography of ectopic pregnancy. Ultrasound Obstet Gynecol 14:348-352

Ordén MR, Gudmundsson S, Kirkinen P (2000) Contrast-enhanced sonography in the examination of benign and malignant adnexal masses. J Ultrasound Med 19:783-788

Ordén MR, Jurvelin JS, Kirkinen PP (2003) Kinetics of a US contrast agent in benign and malignant adnexal tumors. Radiology 226:405-410

Parsons AK, Lense JJ (1993) Sonohysterography for endometrial abnormalities: preliminary results. J Clin Ultrasound 21:87-95

Stein SM, Leifer-Narin S, Jhonson MB et al (1995) Differentiation of benign and malignant adnexal masses: relative value of gray-scale, color Doppler, and spectral Doppler sonography. AJR Am J Roentgenol 164:381-386

Suren A, Osmers R, Kulenkampff D, Kuhn W (1994) Visualization of blood flow in small ovarian tumor vessels by transvaginal color Doppler sonography after echo enhancement with injection of Levovist. Gynecol Obstet Invest 38:210-212

Tekay A., Jouppila P (1992) Validity of pulsatility and resistance indices in classification of adnexal tumors with transvaginal color Doppler ultrasound. Ultrasound Obstet Gynecol 2:338-344

Testa AC, Pomini F, Fattorossi A et al (2003a) Doppler velocimetry and cytofluorimetric analysis in uterine myomas. Gynecol Obstet Invest 56:139-142

Testa AC, Timmerman D, Ferrazzi E, Arduini D (2003b) Preliminary experience with Sono Vue. 13th world congress on ultrasound in obstetrics and gynecology (abstract). 31 Aug-4 Sept, Paris, France

Timmerman D, Valentin L, Testa AC et al (2004) Classifying ovarian masses and lessons from IOTA trial. Ultrasound Obstet Gynecol 24:261

Valentin L (1997) Gray scale sonography, subjective evaluation of the color Doppler image and measurement of blood flow velocity for distinguish benign and malignant tumors of suspected adnexal origin. Eur J Obstet Gynecol 72:63-72

Valentin L (2004) Use of morphology to characterize and manage common adnexal masses. Best Pract Res Clin Obstet Gynaecol 18:71-89

24 Vesicoureteral Reflux

Emilio Quaia

CONTENTS

24.1 Introduction *331*
24.1.1 Technique and Clinical Results *331*
References *334*

24.1
Introduction

Vesicoureteral reflux is the most common urinary tract abnormality in children, with a 1%–2% incidence in the general population (Ascenti et al. 2004; Valentini et al. 2004), and 30%–50% incidence in children with multiple episodes of urinary tract infections. Even though traditional retrograde voiding cystourethrography or radionuclide cystography still remain the reference standard techniques, contrast-enhanced voiding sonocystography now appears as a valuable alternative method, due to the absence of radiation dose and the properties of microbubble-based contrast agents (Mentzel et al. 1999; Darge et al. 2001; Valentini et al. 2004).

Recently, contrast-enhanced voiding sonocystography has been proposed both for the diagnosis and follow-up of vesicoureteral reflux in children (Darge et al. 1999; Ascenti et al. 2004). Several studies have shown the high diagnostic accuracy of contrast-enhanced voiding sonocystography compared to voiding cystourethrography (Berrocal et al. 2001; Valentini et al. 2001) and direct radionuclide cystography (Ascenti et al. 2003) to detect and grade (Darge and Troeger 2002) vesicoureteral reflux in children.

Because of its accuracy, contrast-enhanced voiding sonocystography may replace radiological voiding cystourethrography in the detection of vesicoureteral reflux in girls, the follow-up in boys, and in the management of recurrent infection in children presenting with normal radiological voiding cystourethrography (Galloy et al. 2003).

Further studies have proved the efficacy of voiding sonocystography to detect and grade vesicoureteral reflux also in adult patients who had undergone renal transplantation with previous evidence of urinary tract infection (Kmetec et al. 2001; Valentini et al. 2004).

24.1.1 Technique and Clinical Results

The bladder is emptied after aseptic introduction of a 5- to 8-F infant feeding tube. The bladder is then filled with 200–250 ml of room-temperature saline solution. Microbubble-based contrast agent is administered in a volume of 10% of the bladder volume (Valentini et al. 2004). After microbubble administration, a suspension of a small volume of saline solution is injected in order to push the residual contrast agent through the catheter. In this way, echogenic microbubbles are easily identified in the bladder, which is filled by anechoic saline solution (Fig. 24.1). Harmonic imaging, gray-scale dedicated contrast specific techniques, or pseudo-Doppler contrast specific techniques including stimulated acoustic emission (Riccabona et al. 2003) need to be employed to detect microbubbles.

The microbubbles first reach the ventral region of the bladder creating a posterior strong acoustic shadowing and obscuring the dorsal region of the bladder. By increasing slowly the acoustic power of insonation, microbubbles are distributed into the vesical lumen. Then, acoustic power is switched at the lowest level (mechanical index: 0.04–0.2) to get a satisfactory visualization of microbubbles. During microbubble administration, the bladder, ureter, renal pelvis and calyces are evaluated by color or contrast-specific harmonic US modes. The same evaluation is repeated during the voiding phase.

E. Quaia, MD
Department of Radiology, Cattinara Hospital, University of Trieste, Strada di Fiume 447, Trieste, 34149, Italy

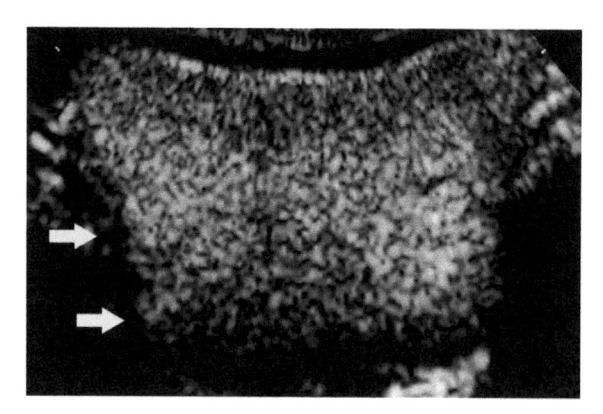

Fig. 24.1. Normal appearance of the bladder (*arrows*) previously filled by microbubble-based agents in a 5-month-old boy. (Image courtesy of Dr. G. Ascenti)

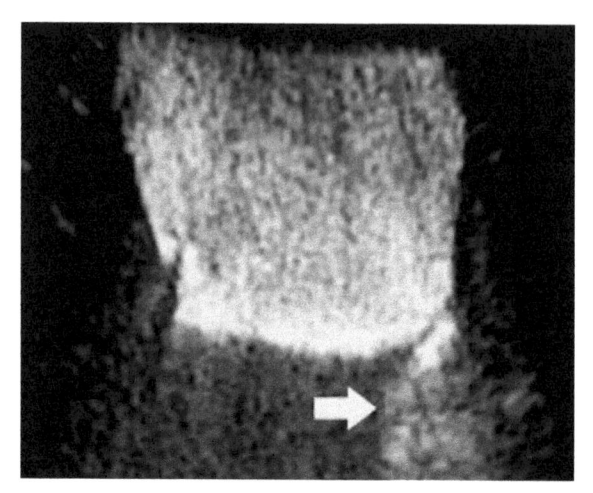

Fig. 24.2. A 2-month-old girl with a grade I vesicoureteric reflux. Bladder fully distended by microbubble-based contrast agent. Minimal vesicoureteric reflux (*arrow*) into the terminal left ureter. [Reproduced with permission from ASCENTI et al. (2004)]

Diagnosis of vesicoureteral reflux is assigned on the basis of echoes refluxing from the bladder to the ureter (Fig. 24.2), renal pelvis, and renal calyces (Fig. 24.3) or when color signals are seen in the urinary tract (VALENTINI et al. 2004). The associated morphologic signs (dilated or nondilated ureter, renal pelvis and calyces) contribute to vesicoureteral reflux assessment with the use of five grades assigned on the basis of contrast-enhanced voiding sonocystography (VALENTINI et al. 2001, 2004), which makes this system comparable to the most frequently used radiographic system of vesicoureteral reflux grading (LEBOWITZ et al. 1985).

Grade I (Fig. 24.2), echoes or color signals in the ureter above the ureteral orifice; grade II (Fig. 24.3a), echoes or color signals extending up to the renal pelvis and calyces, with no ureteral dilatation; grade III, ureter, renal pelvis, and calyces containing echoes or color signals, with mildly dilated ureter (Fig. 24.4); grade IV, echoes or color signals in dilated ureter, renal pelvis and calyces (Fig. 24.5); grade V, echoes or color signals in markedly dilated ureter, renal pelvis and calyces (Fig. 24.6).

Transperineal US was proposed as an imaging modality for studying urethral pathology and the bladder neck (Fig. 24.4c), and thus may complement voiding sonocystography (MATE et al. 2003).

Sensitivity and specificity of contrast-enhanced voiding sonocystography in revealing vesicoureteral reflux in children range from 69% to 100% and from 87% to 100%, respectively (ESCAPE et al. 2001; DARGE et al. 2001; VALENTINI et al. 2002, 2004; ASCENTI et al. 2003; MCEWING et al. 2003; NAKAMURA et al. 2003; UHL et al. 2003; VASSIOU et al. 2004).

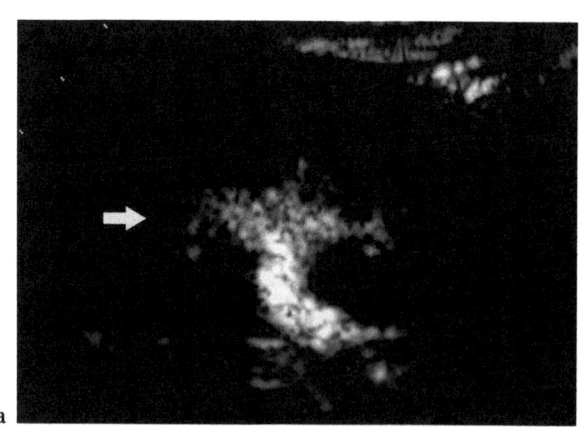

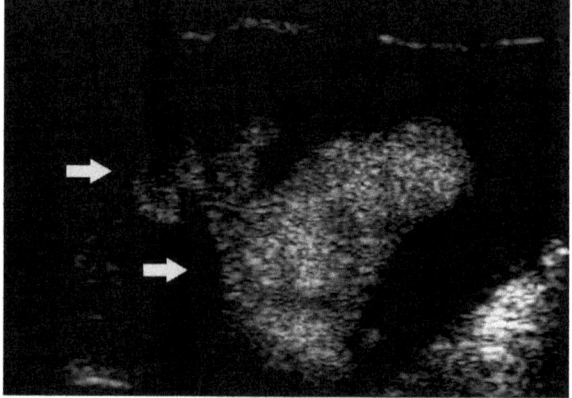

Fig. 24.3a,b. Vesicoureteral reflux diagnosed on the basis of echoes refluxing from the bladder to the ureter, renal pelvis, and renal calyces. Renal pelvis and calyces (*arrow*) present no (a) or marked (b) dilatation. The case in Fig. 24.3a was classified as grade II vesicoureteric reflux. [Reproduced with permission from ASCENTI et al. (2004)]

Vesicoureteral Reflux

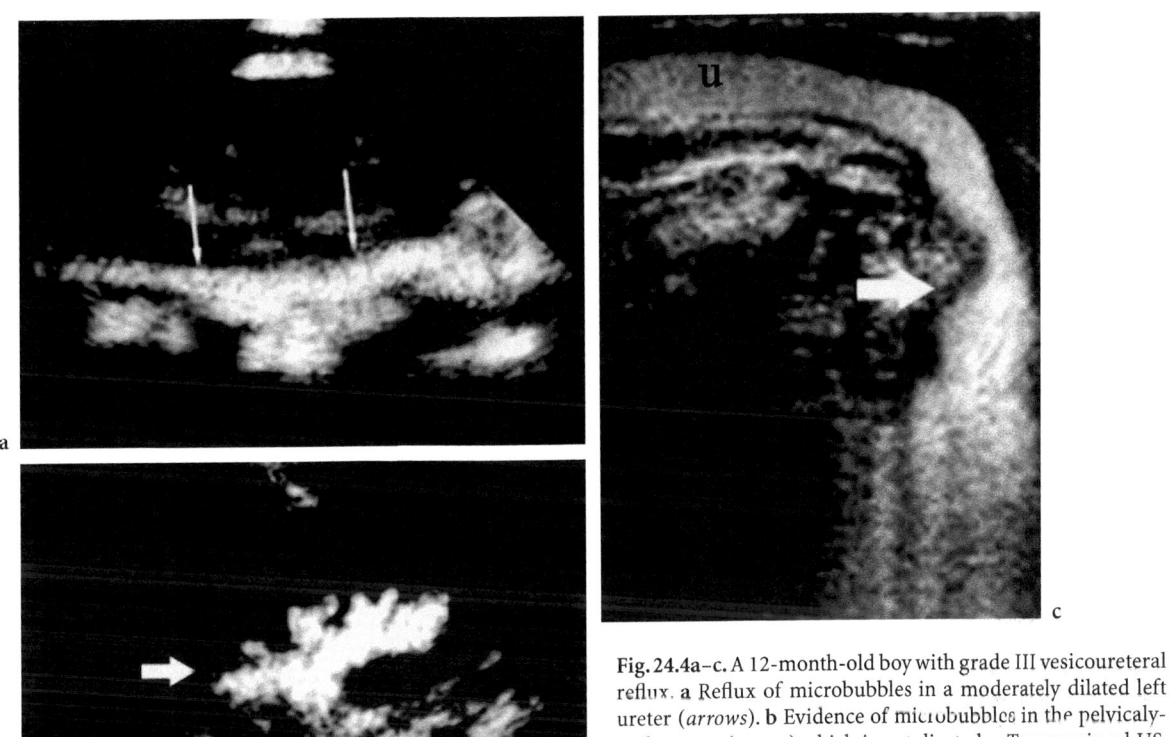

Fig. 24.4a–c. A 12-month-old boy with grade III vesicoureteral reflux. **a** Reflux of microbubbles in a moderately dilated left ureter (*arrows*). **b** Evidence of microbubbles in the pelvicalyceal system (*arrow*) which is not dicated. **c** Transperineal US, complement of voiding sonography. Normal appearance of the urethra (*u*) and the bladder neck (*arrow*) after microbubbles administration by employing the transperineal acoustic window. [Reproduced with permission from Ascenti et al. (2004)]

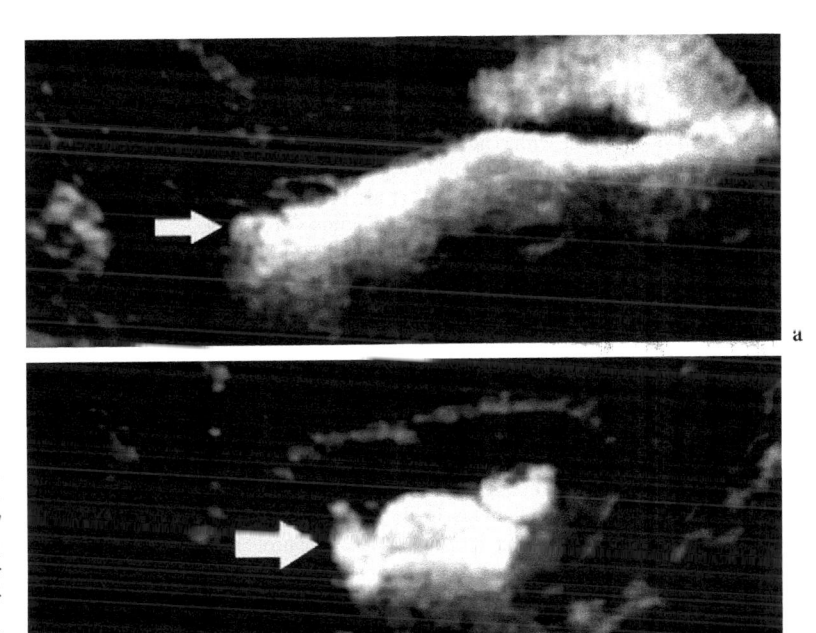

Fig. 24.5a,b. A 4-month-old girl with duplex kidney and a grade IV refluxing in the lower renal pelvis. **a** Reflux of microbubbles in a moderately dilated left ureter (*arrow*). **b** Reflux (*arrow*) of microbubbles into lower two-thirds of the renal pelvis which appears moderately dilated. [Reproduced with permission from Ascenti et al. (2004)]

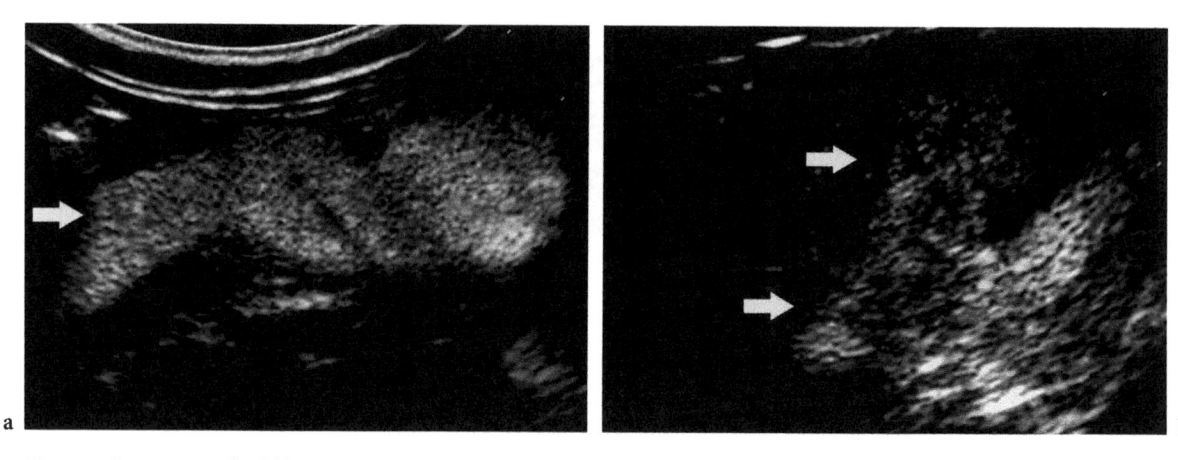

Fig. 24.6a,b. A 12-month-old boy with a grade V vesicoureteral reflux. a Reflux of microbubbles in a markedly dilated left ureter (*arrow*). b Evidence of microbubbles in the dilated renal pelvis and calyceal system (*arrows*). [Reproduced with permission from Ascenti et al. (2004)]

References

Ascenti G, Zimbaro G, Mazziotti S et al (2003) Vesicoureteral reflux: comparison between urosonography and radionuclide cystography. Pediatr Nephrol 18:768-771

Ascenti G, Zimbaro G, Mazziotti S et al (2004) Harmonic US imaging of vesicoureteric reflux in children: usefulness of a second generation US contrast agent. Pediatr Radiol 34:481-487

Berrocal T, Gaya F, Arjonilla A et al (2001) Vesicoureteral reflux: diagnosis and grading with echo-enhanced cystosonography versus voiding cystourethrography. Radiology 221:359-365

Darge K, Troeger J (2002) Vesicoureteral reflux grading in contrast-enhanced voiding urosonography. Eur J Radiol 43:122-128

Darge K, Troeger J, Duetting T et al (1999) Reflux in young patients: comparison of voiding US of the bladder and retrovesical space with echo enhancement versus voiding cystourethrography for diagnosis. Radiology 210:201-207

Darge K, Zieger B, Rohrschneider W et al (2001) Contrast-enhanced harmonic imaging for the diagnosis of vesicoureterorenal reflux in pediatric patients. AJR Am J Roentgenol 177:1411-1415

Escape I, Martinez J, Bastart F et al (2001) Usefulness of echocystography in the study of vesicoureteral reflux. J Ultrasound Med 20:145-149

Galloy MA, Mandry D, Pecastaings M et al (2003) Sonocystography: a new method for the diagnosis and follow-up of vesico-ureteric reflux in children. J Radiol 84:2055-2061

Kmetec A, Bren AF, Kandus A et al (2001) Contrast-enhanced ultrasound voiding cystography as a screening examination for vesicoureteral reflux in the follow-up of renal transplant recipients: a new approach. Nephrol Dial Transplant 16:120-123

Lebowitz RL, Olbing H, Parkkulainen KV et al (1985) International system of radiographic grading of vesicoureteral reflux: international reflux study in children. Pediatr Radiol 15:105-109

Mate A, Bargiela A, Mosteiro S et al (2003) Contrast ultrasound of the urethra in children. Eur Radiol 13:1534-1537

McEwing RL, Anderson NG, Hellewell S, Mitchell J (2003) Comparison of echo-enhanced ultrasound with fluoroscopic MCU for the detection of vesicoureteral reflux in neonates. Pediatr Radiol 32:853-858

Mentzel HJ, Vogt S, Patzer L et al (1999) Contrast-enhanced sonography of vesicoureterorenal reflux in children: preliminary results. AJR Am J Roentgenol 173:737-740

Nakamura M, Shinozaki T, Taniguchi N et al (2003) Simultaneous voiding cystourethrography and voiding urosonography reveals utility of sonographic diagnosis of vesicoureteral reflux in children. Acta Paediatr 92:1422-1426

Riccabona M, Mache CJ, Lindbichler F (2003) Echo-enhanced color Doppler cystosonography of vesicoureteral reflux in children. Improvement by stimulated acoustic emission. Acta Radiol 44:18-23

Uhl M, Kromeier J, Zimmerhackl LB, Darge K (2003) Simultaneous voiding cystourethrography and voiding urosonography. Acta Radiol 44:265-268

Valentini AL, Salvaggio E, Manzoni C et al (2001) Contrast-enhanced gray-scale and color Doppler voiding urosonography versus voiding cystourethrography in the diagnosis and grading of vesicoureteral reflux. J Clin Ultrasound 29:65-71

Valentini AL, de Gaetano AM, Destito C et al (2002) The accuracy of voiding urosonography in detecting vesico-ureteral reflux: a summary of existing data. Eur J Pediatr 161:380-384

Valentini AL, De Gaetano AM, Minordi LM et al (2004) Contrast-enhanced voiding US for grading of reflux in adult patients prior to antireflux ureteral implantation. Radiology 233:35-39

Vassiou K, Vlychou M, Moisidou R et al (2004) Contrast-enhanced sonographic detection of vesicoureteral reflux in children: comparison with voiding cystourethrography. Rofo 176:1453-1457

25 Pancreatic Pathology

Mirko D'Onofrio, Giulia Zamboni, Roberto Malagò, Enrico Martone,
Massimo Falconi, Paola Capelli, and Giancarlo Mansueto

This chapter is dedicated to Professor Carlo Procacci

CONTENTS

25.1 Introduction 335
25.2 Pancreatic Perfusion 335
25.3 Pancreatitis 335
25.3.1 Acute Pancreatitis 335
25.3.2 Pseudocysts 336
25.3.3 Chronic Pancreatitis 336
25.4 Exocrine Tumors 339
25.4.1 Ductal Adenocarcinoma 339
25.4.2 Serous Cystic Tumors 340
25.4.3 Mucin-Producing Cystic Tumors 342
25.5 Endocrine Tumors 343
25.6 Metastases 344
References 346

25.1
Introduction

The innovative use of contrast-enhanced ultrasound (US) in the study of pancreatic pathology creates the necessity of a semiologic definition. A description of the features of pancreatic pathology, diffuse and focal, solid and cystic, tumoral and pseudotumoral, after microbubble-based contrast agents injection, is therefore mandatory.

25.2
Pancreatic Perfusion

The perfusion of the pancreas justifies the semiology of the gland parenchymography at contrast-enhanced US. The differences in semiology between pancreas and liver at contrast-enhanced US (Chap. 11) assessment are substantial. In particular, considering that the blood supply of the pancreas is entirely arterial, the enhancement of the gland begins almost together with the aortic enhancement.

In the pancreas the enhancement reaches its peak between 15 and 20 s after microbubble injection (Fig. 25.1). Pancreatic parenchymography is therefore earlier and shorter than that of the liver, for the absence of a venous blood supply like the portal one (TAKEDA et al. 2003). Afterwards there is a progressive washout of microbubbles with loss of gland echogenicity (Fig. 25.1). For these reasons, it is difficult to obtain a correct characterization of pancreatic lesions for the brief duration of both contrast enhancement (wash-in) and contrast release (wash-out), even though contrast-enhanced US allows the continuous assessment of perfusion of pancreatic lesions (D'Onofrio et al. 2003).

25.3
Pancreatitis

Contrast-enhanced US improves the diagnosis of pancreatic inflammatory diseases (Koito et al. 1997). The identification and differential diagnosis of pancreatic inflammation and its complications, such as pseudocysts, are more reliable at contrast-enhanced US than at baseline US.

25.3.1
Acute Pancreatitis

Acute pancreatitis is an inflammatory process which involves the pancreas and the peri-pancreatic retroperitoneal regions (Klöppel and Schlüter 1999). Acute focal pancreatitis, even when supported by clinical data, frequently needs to be differentiated from pancreatic heteroplastic lesions (Lorèn et al. 1999), and may present a mild or severe form. In mild acute pancreatitis, the gland presents edema and hyperemia. At baseline US, acute focal pancreatitis appears as a segmental volume increase of

---

M. D'Onofrio, MD; G. Zamboni, MD; R. Malagò, MD;
E. Martone, MD; G. Mansueto, MD; M. Falconi, MD
P. Capelli, MD
Department of Radiology, Hospital G. B. Rossi, University of Verona, Piazza L.A. Scuro, 34134 Verona, Italy

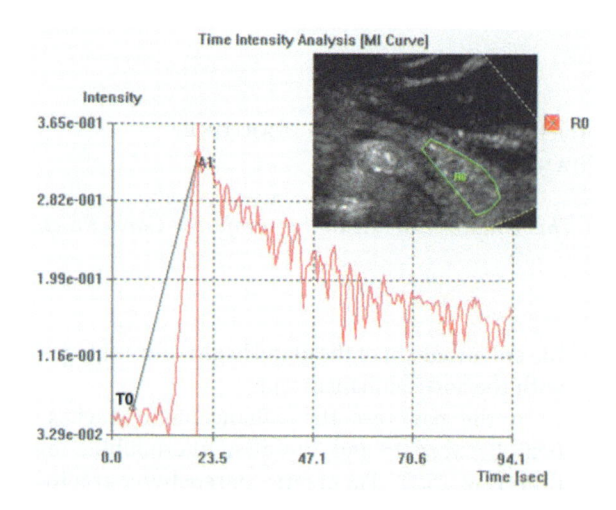

Fig. 25.1. Pancreatic perfusion. Contrast-enhanced US. Time intensity curve of the pancreas, obtained with a region of interest (*R0*) placed at the pancreatic tail, shows the peak of contrast enhancement (*A1*) at about 15 s after injection (*T0*); afterwards a progressive washout of microbubbles occurs

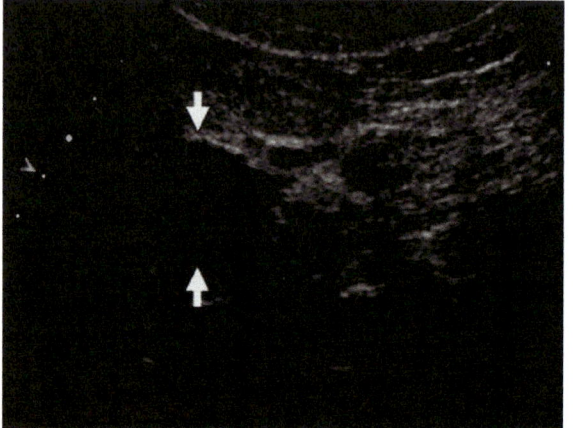

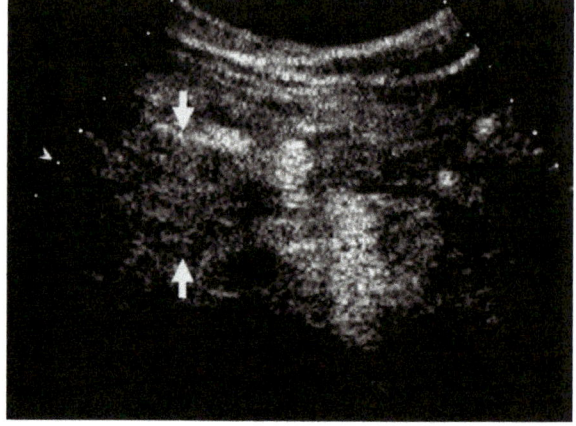

Fig. 25.2a,b. Acute focal pancreatitis. **a** Baseline US. A hypoechoic focal lesion is identified at the pancreatic head (*arrows*). **b** Contrast-enhanced US. The lesion appears hypovascular after microbubble injection with a slight parenchymographic contrast enhancement (*arrows*) in the pancreatic phase

the pancreas (Fig. 25.2), appearing homogeneously hypoechoic (Lorén et al. 1999). At contrast-enhanced US the pancreatic segment affected by inflammation shows diffuse contrast-enhancement (Fig. 25.2).

Severe acute pancreatitis is characterized by the presence of large confluent necrotic areas, the identification of which is important for patient prognosis (Casas et al. 2004). Contrast-enhanced US may improve identification and depiction of regional parenchymal necrosis, which appears as non-vascular areas after microbubble injection.

25.3.2
Pseudocysts

Pseudocysts are the most common cystic lesions of the pancreas (Procacci et al. 2001a). The lesion has a fibrous wall without an epithelial lining (Procacci et al. 2001a). At imaging, whenever inclusions are present, pseudocysts are difficult to differentiate from cystic tumors of the pancreas, especially mucinous cystadenoma (Procacci et al. 2001a).

Pseudocysts, although with a corpuscular and heterogeneous content at baseline US, show absence of contrast enhancement after microbubble injection appearing completely and homogeneously anechoic (Fig. 25.3).

25.3.3
Chronic Pancreatitis

According to the classification of Marseille (Singer et al. 1985), pathological alterations of the pancreatic parenchyma due to chronic pancreatitis are

Pancreatic Pathology

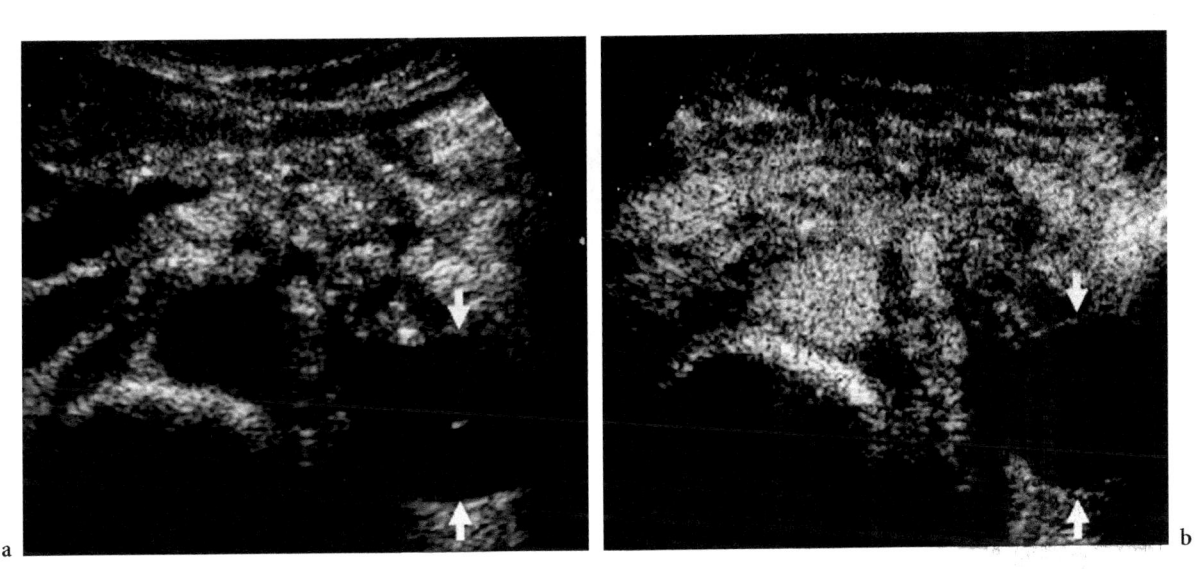

Fig. 25.3a,b. Pancreatic pseudocyst. a Baseline US. A cystic lesion of the pancreatic tail (*arrows*) with intralesional debris. b Contrast-enhanced US. Contrast enhancement is not observed either in the parietal nodules or in the intratumoral septa after microbubble injection, resulting in completely and homogeneously anechoic appearance (*arrows*)

represented by irregular tissue sclerosis with focal, segmentary, or diffuse destruction of exocrine parenchyma. These parenchymal alterations may be associated with various degrees of Wirsung duct dilation and with alterations of the pancreatic perfusion. The inflammatory process increases the blood supply (KOITO et al. 1997) and in the initial phases of the phlogistic process, glandular hyperemia is responsible for the increased gland parenchymography at contrast-enhanced US. However, progression of the chronic inflammatory process induces an increase of the degree of fibrosis with a decrease in hyperemia and, as a consequence, in gland parenchymography (KIM et al. 2001). Contrast-enhanced US is especially useful in the differential diagnosis of mass forming chronic pancreatitis (KOITO et al. 1997).

25.3.3.1
Mass-Forming Chronic Pancreatitis

Mass-forming chronic pancreatitis usually arises in patients with a history of chronic pancreatitis (KIM et al. 2001). Differential diagnosis with a neoplastic disease may be difficult not only due to the very similar features at baseline US (KOITO et al. 1997), but also because mass-forming pancreatitis and pancreatic cancer may present with the same symptoms and signs (VAN GULIK et al. 1997). The main characteristic feature at pathology is progressive interstitial fibrosis with chronic inflammatory infiltrate (KIM et al. 2001). US features of mass-forming pancreatitis are very similar to those of ductal adenocarcinoma (KOITO et al. 1997; KIM et al. 2001), presenting in most cases as a hypoechoic mass in a limited region of the gland, usually at the head, often with enlargement of the gland contour (Fig. 25.4). The presence of small calcifications in the lesion may suggest its inflammatory nature (REMER and BAKER 2002), but this sign is poorly specific.

For the final diagnosis, contrast material-enhanced CT and biopsy are mandatory. Contrast-enhanced US can improve the differentiation between mass-forming pancreatitis and pancreatic adenocarcinoma. Pancreatic ductal adenocarcinoma remains persistently hypoechoic after microbubble injection, due to the intense desmoplastic fibrotic reaction presenting a poor vascular component in the lesion. Mass-forming pancreatitis shows parenchymographic enhancement with isoechoic appearance to the surrounding pancreatic parenchyma in the early phases after microbubble injection (Fig. 25.4), while contrast enhancement decreases with a wash-out rate similar to the pancreatic gland in the late phase.

The presence of a parenchymography similar to the adjacent pancreatic parenchyma after microbubble injection is consistent with an inflammatory origin. The intensity of this parenchymographic contrast enhancement is related to the length of the underlying inflammatory process. It has been observed that, the more the inflammatory process is chronic and long-standing, the less intense the intralesional parenchymography, probably in relation to the entity of the associated fibrosis (KOITO et al. 1997; KIM et al. 2001). Conversely, in mass form-

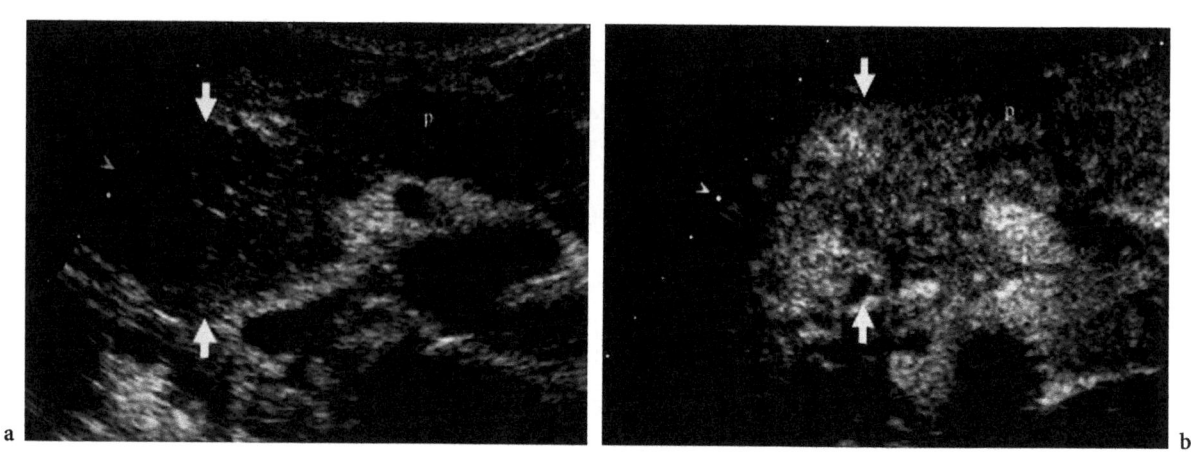

Fig. 25.4a,b. Mass-forming chronic pancreatitis. a Baseline US. A heterogeneous mass (*arrows*) is identified in the head of pancreas (*p*, pancreas body). b Contrast-enhanced US. Diffuse parenchymographic contrast enhancement of the lesion (*arrows*) which appears isoechoic to the adjacent pancreatic parenchyma

ing pancreatitis of more recent onset the enhancement is usually more intense and prolonged.

25.3.3.2
Autoimmune Pancreatitis

Autoimmune chronic pancreatitis is a particular type of chronic pancreatitis, with a very recent pathological definition (FURUKAWA et al. 1998). Autoimmune pancreatitis is characterized by periductal phlogosis, mainly sustained by lymphocytic infiltration, with evolution to fibrosis (FURUKAWA et al. 1998). As opposed to the other forms of chronic pancreatitis, the pancreas is increased in volume, usually in a diffuse way with the typical sausage look, and the main pancreatic duct appears compressed by glandular parenchyma or string-like (FURUKAWA et al. 1998). US features are very similar to those of focal pancreatitis, even though autoimmune pancreatitis may involve the entire gland more frequently, or present a larger extension and ubiquitous localization. US findings are characteristic in the diffuse form when the entire gland is involved.

The echogenicity is markedly reduced, the gland volume is increased, and the Wirsung duct is compressed by the gland parenchyma (Fig. 25.5). Focal autoimmune pancreatitis at the pancreatic head is often characterized by the sole dilation of the common bile duct (NUMATA et al. 2004). The parenchymal vascularization in autoimmune pancreatitis can be demonstrated at contrast-enhanced US (Fig. 25.5), which shows diffuse contrast enhancement (NUMATA et al. 2004) in the early phase (Fig. 25.5). Contrast enhancement appears heterogeneous for a small caliper of the glandular vessels due to thick lymphocytic infiltration and fibrosis.

Microbubble washout is usually slow but progressive. Contrast-enhanced US findings may be especially useful in the study of focal forms of autoimmune chronic pancreatitis, in which the differential diagnosis with ductal adenocarcinoma is very important (KOGA et al. 2002).

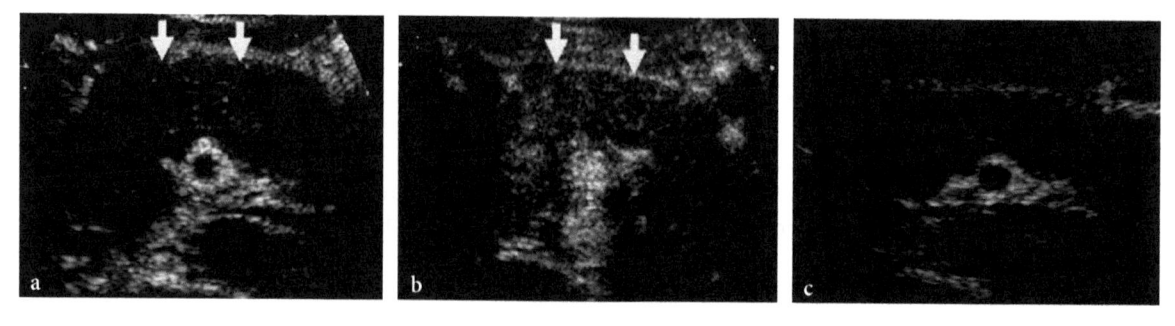

Fig. 25.5a–c. Autoimmune chronic pancreatitis. a Baseline US. The pancreatic gland (*arrows*) appears diffusely hypoechoic and increased in volume, while the Wirsung duct is compressed and not visible. b Contrast-enhanced US. Diffuse heterogeneous contrast enhancement of the pancreatic gland (*arrows*). c Baseline US after steroid therapy. The pancreatic gland presents a normal appearance

25.4
Exocrine Tumors

Pancreatic tumors are classified according to their histological type and grade in the WHO classification (KLÖPPEL et al. 1996). Ductal adenocarcinoma comprises between 80% and 90% of all tumors of the exocrine pancreas.

25.4.1
Ductal Adenocarcinoma

Ductal adenocarcinoma usually presents as a solid mass with infiltrating growth margins. US typically shows a hypoechoic lesion (Fig. 25.6a), with roughly defined margins, confused with the adjacent parenchyma, often altering the gland contour or sometimes completely included in the gland parenchyma (Fig. 25.7a). At histology, the pancreatic ductal adenocarcinoma is characterized by the marked desmoplasia (KLÖPPEL 1984), which determines the hard consistency (Figs. 25.6b,c). The mean vascular density is low (Fig. 25.6d) and often lower than that of the adjacent pancreatic parenchyma.

At contrast-enhanced US ductal adenocarcinoma shows low-grade contrast enhancement during all phases (Figs. 25.6e and 25.7b) for the marked desmoplasia (Fig. 25.6b) and the low mean vascular density of the lesion (Fig. 25.6d). At contrast-enhanced US ductal adenocarcinoma appears as a hypovascular area compared to the adjacent pancreatic parenchyma (Figs. 25.6e and 25.7b) with a clear depiction of tumoral margins and size and a better definition of the relationship with the peri-pancreatic arterial and venous vessels for local staging.

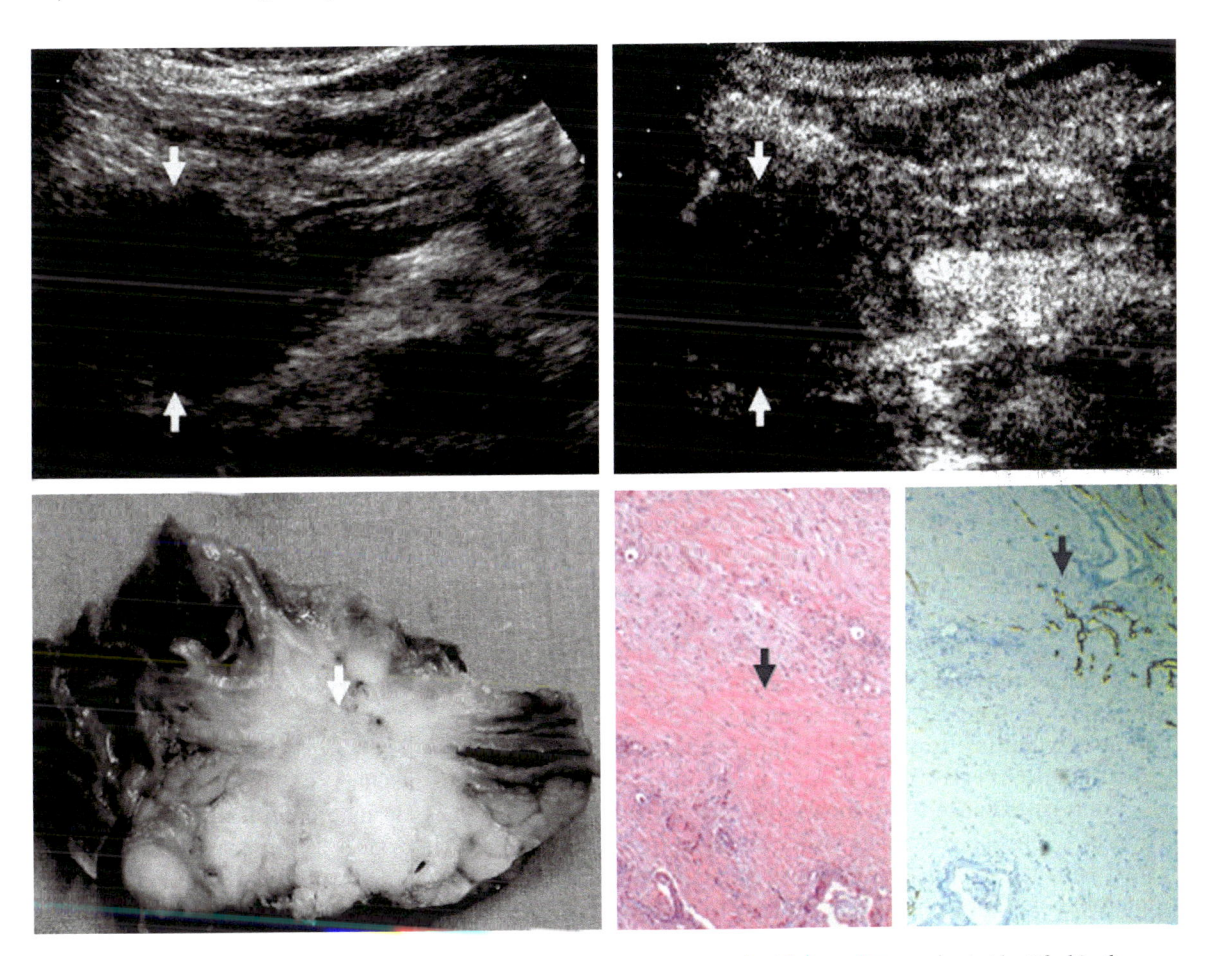

Fig. 25.6a–e. Ductal adenocarcinoma. **a** Baseline US. Hypoechoic mass (*arrows*) with irregular margins is identified in the pancreatic head. **b** Contrast-enhanced US. No contrast enhancement is identified in the pancreatic mass (*arrows*) after microbubble injection, with hypovascular appearance if compared to the rest of the pancreatic parenchyma during the venous contrast enhanced phase. **c** Surgical specimen. Hard tumoral consistency due to the fibrous desmoplastic component (*arrow*) of the tumor which is identified at hematoxylin-eosin staining (**d**). **e** Immunohistochemical analysis of CD34 antigen reveals the low vascular density (*arrow*)

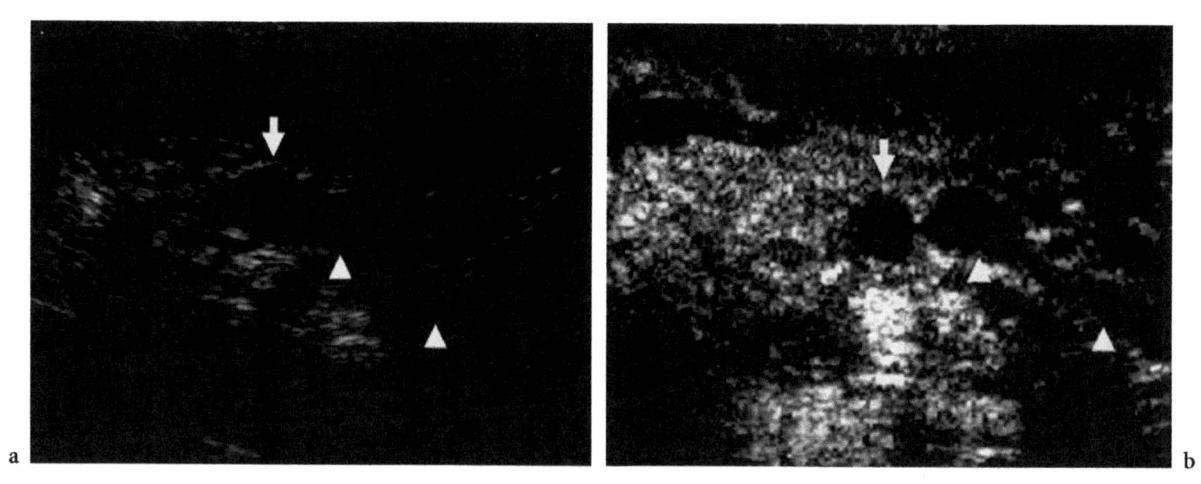

Fig. 25.7a,b. Ductal adenocarcinoma. a Baseline US. A small hypoechoic lesion (*arrow*) is identified at the pancreatic body with upstream main duct dilation (*arrowheads*). b Contrast-enhanced US. No contrast enhancement is identified in the nodule (*arrow*) which appears hypovascular if compared to the rest of the pancreatic parenchyma in the early contrast-enhanced phase

25.4.1.1
Differentiation and Microvascular Density

The differentiation degree of the adenocarcinoma influences its microvascular density. Poorly differentiated adenocarcinoma presents a low microvascular density, high malignancy and regional and distant spread which occur earlier than with ductal adenocarcinoma. Pathology findings are represented by a large soft mass, with central necrotic areas. The appearance of poorly differentiated pancreatic adenocarcinoma at baseline US is not univocal. It appears as a fairly sized hypoechoic lesion (Fig. 25.8a) with central necrotic areas due to the rapid tumoral growth not supported by a sufficient neoangiogenesis. Minute calcifications (Fig. 25.8a) may be present in the intralesional necrotic areas. The tumor grows in all directions, usually in a concentric way (Fig. 25.8a). Color and power Doppler studies have proven to not be so accurate in the identification of tumoral vascularization (Figs. 25.8b,c), while vascular infiltration and regional and hepatic diffusion occur early.

Contrast-enhanced US shows the vascularization of the neoplastic tissue with evidence of contrast enhancement already in the early phase after microbubble injection (Fig. 25.8d). The contrast enhancement in the viable portion of the tumor appears as a shell of solid tissue lining the intratumoral necrotic areas which appear as non-vascular regions (Fig. 25.8d). The viable portion of the tumor appears hypoechoic in the late phase due to microbubble washout.

25.4.1.2
Staging

US staging of ductal adenocarcinoma is accurate (MINNITI et al. 2003). The use of microbubble-based contrast agents may complete the regional staging of pancreatic adenocarcinoma by confirming vascular, arterial, and venous infiltration or involvement by the neoplasm (Fig. 25.9). Contrast-enhanced US also contributes to hepatic staging, increasing sensibility and specificity for liver metastases identification and characterization. After studying the pancreatic lesion in the arterial, pancreatic, and venous phases, liver metastases are sought during the sinusoidal hepatic contrast-enhanced phase (BLOMLEY et al. 1998, 1999; SOLBIATI et al. 2001).

25.4.2
Serous Cystic Tumors

Serous cystoadenoma usually has a benign nature (COMPAGNO and OERTEL 1978a). The typical variety is the microcystic, macroscopically characterized by multiple small cysts (<2 cm) separated by thin septa (PROCACCI et al. 1999a, 2001a). The margins are well-defined and a central scar may be present (PROCACCI et al. 1999a). The intralesional septal enhancement at contrast-enhanced US improves identification of the microcystic features of the lesion (Fig. 25.10). The less common oligocystic or macrocystic types of serous cystadenoma present features indistinguishable from those of the other macrocystic tumors of

Pancreatic Pathology

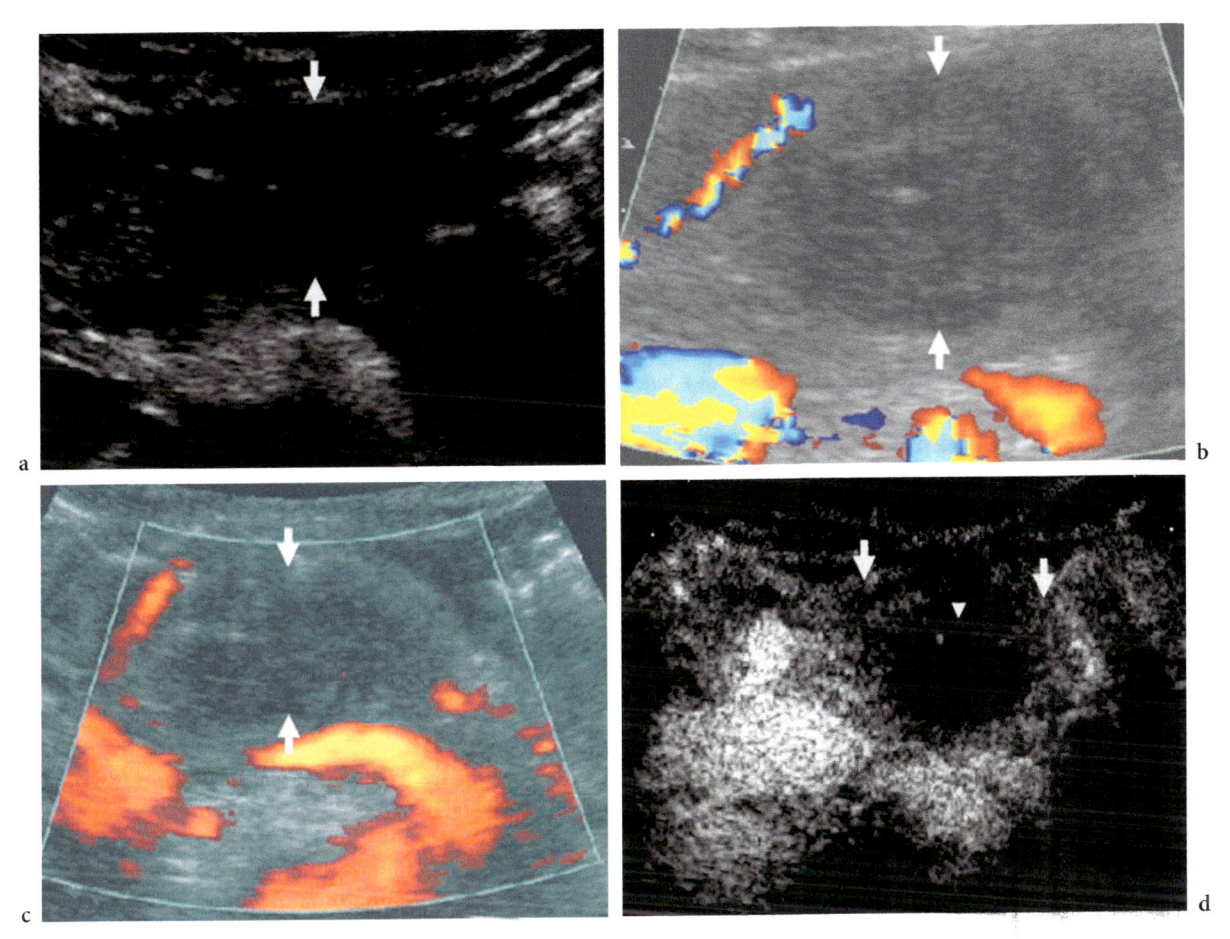

Fig. 25.8a–d. Poorly differentiated pancreatic adenocarcinoma. **a** Baseline US. A hypoechoic mass with diffuse margins (*arrows*) is identified at the pancreatic body. **b,c** Color and power Doppler. No tumoral vessels are identified in the pancreatic mass (*arrows*). **d** Contrast-enhanced US. Contrast enhancement is identified in the viable portion of the tumor, with evidence of a thick tumoral enhancing rim (*arrows*) surrounding a central necrotic area (*arrowhead*)

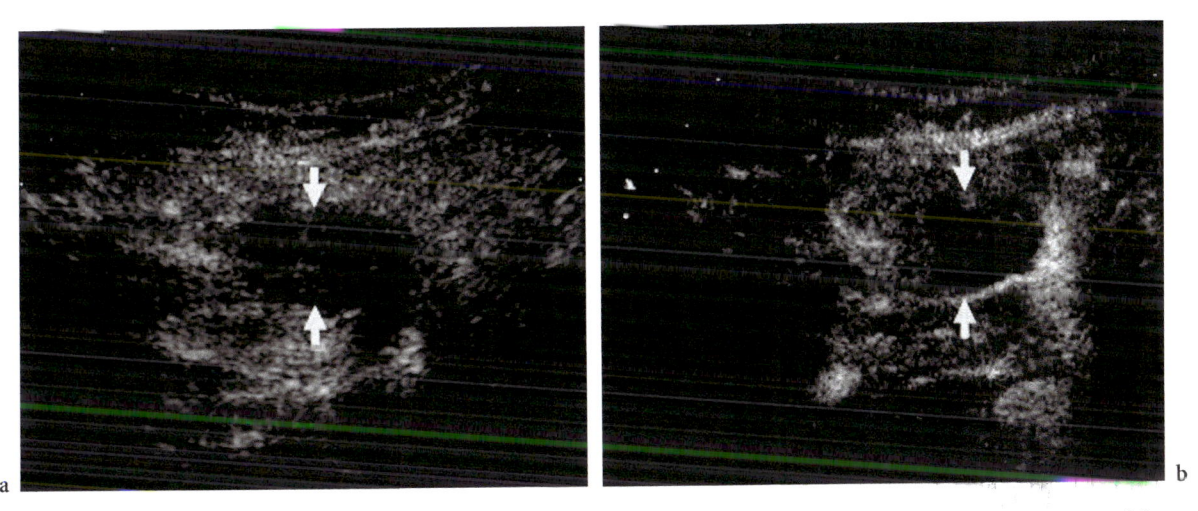

Fig. 25.9a,b. Ductal adenocarcinoma. **a** Baseline US. A hypoechoic mass (*arrows*) is identified at the uncinate process of the pancreas. **b** Contrast-enhanced US. The lesion does not show contrast enhancement (*arrows*) after microbubble injection during the early contrast-enhanced phase. Encasement of the inferior pancreaticoduodenal artery and infiltration of the superior mesenteric artery was shown during the surgical procedure

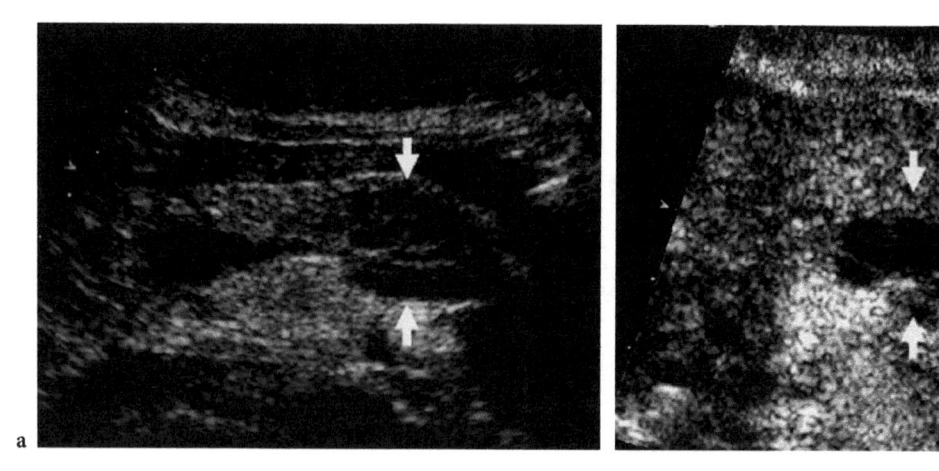

Fig. 25.10a,b. Serous cystadenoma. a Baseline US. Small focal hypoechoic lesion at the pancreatic body (*arrows*). b Contrast-enhanced US. Septal enhancement with microcystic aspect of the lesion (*arrows*) is visualized after microbubble injection in the pancreatic phase

the pancreas (PROCACCI et al. 1997; CARBOGNIN et al. 2003).

25.4.3
Mucin-Producing Cystic Tumors

Mucin-producing tumors of the pancreas may originate either from the peripheral ducts (mucinous cystic tumors) or from the duct of Wirsung and its collateral branches (intraductal papillary mucinous tumors, IPMTs) (PROCACCI et al. 1996).

25.4.3.1
Mucinous Cystic Tumors

Mucinous cystadenoma is a rare primitive pancreatic tumor, even though it is the most common cystic pancreatic tumor (HAMMOND et al. 2002). Mucinous cystadenoma is considered a pre-malignant lesion (COMPAGNO and OERTEL 1978b; PROCACCI et al. 1999a; COHEN-SCALI et al. 2003) and, consequently, the differentiation of mucinous cystadenoma from other cystic pancreatic lesions is important for a correct therapeutic approach. Mucinous cystadenoma presents as a cystic, multilocular or, less often, unilocular round mass, with variable size (range: 2–36 cm) (FUGAZZOLA et al. 1991; BUETOW et al. 1998). The multilocular type is typical, even though it is not pathognomonic (SPERTI et al. 1993). The unilocular appearance is less common and less typical and has to be differentiated from the other cystic lesions of the pancreas (DEMOS et al. 2002), particularly pseudocysts (WARSHAW and RUTLEDGE 1987; SACHS et al. 1989; FUGAZZOLA et al. 1991; SPERTI et al. 1993; BUETOW et al. 1998; KUBA et al. 1998; PROCACCI et al. 1999a; DE LIMA et al. 1999; SCOTT et al. 2000; HAMMOND et al. 2002) and the oligocystic variety of serous pancreatic cystadenoma (COHEN-SCALI et al. 2003).

Mucinous cystadenoma may present calcifications on the wall or the septa (PROCACCI et al. 2001b), parietal nodules and papillary vegetations (FUGAZZOLA et al. 1991). The cystic content of the lesion may be heterogeneous for the presence of mucin or intralesional hemorrhage. At baseline US mucinous cystadenoma presents as a lesion with cystic areas, separated by septa, with corpuscular mucinous content. By using tissue harmonic imaging it is possible to better visualize the cystic walls, septa, nodules and the papillary vegetations (HAMMOND et al. 2002). The content of the mucinous cystadenoma, however, if very corpuscular, may impair identification of parietal nodules, which is fundamental for a radiological diagnosis. Contrast-enhanced US may identify contrast enhancement in nodules and intracystic septa, due to their tumoral nature, after microbubble injection (Fig. 25.11), and improves the differential diagnosis between mucinous cystadenoma and pseudocyst by the identification of contrast enhancement in the inclusions inside the pancreatic cystic masses.

25.4.3.2
Intraductal Papillary-Mucinous Tumors

Intraductal papillary-mucinous tumors are considered rare lesions, but recently they have been reported with increasing frequency (PROCACCI et al. 1996, 1999b, 2001c, 2003). Intraductal papillary-mucinous tumors are macroscopically characterized by their

Pancreatic Pathology

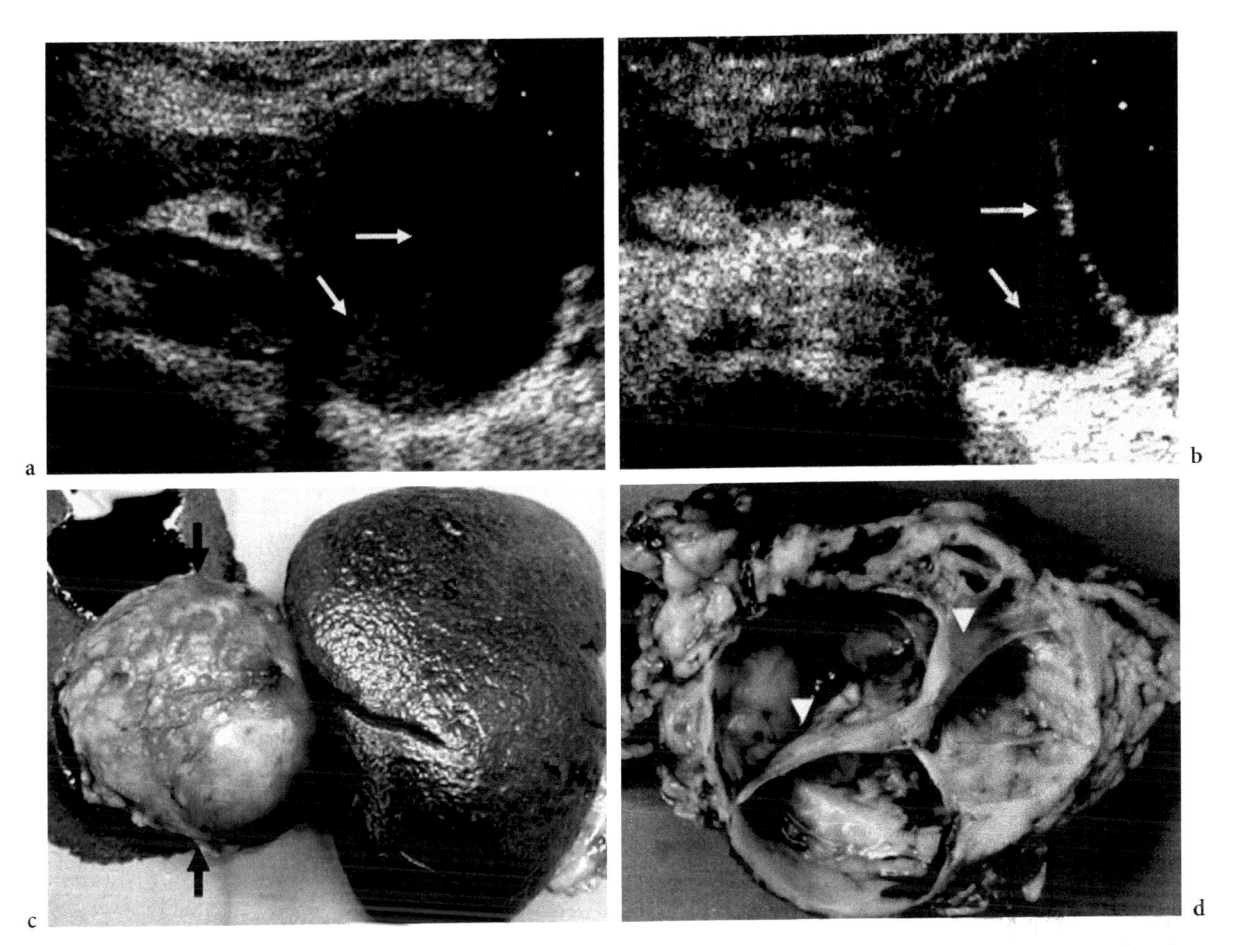

Fig. 25.11a–d. Mucinous cystoadenoma. **a** Baseline US. A cystic mass is identified in the pancreatic tail presenting an intralesional septum and peripheral mural nodules (*arrows*). **b** Contrast-enhanced US. Contrast enhancement is identified in the septa and peripheral mural nodules after microbubble injection (*arrows*). **c,d** Surgical specimen. Mass (*arrows*) of the pancreatic tail resected with the spleen (*s*). Intratumoral septa (*arrowheads*) are evident when the cystic mass is cut

intraductal origin and growth (ZAMBONI et al. 2003) with production of dense mucin filling the Wirsung duct (ductectatic mucin-hypersecreting variant) or with endoluminal papillary proliferation (papillary-villous variant). At baseline US the dilation of the main pancreatic duct is usually demonstrated, while the identification of the lesion depends on its size (Fig. 25.12). Intraductal papillary-mucinous tumors of adequate dimensions appear at baseline US as heterogeneous masses, upstream of the Wirsung dilation (Fig. 25.12). Contrast-enhanced US may allow the identification of intraductal papillary tumoral vegetations, especially in the papillary-villous variant, demonstrating its vascularization after micro bubble injection (Fig. 25.12). However, the definite diagnosis of intraductal papillary-mucinous tumors by demonstrating the communication between the tumor and the pancreatic duct is difficult with US (PROCACCI et al. 2003).

25.5
Endocrine Tumors

Endocrine tumors may induce specific clinical effects due to the hormonal production (functioning endocrine tumors) or aspecific symptoms due to the expansive growth (non-functioning endocrine tumors). Endocrine pancreatic tumors appear hypervascular at contrast material-enhanced CT (PROCACCI et al. 2001d).

Differential diagnosis between non-functioning endocrine pancreatic tumors and ductal pancreatic adenocarcinoma is of fundamental importance for therapeutic strategy and prognosis (PROCACCI et al. 2001d). At color and power Doppler US, a spotted pattern can be demonstrated inside the endocrine tumors (D'ONOFRIO et al. 2004). However, the hypervascular endocrine tumors may reveal no Doppler vascular signal due to the small size of the lesion or the vascular network of the tumor (D'ONOFRIO et al. 2004).

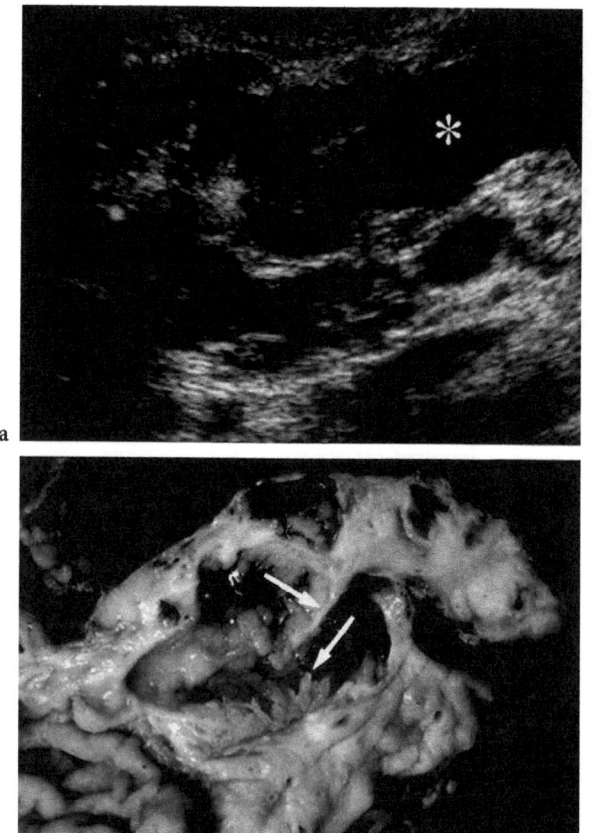

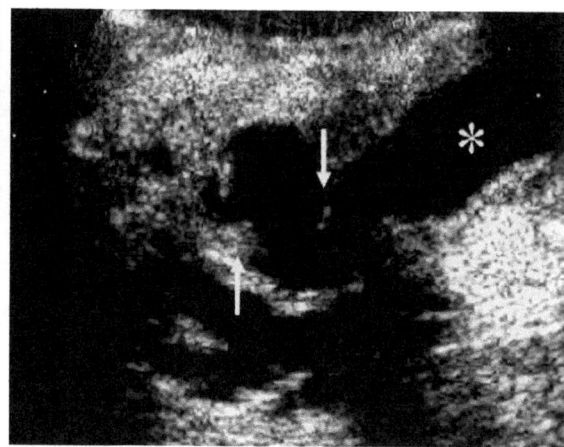

Fig. 25.12a-c. Intraductal papillary-mucinous tumor. a Baseline US. Huge hypoechoic heterogeneous mass of the pancreatic head with upstream main duct dilation (*asterisk*). b Contrast-enhanced US. Intense enhancement of intraductal papillary tumoral vegetations and septa (*arrows*) inside the dilated main pancreatic duct (*asterisk*). c Specimen. Vegetations and septa are identified inside the main pancreatic duct (*arrows*)

At contrast-enhanced US different contrast enhancement patterns may be observed according to the tumoral dimension and tumoral vessels. Huge endocrine tumors show rapid and diffuse contrast enhancement after microbubble injection in the early phases, with the exception of the necrotic intratumoral areas (Fig. 25.13) (D'Onofrio et al. 2004). In moderate-sized neuroendocrine pancreatic tumors a capillary blush enhancement may be identified in the early phase, resembling the most characteristic feature of this tumor at angiography (Rossi et al. 1989), presenting as hypoechoic at late phase (D'Onofrio et al. 2004). Since the characterization of non-functioning endocrine pancreatic tumors is principally linked to frequent tumoral hypervascularization (Procacci et al. 2001d), a high sensitivity of imaging modalities in the detection of macro- and microtumoral circulation is required.

Non-functioning neuroendocrine tumors may be hypovascularized (D'Onofrio et al. 2004). This is directly related to the amount of stroma inside the lesion which is dense and hyalinized. However, in some pancreatic neuroendocrine tumors appearing hypodense at contrast material-enhanced CT, contrast enhancement may be visible after microbubble injection (D'Onofrio et al. 2004). The high capability of contrast-enhanced US in demonstrating endocrine tumor vascularization is due to the high sensitivity of contrast specific modes to the microbubble signal, improving the identification (D'Onofrio et al. 2003) and characterization of pancreatic endocrine tumors (D'Onofrio et al. 2004). Moreover, contrast-enhanced US improves loco-regional (Fig. 25.14) and hepatic staging of pancreatic endocrine tumors (D'Onofrio et al. 2004).

25.6
Metastases

Pancreatic metastases are rare and the most common are those from renal carcinoma. Pancreatic metastases from renal carcinoma, being hypervascular, may show diffuse contrast enhancement after microbubble injection (Fig. 25.15), allowing a characterization and differential diagnosis with pancreatic ductal adenocarcinoma (Flath et al. 2003; Megibow 2003).

Pancreatic Pathology

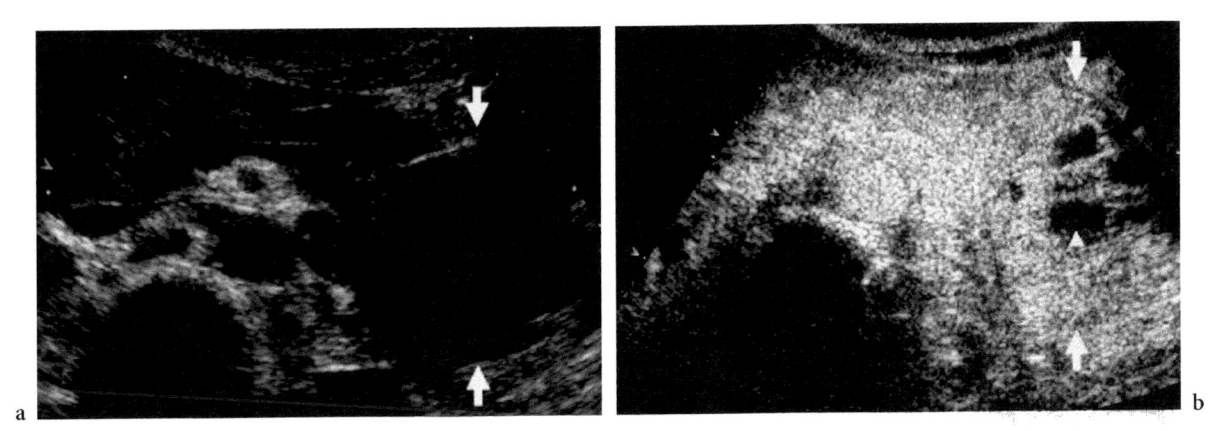

Fig. 25.13a,b. Non-functioning endocrine tumor. **a** Baseline US. Huge heterogeneous mass in the pancreatic tail (*arrows*). **b** Contrast-enhanced US. Diffuse contrast enhancement of the lesion (*arrows*) in the early contrast enhanced phases with evidence of small hypoechoic intratumoral necrotic areas (*arrowhead*)

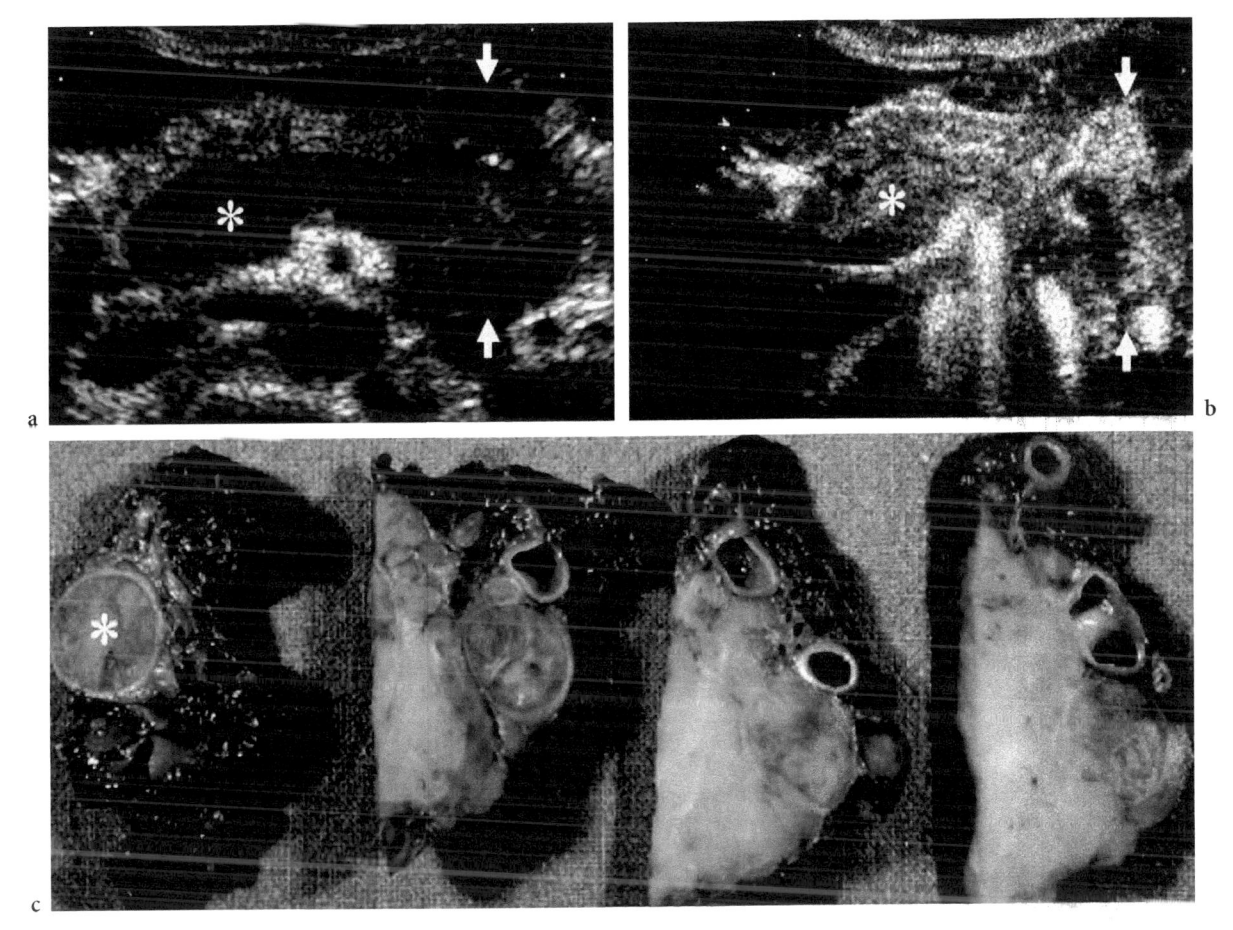

Fig. 25.14a-c. Non-functioning endocrine tumor. **a** Baseline US. Huge hypoechoic heterogeneous mass of the pancreatic body (*arrows*) with associated splenic vein thrombosis (*asterisk*). **b** Contrast-enhanced US. Diffuse contrast enhancement of the tumor (*arrows*) and of the thrombus in the splenic vein (*asterisk*) in the early contrast-enhanced phase. **c** Surgical specimen. Neoplastic infiltration of the splenic vein (*asterisk*)

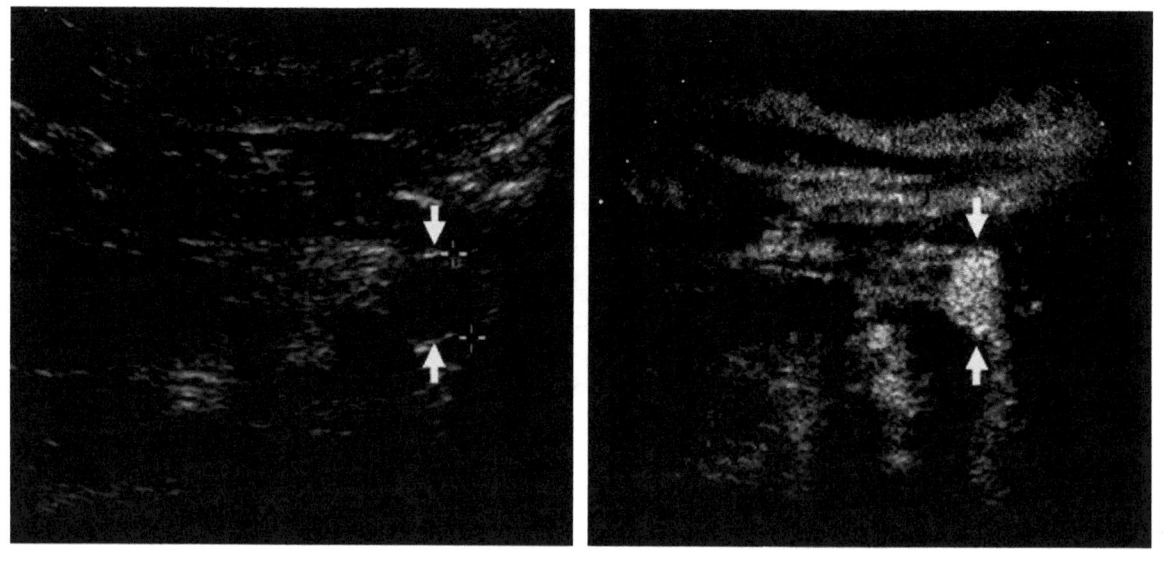

Fig. 25.15a,b. Metastatic renal cell carcinoma. a Baseline US. A small well-defined hypoechoic focal lesion is identified in the pancreatic body (*arrows*). b Contrast-enhanced US. Diffuse and intense contrast enhancement of the lesion (*arrows*) during the arterial phase

References

Blomley MJK, Albrecht T, Cosgrove DO et al (1998) Stimulated acoustic emission in liver parenchyma with Levovist. Lancet 351:568-569

Blomley MJ, Albrecht TA, Cosgrove DO et al (1999) Improved detection of liver metastases with stimulated acoustic emission in late phase of enhancement with the US contrast agent SH U 508: early experience. Radiology 210:409-416

Buetow PC, Rao P, Thompson LDR (1998) Mucinous cystic neoplasm of the pancreas: radiologic-pathologic correlation. Radiographics 18:433-449

Carbognin G, Tapparelli M, Petrella E et al (2003) Serous cystic tumors. In: Procacci C, Megibow AJ (eds) Imaging of the pancreas. Cystic and rare tumors. Springer, Berlin Heidelberg New York, pp 31-57

Casas JD, Diaz R, Valderas G et al (2004) Prognostic value of CT in the early assessment of patients with acute pancreatitis. AJR 182:569-574

Cohen-Scali F, Vilgrain V, Brancatelli G et al (2003) Discrimination of unilocular macrocystic serous cystadenoma from pancreatic pseudocyst and mucinous cystadenoma with CT: initial observations. Radiology 228:727-733

Compagno J, Oertel JE (1978a) Microcystic adenomas of the pancreas (glycogen-rich cystoadenomas). A clinicopathologic study of 34 cases. Am J Clin Pathol 69:289-298

Compagno J, Oertel JE (1978b) Mucinous cystic neoplasm of the pancreas with overt and latent malignancy (cystadenocarcinoma and cystadenoma). A clinicopathologic study of 41 cases. Am J Clin Pathol 69:573-580

De Lima JE Jr, Javitt MC, Mathur SC (1999) Residents' teaching files: mucinous cystic neoplasm of the pancreas. Radiographics 19:807-811

Demos TC, Posniak HV, Harmath C et al (2002) Cystic lesions of the pancreas. AJR 179:1375-1388

D'Onofrio M, Mansueto G, Vasori S et al (2003) Contrast enhanced ultrasonographic detection of small pancreatic insulinoma. J Ultrasound Med 22:413-417

D'Onofrio M, Mansueto G, Falconi M, Procacci C (2004) Neuroendocrine pancreatic tumor: value of contrast enhanced ultrasonography. Abdom Imaging 29:246-258

Flath B, Rickes S, Schweigert M et al (2003) Differentiation of pancreatic metastasis of a renal cell carcinoma from primary pancreatic carcinoma by echo-enhanced power Doppler sonography. Pancreatology 3:349

Fugazzola C, Procacci C, Bergamo Andreis IA et al (1991) Cystic tumors of the pancreas: evaluation by ultrasonography and computer tomography. Gastrointest Radiol 16:53-61

Furukawa N, Muranaka T, Yasumori K et al (1998) Autoimmune pancreatitis: radiologic findings in three histologically proven cases. J Comput Assist Tomogr 22:880-883

Hammond N Miller FH, Sica GT, Gore RM (2002) Imaging of cystic disease of the pancreas. Radiol Clin North Am 40:1243-1262

Kim T, Murakami T, Takamura M et al (2001) Pancreatic mass due to chronic pancreatitis: correlation of CT and MR imaging features with pathologic findings. AJR 177:367-371

Klöppel G (1984) Pancreatic non-endocrine tumors. In: Klöppel G, Heitz PU (eds) Pancreatic pathology. Churchill Livingstone, Edinburgh, pp 87-88

Klöppel G, Schlüter E (1999) Pathology of the pancreas. In: Baert AL, Delorme G, van Hoe L (eds) Radiology of the pancreas, 2nd edn. Springer, Berlin Heidelberg New York, pp 69-100

Klöppel G, Solcia E, Longnecker DS et al (1996) Histological typing of tumors of the exocrine pancreas. International histological classification of tumors, 2nd edn. Springer, Berlin Heidelberg New York

Koga Y, Yamaguchi K, Sugitani A et al (2002) Autoimmune pancreatitis starting as a localized form. J Gastroenterol 37:133-137

Koito K, Namieno T, Nagakawa T, Morita K (1997) Inflammatory pancreatic masses: differentiation from ductal carcinomas with contrast-enhanced sonography using carbon dioxide microbubbles. AJR 169:1263-1267

Kuba H, Yamaguchi K, Shimizu S et al (1998) Chronic asymptomatic pseudocyst with sludge aggregates masquerading as mucinous cystic neoplasm of the pancreas. J Gastroenterol 33:766-769

Lorén I, Lasson A, Fork T et al (1999) New sonographic imaging observations in focal pancreatitis. Eur Radiol 9:862-867

Megibow AJ (2003) Secondary pancreatic tumors: Imaging. In: Procacci C, Megibow AJ (eds) Imaging of the pancreas. Cystic and rare tumors. Springer, Berlin Heidelberg New York, pp 277-288

Minniti S, Bruno C, Biasiutti C et al (2003) Sonography versus helical CT in identification and staging of pancreatic ductal adenocarcinoma. J Clin Ultrasound 31:175-181

Numata K, Ozawa Y, Kobayashi N et al (2004) Contrast enhanced sonography of autoimmune pancreatitis. Comparison with pathologic findings. J Ultrasound Med 23:199-206

Procacci C, Graziani R, Bicego E et al (1996) Intraductal mucin-producing tumors of the pancreas: imaging findings. Radiology 198:249-257

Procacci C, Graziani R, Bicego E et al (1997) Serous cystadenoma of the pancreas: report of 30 cases with emphasis on the imaging findings. J Comput Assist Tomogr 21:373-382

Procacci C, Biasiutti C, Carbognin G et al (1999a) Characterization of cystic tumors of the pancreas: CT accuracy. J Comput Assoc Tomogr 23:906-912

Procacci C, Megibow AJ, Carbognin G, et al (1999b) Intraductal papillary mucinous tumor of the pancreas: a pictorial essay. Radiographics 19:1447-1463

Procacci C et al (2001a) Pancreatic neoplasms and tumor-like conditions. Eur Radiol 11 [Suppl 2]:S167-S192

Procacci C, Carbognin G, Accordini S et al (2001b) CT features of malignant mucinous cystic tumors of the pancreas. Eur Radiol 11:1626-1630

Procacci C, Carbognin G, Biasiutti C et al (2001c) Intraductal papillary mucinous tumors of the pancreas: spectrum of CT and MR findings with pathologic correlation. Eur Radiol 11:1939-1951

Procacci C, Carbognin G, Accordini S et al (2001d) Nonfunctioning endocrine tumors of the pancreas: possibilities of spiral CT characterization. Eur Radiol 11:1175-1183

Procacci C, Schenal G, Della Chiara E et al (2003) Intraductal papillary mucinous tumors: imaging. In: Procacci C, Megibow AJ (eds) Imaging of the pancreas. Cystic and rare tumors. Springer, Berlin Heidelberg New York, pp 97-137

Remer EM, Baker ME (2002) Imaging of chronic pancreatitis. Radiol Clin North Am 40:1229-1242

Rossi P, Allison DJ, Bezzi M et al (1989) Endocrine tumors of the pancreas. Radiol Clin North Am 27:129-161

Sachs JR, Deren JJ, Sohn M, Nusbaum M (1989) Mucinous cystadenoma: pitfalls of differential diagnosis. Am J Gastroenterol 84:811-816

Scott J, Martin I, Redhead D et al (2000) Mucinous cystic neoplasm of the pancreas: imaging features and diagnostic difficulties. Clin Radiol 55:187-192

Singer MW, Gyr K, Sarles H (1985) Revised classification of pancreatitis. Report of the Second International Symposium on the Classification of Pancreatitis in Marseille, France, 28-30 March 1984. Gastroenterology 89:683-685

Solbiati L, Tonolini M, Cova L, Goldberg SN (2001) The role of contrast-enhanced ultrasound in the detection of focal liver lesions. Eur Radiol 11 [Suppl 3]:E15-E26

Sperti C, Cappellazzo F, Pasquali C et al (1993) Cystic neoplasm of the pancreas: problems in differential diagnosis. Am Surg 59:740-745

Takeda K, Goto H, Hirooka Y et al (2003) Contrast enhanced transabdominal ultrasonography in the diagnosis of pancreatic mass lesions. Acta Radiol 44:103-106

Van Gulik TM, Reeders JW, Bosma A et al (1997) Incidence and clinical findings of benign, inflammatory disease in patients resected for pancreatic head cancer. Gastrointest Endosc 46:417-423

Warshaw AL, Rutledge PL (1987) Cystic tumors mistaken for pancreatic pseudocysts. Ann Surg 205:393-398

Zamboni G, Capelli P, Bogina G et al (2003) Pathology of intraductal cystic tumors. In: Procacci C, Megibow AJ (eds) Imaging of the pancreas. Cystic and rare tumors. Springer, Berlin Heidelberg New York, pp 85-94

26 Intestinal Pathology

Giovanni Maconi and Gabriele Bianchi Porro

CONTENTS

26.1 Crohn's Disease 349
26.1.1 Introduction 349
26.1.2 Evaluation of Disease Activity 349
26.1.3 Characterization of Intestinal Strictures 352
26.1.4 Diagnosis of Fistulae and Abscesses 352
26.1.5 Prognostic Aspects and Monitoring of Disease 353
26.2 Neoplastic Diseases 355
26.2.1 Gastric Cancer 355
26.2.2 Colorectal Cancer 356
26.3 Conclusion 357
References 357

26.1 Crohn's Disease

26.1.1 Introduction

Crohn's disease is a heterogeneous chronic disease characterized by acute and chronic inflammation of the wall of the small and large intestines, which is transmural resulting in intestinal fibrosis, luminal stenosis, and fistula formation between adjacent organs and intestinal loops. The role of endoscopy and barium enema in establishing the diagnosis of Crohn's disease is clearly defined by detecting early mucosal and luminal changes. However, computed tomography (CT), magnetic resonance (MR) imaging, and ultrasound (US) have proved to be safe and accurate imaging modalities to evaluate the intestinal wall as well as to reveal classic complications frequently associated with Crohn's disease, such as stenoses, fistulas or fissures, and abscesses. Abdominal US can reliably demonstrate the presence and features of bowel wall thickness, and may be used as the primary imaging method when Crohn's disease is suspected on a clinical basis. Gray-scale US is also useful to detect abdominal complications, to suggest disease activity, and to provide prognostic data concerning clinical and surgical recurrences following surgery.

Since Crohn's disease is associated with a variable degree of vascular changes in the bowel walls, the intestinal microvasculature has been an important field of investigation (Knutson et al. 1968; Wakefield et al. 1989). Evaluation of intestinal vasculature using color and power Doppler US have so far been used in Crohn's disease to identify and characterize pathological wall thickening and its inflammatory nature. However, the exact role of power Doppler US assessment of the bowel wall in Crohn's disease activity remains to be defined. Some authors found that the increased vascularity of the bowel walls, namely the intensity of color signals within the intestinal wall, correlates with Crohn's disease activity, while other authors did not (Tarjan et al. 2000; Spalinger et al. 2000; Esteban et al. 2001).

Power Doppler US may differentiate internal fistulae and inflammatory masses from the intra-abdominal abscesses by revealing color signals within the fistulas and masses, and absence of color signals within the abscesses which show vessel signals only in the periphery. These findings are conceivable if we consider the intrinsic vascular nature of the bowel wall. Even though dedicated contrast-specific techniques should be employed after microbubble injection, microbubble-based contrast agents were used to improve the accuracy of Doppler US in detecting Crohn's disease activity and complications.

26.1.2 Evaluation of Disease Activity

Gray-scale or color Doppler signal may be enhanced after microbubble injection. Color or power Doppler may be employed after microbubble injection, even though they are strongly penalized by artifacts which are almost eliminated with the employment of dedicated contrast-specific techniques. Use of contrast-enhanced power Doppler US can increase the accu-

---

G. Maconi, MD; G. Bianchi Porro, MD
Department of Gastroenterology, L. Sacco University Hospital, Via G.B. Grassi, 74, 20157 Milan, Italy

racy of transabdominal US in the diagnosis of Crohn's disease and also suggests its clinical activity.

It has been shown that the increase in audio Doppler intensity within the bowel wall following intravenous injection of air-filled microbubbles (Levovist; Schering, Berlin, Germany) can differentiate patients with Crohn's disease from healthy controls, in whom contrast enhancement is not detectable. The sensitivity is 97%, compared with transabdominal US alone (70%) or combined with color Doppler without microbubble injection (77%; DI SABATINO et al. 2002).

The usefulness of contrast-enhanced US in the evaluation of Crohn's disease activity is still debatable. To date, two studies have evaluated this topic using comparable methodology and air-filled microbubbles, but they showed contrasting results. In the first study (DI SABATINO et al. 2002), contrast enhancement was detected in 14 of 18 (78%) patients with active Crohn's disease and in 9 of 13 (69%) patients with inactive disease, whereas in the second study (RAPACCINI et al. 2004), contrast enhancement was present in all patients with active disease and in 8 of 26 (31%) with quiescent disease. These findings reflect the variable correlation between the degree of Crohn's disease activity and splanchnic hemodynamics. Hyperdynamic splanchnic circulation has always been shown in active Crohn's disease, while both normal and increased mesenteric blood flow has been found in quiescent Crohn's disease (VAN OOSTAYEN et al. 1994; MACONI et al. 1996, 1998).

Regarding the US assessment of Crohn's disease activity, interesting preliminary data have emerged with sulfur hexafluoride-filled microbubbles (SonoVue, Bracco, Milan, Italy) and dedicated contrast-specific techniques, which allow assessment of the distribution of vascularity within the layers of the bowel wall. Indeed, it is able to reveal whether vascularity is absent or present, and whether it involves the submucosa alone, the submucosa and the mucosa, or the entire bowel wall (Fig. 26.1). Preliminary

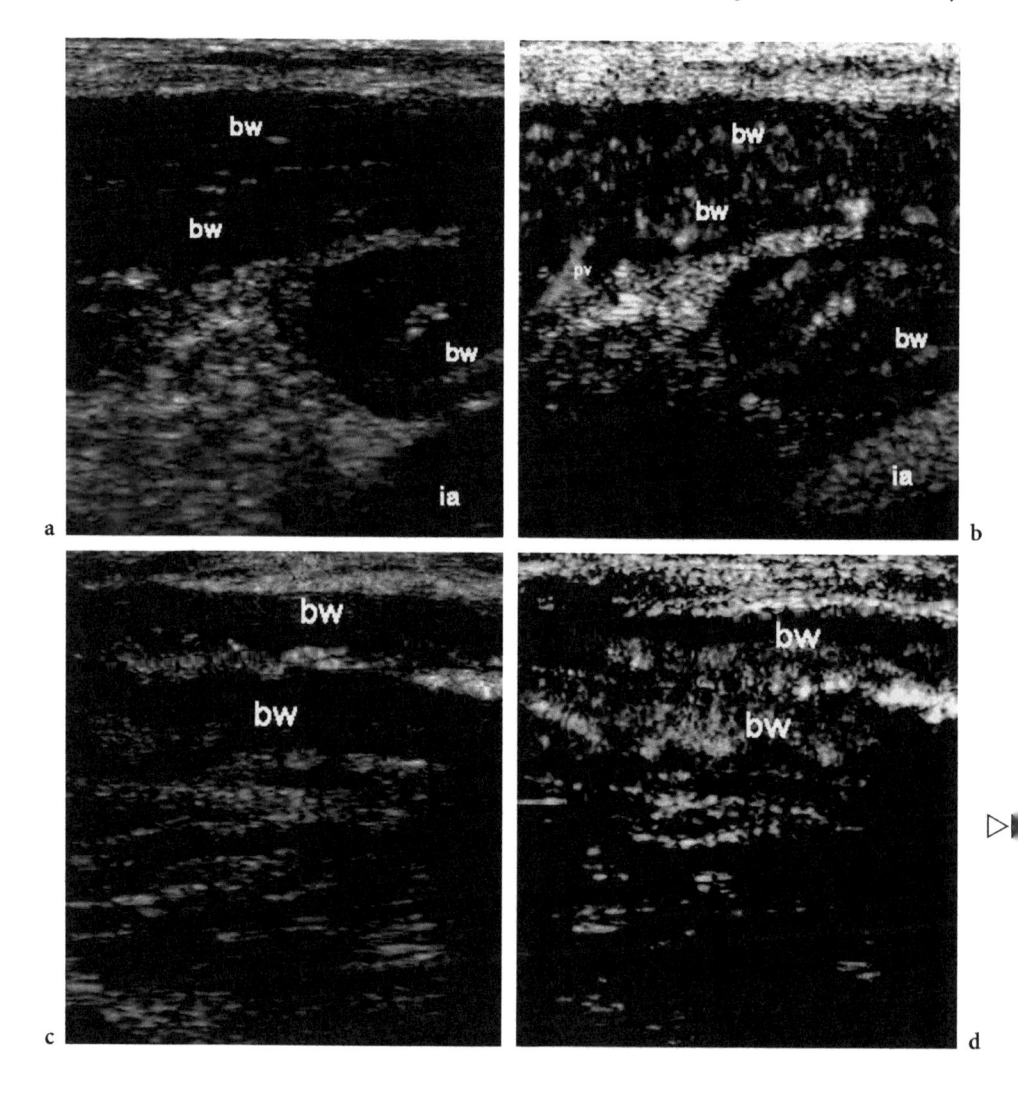

Intestinal Pathology

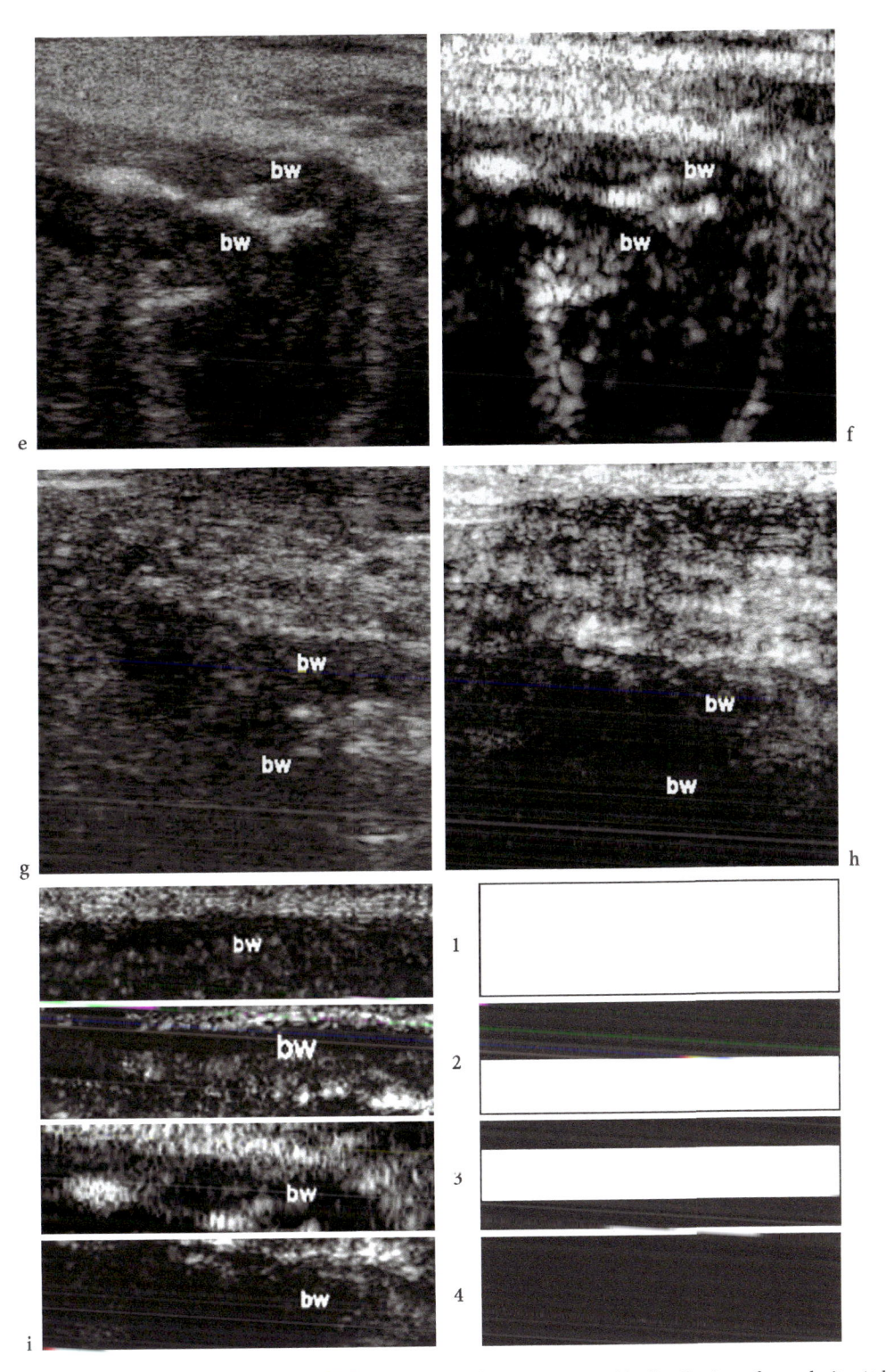

Fig. 26.1a–i. Longitudinal sections of thickened bowel walls showing variable distribution of vascularity. At baseline US scan (**a, c, e, g**) bowel wall shows different grades of thickness, which negatively correlate with the different grades of vascularity (**b, d, f, h**) revealed after microbubble-based contrast agent injection. After microbubble injection, the bowel wall vascularity may appear present (**b, d, f**) or absent (**h**). When vascularity is detectable, enhancement may be observed in the entire bowel wall (**b**), in the superficial layers (mucosa and submucosa; **d**), or within the layer corresponding to the submucosa only (**f**). *ia* iliac vessel, *bw* bowel walls. The scheme of blood flow distribution (**i**) resumes the different grades of vascularity of the bowel wall: *1*=diffuse vascularity; *2*=vascularity detectable in mucosa and submucosa; *3*=vascularity detectable only in submucosa; *4*=absence of vascularity

data suggest that the two last conditions are more frequently found in patients with active Crohn's disease, while the first two are more frequently found in patients with quiescent disease.

A more recent study (ROBOTTI et al. 2004) comprising 52 patients with Crohn's disease evaluated the thickening and the echo texture of the intestinal wall, and the presence or absence of vascular intraparietal signals with contrast-enhanced US after sulfur hexafluoride-filled microbubble injection. Microbubbles were injected at a dose of 4.8 ml and postcontrast images were analyzed by using second harmonic imaging with a low acoustic power (mechanical index=0.09). Data from this study showed that contrast-enhanced US with sulfur hexafluoride-filled microbubbles is of limited value in assessing Crohn's disease activity. In particular, perfect agreement between contrast-enhanced US and clinical and laboratory indexes of activity was 63.4%. Laboratory and clinical tests were indicative of active disease in 42.3% of patients with contrast enhancement and suggestive for inactive disease in 84.6% of patients without evidence of bowel wall contrast enhancement (ROBOTTI et al. 2004).

26.1.3
Characterization of Intestinal Strictures

Strictures occur in about one-third of Crohn's disease patients, and are one of the most frequent reasons for surgery. Even though it is well known that intestinal strictures complicating Crohn's disease usually require surgery, patients may also temporarily benefit from medical treatment such as bowel rest, corticosteroids, and antibiotics which can improve obstructive symptoms and delay the need for surgery. The responsiveness of strictures to medical treatment depends on the severity and histological features, and strictures characterized by severe inflammatory infiltrate are probably more responsive to medical treatment than those with marked fibrosis.

The possibility to discriminate between fibrotic and inflammatory strictures complicating Crohn's disease by means of clinical history and clinical indices, as well as laboratory markers of activity, although widely used, is not completely satisfactory. On the other hand, abdominal US can accurately detect intestinal stenosis in Crohn's disease, and the sonographic assessment of bowel wall echo texture in correspondence of strictures more accurately reflects the pathological features (PARENTE et al. 2002; MACONI et al. 2003). Indeed, the loss of stratification of the bowel wall at the level of the stricture suggests an inflammatory nature with a low degree of fibrosis, while the presence of stratification suggests a higher degree of fibrosis (MACONI et al. 2003). The decreased echogenicity in the hypoechoic echo pattern of strictures is due to hyperemia and neovascularization related to the increased inflammatory response.

It has been shown that vascularity of the bowel walls in Crohn's disease can be better assessed by contrast-enhanced power Doppler US; therefore, this can distinguish between fibrotic and inflammatory strictures and predict the outcome of medical treatment. Power Doppler US with air-filled microbubbles or sulfur hexafluoride-filled microbubbles, combined with real-time US by second harmonic imaging and low acoustic power insonation, can effectively differentiate hypervascularized inflammatory stenoses from those cicatricially transformed characterized by fibrosis, and hypovascularized scar tissue (KRATZER et al. 2002).

26.1.4
Diagnosis of Fistulae and Abscesses

Contrast-enhanced power Doppler US can detect intra-abdominal complications of Crohn's disease and successfully discriminates between abscesses and inflammatory masses, internal fistulae, and peri-intestinal lymph nodes.

It has already been shown that color and power Doppler US can be used to distinguish between phlegmons and abscesses, since abscesses usually present as fluid collections with peripheral flow, while phlegmons appear as a mesenteric mass with increased color signals (MACONI et al. 2002; TARJAN et al. 2000). More recently, it has been shown that power Doppler US with air-filled microbubbles allows diagnosis of inflammatory masses in doubtful cases and to distinguish between small abdominal inflammatory masses and abscesses, both in lesions with evidence of vascularity at power Doppler US and in some lesions showing no vascularity at baseline examination (ESTEBAN et al. 2003). A recent report showed that power Doppler with air-filled microbubbles is highly sensitive and specific in the detection and assessment of abdominal masses associated with Crohn's disease, and can detect abdominal masses of ≥1 cm, being even more accurate than CT which is considered the reference standard (ESTEBAN et al. 2003).

Intestinal Pathology

Inflammatory masses, phlegmons, and intra-abdominal abscesses, identified or suspected at US, may be distinguished or confirmed also using sulfur hexafluoride-filled microbubbles. Following microbubble injection, phlegmons or inflammatory massed show intense vascularization within and in the peripheral soft tissue, while abscesses show vascularization only at their periphery (Fig. 26.2). This is not surprising if we consider that these complications often occur as the result of transmural inflammation that progresses into a fistula and/or abscesses that are characterized by intense neovascularization of the wall (MACONI et al. 2002).

Since the detection of phlegmon in the initial stage allows the effective medical treatment to control progression, contrast-enhanced US can be used before an abscess is evident and surgery is required (SALLOMI 2003).

26.1.5
Prognostic Aspects and Monitoring of Disease

The assessment of color Doppler signals, within the bowel wall, in Crohn's disease has already been used to evaluate disease progression and response to therapy and, in quiescent disease, to assess the risk of clinical relapse (ESTEBAN et al. 2001).

Contrast-enhanced power Doppler can, to a certain extent, indicate the outcome of therapy in Crohn's disease patients. Indeed, patients with clinically active Crohn's disease and higher signal intensity of the thickened bowel walls at baseline and contrast-enhanced color Doppler US show a clear reduction in bowel wall thickening after steroid treatment in most cases. On the other hand, patients with active disease with thickened bowel walls, in whom no signal is detected either before or after microbubble injection,

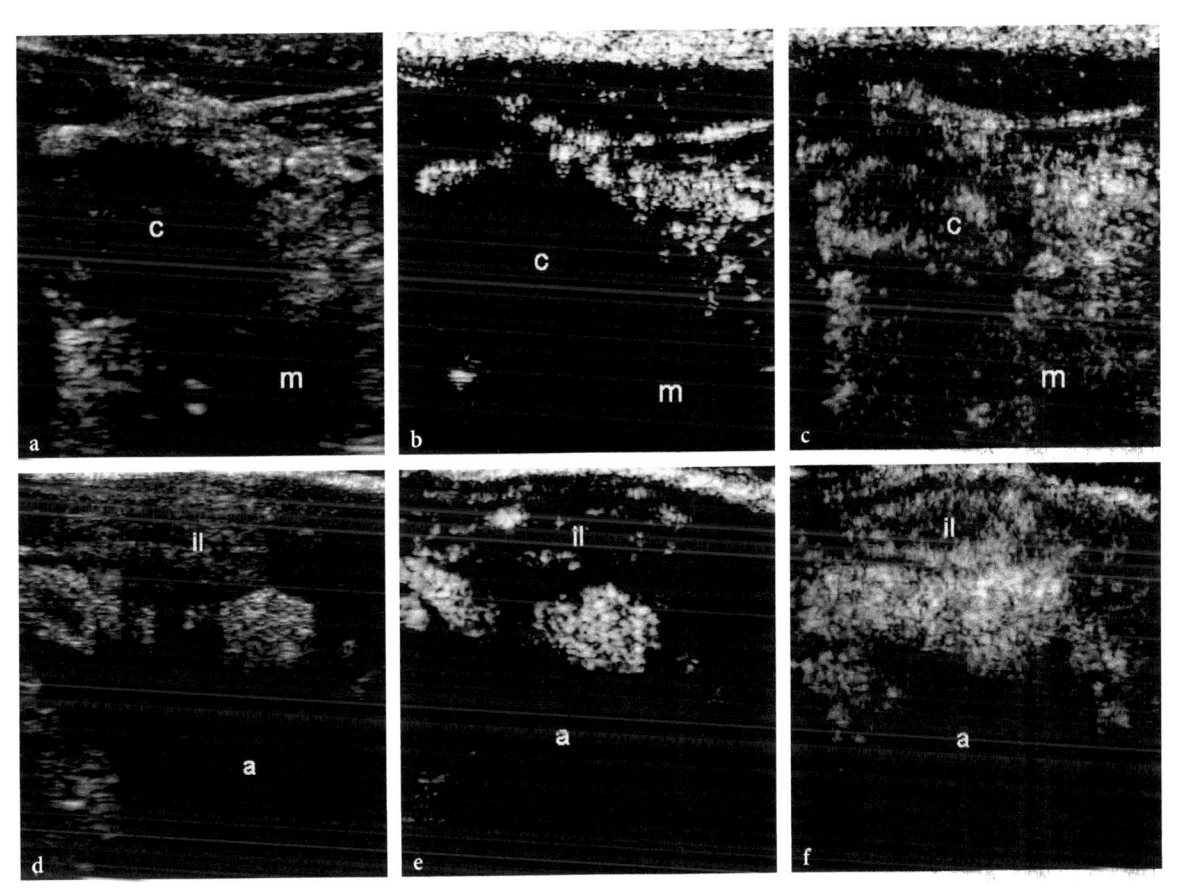

Fig. 26.2 a–f Detection of peri-intestinal inflammatory mass shown by the presence of vascularization within the lesion, following microbubble-based contrast agent injection. Baseline US imaging (**a**) of the lesion, and the same lesion before (**b**) and 23 s after intravenous microbubble injection (**c**) using second harmonic imaging with a low acoustic power insonation. **d–f** Intra-abdominal abscess confirmed by presence of vascularization in the peripheral area of the lesion without enhancement in the lesion center after microbubble-based contrast agent injection. Baseline US scan of the lesion (**d**), and the same lesion before (**e**) and 22 s following intravenous contrast injection (**f**) using second harmonic imaging with a low acoustic power insonation. *m* inflammatory mass, *c* colon, *a* intra-abdominal abscess, *il* ileum

present a disease which is less responsive to steroid therapy and are at higher risk of surgical resection (DI SABATINO et al. 2002; RAPACCINI et al. 2004).

Contrast-enhanced power Doppler US with air-filled microbubbles can also be used to predict early relapse in patients with inactive Crohn's disease. In fact, patients with inactive Crohn's disease with normal or pathological bowel wall thickening (>3 mm), and increased signal intensity after microbubble injection, are at higher risk of early clinical relapse (DI SABATINO et al. 2002; RAPACCINI et al. 2004). Similar results have been shown by using sulfur hexafluoride-filled microbubbles combined with second harmonic imaging with a low acoustic power of insonation. In this context, hypovascularized thickened bowel walls in patients with active Crohn's disease may suggest less responsiveness to anti-inflammatory therapy. On the other hand, in patients with clinical and biochemical remission of Crohn's disease, negative contrast enhancement indicates a stable remission (Fig. 26.3), while a positive contrast enhancement of the thickened bowel walls may suggest a higher risk of relapse and therefore the need of a strict follow-up (Fig. 26.4; ROBOTTI et al. 2004); however, these preliminary data need to be confirmed in prospective controlled trials. In fact, to date, the US assessment of bowel wall vascularity in Crohn's disease is not considered in planning the treatment in active or quiescent disease.

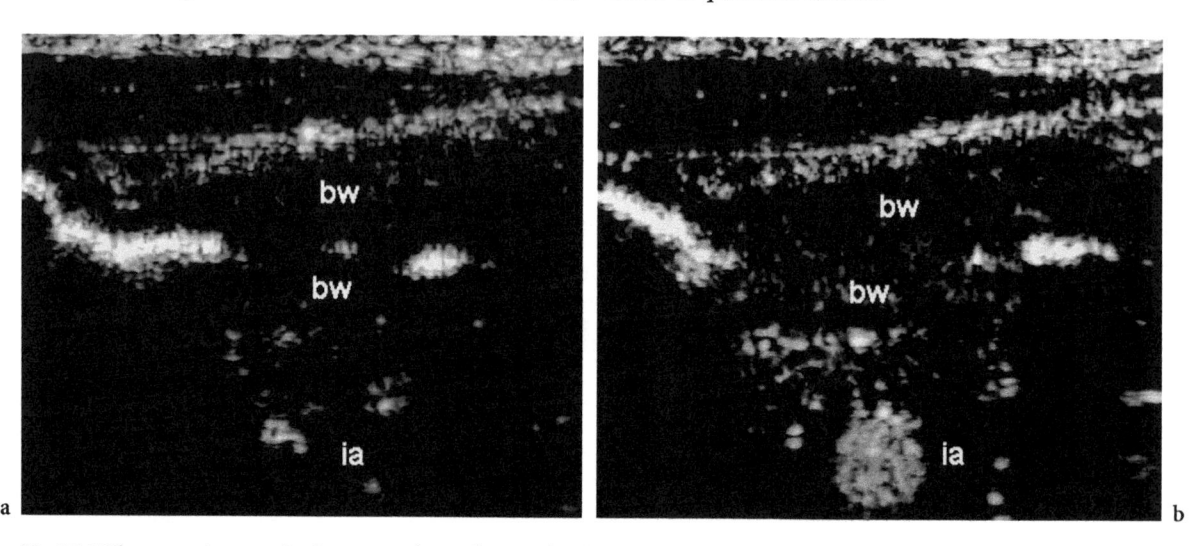

Fig. 26.3 Fibrostenotic stenosis. Contrast-enhanced US with a low transmit power insonation before (a) and 25 s after microbubble-based contrast agent injection (b). *bw* bowel wall, *ia* iliac vessel. Absence of a significant enhancement of the bowel wall at the level of a stricture following intravenous contrast agent injection due to a cicatricially transformed tissue.

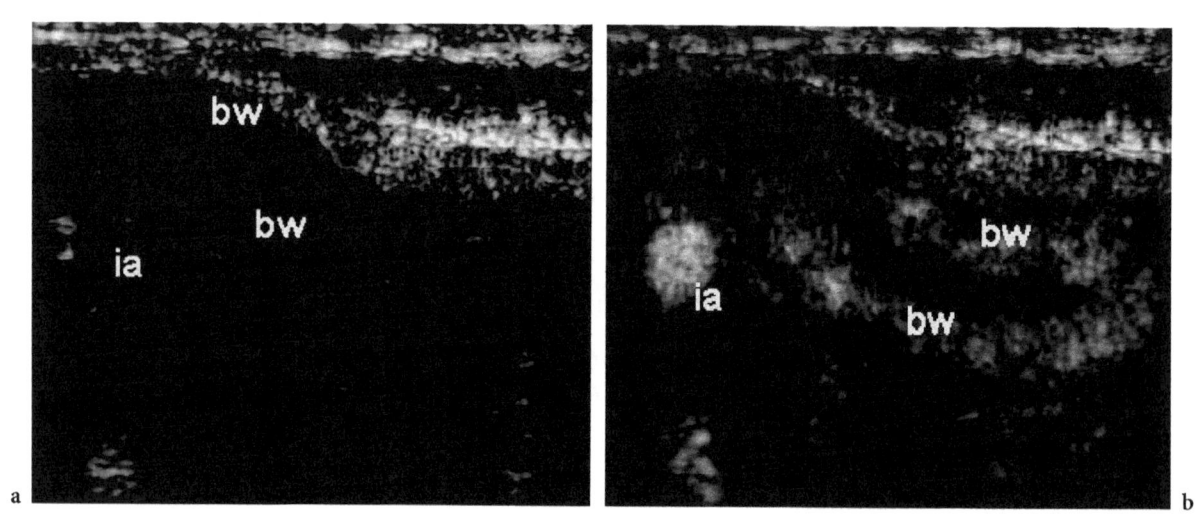

Fig. 26.4 Inflammatory stenosis. Diffuse contrast enhancement of the bowel wall at a stenotic level due to a hypervascularized and inflammatory tissue following intravenous contrast agent injection. Contrast-enhanced US with low transmit power before (a) and 24 s after microbubble-based contrast agent injection (b). *bw* bowel wall, *ia* iliac vessel

Intestinal Pathology

26.2
Neoplastic Diseases

26.2.1
Gastric Cancer

Gastric cancer, particularly if in advanced stage and located in the antrum, may be easily revealed at US as a mass or a variable degree of gastric wall thickening (Fig. 26.5).

Increased vascularity of thickened gastric walls can be assessed by power Doppler US in the majority of patients with gastric adenocarcinoma; however, the clinical importance of this evaluation has not yet been well defined. The exact relationship between vascularity of gastric cancer and gross morphologi-

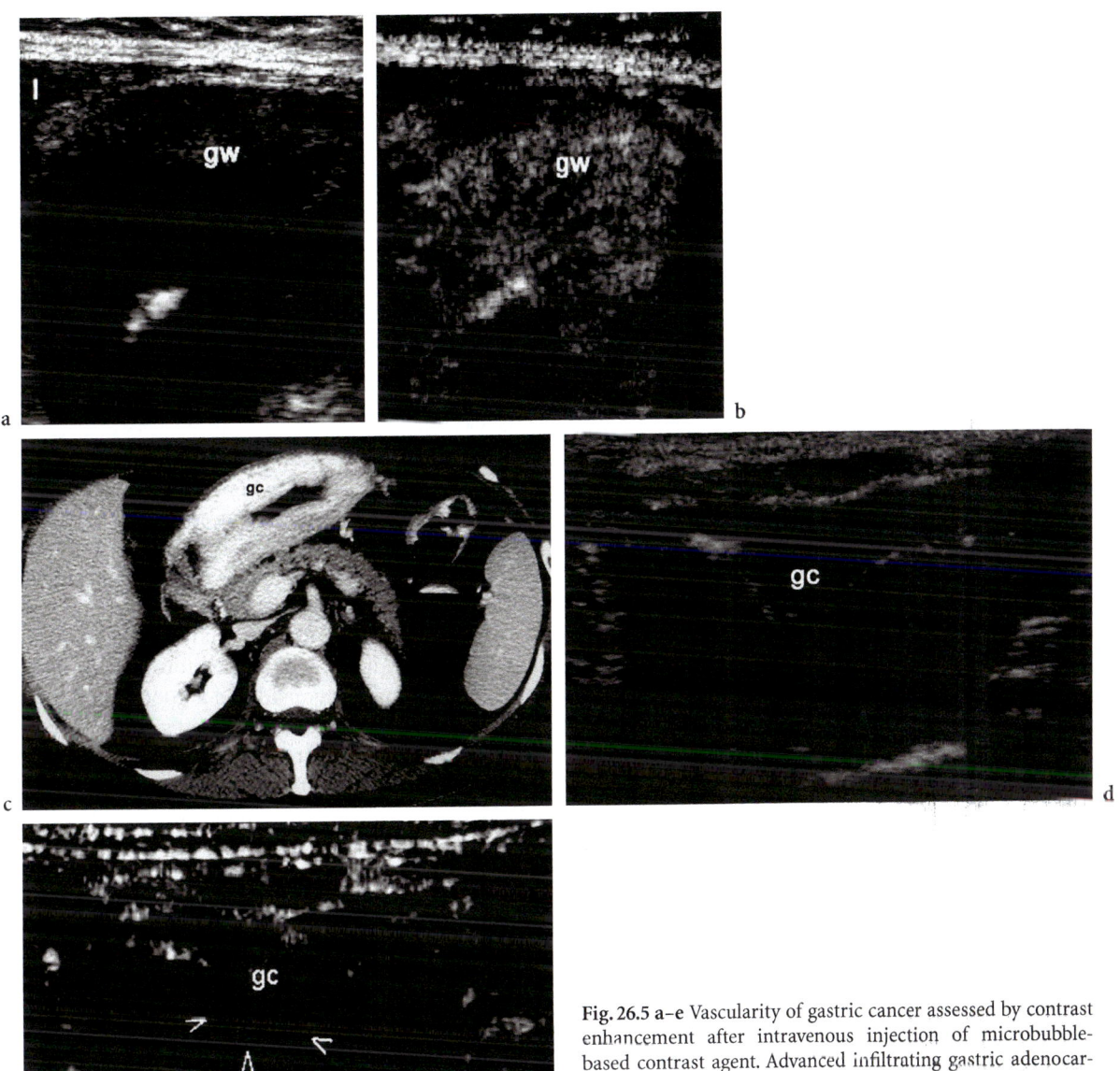

Fig. 26.5 a–e Vascularity of gastric cancer assessed by contrast enhancement after intravenous injection of microbubble-based contrast agent. Advanced infiltrating gastric adenocarcinoma (stage T3). Marked thickening of gastric wall at standard baseline US scan (a) and diffuse contrast enhancement 23 s following microbubble-based contrast agent injection (b). Comparative CT imaging of the same tumor (c). Early gastric adenocarcinoma (stage T1). Focal thickening of gastric wall at baseline US (d) reveals a slight contrast enhancement (*arrowheads*) 25 s after microbubble-based contrast agent injection (e). *gw* gastric wall, *gc* gastric cancer, *ia* iliac vessel

cal and histopathological classification still remains to be fully elucidated (KAWASAKI et al. 2001).

Quantification of the vascular color signals within the gastric cancer, expressed according to CHEN et al. (2002) as color–power Doppler vascularity index (=colored pixels/total pixels), did not show any significant correlation with gross pathological classification, stage, tumor location, or tumor size. On the other hand, color–power Doppler vascularity index was found to be an independent prognostic factor with a significant inverse correlation with the survival rate of patients in patients, and higher values were found in patients with vascular invasion of the tumor and in the diffuse type of gastric cancer (CHEN et al. 2002).

Vascularity of the tumor, assessed by color–power Doppler index, reflects the surface area of intratumoral vessels and may represent the summation effect of biological processes of tumor vascularization, tumor invasiveness and metastasis in gastric cancer. The marked vascularity may predict early death in patients with advanced stage (stage III) gastric cancer (CHEN et al. 2002).

Color Doppler US allows identification of flow signal from larger (≥100 μm in diameter) intratumoral vessels, frequently arterioles, venules, and arteriole-venule shunting (FLEISHER et al. 1999; LASSAU et al. 1999), while it cannot detect the actual neovascularization (vessels ≤15 μm in diameter), which is usually demonstrated by immunohistochemistry. However, microbubble injection coupled with second harmonic imaging technique may be successfully used to assess microcirculation in gastric cancer. Indeed, tumoral enhancement following air-filled microbubble injection shows a significant, strong, positive correlation with gastric cancer vascularity determined by counting stained microvessels in the tumor specimens (OKANOBU et al. 2002). Also, sulfur hexafluoride-filled microbubbles easily reveal the distribution and entity of gastric cancer vascularity with results comparable to those of CT (Fig. 26.5).

Further investigations in larger series of gastric cancer patients are necessary to define the clinical role of US assessment of vascularity in gastric cancer. The possibility to accurately and non-invasively assess tumor vascularity and neoangiogenesis in vivo could provide useful information in defining specific surgical procedures, in planning adjuvant chemotherapy, and in evaluating the efficacy of antiangiogenic therapy. Recent studies in animal tumoral models show that contrast-enhanced power Doppler US is a promising tool for comprehensive monitoring of anti-angiogenic or pro-angiogenic therapies (GEE et al. 2001; KRIX et al. 2003).

26.2.2
Colorectal Cancer

Cancer of the colon or rectum produces a mass or segmental wall thickening that may be revealed with US (LIM 1996). Even though colonoscopy or barium enema are the procedures of choice for the detection and diagnosis of colorectal cancer, abdominal US may be the first test that patients with colon cancer undergo on account of their symptoms. Furthermore, it is the most frequently used procedure for pre-operative staging in patients with colorectal cancer.

At conventional transabdominal US, colorectal cancers may present as either a bulky hypoechoic mass of variable size or segmental thickening of the colonic wall with irregular or lobulated contours and often eccentric. Assessment of colorectal cancer vascularity by transabdominal color or power Doppler US does not provide important insight in the detection, diagnosis, and differential diagnosis of the lesion; however, previous reports showed that assessment of colorectal cancer vascularity by transabdominal color Doppler US with the assessment of the vascularity index according to CHEN et al. (2002) could provide important prognostic parameters.

Colorectal cancer patients with a high vascularity index have a greater prevalence of lymph node metastases, more severe vascular invasion, and, consequently, a high incidence of distant metastasis after curative resection, and thus poorer prognosis than patients with a low vascularity index (CHEN et al. 2000; OGURA et al. 2001); therefore, intra-tumoral vascularity may be considered a good preoperative indicator of recurrence and patient survival in colon cancer, and may be used as a preoperative prognostic indicator in colon cancer, together with staging, to identify patients with poor prognosis and to direct patients for the appropriate neoadjuvant treatment.

Microbubble-based agents may improve the US detection and quantification of vascularity in vivo and optimizes the detection of angiogenesis also in the poorly vascularized tumoral model. Air-filled microbubble injection allows the identification of small intratumoral vessels (<40 μm in diameter; LASSAU et al. 2001). Moreover, contrast-enhanced US with air-filled microbubbles allows detection of areas with high density of vessels or regions with no vascularity at histological analysis. Sulfur hexafluoride-filled microbubbles allow to combine the accuracy in the detection of vascularity with dynamic parameters of vascularity, such as the speed of enhancement, time of onset, and the value of peak signal enhancement, time of decrease of enhancement, as well as enhancement duration. Further studies will establish whether this quantitative analysis would be useful in the differential diagnosis between benign and malignant tumors, and to measure the extent of angiogenesis, the metastatic potential of neoplastic lesions, as well as the effect of treatment.

26.3 Conclusion

The application of microbubble-based agents in intestinal diseases is only at the beginning. Few papers have been published dealing with the usefulness and application of microbubble-based agents in intestinal diseases. The main fields of application are Crohn's disease and malignancies of the gastrointestinal tract.

Microbubble-based contrast agents have been proven to be useful in identifying bowel wall vascularity in Crohn's disease. This frequently correlates with the degree of inflammation in the early stage of the disease and may be useful in detecting the disease and in assessing its clinical activity. The assessment of vascularity of the bowel walls by means of US combined with microbubble-based agents can identify and differentiate between intra-abdominal complications of Crohn's disease, such as fistulae, inflammatory masses, and abscess, and can help to characterize and distinguish between inflammatory and fibrotic stenosis. Furthermore, it is useful in monitoring the course of the disease suggesting early recurrence.

In gastrointestinal malignancies, the assessment of gastrointestinal walls after microbubble-based-agent injection could be used mainly to obtain prognostic parameters regarding tumor invasion and survival of patients; however, the potential of microbubbles to enhance and quantify neoangiogenesis will allow differentiation between benign and malignant tumors, definition of the vascular invasion of gastric and colorectal cancer, the metastatic potential of neoplastic lesions, and quantification of the effect of treatment.

References

Chen CN, Cheng YM, Liang JT et al (2000) Color Doppler vascularity index can predict distant metastasis and survival in colon cancer patients. Cancer Res 60:2892–2897

Chen CN, Cheng YM, Lin MT et al (2002) Association of color Doppler vascularity index and microvessel density with survival in patients with gastric cancer. Ann Surg 235:512–518

Di Sabatino A, Fulle I, Ciccocioppo R et al (2002) Doppler enhancement after intravenous levovist injection in Crohn's disease. Inflamm Bowel Dis 8:251–257

Esteban JM, Maldonado L, Sanchiz V et al (2001) Activity of Crohn's disease assessed by colour Doppler ultrasound analysis of the affected loops. Eur Radiol 11:1423–1428

Esteban JM, Aleixandre A, Hurtado MJ et al (2003) Contrast-enhanced power Doppler ultrasound in the diagnosis and follow-up of inflammatory abdominal masses in Crohn's disease. Eur J Gastroenterol Hepatol 15:253–259

Fleischer AC, Wojcicki WE, Donnelly EF et al (1999) Quantified color Doppler sonography of tumor vascularity in an animal model. J Ultrasound Med 18:547–551

Gee MS, Saunders HM, Lee JC et al (2001) Doppler ultrasound imaging detects changes in tumor perfusion during antivascular therapy associated with vascular anatomic alterations. Cancer Res 61:2974–2982

Kawasaki T, Ueo T, Itani T et al (2001) Vascularity of advanced gastric carcinoma: evaluation by using power Doppler imaging. J Gastroenterol Hepatol 16:149–153

Knutson H, Lunderquist A, Lunderquist A (1968) Vascular changes in Crohn's disease. Am J Roentgenol Radium Ther Nucl Med 103:380–385

Kratzer W, von Tirpitz C, Mason R et al (2002) Contrast-enhanced power Doppler sonography of the intestinal wall in the differentiation of hypervascularized and hypovascularized intestinal obstructions in patients with Crohn's disease. J Ultrasound Med 21:149–157

Krix M, Kiessling F, Vosseler S et al (2003) Comparison of intermittent-bolus contrast imaging with conventional power Doppler sonography: quantification of tumour perfusion in small animals. Ultrasound Med Biol 29:1093–1103

Lassau N, Paturel-Asselin C, Guinebretiere J-M et al (1999) New hemodynamic approach to angiogenesis: color and pulsed Doppler ultrasonography. Invest Radiol 34:194–198

Lassau N, Koscielny S, Opolon P et al (2001) Evaluation of contrast-enhanced color Doppler ultrasound for the quantification of angiogenesis in vivo. Invest Radiol 36:50–55

Lim JH (1996) Colorectal cancer: sonographic findings. Am J Roentgenol 167:45–47

Maconi G, Imbesi V, Bianchi Porro G (1996) Doppler ultrasound measurement of intestinal blood flow in inflammatory bowel disease. Scand J Gastroenterol 31:590–593

Maconi G, Parente F, Bollani S et al (1998) Factors affecting splanchnic haemodynamics in Crohn's disease: a prospective controlled study using Doppler ultrasound. Gut 43:645–650

Maconi G, Sampietro GM, Russo A et al (2002) The vascularity of internal fistulae in Crohn's disease: an in vivo power Doppler ultrasonography assessment. Gut 50:496–500

Maconi G, Carsana L, Fociani P et al (2003) Small bowel stenosis in Crohn's disease: clinical, biochemical and ultrasonographic evaluation of histological features. Aliment Pharmacol Ther 18:749-756

Ogura O, Takebayashi Y, Sameshima T et al (2001) Preoperative assessment of vascularity by color Doppler ultrasonography in human rectal carcinoma. Dis Colon Rectum 44:538-546

Okanobu H, Hata J, Haruma K et al (2002) Preoperative assessment of gastric cancer vascularity by FLASH echo imaging. Scand J Gastroenterol 37:608-612

Parente F, Maconi G, Bollani S et al (2002) Bowel ultrasound in assessment of Crohn's disease and detection of related small bowel strictures: a prospective comparative study versus X-ray and intraoperative findings. Gut 50:490-495

Rapaccini GL, Pompili M, Orefice R et al (2004) Contrast-enhanced power Doppler of the intestinal wall in the evaluation of patients with Crohn disease. Scand J Gastroenterol 39:188-194

Robotti D, Cammarota T, Debani P et al (2004) Activity of Crohn disease: value of color-power Doppler and contrast-enhanced ultrasonography. Abdom Imaging 29(6):648-652

Sallomi DF (2003) The use of contrast-enhanced power Doppler ultrasound in the diagnosis and follow-up of inflammatory abdominal masses associated with Crohn's disease. Eur J Gastroenterol Hepatol 15:249-251

Spalinger J, Patriquin H, Miron MC et al (2000) Doppler US in patients with Crohn's disease: vessel density in the diseased bowel reflects disease activity. Radiology 217:787-791

Tarjan Z, Toth G, Gyorke T et al (2000) Ultrasound in Crohn's disease of the small bowel. Eur J Radiol 35:176-182

Van Oostayen JA, Wasser MN, van Hogezand RA et al (1994) Activity of Crohn's disease assessed by measurement of superior mesenteric artery flow with Doppler US. Radiology 193:551-554

Wakefield AJ, Sawyerr AM, Dhillon AP et al (1989) Pathogenesis of Crohn's disease: multifocal gastrointestinal infarction. Lancet 2:1057-1062

27 Contrast-Enhanced Ultrasound of the Prostate

J. Robert Ramey

CONTENTS

27.1 Introduction 359
27.2 Conventional Gray-Scale Transrectal US and Sextant Biopsy 359
27.3 Prostatic Blood Supply 360
27.4 Prostate Cancer and Angiogenesis 360
27.5 Unenhanced Doppler Imaging 360
27.6 Contrast-Enhanced Transrectal US and Prostate Cancer Detection 360
27.7 Other Imaging Modalities 361
27.8 Conclusion 363
References 363

27.1
Introduction

Adenocarcinoma of the prostate is the most common solid organ malignancy in men. The American Cancer Society estimates 230,110 men will be diagnosed with prostate cancer in 2004 and that approximately 29,900 deaths will occur due to disease over the same time period (Jemal et al. 2004).

Prior to the widespread use of prostate-specific antigen (PSA) screening programs and transrectal ultrasound (US)-guided prostate biopsies, the diagnosis of prostate cancer was made on digital rectal examination and prostatic acid phosphatase. Confirmation was obtained with manually guided, transperineal biopsy. Unfortunately, despite the advances in prostate cancer detection afforded by PSA and transrectal US guided biopsy, a significant number of cancers still go undetected.

J. R. Ramey, MD
Department of Urology, Suite 1100, Jefferson Prostate Diagnostic Center, Thomas Jefferson University, 1015 Walnut Street, Philadelphia, PA 19107, USA

27.2
Conventional Gray-Scale Transrectal US and Sextant Biopsy

The classical description of prostate cancer is that of a hypoechoic lesion in the peripheral zone on conventional gray-scale transrectal US (Fig. 27.1). Hypoechoic lesions represent 60–70% of tumors (Purohit et al. 2003), even though only 17–57% of hypoechoic foci actually harbor a malignancy (Bartsch et al. 1982; Lee et al. 1987; Rifkin et al. 1991; Spencer et al. 1994; Rifkin 1997, 1998; Weaver et al. 1991). Prostate cancer may also appear isoechoic (40% of tumors), occasionally rarely hyperechoic lesions have been reported. As such, <40% of nonpalpable tumors are identifiable sonographically with gray-scale imaging (Shinohara et al. 1989).

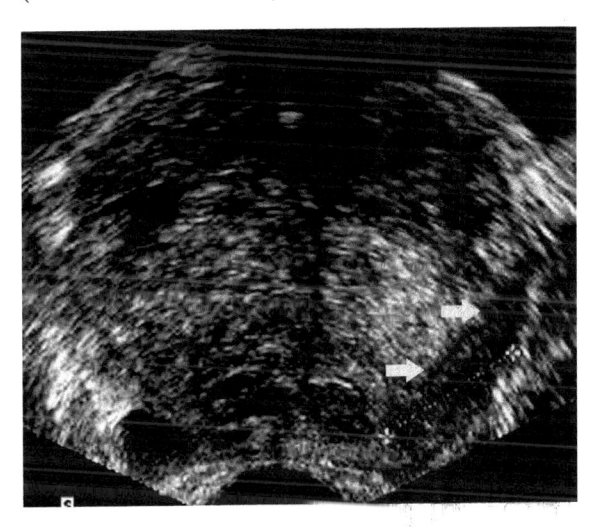

Fig. 27.1 Transverse image of the prostate demonstrates classical hypoechoic lesion in the left mid-gland (*arrows*). Biopsies targeted to this lesion revealed a Gleason-7 adenocarcinoma

Due to the inability of gray-scale transrectal US to accurately identify prostate cancer random systematic biopsy techniques have become routinely employed in the diagnosis of prostate cancer. Introduced by Hodge et al. (1989), transrectal US-guided sextant biopsy has dramatically improved cancer detection but still has a reported false-negative rate of 15–35% (Norberg et al. 1977; Eskew et al. 1997). Various modifications in biopsy core location and number have been subsequently introduced, but none have succeeded in eliminating false-negative results (Eskew et al. 1997; Levine et al. 1998; Babaian et al. 2000; Brossner et al. 2000; Presti et al. 2000; Durkan et al. 2002; Fink et al. 2003). These limitations of conventional gray-scale imaging and systematic random biopsy techniques have led investigators to study the ability of Doppler imaging, microbubble contrast agents, and targeted biopsy protocols to improve prostate cancer detection.

27.3
Prostatic Blood Supply

The paired prostatic arteries arise from the inferior vesical arteries and subsequently divide into two main divisions: (a) the urethral artery; and (b) the capsular artery (Brooks 2002). The capsular arteries course along the posterolateral aspect of the prostate, giving off perforator branches that supply the parenchyma of the gland (Halpern 2002a). These perforators are radially oriented in the transverse plane, producing a symmetric spoke-wheel pattern on Doppler imaging (Lavoipierre et al. 1998).

27.4
Prostate Cancer and Angiogenesis

The increased growth rate of malignant tissue requires increased blood flow to meet the higher metabolic demands. Angioneogenesis has been demonstrated in a variety of malignancies and often corresponds to local aggressiveness and metastatic proclivity (Chodak et al. 1980; Sillman et al. 1981; Weidner et al. 1991). Overexpression of pro-angiogenic growth factors has been implicated in this process and vascular endothelial growth factor, epidermal growth factor, and basic fibroblast growth factor have all been demonstrated to be elevated in prostate tumors (Trojan et al. 2004). Pathologic examinations of prostate tumors from radical prostatectomy specimens have confirmed the presence of angioneogenesis within prostate cancer by demonstrating increased microvessel density compared with surrounding normal parenchyma (Bigler et al. 1993); thus, imaging techniques that provide selective visualization of blood flow within these microvessels should provide the opportunity to significantly improve prostate cancer detection.

27.5
Unenhanced Doppler Imaging

Early attempts to exploit the increased microvascularity of prostate cancers examined the ability of color and power Doppler to identify areas of abnormally increased blood flow within the prostate (Fig. 27.2). Targeted biopsy protocols based on biopsies aimed at areas of abnormal flow have also been developed.

Halpern and Strup (2000) investigated the ability of color and power Doppler imaging to sonographically diagnose carcinoma of the prostate. Using a sextant biopsy protocol, they detected cancer in 211 cores from 85 patients. Doppler imaging prospectively identified 35 of the 211 foci as malignant.

Another recent study compared cancer detection rates between color- and power Doppler-targeted biopsy and sextant biopsy. Confirming previously reported results (Kelly et al. 1993; Rifkin et al. 1993; Newman et al. 1995; Sakarya et al. 1998; Okihara et al. 2000; Shigeno et al. 2000) the positive biopsy rate was improved with targeted cores (13 vs 9.7%). Unfortunately, 33% of patients (6 of 18) diagnosed with cancer had tumors that were undetected by targeted biopsy alone (Halpern et al. 2002a).

27.6
Contrast-Enhanced Transrectal US and Prostate Cancer Detection

The inability of unenhanced transrectal US imaging techniques to accurately identify malignant foci and to reliably detect all tumors with only targeted biopsies has led several groups to study contrast-enhanced transrectal US as a means to improve prostate cancer detection. Microvessels of prostate tumors have been shown to range in diameter from 10–50 µm (Bigler et al. 1993), which is well below the 1-mm-resolution limit of conventional Doppler imaging (Halpern 2002a). This explains the promising yet limited improvements in prostate cancer detection seen with unenhanced Doppler imaging.

Contrast-Enhanced Ultrasound of the Prostate

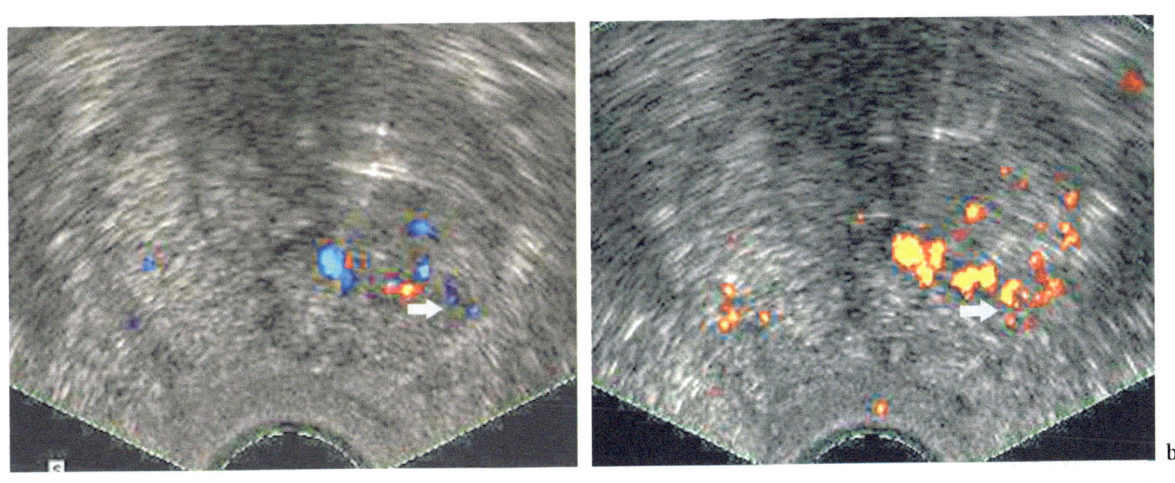

Fig. 27.2a,b. Unenhanced transverse (a) color and (b) power Doppler imaging of a Gleason-7 prostate adenocarcinoma in the left mid to apex of the gland (*arrow*)

Contrast-enhanced transrectal US has been shown to increase the sensitivity of color and power Doppler imaging from 37 to 53% without significantly altering specificity (FRAUSCHER et al. 2002a). The small size of microbubble contrast agents make them ideal for imaging blood flow within the vascular beds of prostate tumors. Microbubbles readily traverse these low-flow, small-diameter vessels amplifying Doppler signals and allowing selective visualization of blood flow within malignant foci (Fig. 27.3).

Initial work by HALPERN et al. (2000) in a phase-II study of the microbubble-based contrast agent Imagent (AFO-150, Imcor Pharmaceutical, San Diego, Calif.) demonstrated the ability to prospectively identify focal areas of enhancement with power Doppler imaging during contrast infusion. These areas of enhancement were all noted to be isoechoic on baseline imaging, but corresponded to foci of cancer on pathologic review of biopsy specimens.

Another early study showed similar success using Levovist (SHU 508 A, Schering, Berlin, Germany) and a color Doppler-based targeted-biopsy protocol. Positive biopsy rates were significantly improved with targeted cores vs sextant cores (13 vs 4.9%, respectively). Furthermore, targeted biopsies detected cancer in 7 patients with negative systematic biopsies while failing to diagnose a cancer detected on sextant biopsy in only one patient (FRAUSCHER et al. 2001).

A recent study of 230 patients utilized contrast-enhanced color Doppler imaging to target biopsies and compared cancer detection rates to sextant biopsies performed in the same subjects. Targeted biopsies were again found to be significantly superior to systematic biopsy with 10.4 vs 5.3% positive cores, respectively (FRAUSCHER et al. 2002b). Several additional studies have further confirmed that contrast-enhanced US improves cancer detection, although none have demonstrated superiority for either color or power Doppler imaging (Fig. 27.4; HALPERN et al. 2001; HALPERN 2002b; ROY et al. 2003).

27.7
Other Imaging Modalities

Newer techniques, such as contrast-enhanced harmonic imaging, have also been evaluated in prostate cancer imaging studies (HALPERN et al. 2000, 2001, 2002b). Using phase-inversion technology, harmonic imaging exploits the nonlinear behavior of the microbubbles to differentiate between vascular echoes and surrounding tissue (FRAUSCHER et al. 2002b).

In a prospective study of the contrast agent Definity (MRX 115, Bristol-Myers Squibb Medical Imaging, North Billerica, Mass.), 60 patients were imaged at baseline and during continuous contrast infusion. Real time and intermittent (scan delays of 0.5, 1.0, 2.0, and 5.0 s) harmonic imaging were performed in addition to power Doppler imaging. The increasing interscan delays during intermittent imaging allow more contrast to enter the prostate between each image producing dramatic enhancement within malignant foci (Fig. 27.5). At baseline cancer was identified at 14 foci in 11 subjects while contrast-enhanced imaging identified cancer at 24 foci in 15 subjects. Sensitivity was significantly improved with contrast-enhanced imaging (65 vs 38%), while specificity was not significantly different (HALPERN et al. 2001).

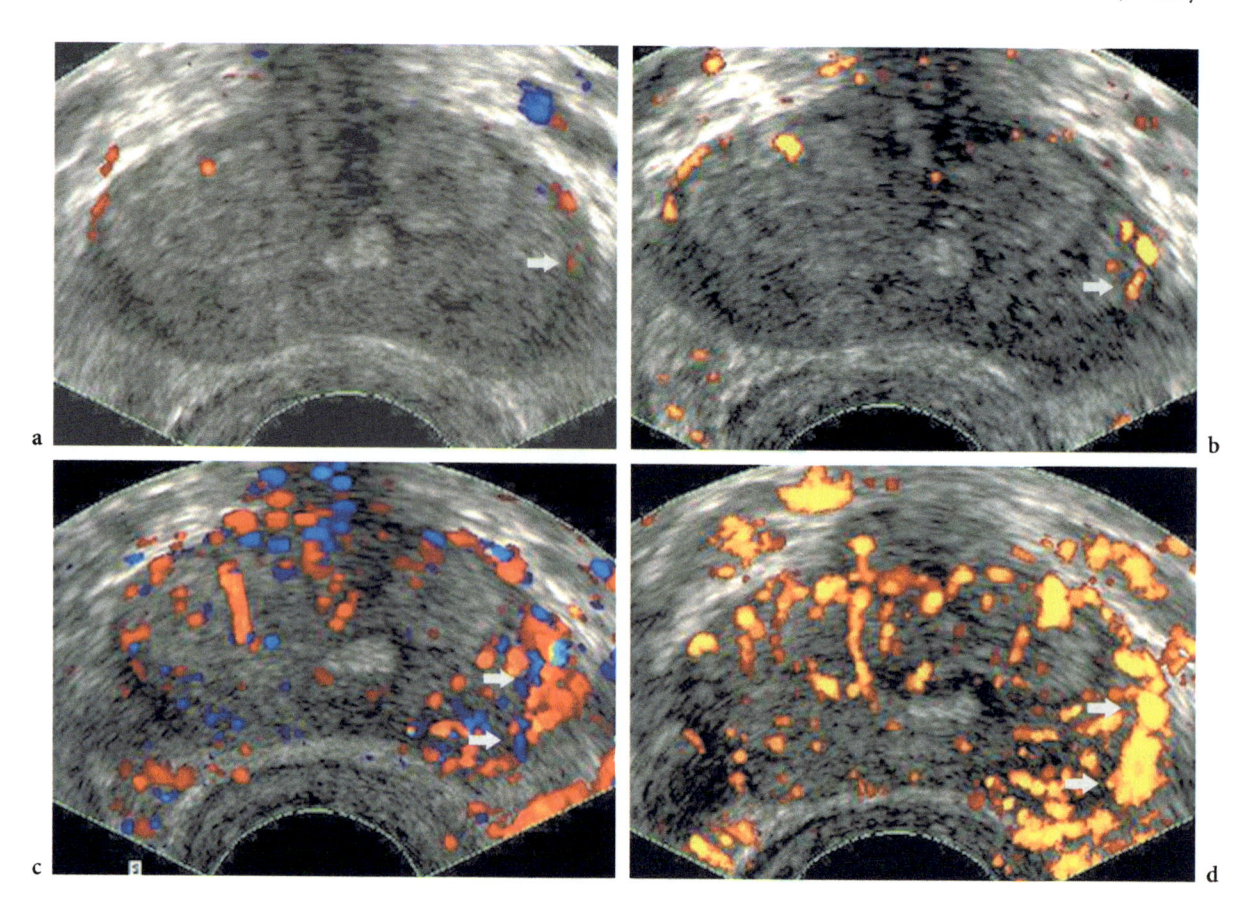

Fig. 27.3 Transverse imaging of a Gleason-6 prostate cancer in the left mid-gland. Baseline unenhanced (**a**) color and (**b**) power Doppler images reveal minimal focus of increased flow (*arrow*), while contrast-enhanced (**c**) color and (**d**) power Doppler images clearly demonstrate diffuse hypervascularity in the site of neoplasia (*arrows*).

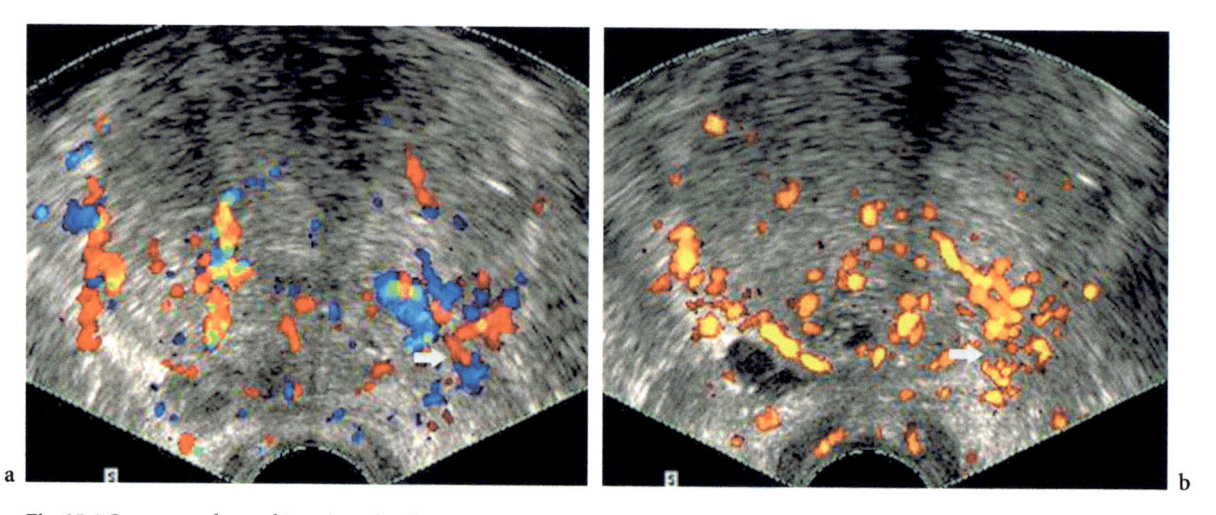

Fig. 27.4 Contrast-enhanced imaging of a Gleason-7 prostate tumor (*arrow*) in the left prostatic base on (**a**) color and (**b**) power Doppler

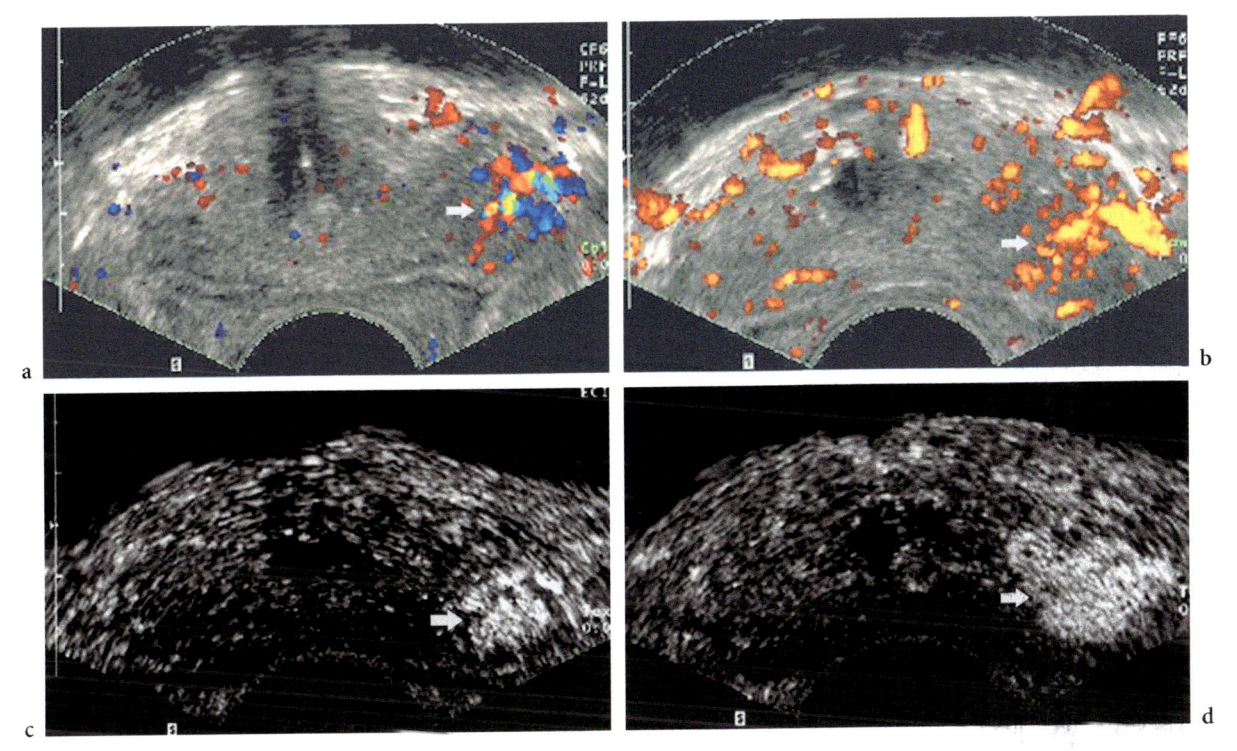

Fig. 27.5 a Color and b power Doppler images of a Gleason-7 adenocarcinoma of the left mid gland (*arrow*). Intermittent harmonic imaging of the same tumor shows increasing enhancement (*arrow*) with increasing interscan delays (c 0.2-s delay and d 1.0-s delay).

27.8 Conclusion

The clear association between increased microvascularity and prostate cancer (BIGLER et al. 1993) suggests that contrast-enhanced transrectal US should significantly improve our ability to detect prostate cancer. Additionally, since increased microvessel density has been correlated with metastatic disease (WEIDNER et al. 1993) and disease-specific survival (LISSBRANT et al. 1997; BORRE et al. 1998), the cancers identified with contrast-enhanced imaging techniques are likely to be more aggressive tumors and thus require treatment. To date, several studies have shown significant improvements in cancer detection using contrast-enhanced imaging and targeted-biopsy protocols. These promising results indicate that further study is clearly warranted to define the clinical role for this imaging modality in our armamentarium of diagnostic tools for prostate cancer detection.

References

Babaian RJ, Toi A, Kamoi K et al (2000) A comparative analysis of sextant and an extended 11-core multisite directed biopsy strategy. J Urol 163:152–157

Bartsch G, Egender G, Hubscher H, Rohr H (1982) Sonometrics of the prostate. J Urol 127:1119–1121

Bigler SA, Deering RE, Brawer MK (1993) Comparison of microscopic vascularity in benign and malignant prostate tissue. Hum Pathol 24:220–226

Borre M, Offersen BV, Nerstrom B, Overgaard J (1998) Microvessel density predicts survival in prostate cancer patients subjected to watchful waiting. Cancer 78:940–944

Brooks JD (2002) Anatomy of the lower urinary tract and male genitalia. In: Walsh PC, Retik AB, Vaughn ED, Wein AJ (eds) Campbell's urology, 8th edn. Saunders, Philadelphia

Brossner C, Bayer G, Madersbacher S et al (2000) Twelve prostate biopsies detect significant cancer volumes (>0.5 ml). Br J Urol Int 85:705–707

Chodak GW, Haudenschild C, Gittes RF, Folkman J (1980) Angiogenic activity as a marker of neoplastic and preneoplastic lesions of the human bladder. Ann Surg 192:762–771

Durkan GC, Sheikh N, Johnson P et al (2002) Improving prostate cancer detection with an extended-core transrectal ultrasonography-guided prostate biopsy protocol. Br J Urol Int 89:33–39

Eskew LA, Bare RL, McCullough DL (1997) Sytematic 5 region prostate biopsy is superior to sextant method for diagnosing carcinoma of the prostate. J Urol 157:199–203

Fink KG, Hutarew G, Pytel A et al (2003) One 10-core prostate biopsy is superior to two sets of sextant biopsies. Br J Urol Int 92:385–388

Frauscher F, Klauser A, Halpern EJ et al (2001) Detection of prostate cancer with a microbubble ultrasound contrast agent. Lancet 357:1849–1850

Frauscher F, Klauser A, Halpern EJ (2002a) Advances in ultrasound for the detection of prostate cancer. Ultrasound Quat 18:135–142

Frauscher F, Klauser A, Volgger H et al (2002b) Comparison of contrast enhanced color Doppler targeted biopsy with conventional systematic biopsy: impact on prostate cancer detection. J Urol 167:1648–1652

Halpern EJ (2002a) Color and power Doppler evaluation of prostate cancer. In: Halpern EJ, Cochlin DL, Goldberg BB (eds) Imaging of the prostate. Dunitz, London, pp 39–50

Halpern EJ (2002b) Advanced sonographic techniques for detection of prostate cancer. In: Halpern EJ, Cochlin DL, Goldberg BB (eds) Imaging of the prostate. Dunitz, London, pp 65–75

Halpern EJ, Strup SE (2000) Using gray-scale and color and power Doppler sonography to detect prostatic cancer. Am J Roentgenol 174:623–627

Halpern EJ, Verkh L, Forsberg F et al (2000) Initial experience with contrast-enhanced sonography of the prostate. Am J Roentgenol 174:1575–1580

Halpern EJ, Rosenberg M, Gomella LG (2001) Prostate cancer: contrast-enhanced US for detection. Radiology 219:219–225

Halpern EJ, Frauscher F, Strup SE et al (2002a) Prostate: high-frequency Doppler US imaging for cancer detection. Radiology 225:71–77

Halpern EJ, Frauscher F, Rosenberg M, Gomella LG (2002b) Directed biopsy during contrast-enhanced sonography of the prostate. Am J Roentgenol 178:915–919

Hodge KK, McNeal JE, Terris MK, Stamey TA (1989) Random systematic versus directed ultrasound guided transrectal core biopsies of the prostate. J Urol 142:71–74

Jemal A, Tiwari RC, Murray T et al (2004) Cancer statistics, 2004. CA Cancer J Clinicians 54:8–29

Kelly IMG, Lees WR, Rickards D (1993) Prostate cancer and the role of color Doppler US. Radiology 189:153–156

Lavoipierre AM, Snow RM, Frydenberg M et al (1998) Prostatic cancer: role of Doppler imaging in transrectal sonography. Am J Roentgenol 171:205–210

Lee F, Littrup PJ, McCleary RD et al (1987) Needle aspiration and core biopsy of prostate cancer: comparative evaluation with biplanar transrectal US guidance. Radiology 163:515–520

Levine MA, Ittman M, Melamed J, Lepor H (1998) Two consecutive sets of transrectal ultrasound guided sextant biopsies of the prostate for the detection of prostate cancer. J Urol 159:471–476

Lissbrant IF, Stattin P, Damber JE, Bergh A (1997) Vascular density is a predictor of cancer-specific survival in prostatic carcinoma. Prostate 33:38–45

Newman JS, Bree RL, Rubin JM (1995) Prostate cancer: diagnosis with color Doppler sonography with histologic correlation of each biopsy site. Radiology 195:86–90

Norberg M, Egevad L, Holmberg L et al (1977) The sextant protocol for ultrasound-guided core biopsies of the prostate underestimates the presence of cancer. Urology 50:562–566

Okihara K, Kojuma M, Nakanouchi T et al (2000) Transrectal power Doppler imaging in the detection of prostate cancer. Br J Urol Int 85:1053–1057

Presti JC, Chang JJ, Bhargava V, Shinohara K (2000) The optimal systematic prostate biopsy scheme should include 8 rather than 6 biopsies: results of a prospective clinical trial. J Urol 163:163–167

Purohit RS, Shinohara K, Meng MV, Carroll PR (2003) Imaging clinically localized prostate cancer. Urol Clin North Am 30:279–293

Rifkin MD (1997) Ultrasound of the prostate. Lippincott-Raven, New York

Rifkin MD (1998) Prostate cancer: the diagnostic dilemma and the place of imaging in detection and staging. World J Urol 16:76–80

Rifkin MD, Alexander AA, Pisarchick J, Matteucci T (1991) Palpable masses in the prostate: superior accuracy of US-guided biopsy compared with accuracy of digitally guided biopsy. Radiology 179:41–42

Rifkin MD, Sudakoff GS, Alexander AA (1993) Prostate: techniques, results, and potential applications of color Doppler US scanning. Radiology 186:509–513

Roy C, Buy X, Lang H, Saussine C, Jacqmin D (2003) Contrast enhanced color Doppler endorectal sonography of the prostate: efficiency for detecting peripheral zone tumors and role for biopsy procedure. J Urol 170:69–72

Sakarya ME, Arslan H, Unal O et al (1998) The role of power Doppler ultrasonography in the diagnosis of prostate cancer: a preliminary study. Br J Urol 82:386–388

Shigeno K, Igawa H, Shiina H et al (2000) The role of colour Doppler ultrasonography in detecting prostate cancer. Br J Urol Int 86:229–233

Shinohara K, Wheeler TM, Scardino PT (1989) The appearance of prostate cancer on transrectal ultrasonography: correlation of imaging and pathological examinations. J Urol 142:76–82

Sillman F, Boyce J, Fruchter R (1981) The significance of atypical vessels and neovascularization in cervical neoplasia. Am J Obstet Gynecol 139:154–159

Spencer JA, Alexander AA, Gomella L et al (1994) Ultrasound-guided four quadrant biopsy of the prostate: efficacy in the diagnosis of isoechoic cancer. Clin Radiol 49:711–714

Trojan L, Thomas D, Knoll T et al (2004) Expression of pro-angiogenic growth factors VEGF, EGF, and bFGF and their topographical relation to neovascularisation in prostate cancer. Urol Res 32:97–103

Weaver RP, Noble MJ, Weigel JW (1991) Correlation of ultrasound guided and digitally guided directed transrectal biopsies of palpable prostatic abnormalities. J Urol 145:516–518

Weidner N, Semple JP, Welch WR, Folkman J (1991) Tumor angiogenesis and metastasis: correlation in invasive breast carcinoma. N Engl J Med 324:1–8

Weidner N, Carroll PR, Flax J et al (1993) Tumor angiogenesis correlates with metastasis in invasive prostate carcinoma. Am J Pathol 142:401–409

28 Contrast-Enhanced Ultrasound in Rheumatic Joint Diseases

Andrea Klauser and Michael Schirmer

CONTENTS

28.1 Introduction 365
28.2 Clinical Applications: Early Disease and Disease Activity 370
28.3 Limitations 375
28.4 Advantages 376
28.5 Conclusion 377
References 377

28.1 Introduction

Arthritis and other rheumatic conditions are the leading cause of disability and constitute a frequent medical disorder accounting for approximately 2.4% of all hospital discharges (MMWR 1999). Rheumatoid arthritis as a subgroup shows a prevalence of 0.5–1% of the population (Alarcon 1995). Clinical and laboratory tests are the first step in the evaluation of patients with inflammatory disease. Because clinical investigation can be insensitive, especially in early rheumatoid arthritis, imaging methods are additionally applied.

a) Conventional radiography. Conventional radiography is the routinely used imaging method for assessing the degree of actual joint destruction, although it has known limited sensitivity and specificity in the investigation of soft tissue inflammation and early disease (Backhaus et al. 1999; Schmidt 2001).

b) Magnetic Resonance Imaging. Magnetic resonance (MR) imaging enables excellent examination of soft tissues (i.e., pannus) and bones, and has been utilised for early detection and characterisation of inflammatory disease (Sugimoto et al. 1996, 2000;

A. Klauser, MD, Associate Professor of Radiology
Department of Radiology II, Medical University Innsbruck, Anichstrasse 35, 6020 Innsbruck, Austria
M. Schirmer, MD
Department of Internal Medicine, Medical University Innsbruck, Anichstrasse 35, 6020 Innsbruck, Austria

Olivieri et al. 1996). Contrast administration is necessary to allow for differentiation between effusion and synovial proliferation. For routine use and especially for follow-up examination MR is still limited by availability, relatively high costs, claustrophobia (as reported in almost 10% of patients) and relatively long examination times for the patients. The early post-gadolinium synovial membrane enhancement, at dynamic contrast material-enhanced MR imaging, has shown promising results in assessing synovial perfusion and disease activity (Gaffney et al. 1998; Hermann et al. 2003).

c) Baseline Ultrasound and Colour Doppler US. Ultrasound (US) allows assessment of erosive changes, and with the imaging capabilities of colour/power Doppler US, it allows detection of vascularity in synovial proliferation, usually caused by inflammatory activity (Bude and Rubin 1996; Balint and Sturrock 1997; Gibbon and Wakefield 1999; Wakefield et al. 2000; Hau et al. 2002). The colour/power Doppler US technique is limited in the detection of slow flow and flow in small vessels as it occurs in angiogenesis (Goldberg et al. 1994; Forsberg et al. 2004).

Angiogenesis is a basic principle of inflammatory disease and refers to the growth of new capillary blood vessels. This is important not only in tumour growth, but also in psoriasis and rheumatoid arthritis (Koch 1998). Microscopic examination of synovial biopsies shows angiogenesis from the earliest beginning of disease. Proliferation of hypervascularised pannus can be seen before joint destruction, correlates with disease activity and appears to be crucial to its invasive and destructive behaviour (Zvaifler and Firestein 1994; FitzGerald and Bresnihan 1995). Serum vascular endothelial growth factor concentrations are elevated in rheumatoid arthritis and are known to correlate with disease activity. Furthermore, a correlation of vascular endothelial growth factor concentration and radiographic progression between first presentation of rheumatoid arthritis patients and the subsequent year has been described. Synovial tissues expressing vascular endothelial growth factor show a significantly higher microvascular density (TAYLOR 2002, 2003); therefore, vascular imaging and serological markers may be more sensitive than clinical assessment of disease activity. Functional imaging of intraarticular vascularisation is thought to improve grading of disease activity. Blood flow at the microvascular level, which is of main interest in inflammatory disease, is at lower velocities and therefore less readily detectable by conventional colour/power Doppler US. Microbubble-based contrast agent administration improves the detection of low-volume blood flow in small vessels by increasing the signal-to-noise ratio (Fig. 28.1; GOLDBERG et al. 1994; BLOMLEY et al. 2001).

d) Contrast-enhanced US. The diagnostic evaluation of tumour-related vascularity has progressed to a new important imaging modality and contrast-enhanced US is used in some organ pathology in daily clinical routine (i.e. liver, kidney, breast, prostate; ALBRECHT et al. 1998; FRAUSCHER et al. 2001; KLAUSER et al. 2002b; RADMAYR et al. 2002; SCHROEDER et al. 2003; PADHANI and DZIK-JURASZ 2004).

The development of novel treatment options (biologicals, tumour necrosis alpha-factor inhibitors), as they target the microvascular level, demands for more sensitive vascular imaging also in the rheumatological field. Treatment follow-up will need sensitive imaging techniques with a good availability in daily routine.

Ultrasound is an imaging modality with good availability and relatively low costs (MANGER and KALDEN 1995; KARIM et al. 2001), and grey-scale or colour Doppler signal may be enhance after microbubble injection. Colour or power Doppler may be employed after microbubble injection, even though they are strongly penalised by artefacts which are almost eliminated with the employment of dedicated contrast-specific techniques.

In a previous study (SCHMIDT et al. 2000) using unenhanced colour Doppler US in patients with knee-joint synovitis the detection of intraarticular flow signals did not correlate with the pathohistological number of vessels. It can be assumed that without contrast administration small microvessels were missed. Using contrast-enhanced colour Doppler US, we were able to detect more vessels in finger joints with active rheumatoid arthritis than without contrast agent (KLAUSER et al. 2002a and 2004). This result supports the hypothesis stated by Schmidt et al., that contrast-enhanced colour Doppler US may increase the detection of even minor perfusion. Our results demonstrated that contrast-enhanced colour Doppler US significantly improved the detection of intraarticular vascularisation. Without the use of

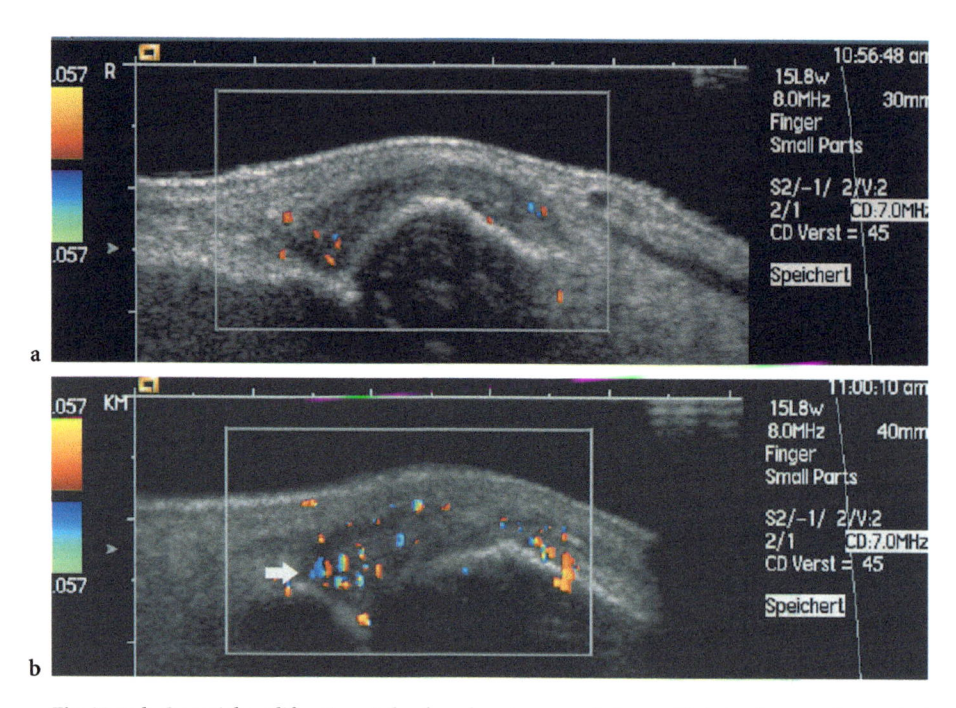

Fig. 28.1a,b. Synovial proliferation at the dorsal metacarpo-phalangeal joint. a Increased vascularity at baseline colour Doppler US. b After microbubble-based contrast agent administration improved vascularity detection (*arrow*). The US equipment settings are maintained constant.

microbubble-based contrast agents, we detected intraarticular vascularisation in only 35% of the 198 joints. Contrast-enhanced colour Doppler US detected flow signals in 78% of the joints. As a result, therapy was modified in 24% of patients studied with contrast-enhanced colour Doppler US.

The following studies address the use of contrast-enhanced colour/power Doppler US in inflammatory disease. CAROTTI et al. (2002) reported that contrast-enhanced power Doppler US was useful in assessing synovial activity and therapeutic response to treatment of synovitis in the knee joints of 42 rheumatoid arthritis patients. A single dose of 2.5 g of Levovist (Schering, Germany) with a concentration of 300 mg/ml was injected by slow flow infusion (1 ml/min) and contrast enhancement was assessed quantitatively by time–intensity curves. A limitation of this study is based on the fact that the contrast agent dynamics were assessed during continuous slow flow infusion with the assessment of time–intensity analysis. Slow flow infusion allows for a longer duration of the contrast enhancement (ALBRECHT et al. 1998). For musculoskeletal applications this is useful for scanning of several joints due to an enlarged time window; however, based on the continuous infusion, only time-to-peak or maximum peak enhancement can be assessed. The washout period of the time–intensity curve can be obtained at the end of the infusion only. The dynamic vascular patterns are optimally observed by the use of a bolus administration. Nonetheless, the authors found an increased area under the curve in active joints and concluded the usefulness of contrast administration to assess synovial activity.

DORIA et al. (2001) assessed 31 knees of patients with juvenile rheumatoid arthritis after a bolus administration of Levovist (Schering, Berlin, Germany). The objective assessment of the overall mean pixel intensity was found to be different in active and inactive disease and therefore helpful in the detection of inflammatory activity in subclinical disease with impact on treatment.

MAGARELLI et al. (2001) evaluated contrast enhancement of a bolus injection of Levovist (Schering, Germany) in different joints of rheumatoid arthritis patients by subjective estimation of power Doppler US signals in 27 knees, showing a good correlation with contrast-enhanced MR. This study included also examination of other joints such as wrists, ankles, elbows, shoulders and hands, where synovial contrast enhancement could be observed with good correlation to MR. As a limitation of this study, the bolus injection technique, which results in initial vascular blooming and in a shorter examination time, was mentioned.

QVISTGAARD et al. (2001) performed contrast-enhanced US examination of finger joints in patients with rheumatoid arthritis by evaluation of resistive index and pulsatility index and after contrast administration by objective quantification of the vascularisation. They found contrast medium helpful in differentiation of fibrous and active synovitis, and concluded that contrast-enhanced US is a reliable tool for assessing synovial activity measured by the degree of vascularisation. FIOCCO et al. (2003) showed a better reproducibility of arthroscopic findings in knee synovitis with a contrast-enhanced power Doppler US signal score compared with the unenhanced method.

Overall, all these studies comparing unenhanced and contrast-enhanced colour/power Doppler US achieved an improved diagnostic accuracy by contrast administration in large and small joints except one study (SZKUDLAREK et al. 2003). This can at least partially be explained by the fact that microbubble administration mode is crucial. Slow microbubble infusion with colour/power Doppler US enables a uniform enhancement with fewer blooming artefacts than bolus administration. The short duration of contrast enhancement obtained by bolus administration and the higher microbubble destruction caused by colour/power Doppler US may result in early microbubble destruction, so that microbubbles cannot enter the small vessels of the synovia. This can explain false-negative contrast-enhanced colour/power Doppler US findings, as resulted in the study by SZKUDLAREK et al. (2003).

In our experience, administration of contrast agent by continuous infusion is preferable when colour/power Doppler US is used. Continuous slow-flow infusion technique with a rate of 1 ml/min reduces the colour Doppler US blooming artefact and enables a mean duration of the contrast agent of about 15–20 min with uniform, subjectively optimal enhancement (KLAUSER et al. 2002a). This allows the microbubbles to enter the small vessels of the synovium, enables the examination of more joints and therefore offers a more cost-effective approach. Using this approach we found contrast-enhanced colour Doppler US a useful method for the detection of early rheumatoid arthritis in finger joints. Examination time of contrast-enhanced colour/power Doppler US with the bolus technique is limited to 3–5 min (ROSENKRANZ et al. 1993).

Development of new contrast-specific techniques that produce images based on nonlinear acoustic effects of US interaction with microbubble-based contrast agents has recently brought attention back to grey-scale US. Contrast-specific imaging techniques, by displaying microbubble enhancement in grey scale, maximise contrast and spatial resolution, and enable the evaluation of the microcirculation, thus prompting the evolution of contrast US from vascular imaging to the imaging of perfused tissues (Fig. 28.2).

The microbubbles bolus administration allows assessment of different parameters in the time–intensity curve, i.e. of time intensity, maximum peak enhancement, area under the curve, time to peak and washout parameters for quantitative assessment. High-frequency probes have become increasingly more optimised for the use of contrast agents and are therefore opening new aspects for the rheumatological field, where the use of higher frequencies is required more than in oncological imaging. The development of microbubble-based contrast agents, especially for high frequencies, could further improve musculoskeletal applications. Newer contrast-specific modes based on the higher harmonic emission capabilities of second-generation contrast agents, such as Contrast Tuned Imaging (Esaote Biomedica, Genoa, Italy), have overcome some of these limitations. Their main advantage is that a lower, non-destructive US power (very low mechanical index: 0.06–0.1) is used, which enables continuous imaging without the need for time intervals between scans for contrast replenishment. Very low acoustic output (1–17 kPq) optimise the detection of microvessel perfusion (Fig. 28.3). Indeed, objective quantitative analysis of vascularisation performed by contrast-enhanced grey-scale mode seems promising in our preliminary and unpublished results of measuring synovial activity.

Using a Technos-MPX (Esaote Biomedica, Genoa, Italy) US unit, equipped with software analysis and automatic quantification of the US signal intensity changes after bolus injection of SonoVue (Bracco, Milan, Italy), the objective quantification of contrast enhancement was determined to be suitable for clinical routine, to improve reproducibility and to be reliable for therapeutic follow-up and in terms for diagnosis of remission (Fig. 28.4). The newest software developments as parametric imaging (Qontrast, Contrast Quantification Tool, AMID and R&D, Bracco, Milan, Italy) impressively show the potential and sensitivity of objective contrast-enhanced imaging (Fig. 28.5). The quantitative analysis has been effective in revealing a significantly higher enhancement slope in shoulders of rheumatoid arthritis patients with erosive disease (HERMANN et al. 2003).

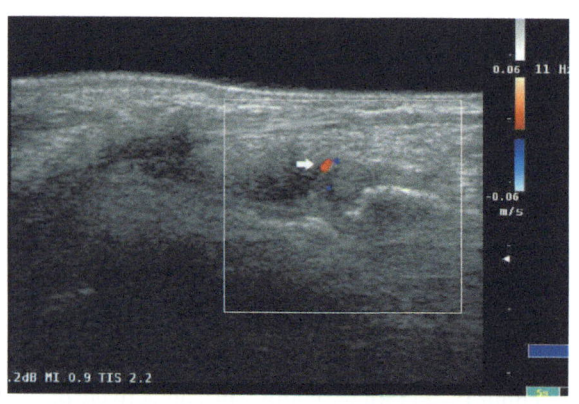

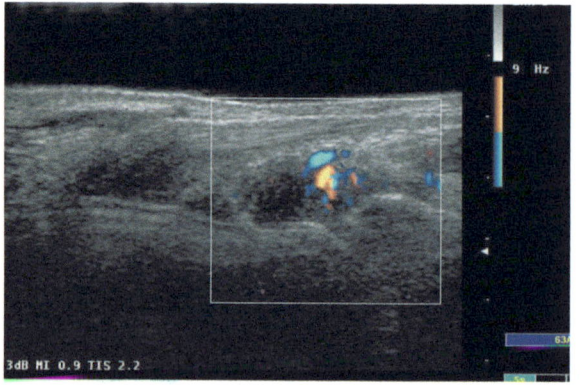

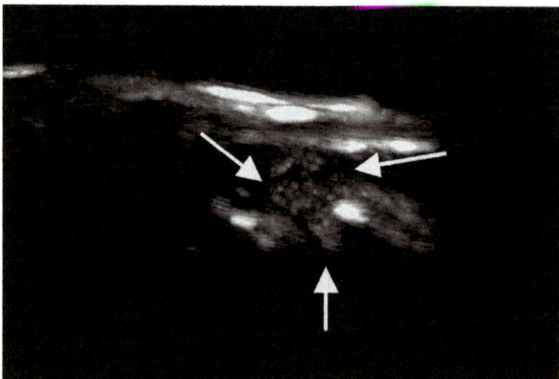

Fig. 28.2a–c. Longitudinal scan of the dorsal radio-carpal joint. a Synovial thickening with one vessel at colour Doppler US (*arrow*). b Improved detection of vascularity at power Doppler US. c After microbubble-based contrast agent administration, further improved detection of the increased synovial perfusion (*arrows*)

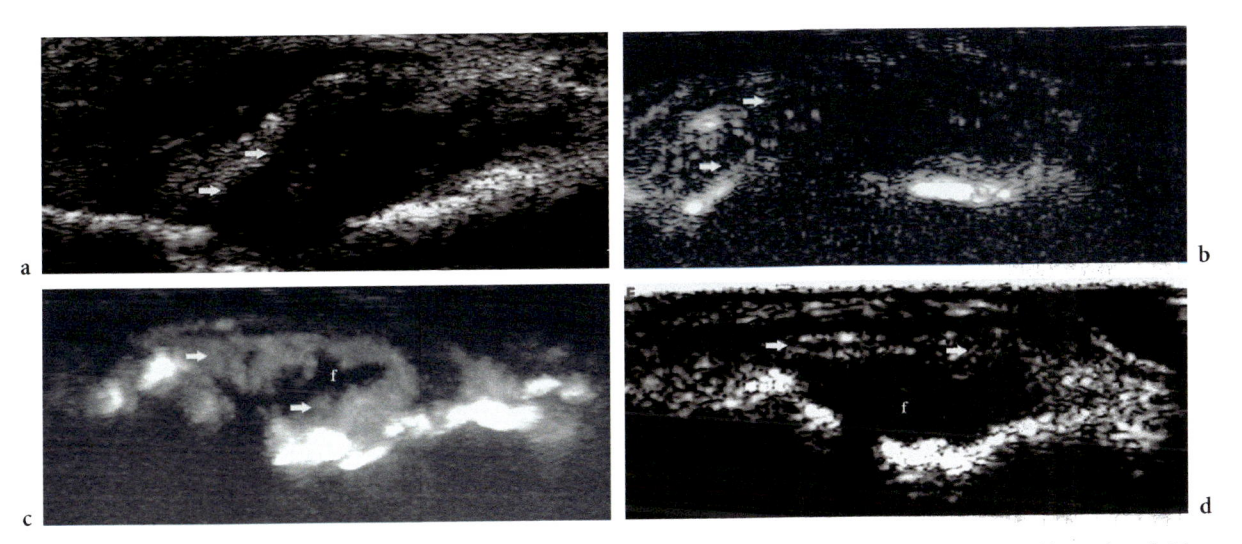

Contrast-Enhanced Ultrasound in Rheumatic Joint Diseases

Fig. 28.3a–d. Longitudinal scan of medial elbow. **a** Synovial proliferation (*arrows*) with mixed echogenicity without clear fluid delineation. **b** Baseline scan before microbubble-based contrast agent with low acoustic power output at contrast-specific mode. **c,d** After microbubble-based contrast agent administration, diffuse enhancement of the synovial proliferation (*arrows*) and improved differentiation of the fluid (*f*) component

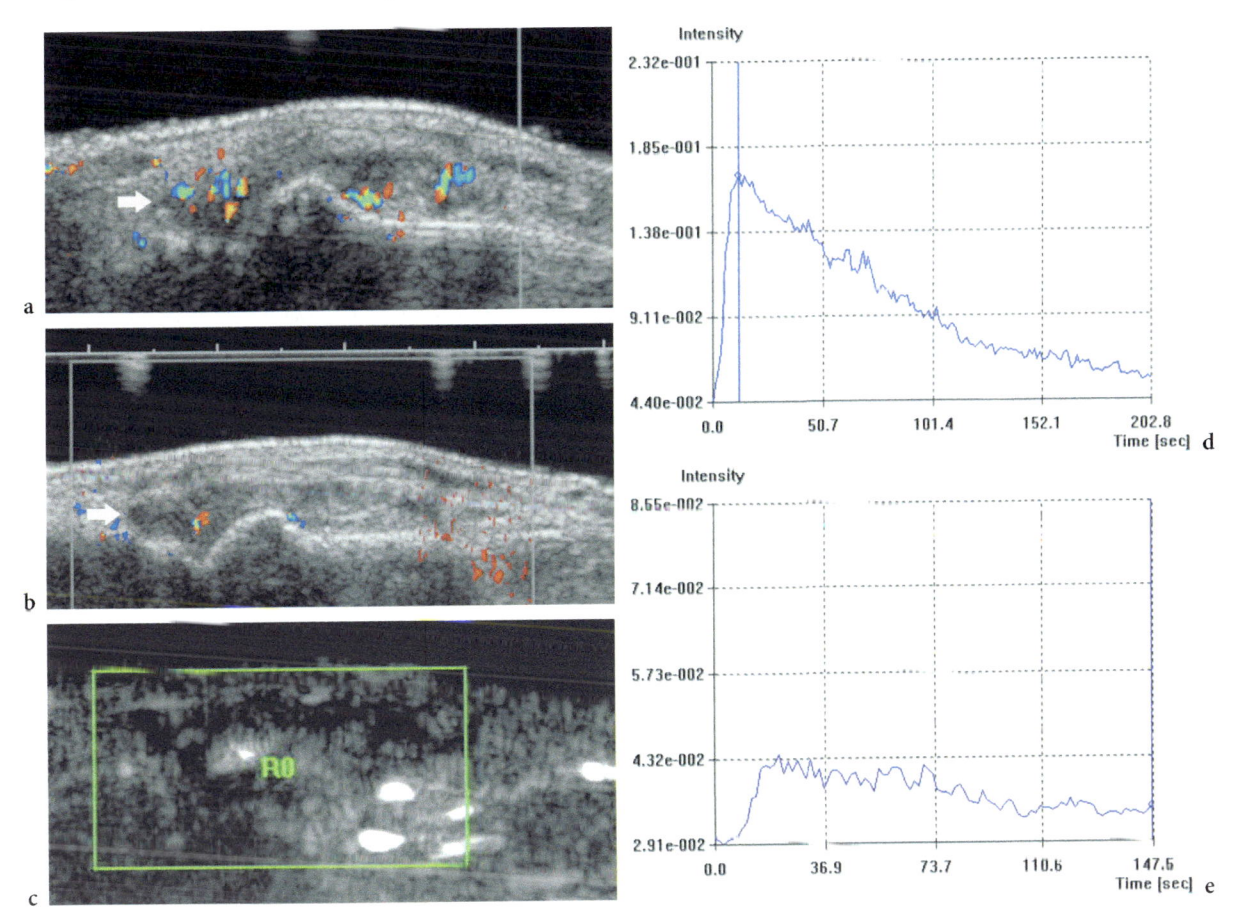

Fig. 28.4a–e. Analysis of the degree of vascularity can be used for therapeutic follow-up. **a** Subjective grading by evaluation of the number of vessels is a tool for daily clinical routine. Synovitis at the dorsal proximal inter-phalangeal joint (*arrow*) with >11 flow signals, corresponding to a grade-3 vascularity. **b** After therapy, one to two vessels are depicted (*arrow*), corresponding to a grade-1 vascularity, well correlating with clinical improvement of the patient. **c** Contrast Tuned Imaging (Esaote Biomedica, Genoa, Italy) as contrast-specific mode with region of interest (*R0*) positioned at synovial proliferation. **d** Time–intensity curve shows early enhancement with a high peak before therapy. **e** Contrast Tuned Imaging with time–intensity curve after therapy shows decreased intensity with a low plateau.

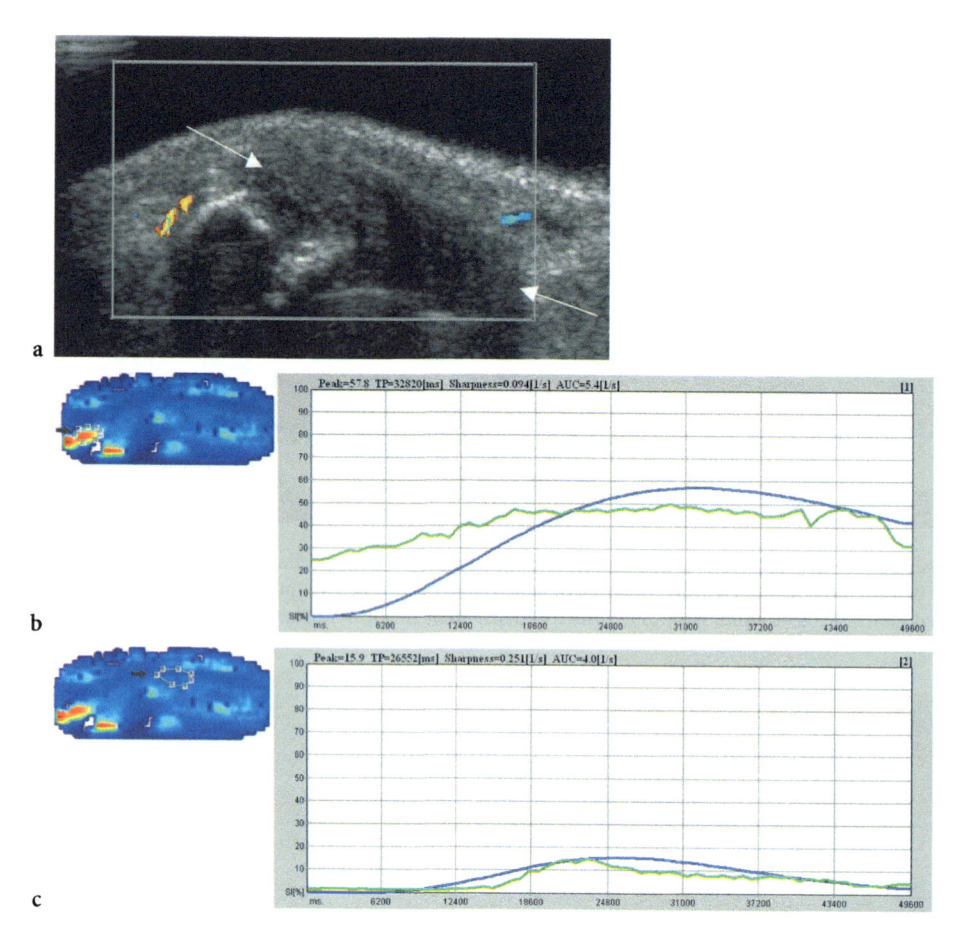

Fig. 28.5a-c. Parametric maps (Qontraxt, AMID and R&D, Bracco, Milan, Italy) allows for objective evaluation of quantitative perfusion parameters during a selected set of frames with assessment of perfusion properties over the entire selected region at once. Patient with early aggressive erosive rheumatoid arthritis under clinical remission. a No visible enhancement at contrast-enhanced colour Doppler US in dorsal metacarpo-phalangeal joint. b Parametric evaluation of the outlined area (*arrow*) shows small high-intensity spots (yellow-reddish colour) in the cortical irregularity, corresponding to vascularised erosions. This is suspicious of latent activity, which could not be detected by subjective evaluation. c Corresponding time-intensity curve for blue area (*arrow*) where no activity could be detected

28.2
Clinical Applications: Early Disease and Disease Activity

a) Differentiation between synovial pannus and fluid. Early diagnosis combined with prompt initiation of appropriate treatment regimen is acknowledged as an important factor in improving clinical outcomes in patients with rheumatoid arthritis. Several MR imaging studies have demonstrated that the presence and amount of synovitis is a prognostic factor for bone damage (OSTERGAARD et al. 1997, 1998, 1999). No bone damage occurs in joints without synovitis, and the presence of pannus is prognostic for bone damage; therefore, early detection of vascularised synovia should be one of the primary goals in assessment of inflammatory disease. Differentiation of synovitis and joint fluid can be difficult because both can show hypoechoic to echoic characteristics on grey-scale US (BREIDAHL et al. 1996). Microbubble-based contrast agent administration allows for differentiation between perfused synovitis and fluid accumulation (Figs. 28.6, 28.7, 28.8).

Analysis of degree of vascularity correlates with disease activity and not necessarily with amount of synovial proliferation and therefore could be helpful for prognosis. Contrast administration can be further helpful in detection of hypervascularization in patients with only small or questionable amount of synovial proliferation (Fig. 28.9).

b) Vascularised erosions. Ultrasound can depict erosions very early before structural damage to the corticalis is visible on X-ray (GRASSI et al. 2001; SCHMIDT

Fig. 28.6a–c. Microbubble-based contrast agent administration allows for differentiation of synovitis and articular fluid. **a** Longitudinal unenhanced grey-scale US shows articular hypoechoic distension (*arrow*) in the volar proximal interphalangeal joint without cortical irregularity in a patient with early rheumatoid arthritis. **b** Unenhanced colour Doppler US with a high-end system shows only one colour signal (*arrow*) near the joint capsule, and no signs of hypervascularised synovia; therefore, the diagnosis is increased joint fluid. **c** Contrast-enhanced colour Doppler US with a continuous infusion of air-filled microbubble contrast agent shows a significant increase of vascularity in the hypoechoic joint thickening (*arrow*), consistent with active synovitis.

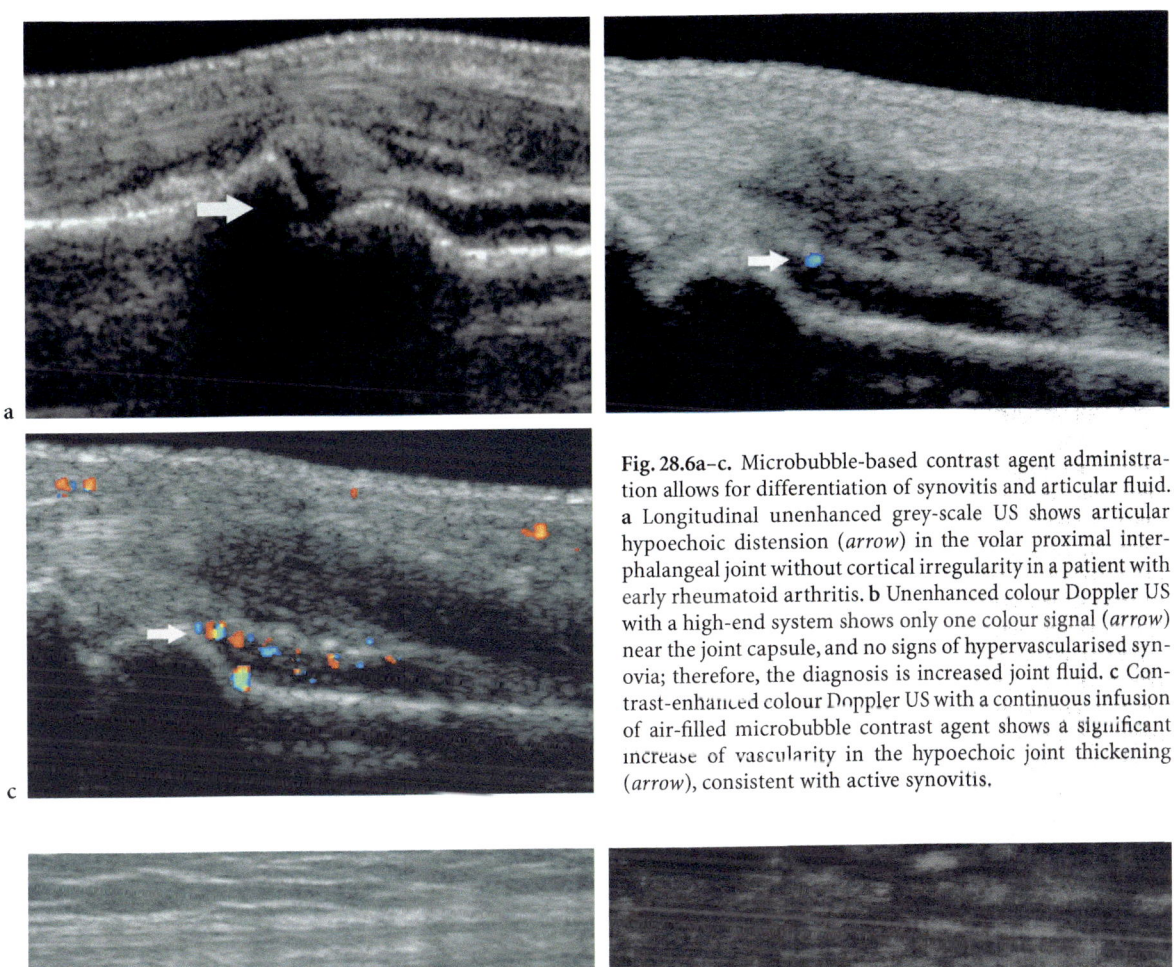

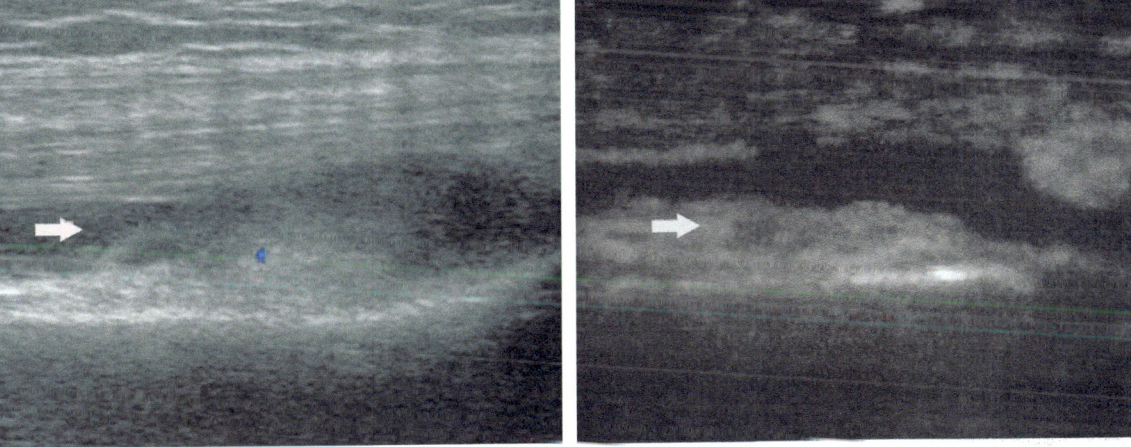

Fig. 28.7a,b. Longitudinal scan of the knee. **a** Increased synovial thickening with mixed echogenicity at the recessus suprapatellaris (*arrow*) with one small vessel in the colour Doppler US examination. **b** After microbubble-based contrast agent administration, clear delineation of a thick perfused peripheral synovitis (*arrow*)

2001). Vascularised erosions can be seen in progressive active disease. In cases of erosive disease, the use of microbubble-based contrast agent will help to ensure lack of vascularity in the present erosions and thus may help to exclude active disease in clinical practice (Fig. 28.10). As shown in MR studies, this has therapeutic impact, as vascularisation of erosions is consistent with aggressive disease (OSTERGAARD et al. 1995).

c) Bursal involvement. Bursae may be involved in rheumatic disease. The Baker's cyst is a common complication in rheumatoid arthritis patients. It is an extraarticular lesion lined by synovial cells. Ultrasound can establish the diagnosis in patients with pain in the popliteal fossa revealing a cystic lesion in its typical location. Contrast administration can show peripheral enhancement in cases with

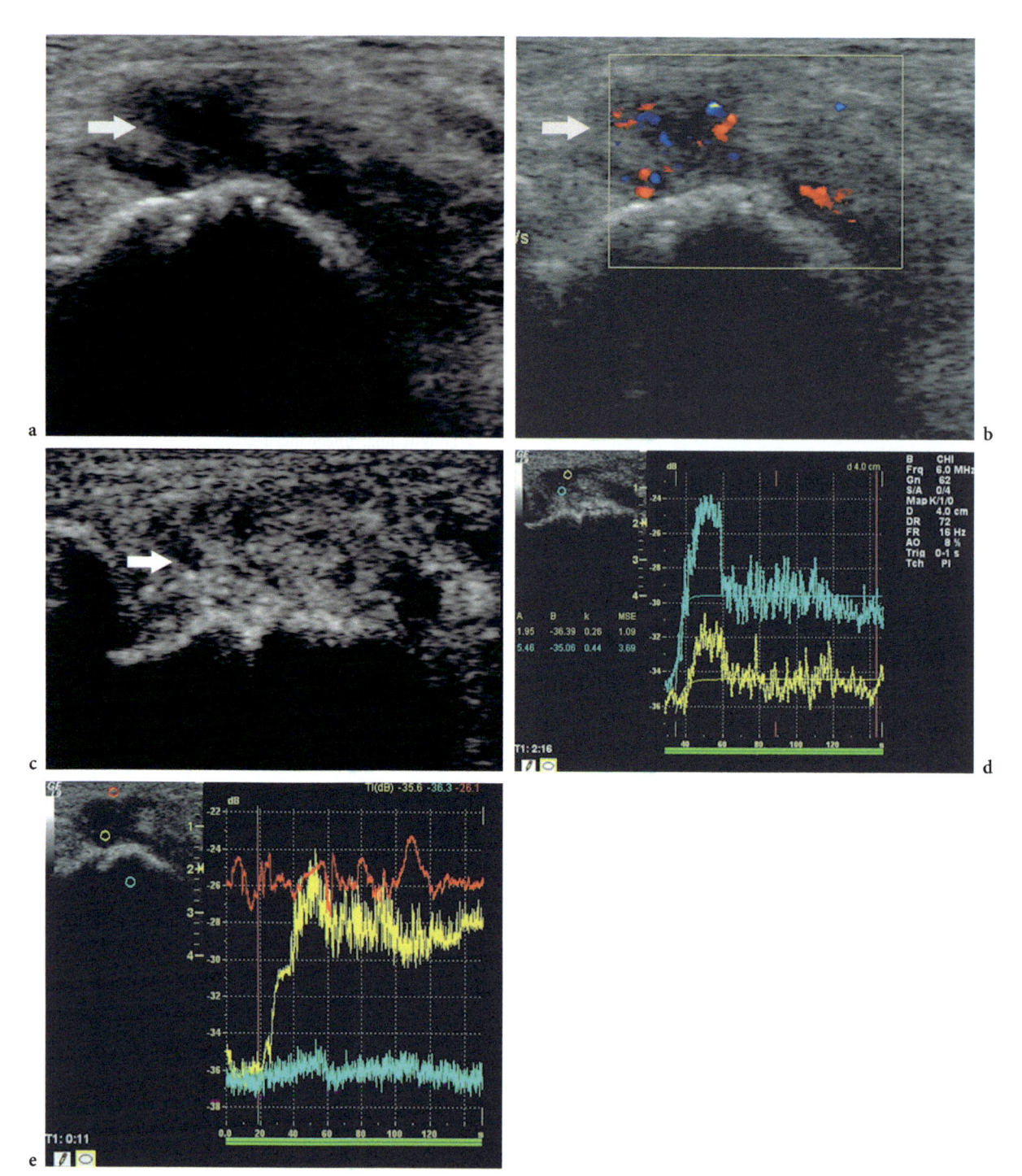

Fig. 28.8a–e. Microbubble-based contrast agent administration can be further helpful in detection of hypervascularisation in patients with clinically only small or questionable amount of synovial proliferation. Six millimetres of joint thickening shows high-grade vascularity in at the dorsal proximal inter-phalangeal joint, consistent with early aggressive synovitis. a Synovial distension (*arrow*) at the lateral malleolus in an untreated patient with early rheumatoid arthritis. b Increased vascularity represents synovial proliferation (*arrow*). c After microbubble-based contrast agent administration, diffuse enhancement of the synovial proliferation (*arrow*). d Time–intensity evaluation shows similar rapid enhancement characteristics with different intensities delineated by different levels of peak enhancement (*yellow*: lower peak, *blue*: higher peak). e Time–intensity evaluation by placing regions of interest in different areas (*yellow*: high peak, regions of interest located in the synovial proliferation, corresponding to synovial activity; *blue*: no enhancement, regions of interest located behind the corticalis; *red*: no peak enhancement, regions of interest located periarticular, where no inflammation can be detected)

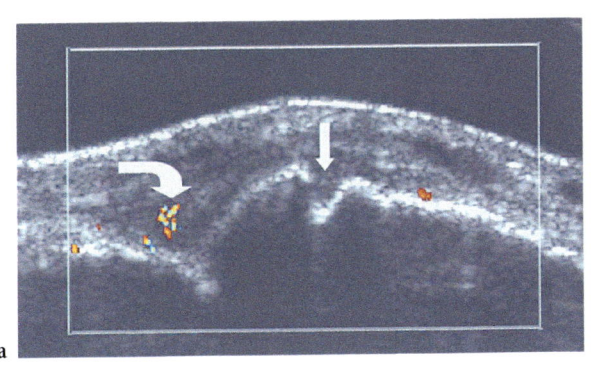

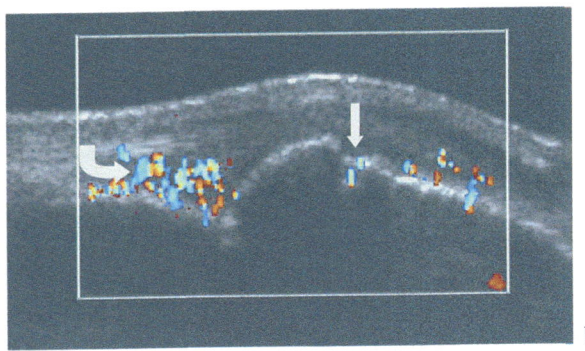

Fig. 28.9a,b. Vascularised erosions. At baseline colour Doppler US (**a**) synovial thickening (*curved arrow*) is revealed but hypervascularisation of the erosion was not detected. Improved detection of vascularity by microbubble-based contrast agent administration (**b**) shows increased vascularity (*straight arrow*) in the dorsal metacarpo-phalangeal joint and vascularisation of the

bursal involvement corresponding to the vascularised synovial lining of the inflamed bursa and can differentiate between fluid, fibrous and hypervascular synovial thickening (Fig. 28.11), although MR has been shown to have some advantages (WAMSER et al. 2003).

d) Therapeutic follow-up. The most pertinent long-term clinical end point is prevention of structural damage. Synovitis is considered the primary abnormality in rheumatoid arthritis. Accurate assessment of synovial vascularity is the first step in establishing diagnosis and initiating early adequate treatment. Treatment is suggested to be successful in case of decreased synovial amount and necrosis of the pannus with regression of vascularity (FIOCCO et al. 1996). In MR imaging fibrotic pannus of patients with burned-out rheumatoid arthritis is known to be hypovascular, contrary to active hypervascularised pannus, which enhances rapidly and intensively after administration of gadolinium (NARVAEZ et al. 2002). On colour/power Doppler US fibrotic pannus shows no vascularity and further lacks enhancement after contrast administration. The distinction between fibrous pannus and residual active synovial proliferation is one of the most important points of interest in therapeutic follow-up, because the volume of synovial proliferation is not related to clinical parameters, as a varying amount of fibrous tissue in synovial membrane can be present (Fig. 28.12).

Quantitative analysis of pannus by MR imaging has been suggested to offer a sensitive method in evaluation of therapeutic response (OSTERGAARD et al. 1995). Analysis of the degree of vascularity relates to synovial proliferation and prognosis and can be used as a tool of therapeutic control (Fig. 28.12).

In oncology various studies recommend the use of colour/power Doppler US with application of contrast agents to document decreasing vascularity under therapy (ECKERSLEY et al. 2002; SCHROEDER et al. 2003). In the rheumatological field sensitive, widely available and cost-effective imaging techniques are required to allow treatment controls especially now, as new potent treatment options are available.

In treated rheumatoid arthritis patients with long-standing disease, serum vascular endothelial growth factor concentrations have been described to be lower than in patients with early rheumatoid arthritis. Furthermore, changes in serum vascular endothelial growth factor concentration and changes in synovial vascularity assessed by power Doppler US in patients receiving tumour necrosis factor alpha inhibitors, in contrast to a group with placebo infusions, have been described (TAYLOR et al. 2002); therefore, power Doppler US seems to be capable of evaluating synovial vascularity for determining prognosis and assessing response to treatment, but up to now few imaging studies are available for the therapeutic follow-up of inflammatory disease.

TERSLEV et al. (2003) found an expected diminishing of colour pixel per region of interest (ROI) as a sign of decreased vascular permeability and vasodilatation in the synovial proliferation after treatment with tumour necrosis factor alpha blockers in 11 patients. Also in the study by HAU et al. (2002) a reduction of power Doppler US flow signals are reported after therapy. These findings may correspond to reported decreased vascularity after treatment with tumour necrosis factor alpha blockers in synovial biopsies (BAETEN et al. 2001).

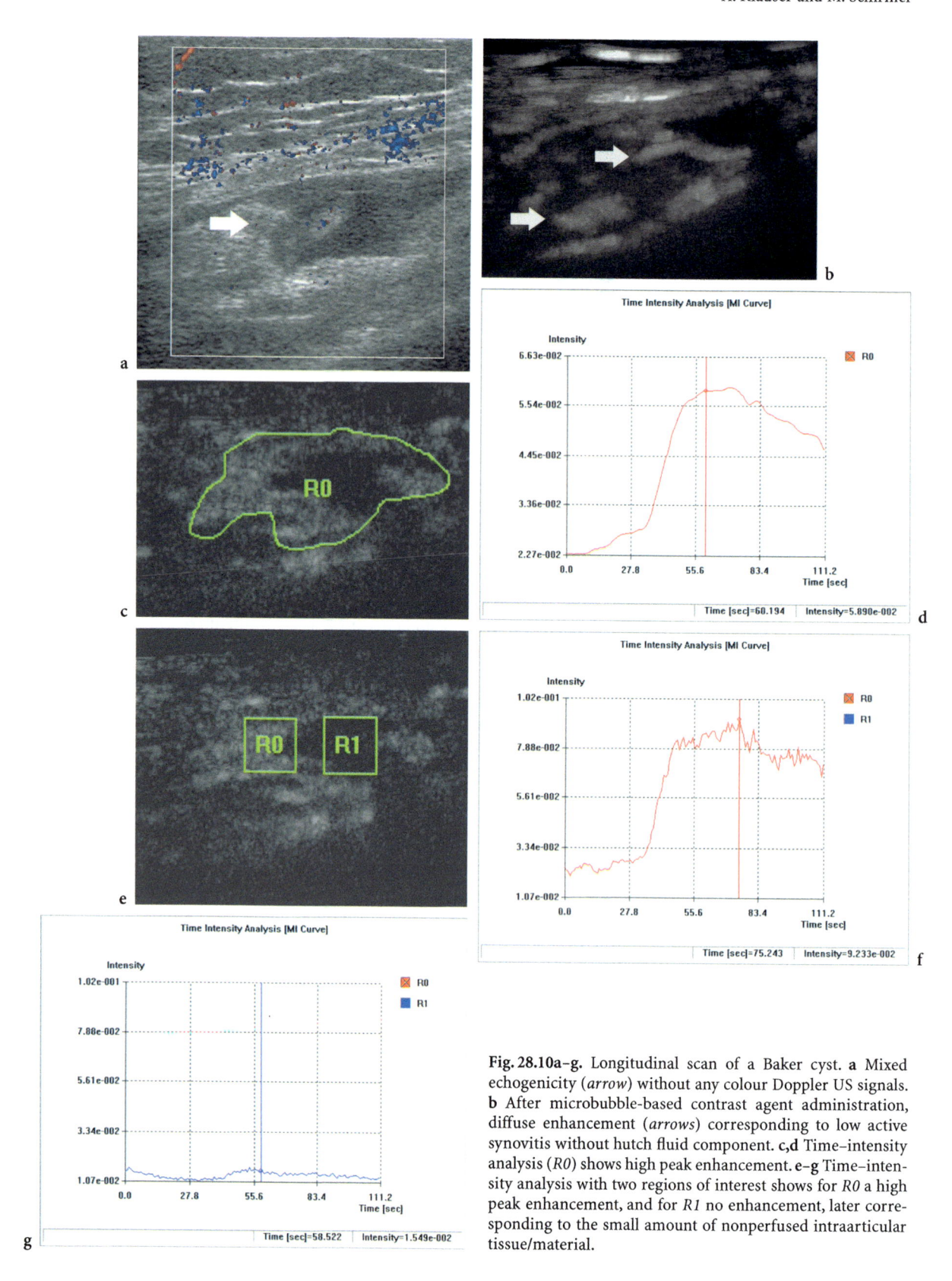

Fig. 28.10a–g. Longitudinal scan of a Baker cyst. **a** Mixed echogenicity (*arrow*) without any colour Doppler US signals. **b** After microbubble-based contrast agent administration, diffuse enhancement (*arrows*) corresponding to low active synovitis without hutch fluid component. **c,d** Time–intensity analysis (*R0*) shows high peak enhancement. **e–g** Time–intensity analysis with two regions of interest shows for *R0* a high peak enhancement, and for *R1* no enhancement, later corresponding to the small amount of nonperfused intraarticular tissue/material.

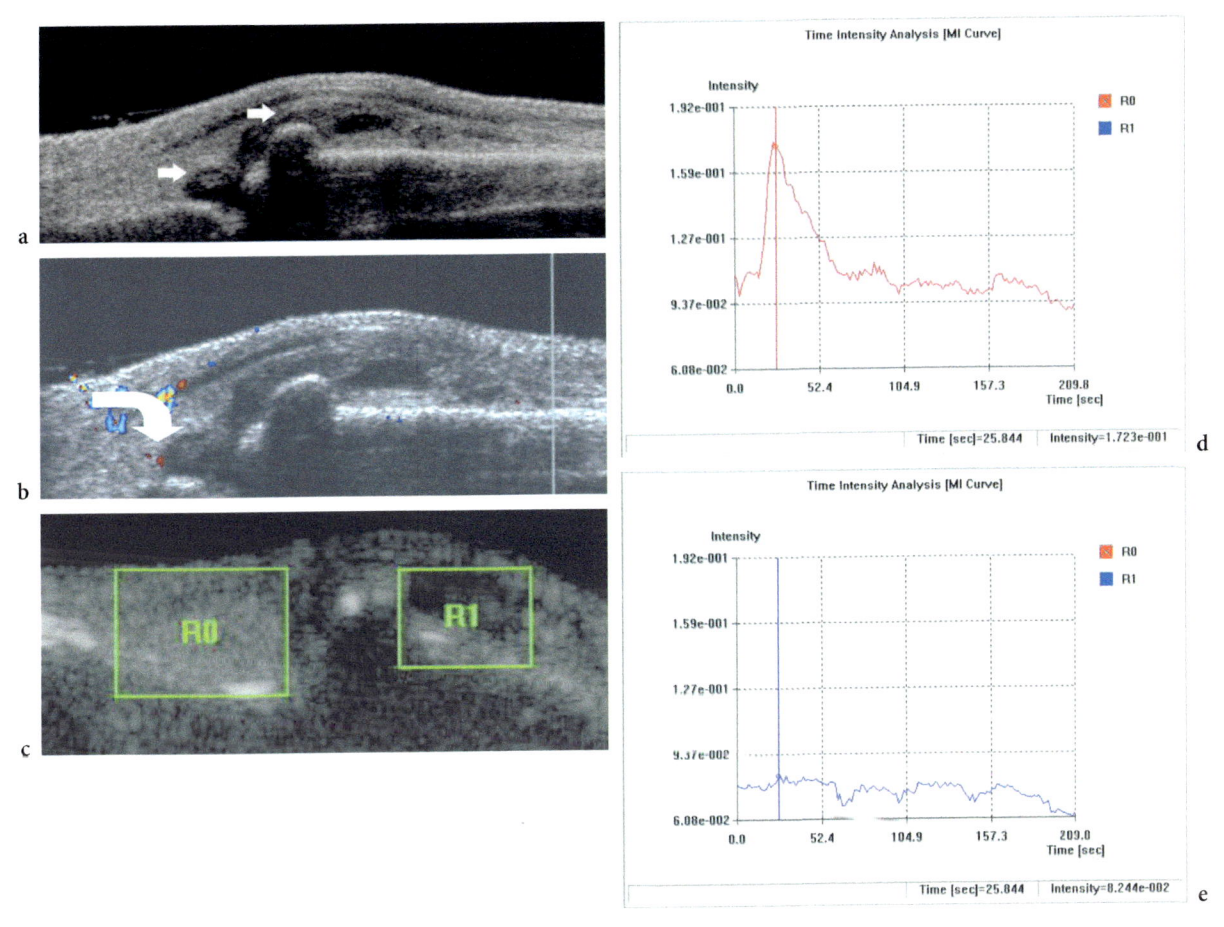

Contrast-Enhanced Ultrasound in Rheumatic Joint Diseases   375

Fig. 28.11a–e. Fibrotic pannus shows no vascularity and further lacks enhancement after contrast administration in the colour Doppler US examination. **a** Extensive synovial thickening (*arrows*) with mixed echo texture at the dorsal proximal inter-phalangeal joint. **b** After microbubble-based contrast agent administration, only one peripheral vessel detectable (*arrow*) consistent with inactive fibrotic pannus. **c–e** After microbubble-based contrast agent administration, confirmation with quantitative time–intensity curves of inactive peripheral synovitis (*R1*), whereas high activity with a high peak enhancement is observed in the joint near synovitis (*R0*).

The value of contrast administration in assisting sensitive evaluation and monitoring of vascularity to ensure a complete therapeutic response should undergo further evaluation.

28.3 Limitations

To ensure usefulness of contrast-enhanced US in daily clinical routine a standardisation of the technique and analysis is required. This is mandatory, not only for reproducibility but also to enable therapeutic follow-up. Results strongly depend on technical equipment, type of transducer, as well as hardware and software of the US unit.

Excessive pressure from the transducer can reduce the blood flow in musculoskeletal applications and result in vessel occlusion and therefore decreased US signals of vascularity. The use of a standoff gel can be helpful.

Movement of the transducer or the patient can result in artefacts by enhancing the Doppler effect, which may compromise interpretation especially in the computer-assisted evaluation. In our experience the subjective grading by evaluation of the number of vessels (Table 28.1) before and after application of contrast is an excellent tool for daily clinical routine to assess contrast enhancement, because it is relatively easy and quick to perform and reliable, when spectral Doppler analysis has confirmed real vascular flow. Subjective grading of vascularity on both pre- and post-therapy images was used and good

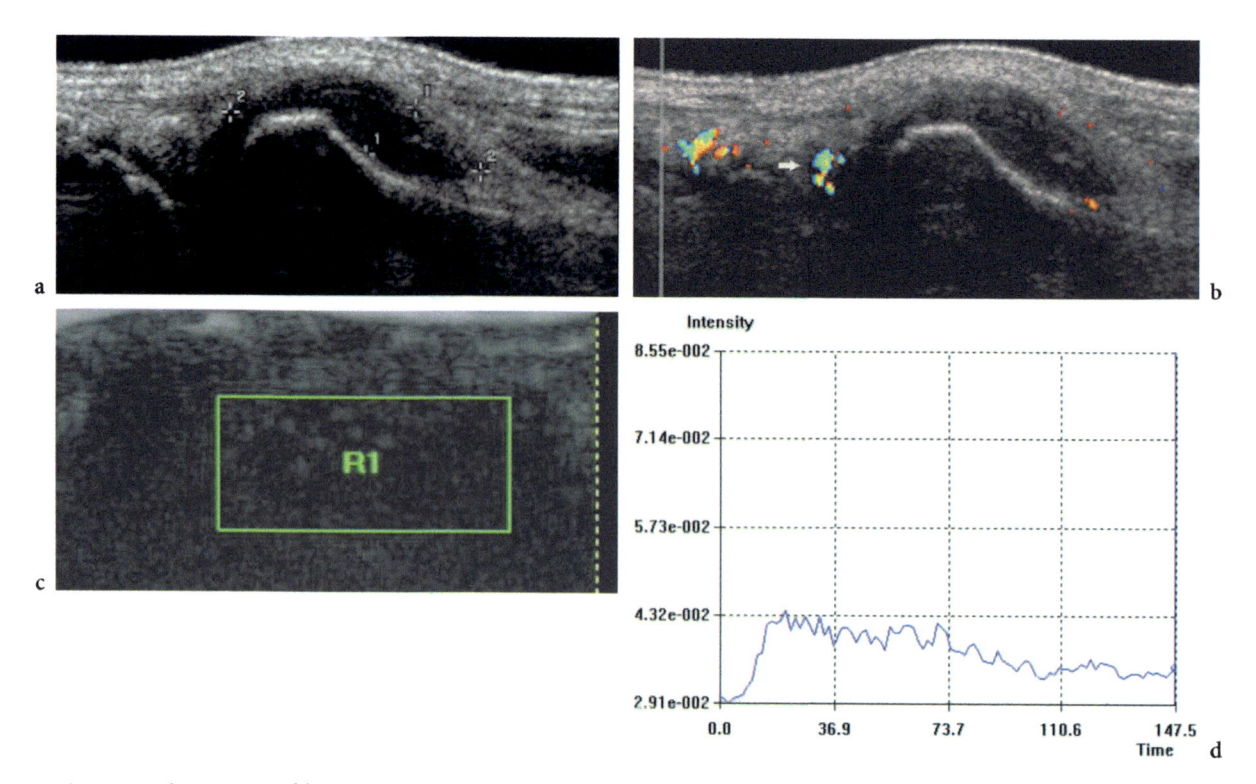

Fig. 28.12a–d. A 41-year-old man with seropositive rheumatoid arthritis and basic therapy for 8 months. Blood test showed a sedimentation rate of 24 (normal: 15–20) and a normal C-reactive protein. **a** Hypoechoic synovial thickening (*callipers*) at the processus styloideus ulnae. **b** Colour Doppler US shows only one peripheral vessel (*arrow*) in the joint capsule. **c,d** After microbubble-based contrast agent administration, a very low and long plateau with low maximal intensity is calculated after placement of region of interest (*R1*), consistent with inflammatory remission under adequate therapy.

Table 28.1 Subjective grading by evaluation of the number of vessels

Grade of vascularity	Colour/power Doppler US
0	No colour intraarticular flow signals
I	1–5 intraarticular colour flow signals
II	6–10 intraarticular colour flow signals
III	>11 intraarticular colour flow signals

results using this technique have been reported (Newman et al. 1996). Good correlation between subjective grading done by the US examiner and histology have been found (Walther et al. 2001). Quantitative computer-based quantification was not found to be superior. These studies were performed without the use of microbubble-based contrast agent. More longitudinal studies should prove the value of vessel counting in terms of reliability of quantification and reproducibility of therapeutic follow-up in rheumatic disease.

Other investigators have used software with digital image analysis to count the number of pixels in chosen regions of interest, resulting in a quantitative score (Hau et al. 1999; Qvistgaard et al. 2001).

Objective quantification of contrast enhancement seems promising for longitudinal assessment and comparison between studies, and standardisation of measurements and especially interpretation of time–intensity curve characteristics needs further investigation.

However, the image acquisition procedure has to be standardised and the quality of the examination is highly dependent on the skill of the operator and the use of optimal equipment. Furthermore, there are potential problems with reproducibility based on intra- and inter-observer variability and the use of different machines.

28.4
Advantages

Ultrasound and therefore also contrast-enhanced US has the advantage of better availability and of being more economical than MR imaging. Ultrasound can be performed as a bedside technique and is greatly appreciated by the patient (Lee 2000).

The aforementioned disadvantages of contrast-enhanced US of costs and time is still lower than those contrast-enhanced MR imaging. If cost-effectiveness has to be considered, costs for contrast-enhanced US are in total still lower than 30–50% compared with those of contrast-enhanced MR imaging. Costs for microbubble-based contrast agent can be reduced by slow-flow infusion with assessment of more joints. To perform a contrast-enhanced US examination with evaluation of time–intensity curves takes <20 min, in our experience.

Furthermore, microbubble-based contrast agents have some advantages over MR contrast agents, since microbubble-based contrast agent are less likely to leak into the synovial fluid and to diffuse into the tissue; therefore, it reflects more accurately changes in the intravascular compartment. Delayed MR sequences can present an enhancement of synovial effusion due diffusion of gadolinium into the intracellular space; therefore, vascularity evaluated by US contrast enhancement cannot be objectively correlated with MR, which is often used as gold standard.

28.5
Conclusion

Sensitive methods for visualising synovial vascularisation are required to improve earlier diagnosis, assess disease activity and to evaluate response to therapy. Because hypervascularisation correlates with disease activity, contrast-enhanced US allows for identification of patients with latent, but aggressive, inflammatory joint disease. Not bony structural damage, which can be detected by radiography, is considered as an early inflammatory stage, but the detection of inflammatory changes are important before structural damage to joints becomes evident on X-ray. This is a worthy goal for early management of patients with inflammatory joint disease and contrast-enhanced US can improve sensitive detection of inflammatory activity.

Determination of early inflammatory stages to prevent structural damage of joints and the follow-up of treatment to determine whether patients are responding to the applied therapy have become realistic goals in the management of patients with rheumatic joint diseases.

All kinds of imaging should be related to clinical settings and how imaging will influence patient management. The development of new therapeutic options with targeting the microvascular level calls for earlier diagnosis and an optimal assessment of disease activity. Imaging can improve prediction of prognosis and therefore influence initiation of aggressive therapy. Contrast-enhanced US offers a promising, new sensitive imaging technology for further clinical trials (Figs. 28.7, 28.8).

For successful assessment of contrast-enhanced US disease activity in early detection and therapeutic follow-up, standardisation of the examination technique is indispensable.

The question of "When to use contrast agent?" was asked a long time ago for MR imaging investigations of inflammatory disease. Beside providing arguments for differential diagnosis, the value for disease activity assessment due to contrast-enhanced MR is now well established, and dynamic MR imaging seems even more promising (HERMANN et al. 2003).

Achieving full remission is a definite aim of treating inflammatory joint disease; therefore, the need for contrast media will increase as soon a sensitive monitoring of decreased vascularity becomes more demanded by the clinician.

In conclusion, contrast-enhanced US is an exciting imaging modality which represents an alternative method to MR imaging and is less expensive and more readily available in clinical routine. The option of contrast administration with improving the detection of low-volume blood flow by increasing the signal-to-noise ratio is opening new horizons in rheumatological imaging to allow for sensitive assessment of disease activity.

References

Alarcon G (1995) Epidemiology of rheumatoid arthritis. Rheum Dis Clin North Am 21:589–604

Albrecht T, Urbank A, Mahler M et al (1998) Prolongation and optimization of Doppler enhancement with a microbubble US contrast agent by using continuous infusion: preliminary experience. Radiology 207:339–347

Backhaus M, Kamradt T, Sandrock D et al (1999) Arthritis of the finger joints: a comprehensive approach comparing conventional radiography, scintigraphy, ultrasound, and contrast-enhanced magnetic resonance imaging. Arthritis Rheum 42:1232–1245

Baeten D, Kruithof E, van den Bosch F et al (2001) Immunomodulatory effects of anti-tumor necrosis factor alpha therapy on synovium in spondylarthropathy: histologic findings in eight patients from an open-label pilot study. Arthritis Rheum 44:186–195

Balint P, Sturrock RD (1997) Musculoskeletal ultrasound imaging: a new diagnostic tool for the rheumatologist? Br J Rheumatol 36:1141–1142

Blomley MJK, Cooke JC, Unger EC et al (2001) Microbubble contrast agents: a new era in ultrasound. Br Med J 322:1222–1225

Breidahl WH, Newman JS, Toljanovic MS, Adler RS (1996) Power Doppler sonography in the assessment of musculoskeletal fluid collections. Am J Roentgenol 166:1443–1446

Bude RO, Rubin JM (1996) Power Doppler sonography. Radiology 2000:21–23

Carotti M, Salaffi F, Manganelli P et al (2002) Power Doppler sonography in the assessment of synovial tissue of the knee joint in rheumatoid arthritis: a preliminary experience. Ann Rheum Dis 61:877–882

Doria AS, Kiss MH, Lotito AP et al (2001) Juvenile rheumatoid arthritis of the knee: evaluation with contrast-enhanced color Doppler ultrasound. Pediatr Radiol 31:524–531

Eckersley RJ, Sedelaar JP, Blomley MJK et al (2002) Quantitative microbubble enhanced transrectal ultrasound as a tool for monitoring hormonal treatment of prostate carcinoma. Prostate 51:256–267

Fiocco U, Cozzi L, Rubaltelli L et al (1996) Long term sonographic follow-up of rheumatoid and psoriatic proliferative knee joint synovitis. Br J Rheumatol 35:155–163

Fiocco U, Ferro F, Cozzi L et al (2003) Contrast medium in power Doppler ultrasound for assessment of synovial vascularity: comparison with artroscopy. J Rheumatol 30:2170–2176

FitzGerald O, Bresnihan B (1995) Synovial membrane cellularity and vascularity. Ann Rheum Dis 54:511–515

Forsberg F, Ro RJ, Potoczek M et al (2004) Assessment of angiogenesis: implications for ultrasound imaging. Ultrasonics 42:325–330

Frauscher F, Klauser A, Halpern EJ et al (2001) Detection of prostate cancer with a microbubble ultrasound contrast agent. Lancet 357:1849–1850

Gaffney K, Cookson J, Blades S et al (1998) Quantitative assessment of the rheumatoid synovial microvascular bed by gadolinium-DTPA enhanced magnetic resonance imaging. Ann Rheum Dis 57:152–157

Gibbon WW, Wakefield RJ (1999) Ultrasound in inflammatory disease. Radiol Clin North Am 37:633–651

Goldberg BB, Liu JB, Forsberg F (1994) Ultrasound contrast agents: a review. Ultrasound Med Biol 20:319–333

Grassi W, Filippucci E, Farina A et al (2001) Ultrasonography in the evaluation of bone erosions. Ann Rheum Dis 60:98–103

Hau M, Schultz H, Tony HP et al (1999) Evaluation of pannus and vascularization of the metacarpophalangeal and proximal interphalangeal joints in rheumatoid arthritis by high-resolution ultrasound (multidimensional linear array). Arthritis Rheum 42:2303–2308

Hau M, Kneitz C, Tony HP et al (2002) High resolution ultrasound detects a decrease in pannus vascularisation of small finger joints in patients with rheumatoid arthritis receiving treatment with soluble tumour necrosis factor alpha receptor (etanercept). Ann Rheum Dis 61:55–58

Hermann KG, Backhaus M, Schneider U et al (2003) Rheumatoid arthritis of the shoulder joint: comparison of conventional radiography, ultrasound, and dynamic contrast-enhanced magnetic resonance imaging. Arthritis Rheum 48:3338–3349

Karim Z, Wakefield RJ, Conaghan PG et al (2001) The impact of ultrasonography on diagnosis and management of patients with musculoskeletal conditions. Arthritis Rheum 44:2932–2933

Klauser A, Frauscher F, Schirmer M et al (2002a) The value of contrast-enhanced color Doppler ultrasound in the detection of vascularization of finger joints in patients with rheumatoid arthritis. Arthritis Rheum 46:647–653

Klauser A, Janetschek G, Helweg G et al (2002b) Small renal masses: value of contrast-enhanced colour Doppler imaging. Eur Radiol 12 (Suppl 1):180

Klauser A, Frauscher F, Schirmer M (2004) Value of contrast-enhanced power Doppler ultrasonography (US) of the metacarpophalangeal joints on rheumatoid arthritis. Eur Radiol 14:545–546

Koch AE (1998) Angiogenesis: implications for rheumatoid arthritis. Arthritis Rheum 41:951–962

Lee FR (2000) The sound of bones. Am J Roentgenol 175:573

Magarelli N, Guglielmi G, Matteo L di et al (2001) Diagnostic utility of an echo-contrast agent in patients with synovitis using power Doppler ultrasound: a preliminary study with comparison to contrast-enhanced MRI. Eur Radiol 11:1039–1046

Manger B, Kalden JR (1995) Joint and connective tissue ultrasonography: A rheumatologic bedside procedure? A German experience. Arthritis Rheum 38:736–742

MMWR (1999) Impact of arthritis and other rheumatic conditions on the Health-Care System-United States, 1997. J Am Med Assoc 281:2177

Narvaez JA, Narvaez J, Roca Y, Aguilera C (2002) MR imaging assessment of clinical problems in rheumatoid arthritis. Eur Radiol 12:1819–1828

Newman JS, Laing TJ, McCarthy CJ, Adler RS (1996) Power Doppler sonography of synovitis: assessment of therapeutic response – preliminary observations. Radiology 198:582–584

Olivieri I, Barozzi L, Favaro L et al (1996) Dactylitis in patients with seronegative spondylarthropathy: assessment by ultrasonography and magnetic resonance imaging. Arthritis Rheum 39:1524–1528

Ostergaard M, Gideon P, Sorensen K et al (1995) Scoring of synovial membrane hypertrophy and bone erosions by MR imaging in clinically active and inactive rheumatoid arthritis of the wrist. Scand J Rheumatol 24:212–218

Ostergaard M, Stoltenberg M, Lovgreen-Neilsen P et al (1997) Magnetic resonance imaging-determined synovial membrane and joint effusion volumes in rheumatoid arthritis and osteoarthritis: comparison with the macroscopic and microscopic appearance of the synovium. Arthritis Rheum 40:1856–1867

Ostergaard M, Stoltenberg M, Lovgreen-Nielsen P et al (1998) Quantification of synovitis by MRI: correlation between dynamic and static gadolinium-enhanced magnetic resonance imaging and microscopic signs of synovial inflammation. Magn Reson Imaging 16:743–754

Ostergaard M, Hansen M, Stoltenberg M et al (1999) Magnetic resonance imaging-determined synovial membrane volume as a marker of disease activity and a predictor of progressive joint destruction in the wrists of patients with rheumatoid arthritis. Arthritis Rheum 42:918–929

Padhani AR, Dzik-Jurasz A (2004) Perfusion MR imaging of extracranial tumor angiogenesis. Top Magn Reson Imaging 15:41–57

Qvistgaard E, Rogind H, Torp-Pedersen S et al (2001) Quantitative ultrasonography in rheumatoid arthritis: evalua-

tion of inflammation by Doppler technique. Ann Rheum Dis 60:690–693
Radmayr C, Klauser A, Pallwein L et al (2002) Contrast-enhanced ultrasonography for the detection of vesicoureteral reflux. J Urol 167:1428–1430
Rosenkranz K, Zendel W, Langer R et al (1993) Contrast-enhanced transcranial Doppler US with a new transpulmonary echo contrast agent based on saccharide microparticles. Radiology 187:439–443
Schmidt WA (2001) Value of sonography in diagnosis of rheumatoid arthritis. Lancet 357:1056–1057
Schmidt WA, Volker L, Zacher J et al (2000) Colour Doppler ultrasonography to detect pannus in knee joint synovitis. Clin Exp Rheumatol 18:439–444
Schroeder RJ, Bostanjoglo M, Rademaker J et al (2003) Role of power Doppler techniques and ultrasound contrast enhancement in the differential diagnosis of focal breast lesions. Eur Radiol 13:68–79
Sugimoto H, Takeda A, Masuyama J, Furuse M (1996) Early-stage rheumatoid arthritis: diagnostic accuracy of MR imaging. Radiology 198:185–192
Sugimoto H, Takeda A, Kyodoh K (2000) Early-stage rheumatoid arthritis: prospective study of the effectiveness of MR imaging for diagnosis. Radiology 216:569–575
Szkudlarek M, Court-Payen M, Strandberg C et al (2003) Contrast-enhanced power Doppler ultrasonography of the metacarpophalangeal joints in rheumatoid arthritis. Eur Radiol 13:163–168
Taylor PC (2003) The value of sensitive imaging modalities in rheumatoid arthritis. Arthritis Res Ther 5:210–213
Taylor PC (2002) VEGF and imaging of vessels in rheumatoid arthritis. Arthritis Res 4 (Suppl 3):99–107
Terslev L, Torp-Pedersen S, Qvisgaard E et al (2003) Effects of treatment with etanercept (Enbrel, TNFR:Fc) on rheumatoid arthritis evaluated by Doppler ultrasonography. Ann Rheum Dis 62:178–181
Wakefield RJ, Gibbon WW, Conaghan PG et al (2000) The value of sonography in the detection of bone erosions in patients with rheumatoid arthritis. Arthritis Rheum 43:2762–2770
Walther M, Harms H, Krenn V et al (2001) Correlation of power Doppler sonography with vascularity of the synovial tissue of the knee joint in patients with osteoarthritis and rheumatoid arthritis. Arthritis Rheum 44:331–338
Wamser G, Bohndorf K, Vollert K et al (2003) Power Doppler sonography with and without echo-enhancing contrast agent and contrast-enhanced MRI for the evaluation of rheumatoid arthritis of the shoulder joint: differentiation between synovitis and joint effusion. Skeletal Radiol 32:351–359
Zvaifler NJ, Firestein GS (1994) Pannus and pannocytes: alternative models of joint destruction in rheumatoid arthritis. Arthritis Rheum 37:783–789

: : # Research Perspectives

29 Quantitative Analysis of Parenchymal Flow at Contrast-Enhanced US

DAVID O. COSGROVE, ROBERT J. ECKERSLEY, and MARTIN J.K. BLOMLEY

CONTENTS

29.1 Introduction 383
29.2 Transit-Time Measurements 384
29.3 Time–Intensity Curve Analysis 387
29.4 Reperfusion Kinetics 388
29.5 Conclusion 390
    References 390

29.1 Introduction

Amongst the various means available for quantification of blood flow, Doppler is the most widely used because it is non-invasive (COSGROVE et al. 2001). Volume flow is calculated as the product of the mean blood velocity and the cross sectional area of the vessel. Unfortunately, estimating both of these is fraught with technical problems: the velocity is not constant, varying across the vessel lumen and over time with the cardiac rhythm; and the mean velocity calculations vary with the make of scanner. Measuring the area is also difficult, especially for small arteries, and this also changes through the cardiac cycle. Taken together, these uncertainties can amount to errors of as much as 100% in estimating volume flow. Transferring this to perfusion is difficult because the tissue volume being supplied is usually not known. In addition, Doppler suffers from a fundamental limitation when slow flow, such as in the microvasculature, is considered because it cannot distinguish blood flow from bulk tissue movement.

The introduction of microbubble contrast agents has opened up new opportunities in this field (JACOBSEN 2001). Not only does the signal boost they produce make Doppler measurements more robust, but they can be used as tracers to enable measurement of flow in novel ways (COSGROVE et al. 2001). The fact that they are strictly intravascular agents, unlike the diffusible agents used in CT and MR, simplifies these calculations; fundamental to these is the ability to quantify the amount of contrast in a region of interest. There are two ways to quantify ultrasound data: work within the scanner with the raw data or use the processed video or audio outputs. The former method requires special software from the manufacturer and many are now beginning to offer such packages; the latter, although less accurate, is more easily implemented on a wide range of scanners. In addition, care must be taken to account for non-linear machine processing of the data.

When using spectral Doppler the loudness of the audio output is proportional to the number of reflectors in the sample volume (Fig. 29.1). The audio signals can be used to generate time–intensity curves to follow the wash-in and wash-out of the microbubble bolus (Fig. 29.2); however, in some cases the small sample volume is a disadvantage of using spectral Doppler.

Working with two-dimensional images reduces this problem and regions selected for measurement can be tailored to the shape of the structure of interest; in addition, two or more regions can be measured simultaneously and tracking algorithms can be deployed to follow movement and keep the region of interest correctly centred on the image (PHILLIPS and GARDNER 2005). The image information can be analysed for grey-scale intensity changes, for example, using the software package NIH-Image (nih-image162_fat.hqz), and this is useful in vitro and in the heart and for parenchymal enhancement when using newer perfluoro-based contrast agents. The same approach can be used for colour Doppler by first removing the black-and-white portions of the image (segmentation) and then analysing the colour segment. For conventional velocity colour Doppler, the colour components can be reverse-mapped to retrieve the original frequency shift values if the look-up table that was used for colour coding is

D. O. COSGROVE, MD, R. J. ECKERSLEY, PhD;
M. J. K. BLOMLEY, MD
Department of Imaging Sciences, Imperial College London, Hammersmith Hospital, Du Cane Road, London, W12 0HS, UK

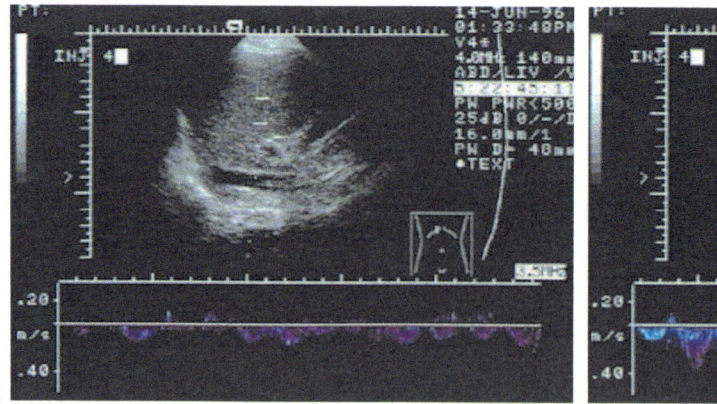

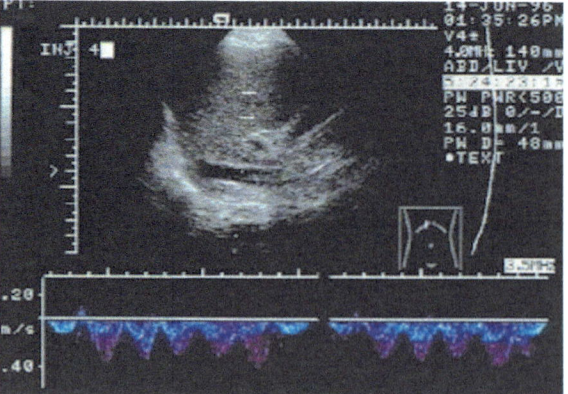

Fig. 29.1a, b. Spectral Doppler for hepatic vein transit-time measurement. The spectral Doppler sample volume is placed on a hepatic vein before injection of the contrast agent, in this case Levovist (**a**), and the time when the signal increases (**b**) is noted. The audio output is fed into a laptop computer and the moment the signal increases consistently above 10% over baseline is taken as the arrival time. The method measures porto-systemic shunting.

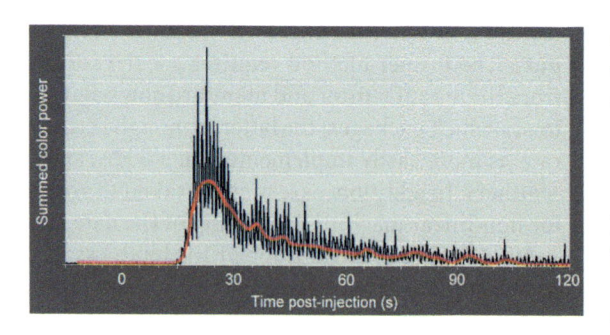

Fig. 29.2 Time–intensity curve. This curve was calculated form power Doppler data form a cine loop after a bolus injection of a contrast agent. The raw data, shown as a *black line*, has a phasic variation caused by cardiac action, and the red line is the result of applying a nine-point smoothing algorithm. Many temporal and quantitative features can be calculated from such curves.

available. In power Doppler, the colours display the signal intensity and provide a direct representation of the main variable that is increased by microbubble enhancing agents. A similar look-up table gives the decibel values throughout the region of interest. At present, these measurements are only available on laboratory systems such as the CQ software (www.kineticimaging.com).

Built-in software packages are now offered on most high-end scanners and they allow the same measurements using either the cleaner, uncompressed and unprocessed data available within the scanner, or at least appropriately corrected post-processed data. They generate the time–intensity curves in real time or at least immediately after the wash-out phase of the transit and can quickly perform calculations such as temporal indices (e.g. arrival time, time-to-peak enhancement) and intensity indices (e.g. peak enhancement, area under the curve; Fig. 29.3).

29.2
Transit-Time Measurements

Tracking the transit of a bolus of microbubbles enables measurements of the physiology of organs. An example is the kidney where the adjacent position of the artery and the vein enables spectral Doppler measurement of the signal rise as the microbubble bolus arrives first in the artery and then in the vein (COSGROVE et al. 2000). The directionality of spectral Doppler allows these two signals to be separated. In the normal kidney the arterial venous transit is approximately 4 s. The true mean transit time can be calculated by plotting the arterial and venous time–intensity curves, applying a gamma-variate fit to select the first pass of the contrast agent, discarding signals from recirculating contrast, and then calculating the difference between the centroids of the two curves. The results correlate closely to those found by more invasive techniques such as magnetic flow meters.

This method has been applied to transplant kidneys in an attempt to distinguish between acute tubular necrosis and rejection. In a preliminary study of 21 patients, a trend to longer arterio-venous transit times was observed in acute rejection, though there was overlap and the difference did not reach statistical significance (HARVEY et al. 2001b). Larger studies are needed to refine the method and

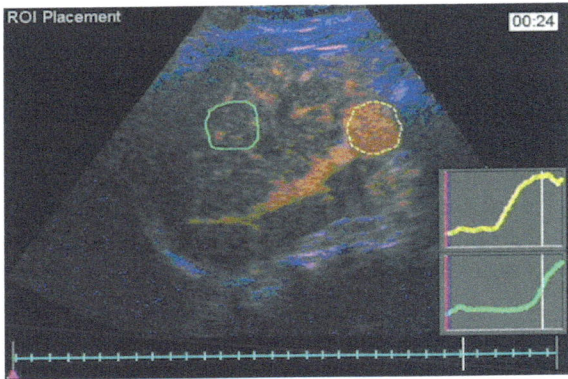

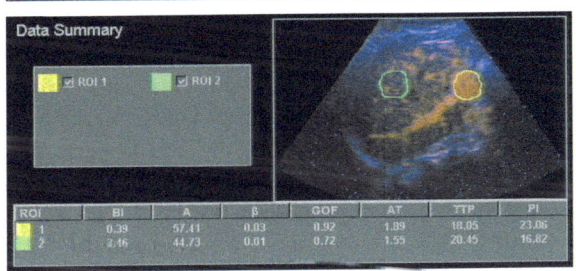

Fig. 29.3a,b. A built-in quantification package (ACQ) was used to calculate perfusion curves for this focal liver lesion (*yellow* region of interest and curve) and an adjacent region of normal liver (*green*) following a bolus injection of the microbubble contrast agent SonoVue (**a**). The software incorporates a tracking mechanism which follows the movement of the liver through breathing and adjusts the position of the regions of interest to maintain their position. Several features from the exponential reperfusion curve are automatically calculated (**b**) including the rate of rise (?) and the maximum level of enhancement reached (*A*). These are two important numbers related to perfusion.

to establish its clinical significance, but the goal of avoiding biopsies remains attractive.

A similar method has been developed for the liver, the goal here being to evaluate arterio-venous shunting (a feature of cirrhosis and malignancies as well as of some rare conditions, such as hereditary haemorrhagic telangiectasia; Blomley et al. 1998). Normally, the hepatic artery supplies approximately 25% of the liver's blood, but this increases in these conditions because of shunts as well as the scarring that increases resistance to portal vein flow in cirrhosis.

The first method developed used spectral Doppler to assess the arrival of Levovist in hepatic veins with the audio output of the scanner fed into a laptop computer (Fig. 29.1; Albrecht et al. 1999). Software to plot the time–intensity curves was developed and the arrival time was defined as a sustained increase in signal strength of 10% over baseline. The time from the bolus injection was measured and, in normal subjects, the multiple microvascular beds that the microbubbles have to traverse before they reach the hepatic veins (lung, splanchnic and hepatic) means that the arrival time is usually around 40 s. (The lower limit of normal was 25 s.) In patients with cirrhosis the arrival could be as early as 5 s and was always <25 s. In addition, the amount of enhancement was also greater, perhaps because less contrast was trapped in the sinusoids of the cirrhotic liver. In a pilot study of 50 patients with diffuse liver diseases of various aetiologies, early arrival times were found in those with cirrhosis but not in those with uncomplicated chronic hepatitis who had arrival times in the normal range (Blomley et al. 2003). There was one exception: a woman with primary biliary cirrhosis who, despite a biopsy that was negative for cirrhosis, had an early arrival time. This could reasonably be attributed to sampling error of the biopsy whereby frankly cirrhotic tissue might have been missed. It is a potential advantage of the arrival-time method that the haemodynamic status of the entire liver be assessed.

A more extensive study focussing on 61 patients with hepatitis C was set up and again showed a good correlation with early arrival times in those with extensive necrosis (fibrosis scores: 6 of 6; Ishak et al. 1995) and late, more normal, arrival in those with no inflammatory change and minimal fibrosis (Ishak et al. 1995: necroinflammatory scores ≤3 of 18; Lim et al. 2005a). Interestingly, in patients with moderately severe disease (Ishak et al. 1995) ≤4 of 18 had significantly early arrival times, suggesting that not only can the arrival time pick out the development of cirrhosis, but that it might also detect pre-cirrhotic changes and thus be of value in decisions about when to offer antiviral treatment.

As part of this study, measurements were repeated in a cohort of 10 patients after a course of treatment with interferon-α and ribavirin. Although still preliminary, there was a trend for normalisation of the arrival time in those patients whose viral load was successfully reduced.

Other centres have performed similar studies and have confirmed these promising results, and hepatologists are now beginning to make use of it, for example, in patients who have refused liver biopsy or in whom there are special contraindications.

In parallel with this, the role of the arrival time in metastatic disease of the liver has been studied. This approach derives from a series of studies pioneered by the Glasgow group on colorectal and other carcinomas using the Doppler Perfusion Index, which assesses the relative contribution of the artery to total liver flow (Leen et al. 2000). It depends on an accurate measurement of the volume flow in both the hepatic artery and portal vein and has been shown to be able to detect not only overt but, importantly, also occult metastatic disease (i.e. disease not detectable at preoperative staging or at laparotomy, which becomes manifest on follow-up). In fact, the basis of this approach was a nuclear medicine finding that the time–activity curve for the liver following a bolus injection of a radio-isotope had two components: an early steep rise, corresponding to the arterial supply; and a later, more gentle rise from the portal supply (Robinson 1991). The first component was found to dominate in patients with liver metastases. For reasons that are unclear, this nuclear medicine test was never widely adopted.

The Doppler Perfusion Index, though very promising, was found to be too technically demanding for general use, so simpler alternatives were sought (Harvey et al. 2001a; Bernatik et al. 2002). Tracking the arrival of a microbubble bolus in the hepatic veins seems to be a feasible alternative that is practical to perform. The earliest technique used spectral Doppler with the sample volume placed on a hepatic vein and the delay from a peripheral intravenous injection to a measured increase in the hepatic vein signal of 10% above baseline was timed.

In a study of 48 patients with colorectal carcinoma, the preoperative hepatic vein transit time was abnormal in 12 who had no definite metastases on CT staging, and of these, 5 had developed overt metastases at their follow-up CT at 1 year (Harvey et al. 2001a). None of those patients with normal hepatic vein transit times developed metastases. If further trials support this finding, the transit time could be useful in selecting patients for adjuvant chemotherapy.

Performing these transit-time studies is cumbersome as it requires at least two operators and dedicated computing equipment. With the advent of perfluoro-gas contrast agents and the development of contrast-specific scanning modes, the possibility of performing the scan in two dimensions became realistic (Fig. 29.4). For this a hepatic vein is targeted with the patient in quiet breathing and the arrival time of contrast in the hepatic arteries is noted with the scanner's timer clock. The delay before the hepatic vein fills is the artery-to-vein transit time (Fig. 29.4). This is shorter than the arm-to-vein transit time used in the previous studies and evaluations of normal volunteers using SonoVue suggests a lower limit than normal of 12 s (Lim et al. 2005b). An advantage of this method is that uninterpretable results where the tracing is flat, which occurs in approximately 10% of cases when using Levovist, are rare; however, the discrimination between the degrees of hepatitis and cirrhosis is a little less clear-cut than with Levovist, perhaps because liver trapping is less marked with SonoVue. Methods to allow the person performing the scan also to give the injection are being explored in a further attempt to simplify the test for routine clinical use, and the most promising is to use an extension tube of the appropriate capacity, preloaded with the contrast agent and the saline flush, such that a single stroke of the plunger pushes the contrast followed by the flush.

All of these studies have focussed on a particular set of large vessels, but it is also possible to measure transit-time curves for regions of tissue. These work best using non-linear modes, such as harmonics, and low-transmit-power methods are preferred because they cause less bubble destruction.

The regional approach has been used mainly for malignancies seeking to improve differential diagnosis by revealing features of neovascularisation, e.g. in the liver (Burns et al. 2000; Harvey and Albrecht 2001; Tanaka et al. 2001). Many studies in the breast show that the arrival time in cancers is earlier than in benign masses, although some cases of benign breast change have been confusing, especially those that have an inflammatory component at histology (Kedar et al. 1996; Albrecht et al. 1998; Baz et al. 2000). Some studies have shown longer persistence of enhancement in cancers, but this has been more variable. The lack of vascularity in mature scars in the breast in comparison to the marked vascularity of tumour recurrence has emerged as a proven clinical tool for this difficult problem (Winehouse et al. 1999).

In the liver, temporal patterns that are generally similar to those seen on triple-phase CT have been described. Malignancies, especially hepatocellular carcinomas, fill from their margin during the arterial phase a few seconds after the injection while regenerating nodules and haemangiomas fill slowly, the latter

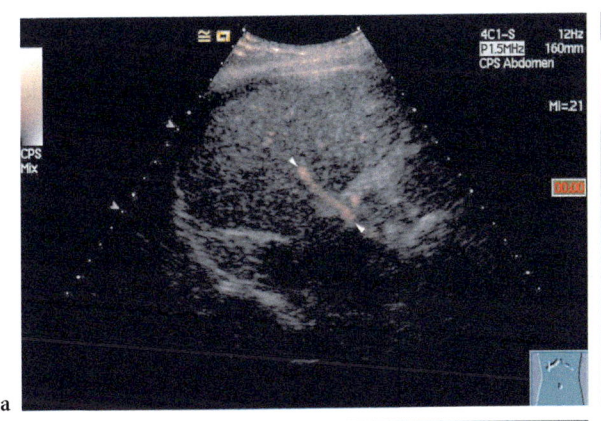

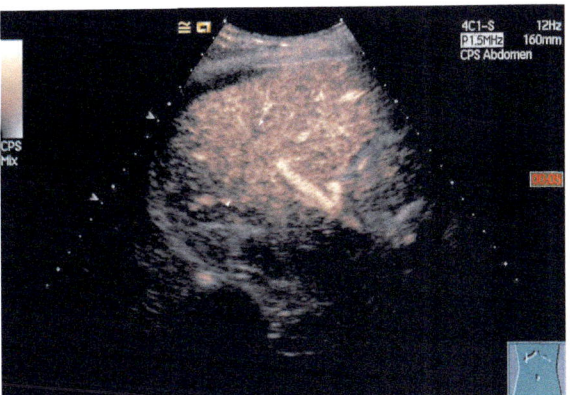

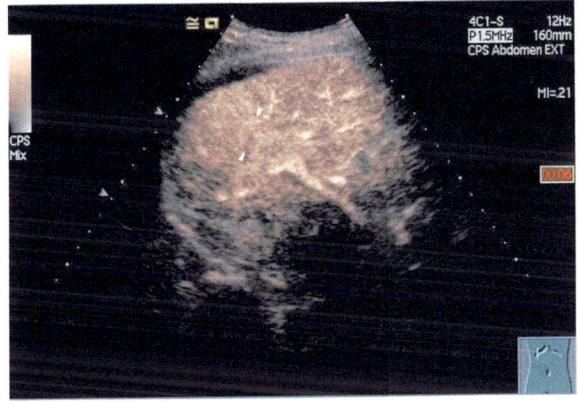

Fig. 29.4a–c. Using a microbubble-specific mode (contrast pulse sequences, in this example), the arrival of the contrast in the hepatic artery can be detected (*arrowheads* in **a**). The timer (highlighted in *red*) is started as soon as this is observed and then attention is focussed on the selected hepatic vein (*arrowheads* in **b**), looking for the arrival of the contrast, which in this patient with hepatitis C occurred at 6 s (*arrowheads* in **c**). This is abnormally early, the normal lower limit being 12 s, and indicates that the liver has arteriovenous shunts which are typical of cirrhosis.

typically from the periphery and usually incompletely. Focal nodular hyperplasia shows similar temporal features to malignancies, although the flow tends to emanate from a central supply artery and their liver-specific phase discriminates them well.

The prostate has also been studied extensively with microbubbles; it has generally been disappointing in cancer detection, although more work is needed here, but the time patterns of treated cancers remains different from benign prostatic hyperplasia, even when the prostate-specific antigen has been reduced to unmeasurable levels, suggesting that the abnormal vascularity persists despite suppression of biochemical activity (ECKERSLEY et al. 1998). Time intensity curves fall rapidly when anti-androgen treatment is administered, as early as day 1, and in a few cases, a rising time–intensity curves value predates escape from hormonal control as judged biochemically and clinically, and this might allow early adjustment of treatment (ECKERSLEY et al. 2002). All of the many indices that can be extracted from these time–intensity curves can also be displayed as colour-coded true functional images which may highlight regional differences in haemodynamics in a useful way.

29.3
Time–Intensity Curve Analysis

The forms of the time–intensity curves contain haemodynamic information which can be revealed using the same mathematics as has classically been applied to radionuclide tracers. In some ways the analyses are simpler because microbubbles are confined to the blood pool and do not diffuse into the interstitial space; however, rigorous analyses are complicated by bubble destruction, non-linearities in the measurements and inhomogeneities in the acoustic fields. The approaches relevant to microbubble time–intensity curves include bolus transit studies in which the true tissue perfusion (i.e. the volume flow per unit of tissue per unit time) is calculated as the ratio of the peak tissue enhancement to the area under the arterial curve (WOLFKIEL and BRUNDAGE 1991). A variant where the peak gradient of the tissue curve is divided by the peak height of the arterial curve has been developed for CT (MILES and BLUMLEY 1997). Provided the necessary arterial and tissue curves could be obtained (and this depends on the particular anatomical arrangements on the organ or lesion), these approaches could be applied to ultrasound.

A somewhat different approach is the Central Volume Theorem in which the perfusion is calculated as the ratio of the central (i.e. fractional vascular) volume to the mean transit time (MAIER and ZIERLER 1954). The mean transit time strictly requires transit curves from the artery and vein, as was described above for renal transplant mean transit time measurements, but approximations to it can be derived from so-called residue functions derived from tissue persistence curves (GOBBEL et al. 1991).

Thus far, there are no reports of attempts to make use of these established methods as experimental or clinical tools using microbubbles.

29.4
Reperfusion Kinetics

The fragility of microbubbles is a feature that can be exploited to obtain a measure of tissue perfusion. First developed for the myocardium (WEI et al. 1998), the method uses a high-power ultrasound beam to destroy the microbubbles within a slice of tissue that corresponds to the orthogonal beam profile.

The destructive pulse creates a negative bolus and "reperfusion kinetics" are used to study the way contrast flows back into the void at a rate that depends on the tissue's perfusion. This refill phase can be assessed in two ways, both of which assume a steady state of blood microbubble concentration which is usually achieved with an infusion pump.

In the first method, developed by WEI et al. (1998), further high-transmit power frames are sent along the same path at progressively increasing intervals, and the signal strength from each is measured. The refill curve has a rising exponential form described by the equation:

$$I = A(1 - e^{-\beta t}),$$

where I–signal intensity and t is the pulsing interval. Its initial exponent (β) is proportional to the speed of microbubble/blood flow into the slice while the peak signal strength, A, is proportional to the fractional vascular volume. The product of these two is an indirect measure of tissue perfusion. In principle, this could be converted to true perfusion if the volume perfused is known, but this is likely to prove elusive since it corresponds to the beam thickness whose shape is complex and dependent on machine settings (e.g. the focus position) and patient variables (e.g. attenuation). The beam's edge is also poorly defined since the energy in it tapers off towards the beam's edges. The consequences of this for microbubble destruction are not well understood. Relative perfusion values are more likely to be achievable. An additional practical problem is tissue movement: if the tissue being insonated moves out of the beam, the signal intensity will be increased artefactually.

Reperfusion kinetics have been applied to the heart (WEI et al. 1998) and the brain (SEIDEL et al. 2002), and the resulting perfusion overlay images are impressive, though it has not yet become routinely accepted.

The original method is time-consuming and this makes it more difficult to keep the probe in the same place over the tissue. A faster and easier method is to switch the scanner to a very low transmit power imaging mode after the destructive burst and observe the reperfusion in real time (Fig. 29.5). This requires a non-linear microbubble-specific mode but, as it only takes a few seconds for most tissues to replenish completely, it can be performed at the plateau of a slow bolus injection. The equation describing the reperfusion and the information that can be extracted from it are identical to the Wei method, although the correspondence between the two has not been investigated systematically; however, this approach does assume that the monitoring mode does not destroy any microbubbles. Just how significant this is, and the fact that the probe needs to stay steadily over the same part of the organ (which applies to both methods), is not yet known. As well as its speed, the real-time reperfusion method has the advantage that in-plane tissue movement can be corrected for by deploying a speckle-tracking method to follow the movement of the region of interest, for example, through the respiratory cycle, provided that the movement is confined to the scan plane. (Out-of-plane movement cannot be tracked.) If three-dimensional acquisition could be achieved, complete tracking should be feasible and the reperfusion could be measured and depicted three-dimensionally.

These reperfusion methods have been applied mainly to the heart in an attempt to quantify myocardial perfusion, and they seem very promising here. In the abdomen, reperfusion has been tried in the kidneys (Fig. 29.6) and liver where, at the least, the method allows a second look at the arterial phase of flow, which is helpful for characterising focal lesions. In the liver, the dual supply means that the reperfusion is not identical to a first-pass bolus because the portal vein supply arrives at the

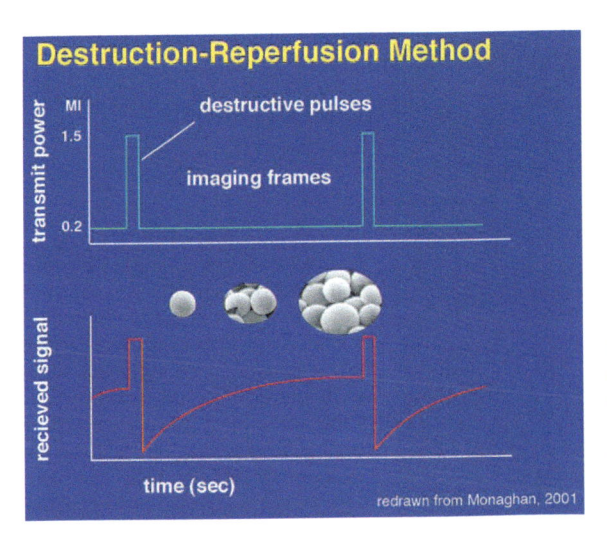

Fig. 29.5 Diagram of pulse sequence for reperfusion kinetics. The high-transmit-power pulses are designed to remove the microbubbles from the scanned plane. The scanner then switches to a low-transmit power mode to follow the exponential reperfusion of the slice from its margins. The curve can then be analysed for features that describe the rate of refill and the maximum signal achieved. (Courtesy of M. Monaghan)

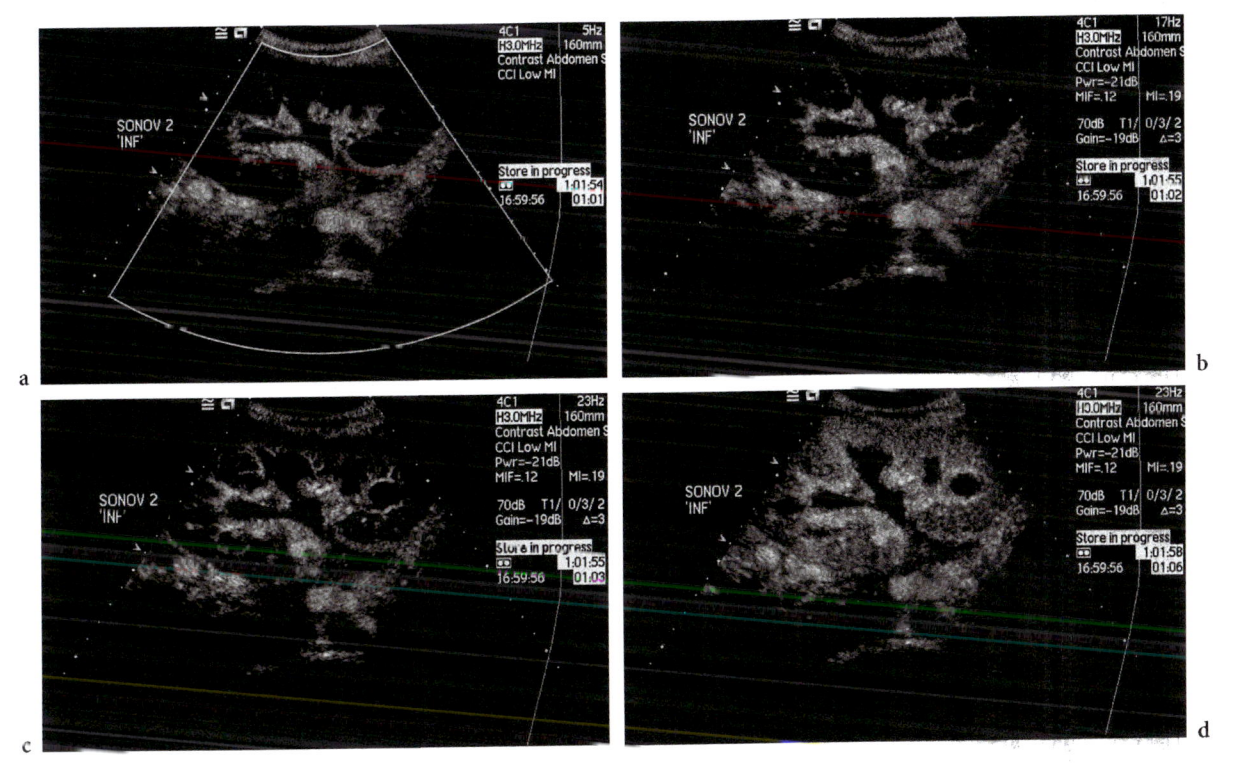

Fig. 29.6a–d. Reperfusion of a renal transplant. The first frame from this cine loop (a) shows the transplant immediately after the destructive frames: the *green box* indicates the area subjected to the high transmit power (mechanical index: 1.5). Thereafter, frames at 1 s (b), 2 s (c) and 5 s (d) show the progressive refill of the main and then the small vessels with eventual filling of the microvasculature throughout the renal cortex.

same time as the hepatic arterial supply without the normal 15- to 30-s delay.

In the kidney a small study using the destruction–reperfusion method with Levovist infusion in normal volunteers showed a good correlation between cortical flow increases produced by administration of dopamine and total renal blood flow measured as the clearance of radio-labelled paramino hippurate (KISHIMOTO et al. 2003). The fractional vascular volume did not change. Although this was a small study, it convincingly demonstrates that non-invasive renal blood flow measurements are feasible.

The opposite approach, known as "diminution kinetics" (METZLER et al. 2003), can also be imple-

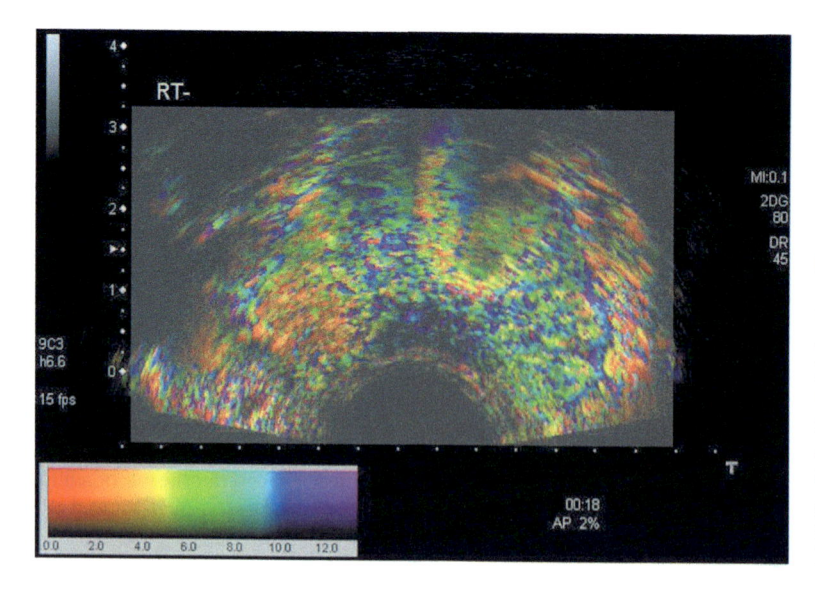

Fig. 29.7 Functional image. The colour scale in this image indicates the arrival time in seconds of a contrast bolus in a transrectal scan of a prostate gland. It was obtained with a phase inversion technique (Aplio US scanner; Pulse Subtract, Toshiba, Tokyo, Japan) by processing the cine loop offline. Functional images may usefully depict the heterogeneity of the circulation in malignancies. (Courtesy of N. Kamiyama, Toshiba, Nasu, Japan.)

mented, i.e. observing the rate of decay of the microbubbles when exposed to a high intensity beam, but this cannot be performed in real time so it has had limited application. This method has been used in the brain to create functional images of time-to-peak enhancement or of relative perfusion, and these seem to be useful in stroke patients because they can be performed at the patient's bedside and can be repeated as often as necessary (MEYER and SEIDEL 2002).

The methods used to create functional images from time–intensity curves can be extended to reperfusion curves in which the product of A and β is plotted to create a map proportional to true perfusion (Fig. 29.7). Although not yet applied clinically, in even small series, this approach is expected to highlight tissues where perfusion is heterogeneous, such as in malignancies.

29.5
Conclusion

Quantification methods can be applied to microbubbles, although the limitations of the non-uniformity of real ultrasound fields in the body must be borne in mind. Measurement of a variety of transit times has been shown to be feasible and they have started to become accepted as clinical tools, especially in the liver. Time–intensity curves can be generated and classical functional analyses applied to them. Functional images can be made from indices derived from them. Perhaps the most interesting approach exploits the fragility of microbubbles to create negative boluses, an approach that is unique in radiology. The subsequent refill of the cleared volume can be used to generate information on tissue perfusion.

References

Albrecht T, Patel N, Cosgrove DO et al (1998) Enhancement of power Doppler signals from breast lesions with the ultrasound contrast agent EchoGen emulsion: subjective and quantitative assessment. Acad Radiol 5 (Suppl 1): S195–S198

Albrecht T, Blomley MJ, Cosgrove DO et al (1999) Non-invasive diagnosis of hepatic cirrhosis by transit-time analysis of an ultrasound contrast agent. Lancet 353:1579–1583

Baz E, Madjar H, Reuss C et al (2000) The role of enhanced Doppler ultrasound in differentiation of benign vs malignant scar lesion after breast surgery for malignancy. Ultrasound Obstet Gynecol 15:377–382

Bernatik T, Strobel D, Hausler J et al (2002) Hepatic transit time of an ultrasound echo enhancer indicating the presence of liver metastases: first clinical results. Ultraschall Med 23:91–95

Blomley MJK, Albrecht T, Cosgrove DO et al (1998) Liver vascular transit time analyzed with dynamic hepatic venography with bolus injections of an US contrast agent: early experience in seven patients with metastases. Radiology 209:862–866

Blomley MJK, Lim AK, Harvey CJ et al (2003) Liver microbubble transit time compared with histology and Child-Pugh score in diffuse liver disease: a cross sectional study. Gut 52:1188–1193

Burns PN, Wilson SR, Simpson DH (2000) Pulse inversion imaging of liver blood flow: improved method for characterizing focal masses with microbubble contrast. Invest Radiol 35:58–71

Cosgrove DO, Kiely P, Williamson R et al (2000) Ultrasonographic contrast media in the urinary tract. Br J Urol Int 86 (Suppl 1):11–17

Cosgrove D, Eckersley R, Blomley M, Harvey C (2001) Quantification of blood flow. Eur Radiol 11:1338–1344

Eckersley R, Butler-Barnes J, Blomley MJK et al (1998) Quantitative microbubble enhanced transrectal ultrasound (TRUS) as a tool for monitoring anti-androgen therapy in prostate carcinoma. Radiology 209:310

Eckersley RJ, Sedelaar JP, Blomley MJK et al (2002) Quantitative microbubble enhanced transrectal ultrasound as a tool for monitoring hormonal treatment of prostate carcinoma. Prostate 51:256–267

Gobbel G, Cann C, Fike J (1991) Measurement of regional cerebral blood flow using ultrafast computed tomography: theoretical aspects. Stroke 22:768–771

Harvey CJ, Albrecht T (2001) Ultrasound of focal liver lesions. Eur Radiol 11:1578–1593

Harvey CJ, Blomley MJK, Cosgrove DO et al (2001a) Liver vascular transit time measured using the carotid delay time with bolus injections of the microbubble Levovist can predict the presence of occult metastases in colorectal cancer. RSNA 2001

Harvey CJ, Lynch M, Blomley MJK (2001b) Quantitation of real-time perfusion with the microbubble optison using power pulsee inversion mode in renal transplants. Eur Radiol 11:103

Ishak K, Baptista A, Bianchi L et al (1995) Histological grading and staging of chronic hepatitis. J Hepatol 22:696–699

Jakobsen JA (2001) Ultrasound contrast agents: clinical applications. Eur Radiol 11:1329–1337

Kedar RP, Cosgrove DO, McCready VR et al (1996) Microbubble contrast agent for color Doppler US: effect on breast masses. Work in progress. Radiology 198:679–686

Kishimoto N, Mori Y, Nishiue T et al (2003) Renal blood flow measurement with contrast-enhanced harmonic ultrasonography: evaluation of dopamine-induced changes in renal cortical perfusion in humans. Clin Nephrol 59:423–428

Leen E, Goldberg JA, Angerson WJ, McArdle CS (2000) Potential role of doppler perfusion index in selection of patients with colorectal cancer for adjuvant chemotherapy. Lancet 355:34–37

Lim AK, Taylor-Robinson SD, Patel N et al (2005a) Hepatic vein transit times using a microbubble agent can predict disease severity non-invasively in patients with Hepatitis C. Gut 54(1):128–133

Lim A, Patel N, Eckersley R et al (2005b) Hepatic vein transit times using SonoVue: a comparative study with Levovist. Hepatology (in press)

Maier P, Zierler K (1954) On the theory of indicator dilution method for the measurement of blood flow and volume. J Appl Physiol 4:308–314

Metzler V, Seidel G, Wiesmann K et al (2003) Perfusion harmonic imaging of the human brain. SPIE 5035:337–348

Meyer K, Seidel G (2002) Transcranial contrast diminution imaging of the human brain: a pilot study in healthy volunteers. Ultrasound Med Biol 28:1433–1437

Miles K, Blomley MJK (1997) Perfusion CT: normal organs. In: Miles K, Dawson P, Blomley MJK (eds) Functional computed tomography. ISIS Medical Media, Oxford

Phillips P, Gardner E (2005) Contrast agent detection and quantification. Eur J Radiol (in press)

Robinson P (1991) Detection of occult hepatic metastases using the hepatic perfusion index. Nucl Med Commun 12:153–158

Seidel G, Meyer K, Metzler V et al (2002) Human cerebral perfusion analysis with ultrasound contrast agent constant infusion: a pilot study on healthy volunteers. Ultrasound Med Biol 28:183–189

Tanaka S, Ioka T, Oshikawa O et al (2001) Dynamic sonography of hepatic tumors. Am J Roentgenol 177:799–805

Wei K, Jayaweera AR, Firoozan S et al (1998) Quantification of myocardial blood flow with ultrasound-induced destruction of microbubbles administered as a constant venous infusion. Circulation 97:473–483

Winehouse J, Douek M, Holz K et al (1999) Contrast-enhanced colour Doppler ultrasonography in suspected breast cancer recurrence. Br J Surg 86:1198–1201

Wolfkiel C, Brundage BH (1991) Measurement of myocardial blood flow by ultrafast computed tomography: towards clinical applicability. Int J Cardiac Imaging 7:89–100

30 Therapeutic Application of Microbubble-Based Agents

Hai-Dong Liang, Martin J. K. Blomley, and David O. Cosgrove

CONTENTS

30.1 Introduction 393
30.2 Targeting and Drug/Gene-Carrying Microbubbles 393
30.3 Gene Delivery 396
30.4 Drug Delivery 397
30.5 Thrombolysis 398
30.6 Tumour Therapy 399
References 400

30.1
Introduction

Encapsulated gas microbubbles have been developed as contrast agents for medical ultrasound (US) imaging. Microbubbles are used not only to image blood pool and tissue perfusion, but they can also be used in therapeutic application such as thrombolysis or drug/gene delivery. Microbubbles are characterized by an average size a little less than that of a red blood cell. As a result, they are capable of penetrating into the microcirculation as well as macrocirculation. Microbubbles can transport bioactive materials such as drug or gene incorporated on or within their shells to a specific site within the body (for instance, an anticancer drug to a specific tumour). Targeted microbubble made by attaching ligands, such as peptides, to their surface can bind specifically to receptors expressed on the blood vessel walls of the target site and cause microbubble accumulation in the target tissue (Klibanov 1999).

H. D. Liang, PhD
Department of Medical Physics and Bioengineering, Bristol General Hospital, Bristol, BS1 6SY, UK
M. J. K. Blomley, MD
Professor of Radiology and Joint Head, Imaging Sciences Department, Faculty of Medicine, Imperial College London, Hammersmith Hospital, Du Cane Road, London, W12 0HS, UK
D. O. Cosgrove, MD
Professor of Clinical Ultrasound, Imperial College London, Hammersmith Hospital, Du Cane Road, London, W12 0HS, UK

Ultrasound is required and used to trace microbubbles. When targeted microbubbles reach the target site, US can be used to disrupt drug-loaded microbubbles to achieve site-specific delivery. Application of US to thin-shelled microbubbles flowing through microvessels is now known to induce vessel wall rupture in vivo (Skyba et al. 1998) large enough to permit extravasation of red blood cells (Price et al. 1998a). In a similar way targeted microbubbles can be disrupted with US, thereby allowing active substance out of the vascular pool and into specific tissue.

Possibilities of targeted delivery of drug-loaded microbubbles and local release by US-triggered bubble destruction are particular assets for microbubbles. The combined capacities of microbubbles for disease detection and assessment, drug and gene targeting, triggered release, and assessment of therapy are unique.

Microbubbles may also provide effective tools for drug development to determine the pharmacokinetics and pharmacodynamics of new molecules, determine dose regimen, and establish therapeutic efficacy.

30.2
Targeting and Drug/Gene-Carrying Microbubbles

Targeting to the diseased tissues can improve the therapeutic effect of any drug by preventing damage of healthy tissues and ensuring high concentration (Fechheimer et al. 1986). Although targeting seems unimportant for intratumoral gene delivery, it becomes crucial when systemic drug/gene delivery is performed. With systemic drug administration, the concentration of drug/gene in the target site is low, and large amount of the drug is needed, which incurs substantial cost. Targeted delivery can reduce the cost by ensuring high concentration in the disease site.

There are broadly two approaches for targeting: nonspecific and specific targeting. The first is the nonspecific targeting. Many microbubbles appear to target certain circulation beds, including the liver, spleen, and activated endothelium. The mechanisms underlying this type of targeting are unclear but almost certainly related to inherent chemical or electrostatic properties of the microbubble shell, resulting in arrest of microbubbles within the microcirculation. This method relies on the disease-related upregulation of receptors that bind non-specifically to either albumin or lipid components of the microbubble shell (LINDNER et al. 2000). The second method, which is referred to as "active targeting" or "specific targeting" (BLOMLEY et al. 2001), uses the deliberate attachment molecular probes, such as ligands, to the microbubble surface, leading to the accumulation of targeted microbubbles at a specific site. Potential ligands include antibodies, peptides, and polysaccharides. Monoclonal antibodies or other ligands that recognize antigens expressed in regions of diseased tissue can be incorporated into or conjugated to the microbubble surface (Figs. 30.1, 30.2).

Chemical spacers (Fig. 30.3a), such as polyethylene glycol (PEG), can be used to project the ligand away from the microbubble surface to allow a greater number of ligand-receptor pairs (KLIBANOV 1999). Monoclonal antibodies against disease antigens can be tagged with biotin. Adhesion to molecules, such as avidin, may then form a bridge between a surface expressing these antigens and biotinylated microbubbles resulting in microbubble aggregation at the site of disease (Fig. 30.3b). Prior to the development of atherosclerosis, endothelial cells express adhesion molecules that mediate monocyte adhesion during atherogenesis. Monoclonal antibodies directed toward one of these endothelial receptors, ICAM-1, have been conjugated to the outer surface of lipid-derived microbubbles (VILLANUEVA et al. 1998). These microbubbles, filled with perfluorobu-

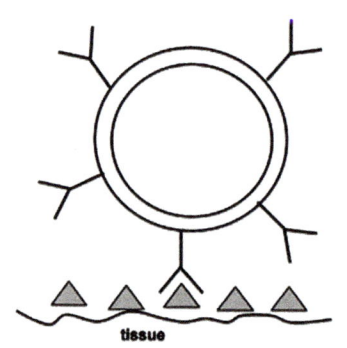

Fig. 30.1 Direct attachment of ligands to microbubble surface

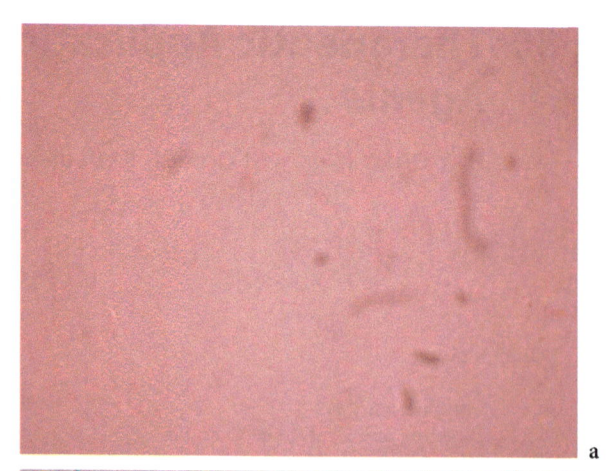

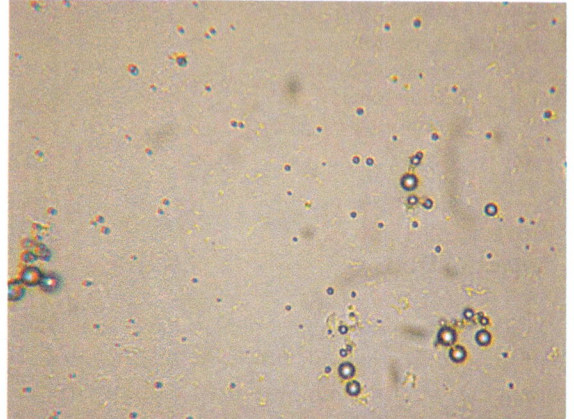

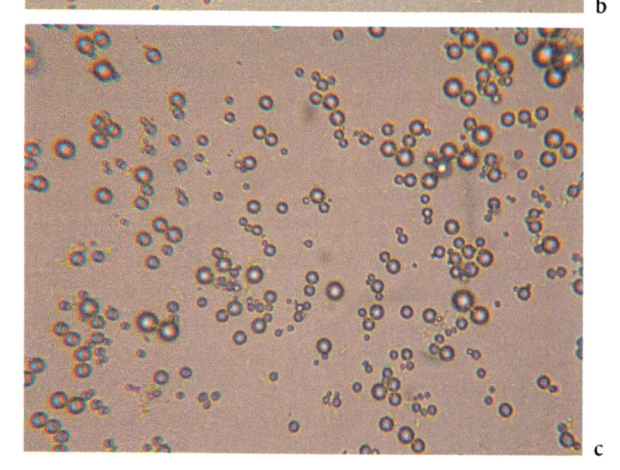

Fig. 30.2a–c. Targeted microbubbles are capable of adhering to sites expressing E-selectin. Specificity of microbubble adhesion was evaluated by dispersing the relevant microbubbles onto recombinant human E-selectin (rHE-selectin) coated plates followed by washing (4°C PBS, 3×) and then visualizing adherent microbubbles by way of an immersion objective (40×). Naked microbubbles bearing no antibody (a) showed no adhesion as compared with isotyped microbubbles bearing a non-specific antibody (b) due to the non-specific binding of the IgG$_1$ Fc portions. Isotyped microbubbles (b) showed lesser adherent microbubbles than targeted microbubbles bearing anti E-selectin antibodies (c). (Courtesy of C. Sennoga)

tane gas, are visible with US and bind specifically to upregulated endothelial cells. Ultrasound therefore has the potential to characterize cell phenotype in vivo.

Targeting ligands called bioconjugates, consisting of a targeting moiety, a linker, and an anchor suitable for incorporation into membranes stabilizing microbubbles, have been developed. The anchor locks the bioconjugate into the membrane surrounding the microbubble and the linker gives the peptide-based targeting ligand enough motional freedom to bind to its target. Thrombus-specific peptides, directed to the activated GPIIb IIIa receptor of platelets, have been evaluated for affinity to bind to activated platelets using photomicrographic images. The prototype bioconjugate, distearyldicarboxyornithine-PEG-CRGDC, can be incorporated into microbubbles. The microbubbles entrapping perfluoropropane gas can be prepared from a blend of phospholipids by agitation. Preliminary in vitro studies have demonstrated binding of these microbubbles to human blood clot (UNGER et al. 2002).

An alternate method for binding microbubbles to disease region has been developed by LANZA et al. (1996). Here an avidin–biotin bridge is used to bind a lipid microemulsion compound to fibrin in a three-step approach (Fig. 30.3b). The initial step of this process is the administration of a biotinylated monoclonal antibody against fibrin followed by administration of avidin, each molecule of which contains four separate binding sites with a very high affinity for biotin (LAVIELLE et al. 1983). Finally, a lipid-perfluorocarbon emulsion that contains a biotinylated phospholipid attaches to the thrombus by means of avidin cross-linking. Although such a technique is somewhat limited by the complexity of administration, the potential to amplify the contrast effect by cross-linking microbubbles to each other via an avidin bridge (microbubble aggregation) may prove advantageous.

There are different ways to transport drug/genes with microbubble. Drugs can be attached to the membrane surface (Fig. 30.4) or embedded into the membrane itself or inside the membrane together with gas. Deoxyribonucleic acid (DNA) may be bound noncovalently to the surface of the microbubbles (UNGER et al. 2002), for example. These microbubbles can be made target specific by using a number of strategies. For example, methods are presently being developed to package hydrophobic drugs into acoustically active microbubbles. One promising avenue for drug delivery is the generation of bilayer-shelled microbubbles made with lipid bilayer that contain concentrated drug between an inner and outer shell. POINT Biomedical (San Carlos, Calif.) has developed a double-shelled microbubble in which the individual shell components can be independently modified to optimize imaging properties, such as sensitivity, resolution, and fragility. The outer shell can be modified to prolong intravascular residence time or to target specific cell-surface receptors. The internal shell, on the other hand, is engineered to respond to specific ultrasound frequencies. Such precise control allows microbubbles to be used as drug-delivery vehicles. Enzymes and a range of different-sized molecules have been successfully inserted.

Microbubbles can only carry limited payloads, as these payloads are generally confined to the bubble shell. Microcapsules with thicker shells, allowing larger drug cargo, could be engineered, but as thicker shells tend to reduce backscatter and susceptibility to acoustic disruption, they are likely to be less effective as acoustically active agent. Dextrose albumin-coated F-butane microbubbles, unlike dextrose albumin-coated air microbubbles, have

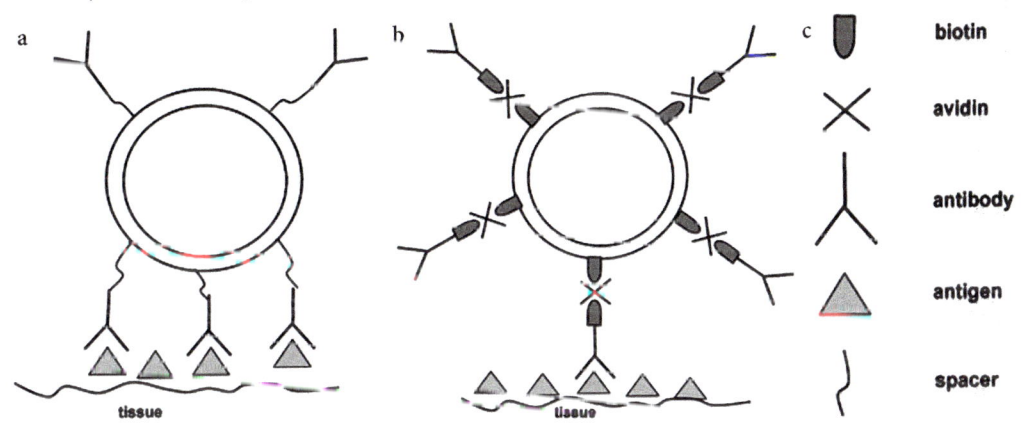

Fig. 30.3 Attachment of ligands to microbubble surface, (a) via flexible spacer and (b) via a avidin bridge.

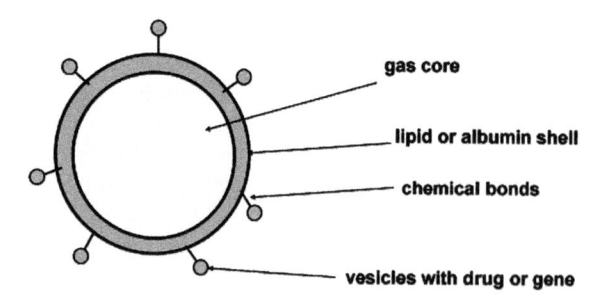

Fig. 30.4 Drug-carrying microbubbles

been reported to preserve albumin's ability to bind synthetic antisense oligonucleotides and allowed their deposition in a specific organ upon insonation (PORTER et al. 1996a). Soybean oil containing *F*-butane microbubbles, proposed to comprise an oil layer inside a phospholipid shell, have been used to deliver paclitaxel (UNGER et al. 1998a). A tenfold reduction in toxicity was observed in mice as compared with free paclitaxel.

30.3
Gene Delivery

In gene therapy, a gene is delivered to cells, allowing them to produce their own therapeutic proteins. The basic concept underlying gene therapy is that human disease might be treated by the transfer of therapeutic nucleotides into specific cells of a patient in order to replace a defective gene or to introduce a new function to the cell. Foreign DNA with appropriate promoters and enhancers is placed into a target cell, and the cellular machinery translates the foreign DNA and manufactures the coded protein. The inserted foreign DNA can therefore be chosen so that the translated protein has some therapeutic value. Gene therapy requires transfection techniques to insert this foreign DNA into the cell.

Transfection generally refers to the uptake and expression of foreign DNA by a cell. Therapeutic genes are macromolecules with several thousand base pairs and molecular weights over 1 million Daltons. These materials, however, are rapidly metabolized by serum esterases after IV injection if they are not encapsulated. Genes are also too large to cross the capillary fenestrations of blood vessels to reach targeted tissue and enter cell without proper delivery method.

Gene delivery by viral vectors can be efficient, but serious problems limit them from use in clinical applications. The problems include immunogenicity of viral proteins, low efficiency for systemic delivery, and potential mutagenicity as a result of viral sequence integration. Non-viral plasmid or "naked" DNA delivery is much safer, but the efficiency is too low to be of clinical value. One alternative for efficient delivery of plasmid DNA is electroporation; however, the electrical power required to create such an effect often causes unacceptable tissue damage, making the technique inappropriate for clinical applications.

Ultrasound has been demonstrated to help deliver fluorescent dextran molecules (FECHHEIMER et al. 1986) and chemotherapeutic compounds (HARRISON et al. 1996) into cells. It has been known since the 1980s that US can enhance gene transfer by increasing cell permeability (FECHHEIMER et al. 1986). Gene transfection can be further potentiated by using microbubbles (PRAT et al. 1993).

While it is evident from existing information that US facilitates delivery of drugs and genes to the interstitial tissue, the physical mechanisms of sonoporation, i.e., transient US-induced perforations in cell membranes by which US affects drug/gene delivery, are not well understood. Currently, acoustic cavitation involving the creation and oscillation of gas bubbles in a liquid has been considered to be the main mechanism. During insonation, dissolved gas and vaporized liquid can form gas bubbles. These bubbles then shrink and grow in size, oscillating in response to the high- and low-pressure portions of the US wave. Further increase of the acoustic pressure will cause the bubbles to implode violently after a few cycles. Such implosion is thought to create holes in the cell membrane ("permeabilization"), which facilitates entry of plasmid DNA into cells. Moreover, membrane permeabilization together with other physical effects of the US, such as transient increase of local temperature and pressure, can be detrimental to cells. The results of such effects on cells varies from being negligible to cell death depending on intensity, duration, and frequency of US, as well as types of cells or tissues (DALECKI et al. 1997a,b; MILLER and GIES 1998). Whereas for some applications, such as cancer therapy, marked cell death may be desirable, therapeutic applications to muscular dystrophy, for example, require minimum cell death with maximum transfection.

With cavitation enhancement, transfection has been demonstrated with low-intensity therapeutic US (i.e., of a few W cm^{-2} as used in physiotherapy; LAWRIE et al. 2000). Because the transfection depends on cavitation activity, the pressure amplitude can be more important than the time-average intensity, which is the critical factor for thermal effects. Diagnostic US can have substantial pulse pressure amplitudes with low time-average intensity, and in vivo transfection has been demonstrated with diagnostic US scanners in the heart with cavitation enhancement (SHOHET et al. 2000; VANNAN et al. 2000).

With intensity values below those for theoretical thermal damage, US has been shown to affect the endothelium by permitting passage of 100 nm macromolecular structures (MR-visible liposomes encapsulating gadopentetate dimeglumine, for example; BEDNARSKI et al. 1997). Microvessel ruptures created by US-triggered microbubble destruction (likely due to cavitation) provide focal delivery of colloidal particles and red blood cells (PRICE et al. 1998b). By applying appropriately timed pulses and levels of energy, US may be used to enhance uptake of DNA into cells and also to induce transfection and ultimately expression of desired gene products. Mechanical insonation with US facilitates transduction of naked plasmid DNA into colon carcinoma cells in vivo (MANOME et al. 2000). The acoustic power required to induce sonoporation was reduced when microbubbles were present (WARD et al. 2000). In vitro experiments on lymphocytes indicated that sonoporation was directly related to microbubble-to-cell ratio and to bubble-to-cell spacing (WARD et al. 2000). Close bubble cell spacing increased the probability of lethal (irreversible) sonoporation.

Ultrasound exposure in the presence of microbubbles has been reported to achieve 300-fold higher transgene expression in vascular cells in vitro than with naked DNA alone. Efficacy of a polyamine transfection agent was also enhanced (LAWRIE et al. 2000). Intrauterine injection of naked DNA-expressing proteins, in combination with perfluorocarbon microbubble-enhanced US, produced protein expression in fetal mice. Luciferase expression increased 1000 fold in comparison with expression after injection of naked DNA alone or naked DNA with US (ENDOH et al. 2002). US-Optison (Amersham Health Inc., Princeton, NJ)-mediated gene transfection has demonstrated the significant prolongation of graft survival by the successful transfection of NFkappaB-decoy into the donor kidney in a rat renal allograft model (AZUMA et al. 2003) and inhibition of renal fibrosis by gene transfer of inducible Smad7 in rat UUO model (LAN et al. 2003).

In vitro US-mediated gene expression and transfection efficiency were enhanced when DNA was incorporated into albumin-coated F-propane microbubbles, as compared with unloaded bubbles mixed with plasmid (FRENKEL et al. 2002). Positively charged microbubbles that bind DNA have also been shown to enhance gene transfection (VANNAN et al. 2002).

Skeletal muscle cell, already known to be one of the few tissues which can be transfected with plasmid DNA, is a particularly promising target for sonoporation strategies. Ultrasound combined with microbubble can enhance muscle gene transfection. Interestingly, in this model, microbubble (Optison and Definity) alone can also induce gene transfection and reduce the damage caused by plasmid injection and application of US (DANIALOU et al. 2002; LU et al. 2003).

30.4
Drug Delivery

The ability of US to release incorporated molecules from solid polymers was first described by LANGER (1990). Increases in release rates are proportional to the intensity of the US beam (KOST et al. 1989). Exposure to US signals induces rupture of drug-containing microbubbles, releasing therapeutic molecules lying as much as 20 cm below the skin surface. Experimental evidence which points to the fact that the effect of US on drug delivery is enhanced in the presence of microbubbles near the target site (PORTER et al. 1996a; PRICE et al. 1998a; MILLER et al. 2000). The US-induced drug delivery will be effective if either microbubble carriers are used (UNGER et al. 2002) or microbubbles are co-delivered with vesicle carriers such as liposomes and micelles (SONG et al. 2002a).

Although vesicles are much more stable in blood compared with encapsulated microbubbles, they interact poorly with ultrasound. To have the increased stability of vesicles and the great echogenicity of microbubbles, drug-containing vesicles should be either injected simultaneously with microbubbles or combined with microbubbles with the formation of microbubble-vesicle aggregates. In both approaches, microbubbles are used as catalysts of acoustic cavitation and possibly the significant deformation of vesicles in the neighbourhood of microbubbles. The increased effect of US on drug delivery by using the former approach has been found experimentally (SONG et al. 2002a).

The drawback to this approach is that the simultaneous injection does not guarantee that microbubbles will be in the immediate vicinity of drug carriers when reaching the target. The drug release can be more effective with the use of microbubble-vesicle aggregates. In this case, vesicles with drugs (1–100 nm in size) are attached to the surface of each encapsulated microbubble through chemical bonds. If the microbubble-vesicle aggregates reach the target blood vessel, microbubbles inside the aggregates will oscillate under the action of US and the possible resulting cavitation might assist in delivering of drugs from vesicles to the interstitial tissue. Such aggregates are under development.

It is possible to achieve tissue-specific drug delivery without targeting of microbubbles via ligand-receptor interactions. Selective tissue insonation may be sufficient. Microbubbles were used to deliver oligonucleotide to some tissues selectively by US activation. Albumin-coated microbubbles were modified with an oligonucleotide derivative and introduced intravenously in the experimental animal. Selective tissue uptake was achieved via US insonation of the tissue of interest (kidney). There was up to ninefold improvement of uptake of the labelled oligonucleotide compared with control non-insonated tissue (PORTER et al. 1996a). A disadvantage of this approach is that if the microbubbles release the drug in the larger vessels during insonation, the drug may be washed away in the flow of blood and not deposited at the insonated tissue. It might be beneficial to attach the bubbles to the surface of the vessels prior to the release of the drug in order to assure its delivery into the tissues via the US pulse (KLIBANOV et al. 2004).

Another form of drug delivery that can also be performed using US and microbubbles is to employ sonosensitizers in sonodynamic therapy (UNGER et al. 2002). Certain compounds, such as lidocaine, cytosine arabinoside, and porfimer sodium (TACHINABA and TACHINABA 1993; TACHINABA et al. 2000), can increase sensitivity to US energy. Sonosensitizers are activated by US and may work similarly to photosensitive agents, except that the method of action uses US rather than light energy. Ultrasound can penetrate tissues much more deeply than light and US energy can be focused. Application of sonodynamic therapy may include tumour ablation and treating vascular disease such as atherosclerotic plaques.

30.5
Thrombolysis

Blood clots in the circulation bed, such as heart, brain, and pulmonary emboli, are a common cause of death. Thrombolysis is the treatment to break up abnormal blood clots that are restricting blood flow. Problems with current thrombolytic therapy include slow and incomplete thrombolysis and frequent bleeding complications. Increasing evidence from in vitro, animal, and initial patient studies (COHEN et al. 2003) indicates that application of US as an adjunct to thrombolytic therapy offers unique potential to improve effectiveness and decrease bleeding complications.

In vitro studies demonstrate that low-intensity US increases enzymatic fibrinolysis through mechanisms that include improving drug transport, reversibly altering fibrin structure, and increasing tPA binding to fibrin. Ultrasound delivered transcutaneously or with an endovascular catheter accelerates thrombolysis in animal models of venous, arterial, and small vessel thrombosis. Ultrasound delivered at higher intensities using either an endovascular vibrating wire or transcutaneously in conjunction with stabilized microbubbles can cause mechanical fragmentation of thrombus without administration of plasminogen activator. Ultrasound at lower frequencies in the range of 20–40 kHz has a greater effect on thrombolysis with improved tissue penetration and less heating. These studies form the basis for clinical trials investigating the potential of US as an adjunct to improve thrombolytic therapy.

Although US intensity, frequency, and methods of exposure have varied among the experiments, the efficiencies of fibrinolytic agents have clearly been increased by nonthermal US energy (LAUER et al. 1992; BLINC et al. 1993; HARPAZ et al. 1993; LUO et al. 1993).

When US and thrombolytics are combined, the improved lysis is thought to be due to better clot penetration by the drug (SIDDIQI et al. 1995). Acoustic cavitation played a major role in increasing the bioavailability of fibrinolytic agents at the surface of the thrombus (ROSENSCHEIN et al. 1994). Cavitation can generate high-velocity jets or a steady flow of fluid known as microstreaming. In addition, microscopic bubbles oscillating during US exposure may increase penetration of fibrinolytic agents into the thrombus and thus accelerate fibrinolysis. APFEL and HOLLAND (1991) reported that albumin microbubbles could lower acoustic cavitation thresholds to as low as one-third of the energy. This phenomenon opens new possibilities for applying microbubble for therapeutic means to induce cavitation with a lower US energy level.

Microbubble lysis works by a different process explained by several potential mechanisms. The combination of thrombolytic drugs and low-frequency US has shown increased lysis, probably due to better penetration of the drug into clot (Luo et al. 1996; Suchkova et al. 2000). High-intensity US causes precavitation and cavitation at the surface of a thrombus that can create sufficient shear stress to lyse the clot. Additionally, the asymmetric collapse of microbubbles during cavitation can create fluid jets that erode the clot surface. With addition of injected microbubbles to those produced by the US there is an increase in the number of bubble–thrombus collisions, and further fragmenting of the thrombus.

The threshold for US-induced cavitation is reduced by the presence of injected microbubbles. These mechanisms produce average thrombus particles of 3.6 μm, similar in size to those obtained with traditional thrombolysis (Wu et al. 1998). Microbubble-augmented low-frequency US clot lysis in animal models has developed from intravenous studies in rabbits with use of very small clots of approximately 0.3 ml volume to moderate-sized clots in the 3–6 ml range with use of direct clot injection of microbubbles in dogs (Porter et al. 1996b; Culp et al. 2001). The combination of microbubbles and US also increases lysis compared with US alone (Porter et al. 1996b). Therapeutic US frequencies from 40 kHz to 2 MHz have been successfully used. Microbubble adheres to the surface of the clot where US destroys the microbubbles. As bubbles fragment, shearing effects mechanically erode the adjacent clot without systemic lysis. Several studies in rabbits where the volume of clot is quite small (<0.3 ml) show reliable lysis of fresh iliac thrombus (Nishioka et al. 1997; Wu et al. 1998).

Microbubble-augmented sonothrombolysis can be enhanced even further by using targeting microbubbles. Unger et al. (1998b), Wright et al. (1998), Takeuchi et al. (1999) and Schumann et al. (2002) demonstrate the efficacy of lipid-shelled microbubble specifically designed to target thrombus. These microbubbles, MRX-408 or MRX-408A1 (ImaRx Inc., Tucson, Ariz.), incorporate the Arg-Gly-Asp (RGD) peptide sequence in the microbubble shell. The RGD sequence is adherent to the receptors for fibrinogen and von Willebrand factor, as well as several other integrins and related heterodimeric proteins (Ruoslahti 1996). MRX-408 is targeted to the GPIIb IIIa binding domain on activated platelets. In vitro 7.5-MHz US studies of artificially generated human thrombus demonstrated that MRX 408 enhanced the detectable extent of the clot an average of approximately ninefold, compared with a control nontargeted agent, and increased the probability of clot detection (Unger et al. 1998b; Wright et al. 1998). MRX-408 has been used to enhance sonothrombolysis (Wu et al. 1998).

30.6
Tumour Therapy

High-intensity focused US has been explored especially for therapy of benign or malignant tumours (Ter Haar 2001; Wu et al. 2001). The primary physical mechanism responsible for ablation of tissue with high-intensity focused US is heating, which kills tissue within small focal volumes. Larger volumes are treated by moving the focal lesion. Ultrasound can also produce bioeffects via nonthermal mechanisms, primarily acoustic cavitation. The initial application of nonthermal therapy was to lithotripsy (Coleman and Saunders 1993), in which widely spaced high-amplitude US pulses with a centre frequency of about 200 kHz pulverize kidney stones. The shock waves can also produce soft tissue damage, such as haemorrhage, that is believed to be due to acoustic cavitations. For lithotripsy treatment, the cavitation threshold has been estimated to be in the range of 1.5–3.5 MPa in human tissue (Coleman et al. 1995). Enhancement of cavitation nucleation by air bubbles can enhance therapeutic efficacy (Prat et al. 1993). Enhancing cavitation nucleation in shock-wave treatment by using gas-body-based microbubble has been explored in mouse tumours (Miller and Song 2002).

The mechanical effects of cavitation can include sonoporation of some surviving cells, which can combine DNA transfer and shock-wave tumour ablation (Bao et al. 1998). This strategy has been tested for shock wave in combination with interleukin-12 gene therapy for the enhancement of the antitumor immune response showing promising results (Song et al. 2002b); however, shock-wave treatment volume could not easily be controlled and it has possible potential for enhanced metastasis of highly malignant tumours. High-intensity focused US at higher frequencies than lithotripter shock waves allows narrow focusing on the volume of interest. Wide range of pulse durations, pulse-repetition frequencies, and intensities can be explored to find optimal conditions. The physical mechanisms of high-intensity focused US for bioeffects range from purely nonthermal to purely thermal. High-intensity focused US has shown promise for DNA transfer. High-intensity focused US at 1.18 MHz compared favourably with lithotripter shock waves for transfection in vitro (HUBER and PFISTERER 2000). In vivo transfection with plasmid DNA has also been demonstrated with high-intensity focused US (at a relatively low 1-MPa pressure amplitude) in a rat tumour model without specific cavitation enhancement (HUBER and PFISTERER 2000), and this treatment method did not appear to increase the incidence of metastases. Intratumoral or intravenous injections of microbubbles combined with high-intensity focused US have been shown to stop tumour growth and enhance gene transfection (MILLER and SONG 2003).

References

Apfel RE, Holland OK (1991) Gauging the likelihood of cavitation from short-pulse, low-duty cycle diagnostic ultrasound. Ultrasound Mod Biol 17(2):179–185

Azuma H, Tomita N, Kaneda Y et al (2003) Transfection of NF kappa B-decoy oligodeoxynucleotides using efficient ultrasound-mediated gene transfer into donor kidneys prolonged survival of rat renal allografts. Gene Ther 10:415–425

Bao SP, Thrall BD, Gies RA, Miller DL (1998) In vivo transfection of melanoma cells by lithotripter shock waves. Cancer Res 58:219–221

Bednarski MD, Lee JW, Callstrom MR, Li KCP (1997) In vivo target-specific delivery of macromolecular agents with MR-guided focused ultrasound. Radiology 204:263–268

Blinc A, Francis CW, Trudnowski JL, Carstensen EL (1993) Characterization of ultrasound-potentiated fibrinolysis in vitro. Blood 81:2636–2643

Blomley MJK, Cooke JC, Unger EC et al (2001) Science, medicine, and the future – microbubble contrast agents: a new era in ultrasound. Br Med J 322:1222–1225

Cohen MG, Tuero E, Bluguermann J et al (2003) Transcutaneous ultrasound-facilitated coronary thrombolysis during acute myocardial infarction. Am J Cardiol 92:454–457

Coleman AJ, Saunders JE (1993) A review of the physical properties and biological effects of the high amplitude acoustic fields used in extracorporeal lithotripsy. Ultrasonics 31:75–89

Coleman AJ, Kodama T, Choi MJ et al (1995) The cavitation threshold of human tissue exposed to 0.2-MHz pulsed ultrasound: preliminary measurements based on a study of clinical lithotripsy. Ultrasound Med Biol 21:405–417

Culp WC, Porter TR, Xie F et al (2001) Microbubble potentiated ultrasound as a method of declotting thrombosed dialysis grafts: experimental study in dogs. Cardiovasc Interv Radiol 24:407–412

Dalecki D, Child SZ, Raeman CH et al (1997a) Ultrasonically induced lung hemorrhage in young swine. Ultrasound Med Biol 23:777–781

Dalecki D, Raeman CH, Child SZ, Carstensen EL (1997b) Effects of pulsed ultrasound on the frog heart. 3. The radiation force mechanism. Ultrasound Med Biol 23:275–285

Danialou G, Comtois AS, Dudley RWR et al (2002) Ultrasound increases plasmid-mediated gene transfer to dystrophic muscles without collateral damage. Mol Ther 6:687–693

Endoh M, Koibuchi N, Sato M et al (2002) Fetal gene transfer by intrauterine injection with microbubble-enhanced ultrasound. Mol Ther 5:501–508

Fechheimer M, Denny C, Murphy RF, Taylor DL (1986) Measurement of cytoplasmic Ph in dictyostelium discoideum by using a new method for introducing macromolecules into living cells. Eur J Cell Biol 40:242–247

Fechheimer M, Boylan JF, Parker S et al (1987) Transfection of mammalian cells with plasmid DNA by scrape loading and sonication loading. Proc Natl Acad Sci USA 84:8463–8467

Frenkel PA, Chen SY, Thai T et al (2002) DNA-loaded albumin microbubbles enhance ultrasound-mediated transfection in vitro. Ultrasound Med Biol 28:817–822

Harpaz D, Chen XC, Francis CW et al (1993) Ultrasound enhancement of thrombolysis and reperfusion in vitro. J Am Coll Cardiol 21:1507–1511

Harrison GH, BalcerKubiczek EK, Gutierrez PL (1996) In vitro mechanisms of chemopotentiation by tone-burst ultrasound. Ultrasound Med Biol 22:355–362

Huber PE, Pfisterer P (2000) In vitro and in vivo transfection of plasmid DNA in the Dunning prostate tumor R3327-AT1 is enhanced by focused ultrasound. Gene Ther 7:1516–1525

Klibanov AL (1999) Targeted delivery of gas-filled microspheres, contrast agents for ultrasound imaging. Adv Drug Deliv Rev 37:139–157

Klibanov AL, Rinkevich D, McConaught JE et al (2004) Ultrasound-triggered release of microbubble-associated material: approaches to site-targeted drug release (abstract). Ultrasound contrast research symposium

Kost J, Leong K, Langer R (1989) Ultrasound-enhanced polymer degradation and release of incorporated substances (controlled release drug delivery systems). Proc Natl Acad Sci USA 86:7663–7666

Lan HY, Mu W, Tomita N et al (2003) Inhibition of renal fibrosis by gene transfer of inducible Smad7 using ultrasound-microbubble system in rat UUO model. J Am Soc Nephrol 14:1535–1548

Langer R (1990) New methods of drug delivery. Science 249:1527–1533

Lanza GM, Wallace KD, Scott MJ et al (1996) A novel site-targeted ultrasonic contrast agent with broad biomedical application. Circulation 94:3334–3340

Lauer CG, Burge R, Tang DB et al (1992) Effect of ultrasound on tissue-type plasminogen-activator induced thrombolysis. Circulation 86:1257–1264

Lavielle S, Chassaing G, Marquet A (1983) Avidin binding of biotinylated analogs of substance-P. Biochim Biophys Acta 759:270–277

Lawrie A, Brisken AF, Francis SE et al (2000) Microbubble-enhanced ultrasound for vascular gene delivery. Gene Ther 7:2023–2027

Lindner JR, Coggins MP, Kaul S et al (2000) Microbubble persistence in the microcirculation during ischemia/reperfusion and inflammation is caused by integrin- and complement-mediated adherence to activated leukocytes. Circulation 101:668–675

Lu QL, Liang HD, Partridge T, Blomley MJK (2003) Microbubble ultrasound improves the efficiency of gene transduction in skeletal muscle in vivo with reduced tissue damage. Gene Ther 10:396–405

Luo H, Steffen W, Cercek B et al (1993) Enhancement of thrombolysis by external ultrasound. Am Heart J 125:1564–1569

Luo H, Nishioka T, Fishbein MC et al (1996) Transcutaneous ultrasound augments lysis of arterial thrombi in vivo. Circulation 94:775–778

Manome Y, Nakamura M, Ohno T, Furuhata H (2000) Ultrasound facilitates transduction of naked plasmid DNA into colon carcinoma cells in vitro and in vivo. Hum Gene Ther 11:1521–1528

Miller DL, Gies RA (1998) Enhancement of ultrasonically induced hemolysis by perfluorocarbon-based compared to air-based echo-contrast agents. Ultrasound Med Biol 24:285–292

Miller DL, Song JM (2002) Lithotripter shock waves with cavitation nucleation agents produce tumor growth reduction and gene transfer in vivo. Ultrasound Med Biol 28:1343–1348

Miller DL, Song JM (2003) Tumor growth reduction and DNA transfer by cavitation-enhanced high-intensity focused ultrasound in vivo. Ultrasound Med Biol 29:887–893

Miller DL, Kripfgans OD, Fowlkes JB, Carson PL (2000) Cavitation nucleation agents for nonthermal ultrasound therapy. J Acoust Soc Am 107:3480–3486

Nishioka T, Luo H, Fishbein MC et al (1997) Dissolution of thrombotic arterial occlusion by high intensity, low frequency ultrasound and dodecafluoropentane emulsion: an in vitro and in vivo study. J Am Coll Cardiol 30:561–568

Porter TR, Iversen PL, Li SP, Xie F (1996a) Interaction of diagnostic ultrasound with synthetic oligonucleotide-labeled perfluorocarbon exposed sonicated dextrose albumin microbubbles. J Ultrasound Med 15:577–584

Porter TR, LeVeen RF, Fox R et al (1996b) Thrombolytic enhancement with perfluorocarbon-exposed sonicated dextrose albumin microbubbles. Am Heart J 132:964–968

Prat F, Chapelon JY, Elfadil FA et al (1993) In vivo effects of cavitation alone or in combination with chemotherapy in a peritoneal carcinomatosis in the rat. Br J Cancer 68:13–17

Price RJ, Skyba DM, Kaul S, Skalak TC (1998a) Delivery of colloidal particles and red blood cells to tissue through microvessel ruptures created by targeted microbubble destruction with ultrasound. Circulation 98:1264–1267

Price RJ, Skyba DM, Skalak TC, Kaul S (1998b) Delivery of colloidal particles and red blood cells to tissue through microvessel ruptures resulting from microbubble destruction by ultrasound. Circulation 98:2999

Rosenschein U, Frimerman A, Laniado S, Miller HI (1994) Study of the mechanism of ultrasound angioplasty from human thrombi and bovine aorta. Am J Cardiol 74:1263–1266

Ruoslahti E (1996) RGD and other recognition sequences for integrins. Annu Rev Cell Dev Biol 12:697–715

Schumann PA, Christiansen JP, Quigley RM et al (2002) Targeted-microbubble binding selectively to GPIIb IIIa receptors of platelet thrombi. Invest Radiol 37:587–593

Shohet RV, Chen SY, Zhou YT et al (2000) Echocardiographic destruction of albumin microbubbles directs gene delivery to the myocardium. Circulation 101:2554–2556

Siddiqi F, Blinc A, Braaten J, Francis CW (1995) Ultrasound increases flow-through fibrin gels. Thromb Haemost 73:495–498

Skyba DM, Price RJ, Linka AZ et al (1998) Direct in vivo visualization of intravascular destruction of microbubbles by ultrasound and its local effects on tissue. Circulation 98:290–293

Song J, Chappell JC, Qi M et al (2002a) Influence of injection site, microvascular pressure and ultrasound variables on microbubble-mediated delivery of microspheres to muscle. J Am Coll Cardiol 39:726–731

Song JM, Tata D, Li L et al (2002b) Combined shock-wave and immunogene therapy of mouse melanoma and renal carcinoma tumors. Ultrasound Med Biol 28:957–964

Suchkova VN, Baggs RB, Francis CW (2000) Effect of 40-kHz ultrasound on acute thrombotic ischemia in a rabbit femoral artery thrombosis model: enhancement of thrombolysis and improvement in capillary muscle perfusion. Circulation 101:2296–2301

Tachibana K, Tachibana S (1993) Use of ultrasound to enhance the local-anesthetic effect of topically applied aqueous lidocaine. Anesthesiology 78:1091–1096

Tachibana K, Uchida T, Tamura K (2000) Enhanced cytotoxic effect of Ara-C by low intensity ultrasound to HL-60 cells. Cancer Lett 149:189–194

Takeuchi H, Ogunyankin K, Pandian NG et al (1999) Enhanced visualization of intravascular and left atrial appendage thrombus with the use of a thrombus-targeting ultrasonographic contrast agent (MRX-408A1): in vivo experimental echocardiographic studies. J Am Soc Echocardiogr 12:1015–1021

Ter Haar GR (2001) High intensity focused ultrasound for the treatment of tumors. Echocardiogr J Cardiovasc Ultrasound Allied Tech 18:317–322

Unger EC, Matsunaga TO, McCreery T et al (2002) Therapeutic applications of microbubbles. Eur J Radiol 42:160–168

Unger EC, McCreery TP, Sweitzer RH et al (1998a) Acoustically active lipospheres containing paclitaxel: a new therapeutic ultrasound contrast agent. Invest Radiol 33:886–892

Unger EC, McCreery TP, Sweitzer RH et al (1998b) In vitro studies of a new thrombus-specific ultrasound contrast agent. Am J Cardiol 81:58G–61G

Vannan M, McCreery T, Li P et al (2002) Ultrasound-mediated transfection of canine myocardium by intravenous administration of cationic microbubble-linked plasmid DNA. J Am Soc Echocardiogr 15:214–218

Villanueva FS, Jankowski RJ, Klibanov S et al (1998) Microbubbles targeted to intercellular adhesion molecule 1 bind to activated coronary artery endothelial cells. Circulation 98:1–5

Ward M, Wu JR, Chiu JF (2000) Experimental study of the effects of Optison (R) concentration on sonoporation in vitro. Ultrasound Med Biol 6:169–175

Wright WH, McCreery TP, Krupinski EA et al (1998) Evaluation of new thrombus-specific ultrasound contrast agent. Acad Radiol 5:S240–S242

Wu F, Chen WZ, Bai J et al (2001) Pathological changes in human malignant carcinoma treated with high-intensity focused ultrasound. Ultrasound Med Biol 27:1099–1106

Wu YQ, Unger EC, McCreery TP et al (1998) Binding and lysing of blood clots using MRX-408. Invest Radiol 33:880–885

Subject Index

A

acoustic power   23, 32, 73, 80, 168, 225, 271, 352
active bleeding   296
ADI, *see* Agent Detection Imaging
agent detection imaging   67, 168
AIP 101   81
Albunex   7, 78-80, 82-83
angiogenesis   303-305, 365
artefact
– conventional sonograms   126
color blooming   26, 109
– jail bar   26
– spikes   25
arterial, phase   129-130
artifact, *see* artefact
autoregulation, myocardium   284
avidin   394

B

background, subtraction   270, 285
backscattering, *see* scattering
Baker's cyst   371
biotin   395
blood, flow   255, 271-272, 278
blood, velocity   255, 271-272, 388
blood volume   255, 271, 278, 282, 388
bolus, administration   71, 91
BR14   10
bulk modulus   19

C

cadence contrast pulse sequence   58, 205
cavitation, inertial and noninertial   77, 78, 399
CCI, *see* Coherent Contrast Imaging
chirp coding   56
clutter   25, 47
coded excitation   55
Coherent Contrast Imaging   54
color Doppler, US or conventional   48, 223, 245, 302, 315, 324, 349, 360, 365, 383
colour Doppler, *see* color Doppler

compound, imaging   126
contrast burst imaging   91
contrast harmonic imaging, *see* harmonic B-mode imaging
contrast echocardiography   267, 271, 277
contrast tuned imaging   368
contusion, parenchymal   295
corticomedullary phase, renal
– arterial, *see* early
– early   224, 248
– late   224, 248

D

damping   18, 20
Definity   10, 82, 126, 225, 361
delayed, phase *see* late, phase
diffusion coefficient   4, 16
Doppler Perfusion Index   386

E

Echogen   11
Echovist   5, 327
enhancement patterns, definition
– absent   132, 236
– central   132
– diffuse   132, 236
– dotted   132
– peripheral nodular   132, 236
– peripheral rim-like   132, 236
– septal   236
epithelioid hemangioendothelioma, liver   159

F

fractional vascular volume, *see* blood volume
fracture, parenchymal   295
fundamental frequency, *see* resonant frequency

G

Gd-BOPTA 132, 139, 143, 167, 176, 181
gene, transfection 396

H

harmonic(s)
- B-mode imaging, second harmonic 44-45, 49, 50, 79, 91, 331
- Doppler 50, 52, 268
- order 46
- tissue, harmonic imaging 47, 126
hematoma 295
hepatocellular carcinoma
- ablation 189
- characterization 151
- detection 178

I

ICAM-1 394
Imagent, *see* Imavist
Imavist 10, 82, 361
infusion 71-72, 91, 119

L

laceration, parenchymal 295
late, phase 129, 167
Levovist 6, 73, 79-80, 126-127, 132, 140, 167 205, 350, 361, 367, 385, 389
Levovist, late phase 167
loss of correlation 51, 91
LOC, *see* loss of correlation
lymphoma
- liver 159
- spleen 212

M

mechanical index 23, 72, 79, 127, 206, 225, 257, 352
metastases, liver
- ablation 191
- characterization 154
- detection 167
metastases, renal 232
metastases, spleen 214
MI, *see* mechanical index
microbubble-based contrast agents
- coalescence 24
- destruction 24, 256, 268
- fragmentation 24, 256
- reticuloendothelial system uptake, hepatospleno-specific 7, 8, 10, 167-168, 205
- Kupffer cells, *see* reticuloendothelial system
- safety profile 12
microbubbles, *see* microbubble-based contrast agents
microvessel density, *see* angiogenesis
monoclonal antibodies 394
Myomap 7

O

Optison (Amersham Health Inc., Princeton, NJ) 10, 79-80, 82, 225, 397
Ostwald, coefficient 16

P

parasitic cysts, spleen 208-209
parenchymal, phase *see* late phase
perflubron 9
perflutren 10
perfluorobutane, *see* peflutren
perfluorooctyl bromide, *see* perflubron
perfusion, parenchymal 255-256, 388
PESDA 6 (table 1.3), 79
portal, phase 132
power Doppler 48, 223, 245, 256, 315, 324, 349, 360, 365
power modulation 57
power pulse inversion 28, 55, 257
pressure amplitude(s) *see* acoustic power
prostate cancer 359
pseudoaneurysm, intraparenchymal 296
pulsatility, index 316
pulse inversion 28, 32, 53, 91, 168, 257
pulse inversion Doppler 63
pulse inversion with three transmissions, *see* power pulse inversion

Q

Quantison 7

R

Rayleigh-Plesset, equation 19
resistivity, index 316,
resonant frequency 17, 18, 44, 46

S

scattering 46
scattering cross section 20
Stimulated Acoustic Emission 51, 91

Subject Index

SAE, *see* Stimulated Acoustic Emission
shell, microbubble
– composition   4, 33, 37
– elasticity   19, 33
– viscosity   18, 20, 33
SH U 454, *see* Echovist
SH U 508, *see* Levovist
SH U 563A, *see* Sonavist
Sonavist   8, 73, 127, 132, 140, 167, 205
Sonazoid   10, 132, 126, 168, 205
SonoVue   11, 126, 168, 205-207, 225, 304, 324, 327, 350, 368
speckles   126, 256
SPIO, Kupffer cells agents   168, 176, 181
splenunculus   207-208
subharmonic imaging   68
surface tension, microbubble   16, 268

T

tear, parenchymal *see* laceration, parenchymal
time-intensity curve   307, 368, 387
time variance imaging   91
thrombus, renal tumour   232
transit time   256, 384

V

vascular, phase *see* arterial, phase
vascular recognition imaging   64, 206
vectors   396

List of Contributors

TOMMASO V. BARTOLOTTA, MD
Assistant professor of Radiology
Department of Radiology
University of Palermo
Via Del Vespro 127
90127 Palermo
Italy

GIUSEPPE BELLISSIMA, MD
Department of Radiology
University of Palermo
Via Del Vespro 127
90127 Palermo
Italy

GABRIELE BIANCHI PORRO, MD
Department of Gastroenterology
Luigi Sacco University Hospital
University of Milan
Via Giovan Battista Grassi 74
20157 Milan
Italy

MARTIN J.K. BLOMLEY, MD, FRCR
Professor of Radiology
Department of Imaging
Imaging Science Department
Hammersmith Hospital
Imperial College School of Medicine
150 Du Cane Road
London W12 0HS
UK

GIUSEPPE BRANCATELLI, MD
Department of Radiology
University of Palermo
Via Del Vespro 127
90127 Palermo
Italy

ANTONIO CALGARO, MD
Department of Radiology
Cattinara Hospital
University of Trieste
Strada di Fiume 447
34149 Trieste
Italy

FABRIZIO CALLIADA, MD
Professor of Radiology
Department of Radiology
San Matteo Hospital
University of Pavia
Piazzale Golgi 1
Pavia
Italy

PAOLA CAPELLI, MD
Department of Pathology
Hospital G.B. Rossi, University of Verona
Piazza L.A. Scuro
37134 Verona
Italy

GIUSEPPE CARUSO, MD
Professor of Radiology
Department of Radiology
University of Palermo
Via del Vespro, 127
90127 Palermo
Italy

ROBERTA CHERSEVANI, MD
Department of Diagnostic Imaging
General Hospital
Via Vittorio Veneto 171
34170 Gorizia
Italy

DANIA CIONI, MD
Assistant professor of Radiology
Division of Diagnostic and Interventional Radiology
Department of Oncology, Transplants, and Advanced
Technologies in Medicine
University of Pisa
Via Roma 67
56126 Pisa
Italy

DAVID O. COSGROVE, FRCP FRCR
Professor of Clinical Ultrasound
Department of Radiology
Hammersmith Hospital
Imperial College School of Medicine
150 Du Cane Road
London W12 0HS
UK

MARIA COVA, MD
Professor of Radiology
Department of Radiology
Cattinara Hospital
University of Trieste
Strada di Fiume 447
34149 Trieste
Italy

DIANE DALECKI, PhD
Assistant Professor
Department of Biomedical Engineering
and the Rochester Center for Biomedical Ultrasound
University of Rochester
309 Hopeman Building,
P.O. Box 270168
Rochester, NY 14627
USA

MIRKO D'ONOFRIO, MD
Assistant Professor of Radiology
Department of Radiology
Hospital G.B. Rossi, University of Verona
Piazza L.A. Scuro
37134 Verona
Italy

ROBERT ECKERSLEY, PhD
Department of Radiology
Hammersmith Hospital
Imperial College School of Medicine
150 Du Cane Road
London W12 0HS
UK

CATERINA EXACOUSTOS, MD
Department of Surgery, Obstetrics and Gynecology Unit
University of Rome "Tor Vergata"
Rome
Italy

MASSIMO FALCONI, MD
Department of Surgery
Hospital G.B. Rossi, University of Verona
Piazza L.A. Scuro
37134 Verona
Italy

GABRIELLA FERRANDINA, MD
Gynecologic Oncology Unit
Catholic University of Sacred Heart
L.go A. Gemelli 8
00168 Rome
Italy

ERIKA FRUSCELLA, MD
Gynecologic Oncology Unit
Catholic University of Sacred Heart
L.go A. Gemelli 8
00168 Rome
Italy

CHRISTOPHER J. HARVEY, MRCP FRCR
Consultant Radiologist
Department of Imaging, Imaging Sciences Department,
Hammersmith Hospital, Imperial College Faculty of
Medicine,
150 Du Cane Road
London W12 0HS
UK

SAUL KALVAITIS, MD
Cardiac Imaging Center, Cardiovascular Division
University of Virginia School of Medicine
Charlottesville, VA 22908-0158
USA

ANDREA KLAUSER, MD
Associate Professor of Radiology
Department of Radiology II
Medical University Innsbruck
Anichstrasse 35
6020 Innsbruck
AUSTRIA

ROBERTO LAGALLA, MD
Professor of Radiology
Department of Radiology
University of Palermo
Via Del Vespro 127
90127 Palermo
Italy

RICCARDO LENCIONI, MD
Professor of Radiology
Division of Diagnostic and Interventional Radiology
Department of Oncology, Transplants and Advanced
Technologies in Medicine
University of Pisa
Via Roma 67
56126 Pisa
ITALY

HAI-DONG LIANG, PhD
Research Fellow
Department of Medical Physics and Bioengineering
Bristol General Hospital
Bristol BS1 6SY
UK

ADRIAN K. P. LIM, MRCP FRCR
Consultant Radiologist
Department of Imaging, Imaging Sciences Department,
Hammersmith Hospital, Imperial College Faculty of
Medicine,
150 Du Cane Road
London W12 0HS
UK

MADELINE LYNCH, MSc
Senior Sonographer
Department of Imaging, Imaging Sciences Department,
Hammersmith Hospital, Imperial College Faculty of
Medicine,
150 Du Cane Road
London W12 0HS
UK

GIOVANNI MACONI, MD
Assistant professor of Radiology
Department of Gastroenterology
Luigi Sacco University Hospital
University of Milan
Via Giovan Battista Grassi 74
20157 Milan
Italy

MARINELLA MALAGGESE, MD
Gynecologic Oncology Unit
Catholic University of Sacred Heart
L.go A. Gemelli 8
00168 Rome
Italy

ROBERTO MALAGÒ, MD
Department of Radiology
Hospital G.B. Rossi, University of Verona
Piazza L.A. Scuro
37134 Verona
Italy

GIANCARLO MANSUETO, MD
Professor of Radiology
Department of Radiology
Hospital G.B. Rossi, University of Verona
Piazza L.A. Scuro
37134 Verona
Italy

ENRICO MARTONE, MD
Department of Radiology
Hospital G.B. Rossi, University of Verona
Piazza L.A. Scuro
37134 Verona
Italy

MASSIMO MIDIRI, MD
Professor of Radiology
Department of Radiology
University of Palermo
Via Del Vespro 127
90127 Palermo
Italy

ANTONIO NICOSIA, MD
Department of Radiology
University of Palermo
Via Del Vespro 127
90127 Palermo
Italy

ALESSANDRO PALUMBO, MD
Department of Radiology
Cattinara Hospital
University of Trieste
Strada di Fiume 447
34149 Trieste
Italy

FABIO POZZI MUCELLI, MD
Department of Radiology
Cattinara Hospital
University of Trieste
Strada di Fiume 447
34149 Trieste
Italy

ROBERTO POZZI MUCELLI, MD
Professor of Radiology
Department of Radiology
Hospital GB Rossi
University of Verona
Piazza L.A. Scuro 10
37134 Verona
Italy

EMILIO QUAIA, MD
Assistant Professor of Radiology
Department of Radiology
Cattinara Hospital
University of Trieste
Strada di Fiume 447
34149 Trieste
Italy

GITA RALLEIGH, MD
Department of Radiology
King's College Hospital
Denmark Hill,
London, SE5 9RS
UK

J. ROBERT RAMEY, MD
Jefferson Prostate Diagnostic Center
Department of Urology
Thomas Jefferson University
1015 Walnut Street, Suite 1100
Philadelphia, PA 19107
USA

GIORGIO RIZZATTO, MD
Department of Diagnostic Imaging
General Hospital
Via Vittorio Veneto 171
34170 Gorizia
Italy

SANDRO ROSSI, MD
Operative Unit for Interventional US,
San Matteo Hospital, University of Pavia,
Piazzale Golgi 1
Pavia
Italy

LEOPOLDO RUBALTELLI, MD
Associate Professor of Radiology
Department of Medical Diagnostic Sciences and Special Therapies
University of Padova
Via Giustiniani 2
35128 Padua
Italy

GIUSEPPE SALVAGGIO, MD
Department of Radiology
University of Palermo
Via del Vespro, 127
90127 Palermo
Italy

GIOVANNI SCAMBIA, MD
Oncology Department
Catholic University of Sacred Heart
Centro di Ricerca e formazione ad alta tecnologia nelle
Scienze Biomediche
Campobasso
Italy

MICHAEL SCHIRMER, MD
Department of Internal Medicine
Medical University Innsbruck
Anichstrasse 35
6020 Innsbruck
AUSTRIA

SALVATORE SIRACUSANO, MD
Department of Urology
Cattinara Hospital
University of Trieste
Strada di Fiume 447
34149 Trieste
Italy

FORTUNATO SORRENTINO, MD
Department of Radiology
University of Palermo
Via del Vespro, 127
90127 Palermo
Italy

ROBERTO STRAMARE, MD
Department of Medical Diagnostic Sciences and Special
Therapies
University of Padova
Via Giustiniani 2
35128 Padua
Italy

ELEANOR STRIDE, PhD
Department of Mechanical Engineering
University College London
Torrington Place
London WC1E 7JE
UK

ANTONIA CARLA TESTA, MD
Gynecologic Oncology Unit
Catholic University of Sacred Heart
L.go A. Gemelli 8
00168 Rome
Italy

ALBERTO TREGNAGHI, MD
Department of Medical Diagnostic Sciences and Special
Therapies
University of Padova
Via Giustiniani 2
35128 Padua
Italy

MAJA UKMAR, MD
Department of Radiology
Cattinara Hospital
University of Trieste
Strada di Fiume 447
34149 Trieste
Italy

KEVIN WEI, MD
Assistant Professor of Internal Medicine
Cardiac Imaging Center, Cardiovascular Division
University of Virginia School of Medicine
P.O. Box 800158
Charlottesville, VA 22908-0158
USA

TOMAS ANTHONY WHITTINGHAM, PhD
Regional Medical Physics Department
Newcastle General Hospital
Westgate Road
Newcastle Upon Tyne NE4 6BE
UK

GIULIA ZAMBONI, MD
Department of Radiology
Hospital G.B. Rossi, University of Verona
Piazza L.A. Scuro
37134 Verona
Italy

MEDICAL RADIOLOGY Diagnostic Imaging and Radiation Oncology

Titles in the series already published

DIAGNOSTIC IMAGING

Innovations in Diagnostic Imaging
Edited by J. H. Anderson

Radiology of the Upper Urinary Tract
Edited by E. K. Lang

The Thymus - Diagnostic Imaging, Functions, and Pathologic Anatomy
Edited by E. Walter, E. Willich, and W. R. Webb

Interventional Neuroradiology
Edited by A. Valavanis

Radiology of the Pancreas
Edited by A. L. Baert,
co-edited by G. Delorme

Radiology of the Lower Urinary Tract
Edited by E. K. Lang

Magnetic Resonance Angiography
Edited by I. P. Arlart, G. M. Bongartz, and G. Marchal

Contrast-Enhanced MRI of the Breast
S. Heywang-Köbrunner and R. Beck

Spiral CT of the Chest
Edited by M. Rémy-Jardin and J. Rémy

Radiological Diagnosis of Breast Diseases
Edited by M. Friedrich
and E.A. Sickles

Radiology of the Trauma
Edited by M. Heller and A. Fink

Biliary Tract Radiology
Edited by P. Rossi,
co-edited by M. Brezi

Radiological Imaging of Sports Injuries
Edited by C. Masciocchi

Modern Imaging of the Alimentary Tube
Edited by A. R. Margulis

Diagnosis and Therapy of Spinal Tumors
Edited by P. R. Algra, J. Valk, and J. J. Heimans

Interventional Magnetic Resonance Imaging
Edited by J.F. Debatin and G. Adam

Abdominal and Pelvic MRI
Edited by A. Heuck and M. Reiser

Orthopedic Imaging
Techniques and Applications
Edited by A. M. Davies
and H. Pettersson

Radiology of the Female Pelvic Organs
Edited by E. K.Lang

Magnetic Resonance of the Heart and Great Vessels
Clinical Applications
Edited by J. Bogaert, A.J. Duerinckx, and F. E. Rademakers

Modern Head and Neck Imaging
Edited by S. K. Mukherji
and J. A. Castelijns

Radiological Imaging of Endocrine Diseases
Edited by J. N. Bruneton
in collaboration with B. Padovani and M.-Y. Mourou

Trends in Contrast Media
Edited by H. S. Thomsen,
R. N. Muller, and R. F. Mattrey

Functional MRI
Edited by C. T. W. Moonen
and P. A. Bandettini

Radiology of the Pancreas
2nd Revised Edition
Edited by A. L. Baert
Co-edited by G. Delorme
and L. Van Hoe

Emergency Pediatric Radiology
Edited by H. Carty

Spiral CT of the Abdomen
Edited by F. Terrier, M. Grossholz, and C. D. Becker

Liver Malignancies
Diagnostic and
Interventional Radiology
Edited by C. Bartolozzi
and R. Lencioni

Medical Imaging of the Spleen
Edited by A. M. De Schepper
and F. Vanhoenacker

Radiology of Peripheral Vascular Diseases
Edited by E. Zeitler

Diagnostic Nuclear Medicine
Edited by C. Schiepers

Radiology of Blunt Trauma of the Chest
P. Schnyder and M. Wintermark

Portal Hypertension
Diagnostic Imaging-Guided Therapy
Edited by P. Rossi
Co-edited by P. Ricci and L. Broglia

Recent Advances in Diagnostic Neuroradiology
Edited by Ph. Demaerel

Virtual Endoscopy and Related 3D Techniques
Edited by P. Rogalla, J. Terwisscha Van Scheltinga, and B. Hamm

Multislice CT
Edited by M. F. Reiser, M. Takahashi, M. Modic, and R. Bruening

Pediatric Uroradiology
Edited by R. Fotter

Transfontanellar Doppler Imaging in Neonates
A. Couture and C. Veyrac

Radiology of AIDS
A Practical Approach
Edited by J.W.A.J. Reeders
and P.C. Goodman

CT of the Peritoneum
Armando Rossi and Giorgio Rossi

Magnetic Resonance Angiography
2nd Revised Edition
Edited by I. P. Arlart,
G. M. Bongratz, and G. Marchal

MEDICAL RADIOLOGY   Diagnostic Imaging and Radiation Oncology
Titles in the series already published

Pediatric Chest Imaging
Edited by Javier Lucaya
and Janet L. Strife

**Applications of Sonography
in Head and Neck Pathology**
Edited by J. N. Bruneton
in collaboration with C. Raffaelli
and O. Dassonville

Imaging of the Larynx
Edited by R. Hermans

3D Image Processing
Techniques and Clinical Applications
Edited by D. Caramella
and C. Bartolozzi

**Imaging of Orbital and
Visual Pathway Pathology**
Edited by W. S. Müller-Forell

Pediatric ENT Radiology
Edited by S. J. King
and A. E. Boothroyd

**Radiological Imaging
of the Small Intestine**
Edited by N. C. Gourtsoyiannis

Imaging of the Knee
Techniques and Applications
Edited by A. M. Davies
and V. N. Cassar-Pullicino

Perinatal Imaging
From Ultrasound to MR Imaging
Edited by Fred E. Avni

**Radiological Imaging
of the Neonatal Chest**
Edited by V. Donoghue

**Diagnostic and Interventional
Radiology in Liver Transplantation**
Edited by E. Bücheler, V. Nicolas,
C. E. Broelsch, X. Rogiers,
and G. Krupski

Radiology of Osteoporosis
Edited by S. Grampp

Imaging Pelvic Floor Disorders
Edited by C. I. Bartram
and J. O. L. DeLancey
Associate Editors: S. Halligan,
F. M. Kelvin, and J. Stoker

Imaging of the Pancreas
Cystic and Rare Tumors
Edited by C. Procacci
and A. J. Megibow

**High Resolution Sonography
of the Peripheral Nervous System**
Edited by S. Peer and G. Bodner

Imaging of the Foot and Ankle
Techniques and Applications
Edited by A. M. Davies,
R. W. Whitehouse,
and J. P. R. Jenkins

Radiology Imaging of the Ureter
Edited by F. Joffre, Ph. Otal,
and M. Soulie

Imaging of the Shoulder
Techniques and Applications
Edited by A. M. Davies and J. Hodler

Radiology of the Petrous Bone
Edited by M. Lemmerling
and S. S. Kollias

Interventional Radiology in Cancer
Edited by A. Adam, R. F. Dondelinger,
and P. R. Mueller

**Duplex and Color Doppler Imaging
of the Venous System**
Edited by G. H. Mostbeck

Multidetector-Row CT of the Thorax
Edited by U. J. Schoepf

Functional Imaging of the Chest
Edited by H.-U. Kauczor

**Radiology of the Pharynx
and the Esophagus**
Edited by O. Ekberg

**Radiological Imaging
in Hematological Malignancies**
Edited by A. Guermazi

**Imaging and Intervention in
Abdominal Trauma**
Edited by R. F. Dondelinger

Multislice CT
2nd Revised Edition
Edited by M. F. Reiser, M. Takahashi,
M. Modic, and C. R. Becker

**Intracranial Vascular Malformations
and Aneurysms**
From Diagnostic Work-Up
to Endovascular Therapy
Edited by M. Forsting

Radiology and Imaing of the Colon
Edited by A. H. Chapman

Coronary Radiology
Edited by M. Oudkerk

**Dynamic Contrast-Enhanced Magnetic
Resonance Imaging in Oncology**
Edited by A. Jackson, D. L. Buckley,
and G. J. M. Parker

**Imaging in Treatment Planning
for Sinonasal Diseases**
Edited by R. Maroldi and P. Nicolai

Clinical Cardiac MRI
With Interactive CD-ROM
Edited by J. Bogaert,
S. Dymarkowski, and A. M. Taylor

Focal Liver Lesions
Detection, Characterization,
Ablation
Edited by R. Lencioni, D. Cioni,
and C. Bartolozzi

Multidetector-Row CT Angiography
Edited by C. Catalano
and R. Passariello

**MR Imaging in White Matter Diseases of
the Brain and Spinal Cord**
Edited by M. Filippi, N. De Stefano,
V. Dousset, and J. C. McGowan

Paediatric Musculoskeletal Diseases
With an Emphasis on Ultrasound
Edited by D. Wilson

Contrast Media in Ultrasonography
Basic Principles and Clinical Applications
Edited by Emilio Quaia

Springer

MEDICAL RADIOLOGY Diagnostic Imaging and Radiation Oncology

Titles in the series already published

RADIATION ONCOLOGY

Lung Cancer
Edited by C. W. Scarantino

Innovations in Radiation Oncology
Edited by H. R. Withers
and L. J. Peters

**Radiation Therapy
of Head and Neck Cancer**
Edited by G. E. Laramore

**Gastrointestinal Cancer –
Radiation Therapy**
Edited by R.R. Dobelbower, Jr.

**Radiation Exposure
and Occupational Risks**
Edited by E. Scherer, C. Streffer,
and K.-R. Trott

**Radiation Therapy of Benign Diseases
A Clinical Guide**
S. E. Order and S. S. Donaldson

**Interventional Radiation
Therapy Techniques – Brachytherapy**
Edited by R. Sauer

Radiopathology of Organs and Tissues
Edited by E. Scherer, C. Streffer,
and K.-R. Trott

**Concomitant Continuous Infusion
Chemotherapy and Radiation**
Edited by M. Rotman
and C. J. Rosenthal

**Intraoperative Radiotherapy
Clinical Experiences and Results**
Edited by F. A. Calvo, M. Santos,
and L.W. Brady

**Radiotherapy of Intraocular
and Orbital Tumors**
Edited by W. E. Alberti and
R. H. Sagerman

**Interstitial and Intracavitary
Thermoradiotherapy**
Edited by M. H. Seegenschmiedt
and R. Sauer

**Non-Disseminated Breast Cancer
Controversial Issues in Management**
Edited by G. H. Fletcher and
S.H. Levitt

**Current Topics in
Clinical Radiobiology of Tumors**
Edited by H.-P. Beck-Bornholdt

**Practical Approaches to
Cancer Invasion and Metastases
A Compendium of Radiation
Oncologists' Responses to 40 Histories**
Edited by A. R. Kagan with the
Assistance of R. J. Steckel

Radiation Therapy in Pediatric Oncology
Edited by J. R. Cassady

Radiation Therapy Physics
Edited by A. R. Smith

Late Sequelae in Oncology
Edited by J. Dunst and R. Sauer

Mediastinal Tumors. Update 1995
Edited by D. E. Wood
and C. R. Thomas, Jr.

**Thermoradiotherapy
and Thermochemotherapy**

Volume 1:
Biology, Physiology, and Physics

Volume 2:
Clinical Applications

Edited by M. H. Seegenschmiedt,
P. Fessenden, and C.C. Vernon

**Carcinoma of the Prostate
Innovations in Management**
Edited by Z. Petrovich, L. Baert,
and L.W. Brady

**Radiation Oncology
of Gynecological Cancers**
Edited by H.W. Vahrson

**Carcinoma of the Bladder
Innovations in Management**
Edited by Z. Petrovich, L. Baert,
and L. W. Brady

**Blood Perfusion and
Microenvironment of Human Tumors
Implications for
Clinical Radiooncology**
Edited by M. Molls and P. Vaupel

**Radiation Therapy of Benign Diseases
A Clinical Guide
2nd Revised Edition**
S. E. Order and S. S. Donaldson

**Carcinoma of the Kidney and Testis, and
Rare Urologic Malignancies
Innovations in Management**
Edited by Z. Petrovich, L. Baert,
and L.W. Brady

**Progress and Perspectives in the
Treatment of Lung Cancer**
Edited by P. Van Houtte,
J. Klastersky, and P. Rocmans

**Combined Modality Therapy of
Central Nervous System Tumors**
Edited by Z. Petrovich, L. W. Brady,
M. L. Apuzzo, and M. Bamberg

**Age-Related Macular Degeneration
Current Treatment Concepts**
Edited by W. A. Alberti, G. Richard,
and R. H. Sagerman

**Radiotherapy of Intraocular
and Orbital Tumors
2nd Revised Edition**
Edited by R. H. Sagerman,
and W. E. Alberti

**Modification of Radiation Response
Cytokines, Growth Factors,
and Other Biolgical Targets**
Edited by C. Nieder, L. Milas,
and K. K. Ang

Radiation Oncology for Cure and Palliation
R. G. Parker, N. A. Janjan,
and M. T. Selch

**Clinical Target Volumes in
Conformal and Intensity Modulated
Radiation Therapy
A Clinical Guide to Cancer
Treatment**
Edited by V. Grégoire, P. Scalliet,
and K. K. Ang

**Advances in Radiation Oncology
in Lung Cancer**
Edited by Branislav Jeremić

Springer

Printing and Binding: Stürtz GmbH, Würzburg

9783540407409